Bovine Tuberculosis

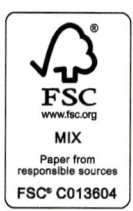

Bovine Tuberculosis

―――――――

Edited by

Mark Chambers

University of Surrey, UK

Stephen Gordon

University College Dublin, Ireland

Francisco Olea-Popelka

Colorado State University, USA

and

Paul Barrow

University of Nottingham, UK

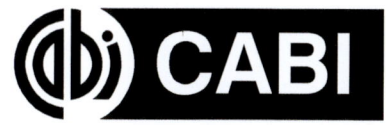

CABI is a trading name of CAB International

CABI
Nosworthy Way
Wallingford
Oxfordshire OX10 8DE
UK

Tel: +44 (0)1491 832111
Fax: +44 (0)1491 833508
E-mail: info@cabi.org
Website: www.cabi.org

CABI
745 Atlantic Avenue
8th Floor
Boston, MA 02111
USA

Tel: +1 (617)682-9015
E-mail: cabi-nao@cabi.org

© CAB International 2018. All rights reserved. No part of this publication may be reproduced in any form or by any means, electronically, mechanically, by photocopying, recording or otherwise, without the prior permission of the copyright owners.

A catalogue record for this book is available from the British Library, London, UK.

Library of Congress Cataloging-in-Publication Data

Names: Gordon, Stephen B., editor. | Barrow, Paul, editor.
Title: Bovine tuberculosis / edited by Mark Chambers, University of Surrey, UK, Stephen Gordon, University College, Dublin, Ireland, Francisco Olea-Popelka, Colorado State University, USA and Paul Barrow, University of Nottingham, UK.
Description: Wallingford, Oxfordshire, UK ; Boston, MA, USA : CABI, [2018] | Includes bibliographical references and index.
Identifiers: LCCN 2017050595 (print) | LCCN 2017054340 (ebook) | ISBN 9781786391537 (epdf) | ISBN 9781786391544 (epub) | ISBN 9781786391520 (hardcover : alk. paper)
Subjects: LCSH: Tuberculosis in cattle. | Cattle--Diseases.
Classification: LCC SF967.T8 (ebook) | LCC SF967.T8 B685 2018 (print) | DDC 636.2089/995--dc23
LC record available at https://lccn.loc.gov/2017050595

ISBN-13: 9781786391520

Commissioning editor: Caroline Makepeace
Editorial assistant: Alexandra Lainsbury
Production editor: Marta Patiño

Typeset by AMA DataSet Ltd, Preston, UK.
Printed and bound in the UK by CPI Group (UK) Ltd, Croydon, CR0 4YY.

Contents

	Preface	vii
	Contributors	ix
	List of figures	xii
1	**Bovine Tuberculosis: Worldwide Picture** *Lina Awada, Paolo Tizzani, Elisabeth Erlacher-Vindel, Simona Forcella and Paula Caceres*	1
2	***Mycobacterium bovis* as the Causal Agent of Human Tuberculosis: Public Health Implications** *Francisco Olea-Popelka, Anna S. Dean, Adrian Muwonge, Alejandro Perera, Mario Raviglione and Paula I. Fujiwara*	16
3	**Economics of Bovine Tuberculosis: A One Health Issue** *Hind Yahyaoui Azami and Jakob Zinsstag*	31
4	**The Epidemiology of *Mycobacterium bovis* Infection in Cattle** *Andrew J.K. Conlan and James L.N. Wood*	43
5	***Mycobacterium bovis* Molecular Typing and Surveillance** *Robin A. Skuce, Andrew W. Byrne, Angela Lahuerta-Marin and Adrian Allen*	58
6	**Bovine Tuberculosis in Other Domestic Species** *Anita L. Michel*	80
7	**Role of Wildlife in the Epidemiology of *Mycobacterium bovis*** *Naomi J. Fox, Paul A. Barrow and Michael R. Hutchings*	93
8	**Molecular Virulence Mechanisms of *Mycobacterium bovis*** *Alicia Smyth and Stephen V. Gordon*	106

9	The Pathology and Pathogenesis of *Mycobacterium bovis* Infection *Francisco J. Salguero*	122
10	**Innate Immune Response in Bovine Tuberculosis** *Jacobo Carrisoza-Urbina, Xiangmei Zhou and José A. Gutiérrez-Pabello*	140
11	**Adaptive Immunity** *Jayne Hope and Dirk Werling*	154
12	**Immunological Diagnosis** *Ray Waters and Martin Vordermeier*	173
13	**Biomarkers in the Diagnosis of *Mycobacterium tuberculosis* Complex Infections** *Sylvia I. Wanzala and Srinand Sreevatsan*	191
14	**Vaccination of Domestic and Wild Animals Against Tuberculosis** *Bryce M. Buddle, Natalie A. Parlane, Mark A. Chambers and Christian Gortázar*	206
15	**Managing Bovine Tuberculosis: Successes and Issues** *Paul Livingstone and Nick Hancox*	225
16	**Perspectives on Global Bovine Tuberculosis Control** *Francisco Olea-Popelka, Mark A. Chambers, Stephen Gordon and Paul Barrow*	248
Index		**255**

Preface

Bovine tuberculosis (bTB) remains a major endemic infectious disease in cattle worldwide and a serious zoonosis. It remains a source of economic loss in several countries, even in those that introduced comprehensive control and eradication schemes many decades ago. In countries that do not currently have the infrastructure to introduce national control measures, zoonotic transmission of infection continues to inflict morbidity and mortality in humans of all ages.

Despite the recent publication of a number of books covering bTB, these have emphasized the diagnosis and epidemiology of *Mycobacterium bovis* in different countries (Thoen *et al.*, 2006, ISBN-13: Ib. 978-0813809199; 2014, ISBN: 978-1-118-47429-7), or include *M. bovis* amongst other mycobacteria such as *M. tuberculosis* and *M. leprae* (Mukundan *et al.*, 2015, ISBN-13: 978-1780643960). We felt that there was need for a book covering all aspects of *M. bovis* biology and infection: epidemiological, pathological, microbiological, genomic and immunological together with a comparative approach to the different control schemes being undertaken in different countries. Indeed, despite the well-known threat of *M. bovis* to human health, zoonotic tuberculosis in humans has long been neglected. For this reason, in October 2017, a Zoonotic Tuberculosis Roadmap was launched as a joint effort between the World Health Organization (WHO), The International Union Against Tuberculosis and Lung Disease (The Union), the World Health Organization for Animal Health (OIE), and the Food and Agricultural Organization (FAO) to address the prevention, control, and treatment challenges faced by communities at higher risk of contracting zoonotic tuberculosis. This roadmap recognizes 'the interdependence of the health of people and animals, and the importance of a One Health approach to zoonotic TB, which draw on expertise and collaborative relationships across different sectors and disciplines'. We therefore see the publication of this book as timely, bringing together international experts to provide a current synthesis of the key issues facing us in the control of bTB.

Huge progress has been made in controlling bTB in the last 100 years. In the late 19th century and early years of the 20th century, comprehensive pathological and microbiological analysis of bovine and human disease demonstrated that *M. bovis* could cause generalized disease in man. Initial control of zoonotic infection involved milk pasteurization. National control schemes were introduced in the early 20th century in many European countries, North America and Australasia, which resulted in ever-increasing areas within individual countries with ever-decreasing levels of infection. Many developed countries are now 'officially' TB free. This has all been done through the use of the tuberculin skin test, relying as it does on a relatively crude antigen preparation that is difficult to standardize. Demands for more sensitive and specific diagnostic methods will need to be met in the coming years.

Historically, the use of vaccines for controlling bTB was not pursued, with reliance instead on the currently accepted methods of tuberculin test-and-slaughter. However, the persistence of infection in wildlife reservoirs, some of which are protected by law, is driving research towards vaccine development and deployment, including approaches that would allow differentiation between vaccinated animals and those infected with *M. bovis* or with other mycobacteria. These requirements underlie the drive for detailed understanding of the immunological responses of cattle, and of key wildlife species such as badgers, possums, white tailed deer and wild boars, to infection with *M. bovis*.

The availability of the first genome sequence of *M. bovis* in 2003, coupled with transcriptional analysis at the level of the genome, has led to huge strides in understanding the metabolism and virulence of this organism and how it differs from *M. tuberculosis* and the attenuated *M. bovis* bacillus Calmette–Guérin vaccine. Whole genome sequencing of multiple *M. bovis* isolates is now leading to a better understanding of the global population structure and has been adapted for strain typing purposes, an area already supplying insights into *M. bovis* transmission dynamics. An improved understanding of *M. bovis* virulence genes could identify targets to be exploited in development of the next generation of live vaccines.

We have divided this book into separate sections with cross-referencing, where appropriate. Chapters 1 to 7 cover the global situation, public health and economic significance and epidemiology of TB cattle, other species and wildlife. Chapters 8 and 9 cover the mechanism of disease, namely the molecular basis of virulence, pathogenesis and pathology. Chapters 10 and 11 cover innate and adaptive immunity. Chapters 12 to 15 include approaches to surveillance (immunological and molecular diagnosis) and control (vaccination and other approaches to control). Finally, in Chapter 16 the editors have synthesized the main findings from the chapters with a look forward to the future.

It is over 110 years since Theobald Smith first differentiated the human and bovine tubercle bacilli. We hope that the comprehensive update on *M. bovis* and bTB delivered in this book will provide the reader with a feeling for this fascinating organism, a pathogen that still challenges at the nexus of animal and human medicine.

Paul Barrow
Mark Chambers
Stephen Gordon
Francisco Olea-Popelka

Contributors

Adrian Allen, Veterinary Sciences Division, Agrifood and Biosciences Institute, Belfast, BT4 3SD, UK. E-mail: adrian.allen@afbini.gov.uk

Lina Awada, World Organisation for Animal Health (OIE), Paris, 12 Rue de Prony, 75017, France. E-mail: L.Awada@oie.int

Paul A. Barrow, School of Veterinary Medicine and Science, University of Nottingham, Sutton Bonington Campus, Sutton Bonington, Loughborough, LE125RD, UK. E-mail: paul.barrow@nottingham.ac.uk

Bryce M. Buddle, AgResearch, Hopkirk Research Institute, Palmerston North, New Zealand. E-mail: bryce.buddle@agresearch.co.nz

Andrew W. Byrne, School of Biological Sciences, Queens University Belfast, AgriFood and Biosciences Institute, Belfast BT4 3SD, UK. E-mail: andrew.byrne@afbini.gov.uk

Paula Caceres, World Organisation for Animal Health (OIE), Paris, 12 Rue de Prony, 75017, France. E-mail: p.caceres@oie.int

Jacobo Carrisoza-Urbina, Departamento de Microbiología e Inmunología, Facultad de Medicina Veterinaria y Zootecnia, Universidad Nacional Autónoma de México, Mexico City, 04510, Mexico.

Mark A. Chambers, Animal and Plant Health Agency, Woodham Lane, Addlestone, KT153NB, UK; School of Veterinary Medicine, Faculty of Health and Medical Sciences, University of Surrey, UK. E-mail: m.chambers@surrey.ac.uk

Andrew J.K. Conlan, Department of Veterinary Medicine, University of Cambridge, Madingley Road, Cambridge, UK. E-mail: ajkc2@cam.ac.uk

Anna S. Dean, Global TB Programme, World Health Organization, Geneva, Switzerland. E-mail: deanan@who.int

Elisabeth Erlacher-Vindel, World Organisation for Animal Health (OIE), Paris, 12 Rue de Prony, 75017, France. E-mail: E.Erlacher-Vindel@oie.int

Simona Forcella, World Organisation for Animal Health (OIE), Paris, 12 Rue de Prony, 75017, France. E-mail: S.Forcella@oie.int

Naomi J. Fox, Animal and Veterinary Sciences, SRUC, Roslin Institute Building, Easter Bush, Midlothian, EH25 9RG, UK. E-mail: naomi.fox@sruc.ac.uk

Paula I. Fujiwara, International Union Against Tuberculosis and Lung Disease, Boulevard Saint Michel, 75006, Paris, France. E-mail: pfujiwara@theunion.org

Stephen V. Gordon, School of Veterinary Medicine, University College Dublin, Dublin, D04 W6F6, Ireland. E-mail: stephen.gordon@ucd.ie

Christian Gortázar, SaBio - Instituto de Investigación en Recursos Cinegéticos IREC, Universidad de Castilla-La Mancha and CSIC, Ciudad Real, Spain. E-mail: Christian.Gortazar@uclm.es

José A. Gutiérrez-Pabello, Departamento de Microbiología e Inmunología, Facultad de Medicina Veterinaria y Zootecnia, Universidad Nacional Autónoma de México, Mexico City, 04510, Mexico. E-mail: jagp@unam.mx

Nick Hancox, OSPRI New Zealand Limited, Level 9, 15 Willeston Street, PO Box 3412, Wellington 6140, New Zealand. E-mail: nick.hancox@tbfree.org.nz

Jayne Hope, Roslin Institute, University of Edinburgh, Easter Bush, Midlothian, EH25 9RG, UK. E-mail: jayne.hope@roslin.ed.ac.uk

Michael R. Hutchings, Animal and Veterinary Sciences, SRUC, Roslin Institute Building, Easter Bush, Midlothian, EH25 9RG, UK. E-mail: mike.hutchings@sruc.ac.uk

Angela Lahuerta-Marin, Veterinary Sciences Division, Agrifood and Biosciences Institute, Belfast, BT4 3SD, UK. E-mail: angel.marin@afbini.gov.uk

Paul Livingstone, TB Consultant, Domestic Animals and Wildlife, New Zealand. E-mail: consultantbtb@gmail.com

Anita L. Michel, Department Veterinary Tropical Diseases, Bovine Tuberculosis and Brucellosis Research Programme, Faculty of Veterinary Science, University of Pretoria, Onderstepoort, South Africa. E-mail: Anita.Michel@up.ac.za

Adrian Muwonge, Genetics and Genomics, Roslin Institute, Royal (Dick) School of Veterinary Studies, University of Edinburgh, Edinburgh, UK. E-mail: adrian.muwonge@roslin.ed.ac.uk

Francisco Olea-Popelka, College of Veterinary Medicine and Biomedical Sciences, Department of Clinical Sciences and Mycobacteria Research Laboratories, Colorado State University, Fort Collins, Colorado, USA. E-mail: folea@colostate.edu

Natalie A. Parlane, AgResearch, Hopkirk Research Institute, Palmerston North, New Zealand. E-mail: natalie.parlane@agresearch.co.nz

Alejandro Perera, United States Embassy, Mexico City, US Department of Agriculture, Animal and Plant Health Inspection Service, Mexico City, Mexico. E-mail: Alejandro.Perera@aphis.usda.gov

Mario Raviglione, Global TB Programme, World Health Organization, Geneva, Switzerland. E-mail: raviglione@who.int

Francisco J. Salguero, Department of Pathology and Infectious Diseases, School of Veterinary Medicine, University of Surrey, Guildford, GU2 7AL, UK. E-mail: f.salguerobodes@surrey.ac.uk

Robin A. Skuce, Veterinary Sciences Division, Agrifood and Biosciences Institute, Belfast, BT4 3SD, UK; Queens University Belfast, University Road, Belfast, BT9 1NN, UK. E-mail: robin.skuce@afbini.gov.uk

Alicia Smyth, School of Veterinary Medicine, University College Dublin, Dublin, D04 W6F6, Ireland. E-mail: alicia.smyth@ucd.ie

Srinand Sreevatsan, Pathobiology and Diagnostic Investigation, College of Veterinary Medicine, Michigan State University, Michigan, USA. E-mail: sreevats@msu.edu

Paolo Tizzani, World Organisation for Animal Health (OIE), Paris, 12 Rue de Prony, 75017, France. E-mail: P.Tizzani@oie.int

Martin Vordermeier, Tuberculosis Research Group, Animal and Plant Health Agency, Woodham Lane, Addlestone, KT15 3NB, UK. E-mail: Martin.Vordermeier@apha.gsi.gov.uk

Sylvia I. Wanzala, Department of Pathobiology and Diagnostic Investigation, Michigan State University, 784 Wilson Road, F130G, East Lansing, Michigan, 48824 USA. E-mail: wanza003@umn.edu

Ray Waters, National Animal Disease Center, Agricultural Research Service, United States Department of Agriculture, Ames, Iowa, USA. E-mail: wwaters@iastate.edu

Dirk Werling, Royal Veterinary College, Hawkshead Campus, Hatfield, AL97TA, UK. E-mail: dwerling@rvc.ac.uk

James L.N. Wood, Department of Veterinary Medicine, University of Cambridge, Madingley Road, Cambridge, UK. E-mail: jlnw2@cam.ac.uk

Hind Yahyaoui Azami, Institut Agronomique et Vétérinaire Hassan II, Rabat, Morocco; Swiss Tropical and Public Health Institute, Basel, Switzerland; University of Basel, Basel, Switzerland. e-mail: yahyaouiazamihind@gmail.com

Xiangmei Zhou, Veterinary Pathology Department, College of Veterinary Medicine, China Agricultural University, Yuanmingyuan West Road No.2, Haidian District, Beijing 100193, P.R. China. E-mail: zhouxm@cau.edu.cn

Jakob Zinsstag, Swiss Tropical and Public Health Institute, Basel, Switzerland; University of Basel, Basel, Switzerland. E-mail: jakob.zinsstag@swisstph.ch

List of Figures

Fig. 1.1. Statistics on animal tuberculosis published in the Bulletin of the Office International des Epizooties, July 1927–June 1928.

Fig. 1.2. Percentage of the reporting countries for each year between 1986 and 2015 that notified bovine tuberculosis present, with the 95% confidence interval, and simple linear regression trend line.

Fig. 1.3. Percentage of the reporting countries by region for each year between 1986 and 2015 that notified bovine tuberculosis present.

Fig. 1.4. Trend in the average number of cases reported to the OIE since 2005 by the countries in Group C. The linear regression is reported on the graph.

Fig. 1.5. Trend in the average number of cases reported to the OIE since 2005 by the countries in Group D. The linear regression is reported on the graph.

Fig. 1.6. Trend in the average number of cases reported to the OIE since 2005 in the Americas and Europe.

Fig. 1.7. Trend in the average number of cases reported to the OIE since 2005 in Africa, Asia and Oceania.

Fig. 1.8. Distribution of bovine tuberculosis in domestic animals in 2015, as reported to the OIE up to 4 May 2016.

Fig. 1.9. Distribution of bovine tuberculosis in wildlife in 2015, as reported to the OIE up to 4 May 2016.

Fig. 3.1. Schematic diagram of the bovine TB cattle–human transmission model for Morocco (Abakar *et al.*, 2017).

Fig. 4.1. Conceptual model of progression of bovine tuberculosis infection and relationship of model compartments to surveillance and control measures. S, susceptible; O, occult/unreactive; R, reactive; I, infectious; A, anergic.

Fig. 4.2. (a) Average percentage of animals reacting to the tuberculin skin test with increasing herd size. (b) Estimated reproduction ratio based upon the apparent average prevalence of tuberculin reactors within these coarse herd size ranges. Adapted from Francis, J. (1947) *Bovine Tuberculosis*, Table XI.

Fig. 4.3. (a) Percentage of animals reacting to skin test within coarse age groups (b) Estimated force of infection within the same age groups. Adapted from Francis, J. (1947) *Bovine Tuberculosis*, Table I.

Fig. 4.4. Distribution of reactor animals disclosed at the beginning of a herd breakdown in PTI 1, 2 and 4 historical testing areas in Great Britain (2003–2005).

Fig. 9.1. Gross pathology of *Mycobacterium bovis* infection in cattle. (a) Multiple sub-pleural lesions can be observed in the dorsal part of the right middle lung lobe. (b) After sectioning, multiple coalescing granulomatous lesions observable with caseous necrosis in the centre and inflammatory reaction surrounding the areas of necrosis.

Fig. 9.2. (a) Stage I granuloma showing clustered epithelioid macrophages with some Langhans-type multi-nucleated giant cells (MNGCs). (H&E, 200×) (b) Stage II granuloma with abundant epithelioid macrophages, visible MNGCs and an incomplete fibrous capsule. (H&E, 100×) (c) Stage III granuloma showing a complete fibrous capsule and central necrosis. (H&E, 40×) (d) Stage IV granuloma with a complete fibrous encapsulation, extensive central necrosis and mineralization. (H&E, 40×)

Fig. 9.3. Acid-fast bacilli within the cytoplasm of a MNGC. (Ziehl-Neelsen, 600×)

Fig. 9.4. CD68+ staining in stage I and II granulomas in the lung of a cow experimentally infected with *M. bovis*. Heavy positive staining can be observed within the cytoplasm of macrophages and multi-nucleated giant cells. (IHC, 100×)

Fig. 9.5. CD3+ staining in stage IV granulomas in the lung of an infected cow with *M. bovis*. Abundant positive T cells can be observed mostly in the outer layers of the granulomas. (IHC, 100×)

Fig. 9.6. CD79a+ staining in stage I, II and IV granulomas in the lung of a cow experimentally infected with *M. bovis*. Scattered CD79a+ cells can be observed within the rim of inflammatory cells surrounding the necrotic core of the stage IV granuloma and interspersed within the stage I and II granulomas. The formation of a nest of B cells can be observed in the lesion with a high number of CD79a+ cells. (IHC, 100×)

Fig. 9.7. Staining of INF-γ in a stage II granuloma from the mediastinal lymph node of a cow experimentally infected with *M. bovis*. Abundant IFN-γ positive cells can be observed within the granuloma. (IHC, 400×)

Fig. 9.8. Staining of TNF-α in a stage IV granuloma from the lung of a cow experimentally infected with *M. bovis*. The expression of TNF-α can be observed within the cytoplasm of few epithelioid macrophages and a multi-nucleated giant cell. (IHC, 400×)

Fig. 9.9. Staining of TGF-β in a stage IV granuloma from the mediastinal lymph node of a cow experimentally infected with *M. bovis*. Abundant epithelioid macrophages are expressing TGF-β within a rim of inflammatory cells adjacent to the necrotic core. (IHC, 40×)

Fig. 9.10. (a) Granulomatous disorganized and diffuse lesion, poorly demarcated within the lung of a mouse experimentally infected with *M. bovis*. (H&E, 100×) (b) Abundant AFBs within the cytoplasm of 'foamy' macrophages at the periphery of the granulomatous lesion. (Ziehl-Neelsen, 600×)

Fig. 9.11. Multifocal granulomas within the lung of a guinea pig infected with *M. tuberculosis*. The granulomas are in different stages of development showing solid lesions with no necrosis (small) and extensive necrosis and fibrotic capsule (large). (H&E, 20×)

Fig. 9.12. (a) Pyogranulomatous severe panniculitis from a cat naturally infected with *M. bovis*. (b) Skin lesion from a cat infected with *M. bovis*, showing extensive dermatitis and inflammatory cell infiltration in the subcutis, with disruption of the normal epithelium, close to a fistula. (H&E, 40×) (c) Granulomatous inflammation within extensive necrotic core within the axillar lymph node. (HE, 40×) (d) Abundant acidfast bacilli within the necrotic centre of the lymph node. (Ziehl-Neelson, 400×; inset, 1000×)

Fig. 9.13. (a) Detail of the outer layer of a granuloma from the mesenteric lymph node of an alpaca infected with *M. bovis*. The necrotic area (upper part of Fig) is surrounded by abundant inflammatory infiltrate, mostly composed of lymphocytes, a few macrophages and no multi-nucleated giant cells. (inset) Extensive necrotic core of the lesion. (H&E, 200×; inset 20×) (b) Few acid-fast bacilli (arrows) are observed within the necrotic centre of the lymph node. (Ziehl-Neelson, 600×)

Fig. 9.14. Multifocal granulomas at different stage of development in a badger infected with *M. bovis*. Some of the lesions are small and solid, while other show a central area of necrosis surrounded by a rim of epithelioid cells, no multinucleated giant cells and lymphocytes at the outer layers of the lesion. No evident capsule can be identified. (H&E, 40×)

Fig. 9.15. Large coalescent caseous granulomas in the lung of a fallow deer infected with *M. bovis*. Yellowish creamy material can observed within the lesion. Courtesy of 'Red de Recursos Faunisticos' group, University of Extremadura, Spain.

Fig. 9.16. Solid well-encapsulated lesion in the mandibular lymph node from a wild boar infected with *M. bovis*. The lesion is also heavy mineralized and 'gritty' on sectioning. Courtesy of 'Red de Recursos Faunisticos' group, University of Extremadura, Spain.

Fig. 12.1. Hierarchy of T-cell responses to 626 *M. bovis*/*M. tuberculosis* proteins. Results are shown as responder frequencies (proportion of tested animals responding to a given protein). Responses were established using whole blood cultures from *M. bovis*-infected cattle to measure antigen-specific IFN-γ responses.

Fig. 15.1. Direct and indirect pathways for spread of bovine tuberculosis between and within species in New Zealand. Bold arrows indicate a main source or route of infection; brown depicts direct transmission, green depicts indirect transmission via scavenging or investigation of tuberculous carcasses and offal, red indicates that the source of infection is unknown but is likely to be by direct means. This figure is reproduced with permission of the Editor, New Zealand Veterinary Journal, where it was first published as Figure 2 in the following paper: P.G. Livingstone, N. Hancox, G. Nugent, G.W. de Lisle (2015) Toward eradication: the effect of *Mycobacterium bovis* infection in wildlife on the evolution and future direction of bovine tuberculosis management in New Zealand. *New Zealand Veterinary Journal* 63 (S1), p7.

1 Bovine Tuberculosis: Worldwide Picture

Lina Awada, Paolo Tizzani, Elisabeth Erlacher-Vindel,
Simona Forcella and Paula Caceres*

World Organisation for Animal Health (OIE), Paris, France

1.1 Introduction

Bovine tuberculosis caused by *Mycobacterium bovis* is a disease of livestock and wildlife and causes global economic losses, including those resulting from trade barriers (OIE, 2015), estimated at several billion USD annually despite widespread control efforts (Schiller *et al.*, 2010).

The objective of this chapter is to provide information on the worldwide bovine tuberculosis situation, using data from the OIE. The OIE's World Animal Health Information System (WAHIS), is a reference for conducting global analyses in this field.

1.1.1 The World Organisation for Animal Health and the World Health Information System

The dissemination of rinderpest in Europe in 1920, resulting from a shipment of infected zebu cattle originating from India and destined for Brazil transiting through the Belgium port of Antwerp, alerted a group of countries to the need to organize themselves to notify the sanitary status of their animals and animal products prior to commercialization. The resurgence of rinderpest in Europe, from whence it had been eradicated, highlighted the need for international collaboration to control major infectious animal diseases. Concern over the resulting international spread of rinderpest led to an international conference of Chief Veterinary Officers from various countries in May 1921 in Paris. This eventually led to the creation in 1924 of the Office International des Epizooties (OIE), founded by 28 Member Countries, under the terms of the International Agreement signed on 25 January 1924 (OIE, 2011). The exchange of information on animal diseases between countries was one of the prime reasons for creating the OIE, with the ultimate aim of ensuring transparency of the animal health situation worldwide.

In May 2003 the Office became the World Organisation for Animal Health but kept its historic acronym 'OIE'. The OIE is the intergovernmental organization responsible for improving animal health worldwide. It is recognized as the reference organization by the World Trade Organization (WTO) in this domain and in 2016 had a total of 180 member countries. The OIE maintains permanent relations with 71 other international and regional organizations and has regional and sub-regional offices on every continent. The missions of the OIE are as follows:

- Ensuring transparency in the global animal disease situation.

---

* Email: p.caceres@oie.int

© CAB International 2018. *Bovine Tuberculosis*
(eds M. Chambers, S. Gordon, F. Olea-Popelka, P. Barrow)

- Collecting, analysing and disseminating veterinary scientific information.
- Encouraging international solidarity in the control of animal diseases.
- Safeguarding world trade by publishing health standards for international trade in animals and animal products.
- Improving the legal framework and resources of national Veterinary Services for a good sanitary governance.
- Providing a better guarantee of the safety of food of animal origin and promoting animal welfare through a science-based approach.

Within the framework of the OIE's first mandatory mission ('ensuring transparency in the global animal disease situation'), each member country undertakes to report the animal diseases, including those transmissible to humans, that it detects on its territory. This applies both to naturally occurring and deliberately caused disease events. The OIE then disseminates the information to other countries, which can then take any necessary preventive actions. Information is sent out immediately or periodically depending on the seriousness of the disease.

In 2006, to help its member countries fulfil their reporting obligations, the OIE launched the WAHIS, a secure computer system accessible via the Internet that enables member countries to enter, store and view data on animal diseases, including zoonoses, in the OIE's three official working languages (English, French and Spanish). WAHIS replaced the former system (Handistatus), which was the first online reporting system. Access to this secure system is only available to authorized users, namely the delegates of OIE member countries and their authorized representatives. After this information has been verified and validated by the OIE, it is published on the public WAHIS portal (OIE, 2016a).

WAHIS consists of four inter-related components (see OIE, 2015):

- The early warning system, the main component dedicated to animal health events notifiable within 24 hours of confirmation, which allows other countries to take appropriate measures to prevent the spread of animal diseases with a significant impact. The early warning system includes the notification of more than 100 OIE-listed diseases and other emerging diseases in domestic animals and wildlife.
- The monitoring system, which enables countries to notify every 6 months the presence or absence of more than 100 diseases listed by the OIE, and includes several types of reports on terrestrial and aquatic animal diseases in domestic animals and wildlife.
- The annual report, through which important additional information on the national veterinary services and other relevant details about the country are collected once a year (zoonotic diseases transmitted to humans, animal population figures, veterinary staff, vaccine production, etc.).
- The 'Wild' annual report, which enables countries to notify information on more than 50 diseases in wildlife that are not listed by the OIE. This report is submitted by member countries on a voluntary basis.

1.2 Bovine Tuberculosis Notification Since the Creation of the OIE

At the creation of the OIE and as per its Organic Statutes (OIE, 1924), signed on 25 January 1924, member countries had a legal obligation to forward to the Organisation information on the presence and distribution of the following nine diseases: anthrax, contagious pleuropneumonia, dourine, glanders, foot and mouth disease, rabies, rinderpest, sheep pox and swine fever.

However, even though animal tuberculosis (including both bovine and avian tuberculosis) was not listed at that time, information that had been provided for this disease was published in 1927 in the Bulletin of the Office International des Epizooties. This issue of the OIE Bulletin contained statistics on animal health status worldwide (Fig. 1.1). This is the first notification of animal tuberculosis recorded in the OIE archives.

Bovine tuberculosis was included among the OIE-listed diseases in May 1964, when the list of notifiable diseases was revised by the International Committee[1] of the OIE. This revision took into consideration changes in the national zoosanitary legislation of member countries during the previous 40 years, the large number

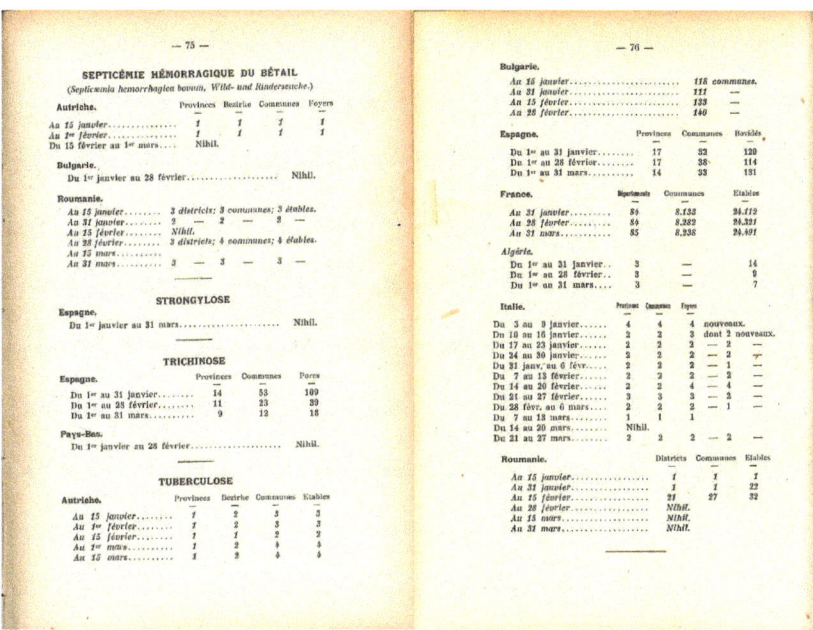

Fig. 1.1. Statistics on animal tuberculosis published in the Bulletin of the Office International des Epizooties, July 1927–June 1928.

of different diseases that were now included in national sanitary legislation, and the specific request by some international organizations, such as the Food and Agriculture Organization of the United Nations (FAO), the Organisation for Economic Co-operation and Development and the European Economic Community, that the OIE establish a new list of diseases.[2]

Bovine tuberculosis was initially included in List B,[3] comprising diseases reportable annually to the OIE. This list included all the transmissible diseases that were considered to be of socio-economic or public health importance within countries and that were significant in the international trade of animals and animal products. In contrast, List A[4] comprised compulsorily notifiable diseases to be reported monthly or fortnightly to the OIE. This list included all the transmissible diseases that were potentially able to spread across national borders very rapidly with serious socio-economic or public health effects and that are of major significance for international trade in animals and their products. In 1996, the launch of the OIE Handistatus online reporting system enabled member countries to provide information in a digital form.

In 2004, the International Committee of the OIE passed resolutions that, together with the recommendations of the Regional Commissions of the OIE, instructed OIE Headquarters to establish one list of notifiable terrestrial and aquatic animal diseases that would replace Lists A and B produced formerly, which included 15 and 93 diseases, respectively. The OIE developed criteria to identify diseases that would be included in this OIE single list. These criteria were approved in May of that year and in 2005 this first single list came into effect (see OIE, 2015). The criteria relate to the risks of spread of the infectious microorganism internationally, together with the consequences for humans, for domestic livestock and wildlife and the of reliable methods for diagnosis and detection.

In parallel with the implementation of this list, the launch of WAHIS meant that member countries could now generate information on diseases on this OIE list in a standardized format. Several improvements to WAHIS then enabled member countries to provide more detailed information on OIE-listed diseases, in particular for wildlife. Thus, since 2009 it has been possible to report the occurrence of diseases in domestic animals and in wildlife separately and, since 2012, to provide both the scientific and common names of the wildlife species affected. Bovine tuberculosis has been listed by the OIE since 1964.

1.3 Trend in the Presence of Bovine Tuberculosis over the Past 30 Years

This section presents the results of an analysis of changes in the presence of bovine tuberculosis over the past 30 years, based on data collected by the OIE. From 1986 to 1995, the annual occurrence of bovine tuberculosis in member countries was compiled in the annual OIE publication *World Animal Health*. Thereafter, the data were digitized and from 1996 to 2004 they were recorded in the 'Handistatus' information system. Since 2005, they have been collected through WAHIS.

For each year between 1986 and 2015, the annual percentage of affected countries among those providing the OIE with information was calculated, as well as the 95% confidence interval (Fig. 1.2).

The number of OIE member countries varied during the period of the analysis, increasing from 103 in 1986 to 180 in 2015. The historical trend in the presence of bovine tuberculosis is therefore influenced by the variation in the number of reporting member countries throughout the years.

The percentage of reporting countries that notified bovine tuberculosis present decreased between 1986 and 2015, from 84% (CI95% = 80%–88%) to 50% (CI95% = 46%–54%) (Spearman's rank correlation = 8764, $p < 0.001$; rho = −0.95), indicating a general improvement in the global situation over the past 30 years. This trend followed a simple linear model ($R^2 = 0.9$; $p < 0.001$). Even if the data present a high degree of variability among the different years, the overall tendency is clearly shown by the regression model. Variability in the observed trend can be explained by different levels of accuracy and quality of the information provided to the OIE by member countries. The diagnostic capabilities and the degree of preparedness of the veterinary services may vary from month to month during the year and among the countries. These differences should be considered when assessing historical trends in disease.

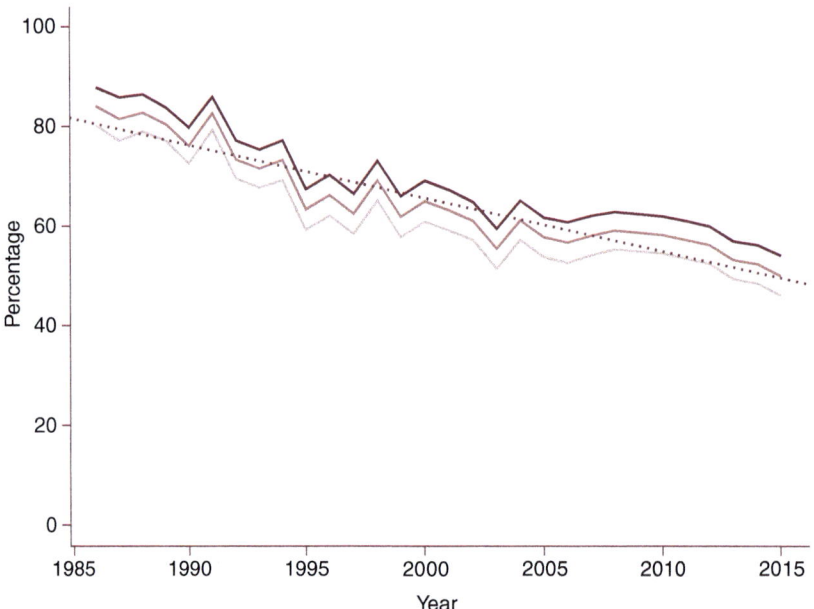

Fig. 1.2. Percentage of the reporting countries for each year between 1986 and 2015 that notified bovine tuberculosis present, with the 95% confidence interval, and simple linear regression trend line.

In order to analyse and compare regional differences, reporting countries are categorized by geographical region and the trend was calculated by each region. Regional trends are presented in Fig. 1.3. In all regions, the percentage of reporting countries notifying bovine tuberculosis decreased significantly from 1986 to 2015.

The most rapid decrease was observed in Oceania and Europe, changing by more than 45% during the 30-year period. In Oceania, the actual percentage decreased from 75% (CI95%=53–97%) to 27% (CI95%=14%–41%) (Spearman's rank correlation=7595, $p<0.001$; rho=–0.68), while in Europe it decreased from 84% (CI95%=78%–89%) to 38% (CI95%=31%–45%) (Spearman's rank correlation=8767, $p<0.001$; rho=–0.95).

A rapid change was also observed in Asia, with a 38% decrease over the 30-year period. The actual percentage decreased from 80% (CI95%=67%–93%) to 42% (CI95%=33%–51%) (Spearman's rank correlation=7919, $p<0.001$; rho=–0.76).

Finally, the change in disease notification was slower in Africa and the Americas, with a decrease of 25% and 18%, respectively, over the 30-year period. In Africa, it decreased from 85% (CI95%=78%–92%) to 67% (CI95%=59%–75%) (Spearman's rank correlation=8514, $p<0.001$; rho=–0.89), while in the Americas it decreased from 91% (CI95%=82%–100%) to 66% (CI95%=57%–74%) (Spearman's rank correlation=6471, $p=0.01$; rho=–0.44).

The results presented in this section clearly show a regular and significant improvement in the global bovine tuberculosis situation. The percentage of affected countries decreased by more than 30% in 30 years, which is a considerable positive change. In addition, this decrease was observed in all geographical regions, albeit with differences in the rate of decrease. Nevertheless, more than half of the reporting countries still notified the presence of the disease in 2015, which indicates that efforts to achieve global control still need to be pursued.

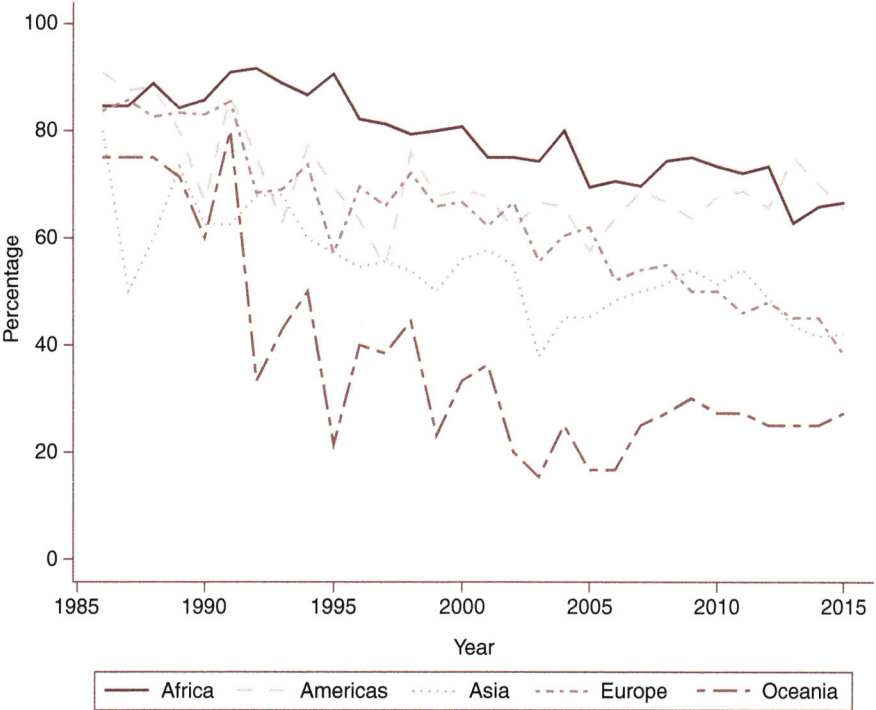

Fig. 1.3. Percentage of the reporting countries by region for each year between 1986 and 2015 that notified bovine tuberculosis present.

1.4 Detailed Trend in Cattle Since 2005, Based on Annual Incidence

The evaluation of the percentage of affected countries presented in the previous section provides interesting qualitative information about the trend of the disease in the last 30 years. Further information about the historical trend of the disease can be derived by analysing the quantitative data reported to the OIE. As well as reporting qualitative information to the OIE about the presence or absence of the disease, member countries can also provide quantitative details, such as the number of susceptible animals, cases, dead animals, slaughtered animals and destroyed animals.

This section presents the results of an analysis of the evolution of bovine tuberculosis in cattle over the past 11 years, based on data collected by the OIE.

The OIE does not collect information about herd prevalence; therefore, to measure the quantitative trend of bovine tuberculosis in cattle, the number of new cases yearly (i.e. annual incidence) has been used. Although quantitative information is very informative, not all countries have the capacity to monitor the evolution of the disease with this level of detail and to provide the OIE with the corresponding data. Therefore, the data presented in this section include only those provided by countries that submitted regular quantitative information to the OIE. Moreover, the annual incidence trend was analysed starting from 2005 in order to present information collected using the same standard format (WAHIS platform). This helped to avoid potential inconsistencies related to the methodology of data collection.

During the period (2005–2015), 142 countries reported complete quantitative information regarding the annual incidence of bovine tuberculosis in cattle. Around two million cases of bovine tuberculosis in cattle were reported to the OIE, with countries presenting different epidemiological situations (epizootic, enzootic). For a better evaluation of the trend of the disease, the reporting countries were assigned to four different groups, according to the number of cases reported each year:

- **Group A:** composed of 62 countries that reported the disease absent for the entire period;
- **Group B:** composed of 19 countries that reported fewer than 100 cases for the entire period;
- **Group C:** composed of 22 countries that reported between 101 and 1000 cases for the entire period; and
- **Group D:** composed of 39 countries that reported more than 1000 cases for the entire period.

The most important groups from a quantitative perspective were Groups C and D. In particular, Group D alone represented 99.5% of the total number of cases reported during the period, while Group C represented 0.4% of the total number of cases. Group D comprises 12 countries in Europe, 11 in Africa, 9 in the Americas, 6 in Asia and 1 in Oceania.

The average number of cases reported in cattle was calculated by group and by year. Considering quantitative data at group level, there was no obvious trend for Group B, while Groups C and D showed a significant decrease in the average number of cases reported over the years (Group C: Spearman's rank correlation test: rho = −0.74, $p < 0.01$; Group D: rho = −0.8, $p < 0.005$; Figs 1.4 and 1.5).

For Group C, the average number of cases reported in cattle decreased slightly, from 72 cases/year in 2006 to 26 cases/year in 2015. For Group D, the average number of cases reported decreased from a peak of 6645 cases/year in 2006 to 3903 cases/year in 2015.

The Americas and Europe represented 89% of the total reported cases, most likely due to a better quality of information provided by these regions in comparison with other regions. Considering the same trend in the average number of cases reported at regional level, the Americas and Europe showed a strong decrease over the years (rho = −0.75 and −0.72, respectively; $p < 0.05$). The largest decrease was observed in the Americas, where the yearly average number of cases decreased from a peak of 15,381 in 2007 to 6,093 in 2015 (reduction of 60% in eight years; Fig. 1.6).

A similar trend was observed in Oceania, with a significant decrease in the number of cases reported (Spearman's rank correlation

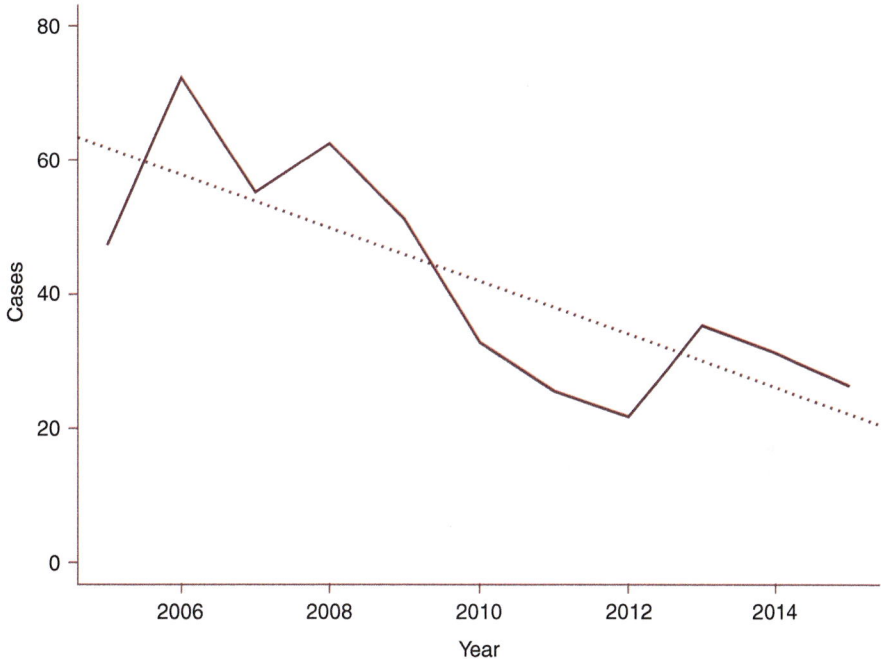

Fig. 1.4. Trend in the average number of cases reported to the OIE since 2005 by the countries in Group C. The linear regression is reported on the graph.

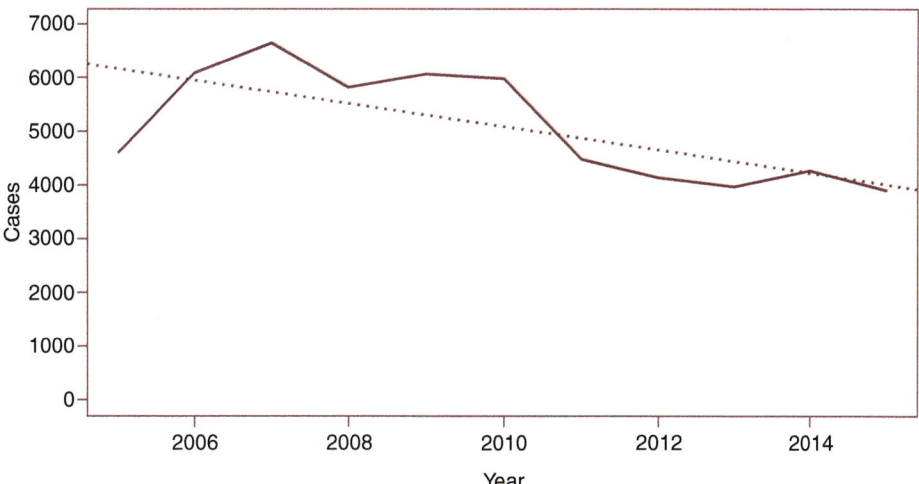

Fig. 1.5 Trend in the average number of cases reported to the OIE since 2005 by the countries in Group D. The linear regression is reported on the graph.

test: rho = −0.72, $p < 0.05$). Finally, a completely different situation was observed in the other regions, with a significant increase in the number of cases reported (rho value = 0.55 (Africa) and 0.71 (Asia); $p < 0.1$ (Africa) and $p < 0.05$ (Asia); Fig. 1.7).

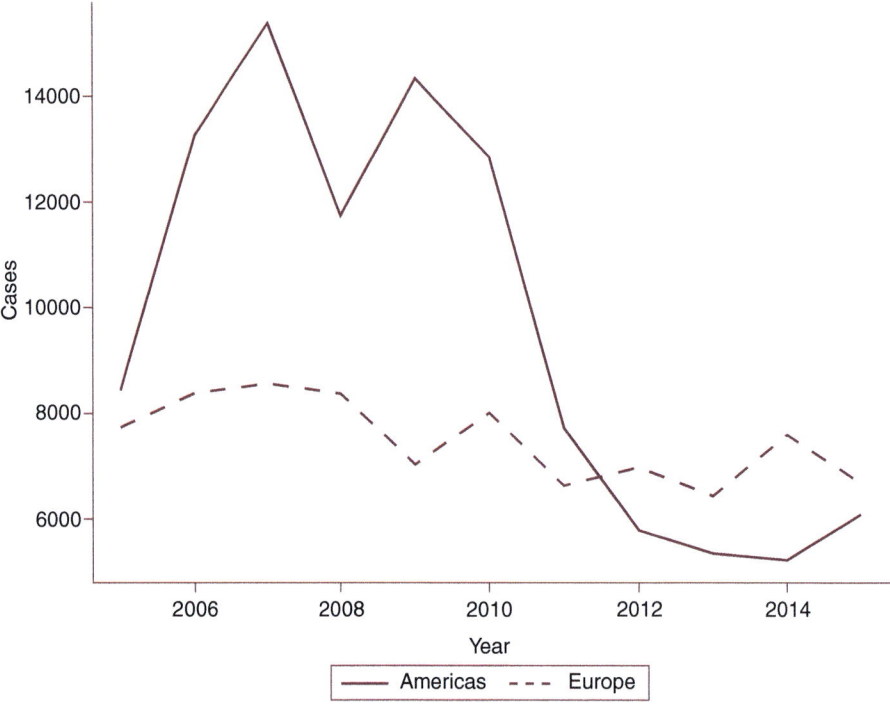

Fig. 1.6. Trend in the average number of cases reported to the OIE since 2005 in the Americas and Europe.

The control of bovine tuberculosis in cattle is a major animal health issue in many parts of the world. The analysis of the detailed quantitative data in the WAHIS database provides interesting information on the success of eradication programmes (Knobler *et al.*, 2005). It is clear from the yearly incidence trend that the global impact of bovine tuberculosis decreased considerably between 2005 and 2015 (from an average of 1276 cases/year reported in 2005 to an average of 1082 cases/year in 2015). These quantitative results strengthen the findings of the qualitative analysis, which showed a decreasing trend over the past 30 years in the percentage of reporting countries that declared bovine tuberculosis present.

However, the decrease shows strong regional differences. In America, Europe and Oceania, the eradication plans seem to have been implemented efficiently, leading to the control of the bovine tuberculosis situation. In contrast, in other regions the disease has been spreading and the impact on animal populations (number of cases reported) remains very high.

1.5 The Situation in 2015: The Worldwide Distribution in Domestic Animals and in Wildlife

This section presents the worldwide distribution of bovine tuberculosis in 2015, firstly for domestic animals and secondly for wildlife, based on data collected by the OIE through WAHIS.

As of 4 May 2016, 165 countries had provided information for bovine tuberculosis in domestic animals in 2015 and 50% of them reported the disease present (Fig. 1.8). A total of 108 countries provided information for bovine tuberculosis in wildlife and 25% of them reported the disease present (Fig. 1.9). In all cases the situation was reported to the OIE as being stable, since in 2015 no alert was submitted to the OIE for an exceptional epidemiological event involving bovine tuberculosis.

As shown in Fig. 1.8, the global coverage of information on the bovine tuberculosis situation in domestic animals in 2015 is satisfactory, as a very large proportion of countries in the world

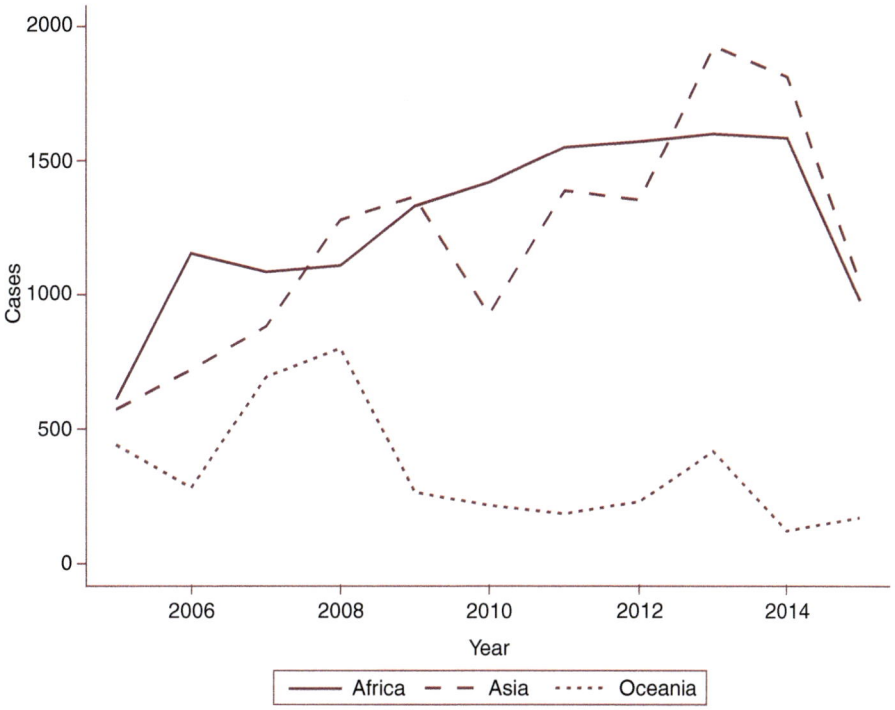

Fig. 1.7. Trend in the average number of cases reported to the OIE since 2005 in Africa, Asia and Oceania.

were able to describe their situation. Conversely, and as shown in Fig. 1.9, the global coverage of information on the bovine tuberculosis situation in wildlife is limited, with important gaps of information in some developing countries, in particular those in Africa, Asia and South America. This lack of information is a cause for concern from an epidemiological point of view as the presence of the disease in wildlife reservoirs presents significant challenges for disease management, particularly in areas where the infection is able to circulate among a community of wild mammal hosts, with the potential for onward spread to cattle and consequent limitation of progress towards eradication (Gortazar et al., 2014).

Countries notified the detection of bovine tuberculosis in a total of 19 wild species in 2015, with the highest number of cases at global level reported in wild boar (*Sus scrofa*), European badger (*Meles meles*) and African buffalo (*Syncerus caffer*), which appear to be the main reservoir species, as also described in the scientific literature (Fitzgerald and Kaneene, 2013). For more details about bovine tuberculosis in wildlife species see Chapter 7, this volume.

1.6 OIE Standards Relating to Bovine Tuberculosis

The OIE *Terrestrial Animal Health Code* sets out standards for the improvement of animal health and welfare and veterinary public health worldwide, including through standards for safe international trade in terrestrial animals (mammals, birds and bees) and their products. The health measures in the *Terrestrial Animal Health Code* should be used by the veterinary authorities of importing and exporting countries to provide for early detection, reporting and control of agents that are pathogenic to animals or humans, and to prevent their transfer via international trade in animals and animal products, while avoiding unjustified sanitary barriers to trade.

The health measures in the *Terrestrial Animal Health Code* have been formally adopted by

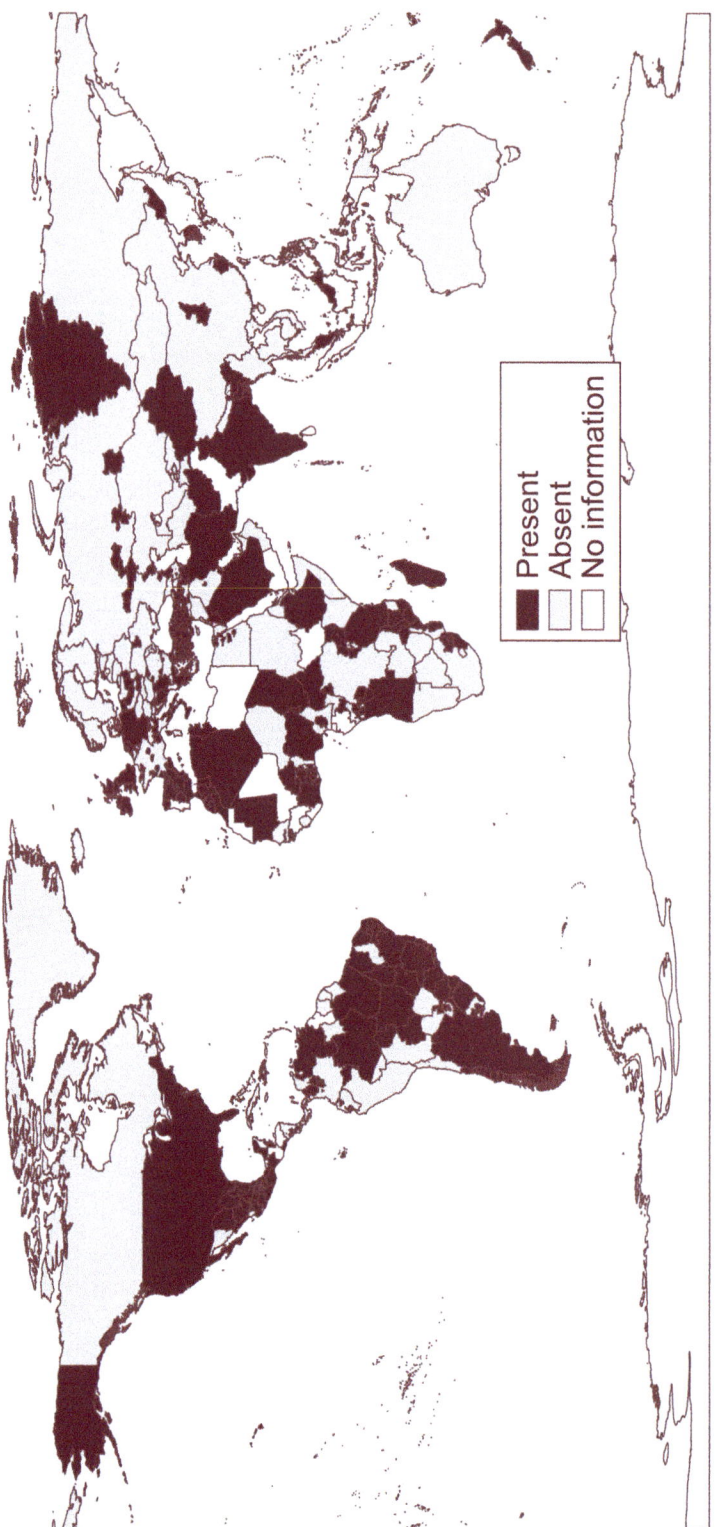

Fig. 1.8. Distribution of bovine tuberculosis in domestic animals in 2015, as reported to the OIE up to 4 May 2016.

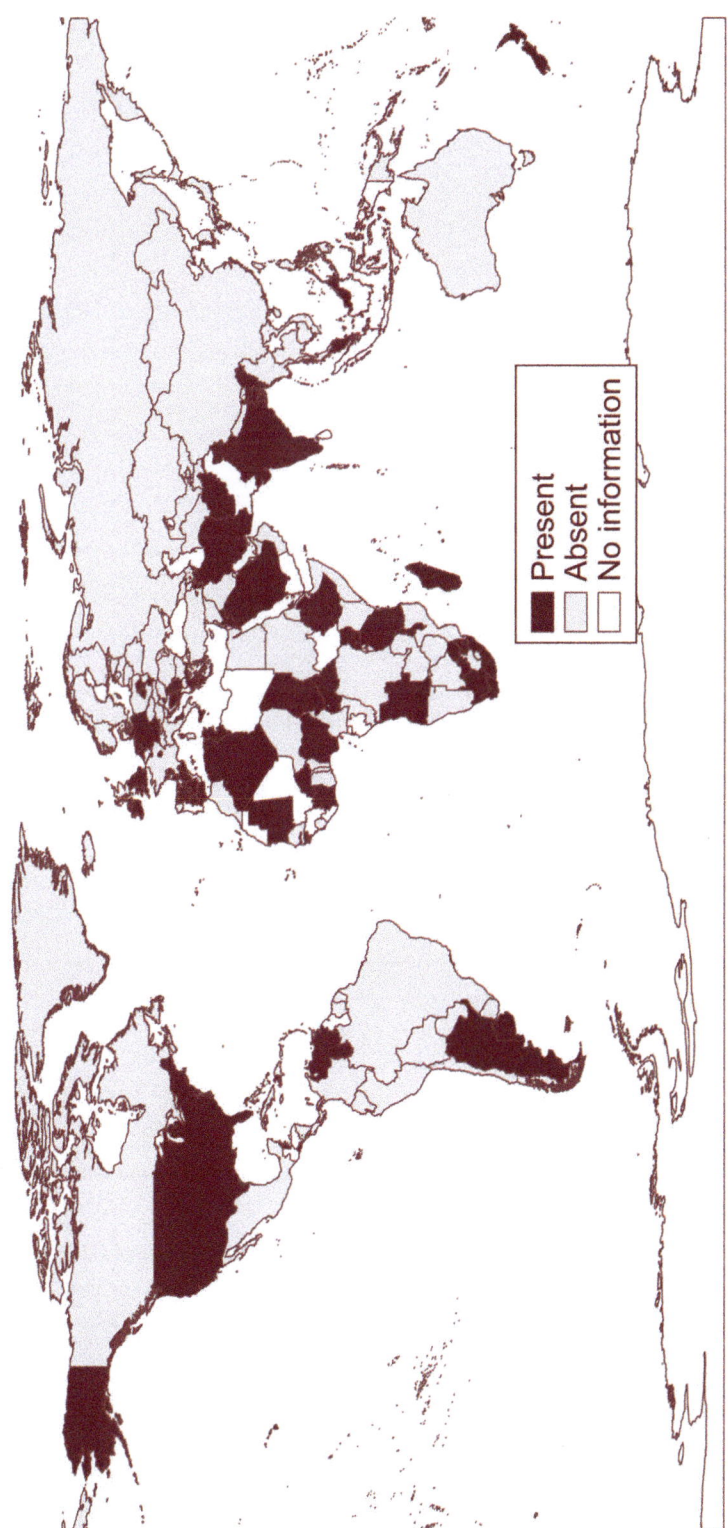

Fig. 1.9. Distribution of bovine tuberculosis in wildlife in 2015, as reported to the OIE up to 4 May 2016.

the World Assembly of Delegates of the OIE. The development of these standards and recommendations is the result of the continuous work since 1960 of two of the OIE's specialist commissions, namely the OIE Scientific Commission for Animal Diseases and the Terrestrial Animal Health Standards Commission. The first *Terrestrial Animal Health Code* was published in 1968. The Terrestrial Animal Health Standards Commission draws upon the expertise of internationally renowned specialists to prepare draft texts for new articles of the *Terrestrial Animal Health Code* or revise existing articles in the light of advances in veterinary science.

The value of the *Terrestrial Animal Health Code* is twofold: that the measures published in it are the result of consensus among the veterinary authorities of OIE member countries, and that it constitutes a reference within the World Trade Organization Agreement on the Application of Sanitary and Phytosanitary Measures as an international standard for animal health and zoonoses.

As of May 2016, in Chapter 11.5 of the *Terrestrial Animal Health Code*, the OIE provides recommendations on managing the human and animal health risks associated with *M. bovis* infection in domestic bovines, including cattle, water buffaloes and wood bison. In Chapter 11.6 of the same document, the OIE provides recommendations on managing risks in domestic (permanently captive and owned free-range) farmed Cervidae.

These two chapters list the requirements that should be satisfied for a country, a zone or a compartment to qualify as free from bovine tuberculosis. These requirements mainly relate to surveillance, regular and periodic testing of animals and control at borders. The chapters also describe the requirements that should be satisfied for a herd to qualify as free from bovine tuberculosis. Finally, these chapters provide recommendations for the importation of animals and animal products.

In addition, the OIE *Manual of Diagnostic Tests and Vaccines for Terrestrial Animals* (OIE, 2016b) aims to facilitate international trade in animals and animal products and to contribute to the improvement of animal health services worldwide. The principal target readership is laboratories carrying out veterinary diagnostic tests and surveillance, as well as vaccine manufacturers and regulatory authorities in member countries. The objective is to provide internationally agreed diagnostic laboratory methods and requirements for the production and control of vaccines and other biological products.

The *Manual of Diagnostic Tests and Vaccines for Terrestrial Animals*, covering infectious and parasitic diseases of mammals, birds and bees, was first published in 1989. Each successive edition has extended and updated the information provided. The chapter on bovine tuberculosis provides standards for diagnostic techniques and for vaccines and diagnostic biologicals for bovine tuberculosis.

As of May 2016, the diagnostic techniques described in the *Manual of Diagnostic Tests and Vaccines for Terrestrial Animals* are classified as follows:

- identification of the agent: microscopic examination, culture and nucleic acid recognition methods;
- delayed hypersensitivity test: tuberculin test; and
- blood-based laboratory tests: gamma-interferon assay, lymphocyte proliferation assay and enzyme-linked immunosorbent assay.

The tuberculin test is recommended as the prescribed test for international trade, while the gamma-interferon assay is listed as the alternative test for international trade.

The requirements for vaccines and diagnostic biologicals cover the production of tuberculin, with a detailed description of seed management, method of manufacture, in-process control, batch control and tests on the final product.

1.7 The Importance of Controlling Zoonotic Tuberculosis in Animals

Although *M. tuberculosis* is recognized as the primary causal agent of human tuberculosis, WHO estimates that around 149,000 incident cases of zoonotic tuberculosis are caused by foodborne *M. bovis* each year (World Health Organization, 2015). Risk factors for the human population include close physical contact with infected animals and consumption of animal products (unpasteurized milk and untreated animal products) (Cosivi *et al.*, 1998). For more details about the public health impact of *M. bovis*, see Chapters 2 and 6, this volume.

Bovine tuberculosis is a disease of livestock and wildlife and causes global economic losses, including those resulting from trade barriers (OIE, 2015), estimated at several billion USD annually despite widespread control efforts (Schiller *et al.*, 2010).

Bovine tuberculosis in humans cannot be adequately addressed without considering the burden of disease in the animal reservoir and the risk pathways for transmission at the animal–human interface. The reduced productivity within livestock populations caused by *M. bovis* impacts on livelihoods in poor and marginalized communities. Appropriate control of bovine tuberculosis in animals allows early intervention and prevention of spread from domestic animals to wildlife, minimizing risks of infection to the human population, avoiding economic losses for poor communities and increasing opportunities for trade.

The OIE is the WTO's reference intergovernmental organization for animal health and welfare. As such, it is responsible for developing, publishing and constantly reviewing intergovernmental regulations and standards, not only for disease prevention and control methods, but also regarding the quality of national animal and veterinary public health systems.

Coordinating the effective implementation of these standards at the national, regional and global level with efficient cooperation between veterinary and public health services is one of the most critical factors for controlling health hazards worldwide, including zoonotic tuberculosis.

In this context, the OIE, jointly with WHO and the World Bank, has released a guide for national public health authorities and national animal health authorities (represented by the veterinary services) outlining methods for strengthening the good governance of health systems worldwide.

Within the 'One Health' framework, the Tripartite Alliance (the FAO, OIE and WHO) recognize their respective responsibilities in fighting diseases, including zoonoses, that can have a serious health and economic impact. The three organizations have been working together to prevent, detect, control and eliminate disease risks to humans originating directly or indirectly from animals. In 2010, the FAO/OIE/WHO Tripartite Concept Note (April 2010) officially recognized this close collaboration with the objective of sharing responsibilities and coordinating global activities to address health risks at the human–animal–ecosystem interface.

In February 2016, the Tripartite gave a commitment to define a common strategy to increase awareness and knowledge of the burden of zoonotic tuberculosis and to advocate for the control of the disease at the animal source.

1.8 Conclusion

Bovine tuberculosis has been of great interest to OIE member countries for a very long time, and especially since it was incorporated into the OIE List of Notifiable Diseases in 1964. In fact, the OIE's first records of national statistics on bovine tuberculosis date back to 1927.

As presented in this chapter, the results of the trend analysis of the presence of bovine tuberculosis over the past 30 years show a regular and significant improvement in the global situation, with a percentage of affected countries that decreased by about 30% during this period. Similarly, the analysis of detailed quantitative data in WAHIS points to the success of eradication programmes, with a significant decrease in the global yearly incidence trend between 2005 and 2015. However, the results presented also highlight regional differences, with a high degree of variability in disease presence worldwide, in the ability of countries to report information, and in the outcome of eradication programmes.

In 2015, a very large proportion of countries in the world were able to describe their bovine tuberculosis situation in domestic animals. However, major information gaps were observed for wildlife in some developing countries, in particular those in Africa, Asia and South America. Therefore, more efforts are needed in the monitoring, control and eradication of bovine tuberculosis worldwide, as 50% of the reporting countries reported bovine tuberculosis present in domestic animals in 2015 and 25% reported the disease present in wildlife.

To guide countries in the control and eradication of bovine tuberculosis, the OIE provides standards in its *Terrestrial Animal Health Code*. These health measures should be used by the veterinary authorities of importing and exporting countries to provide for early detection, reporting and control of agents that are pathogenic to animals or humans, and to prevent their transfer via international trade in animals and animal products, while avoiding unjustified sanitary barriers to trade. In addition, the OIE *Manual of Diagnostic Tests and Vaccines for Terrestrial Animals* aims to facilitate international trade in animals and animal products and to contribute to the improvement of animal health services worldwide. The objective is to provide internationally agreed diagnostic laboratory methods and requirements for the production and control of vaccines and other biological products.

The OIE is promoting a collaborative 'One Health' approach at international and national levels for the control of zoonotic diseases, including bovine tuberculosis. This will result in deeper and sustainable political support for the coordinated prevention of diseases with a high impact on public health and animal health at the human–animal interface. This approach is also promoted within the framework of the Tripartite Alliance by the FAO, OIE and WHO.

Notes

[1] Currently named 'World Assembly of Delegates'.

[2] Report of the Director on the Scientific and Technical Activities of the Office International des Epizooties from May 1963 to May 1964, by Dr R. Vittoz.

[3] List B in 1964: anaplasmosis, atrophic rhinitis, Aujeszky's disease, babesioses, bovine and avian tuberculosis, bovine vibriosis, brucelloses, contagious agalactia, contagious pleuropneumonia of small ruminants, contagious pustular dermatitis of sheep, epizootic lymphangitis, equine encephalomyelitis, European foul brood, acariasis of bees, furunculosis of Salmonidae, heartwater, infectious dropsy of carp, infectious equine anaemia, infectious respiratory diseases of poultry, Johne's disease, leptospirosis, leukaemia in cattle, malignant foul brood (American), mange and scab, mastitis, myxomatosis, nosemosis of bees, *Nuttallia equi* infection, psittacosis-ornithosis, Q fever, Rift Valley fever, salmonellosis, theileriases, trichinosis, trichomonas infection, *Trypanosoma brucei* infection, *Trypanosoma evansi*, tularaemia, vesicular stomatitis and viral haemorrhagic septicaemia of rainbow trout.

[4] List A in 1964: African horse sickness, African swine fever, anthrax, blue tongue, bovine contagious pleuropneumonia, exanthema coitale paralyticum, foot and mouth disease, fowl plague, glanders and farcy, lumpy skin disease, Newcastle disease, rabies, rinderpest, sheep pox, swine fever (hog cholera) and Teschen disease.

References

Cosivi, O., Grange, J.M., Daborn, C.J., Raviglione, M.C., Fujikura, T., *et al.* (1998) Zoonotic tuberculosis due to *Mycobacterium bovis* in developing countries. *Emerging Infectious Diseases* 4(1), 59–70.

Fitzgerald, S.D. and Kaneene, J.B. (2013) Wildlife reservoirs of bovine tuberculosis worldwide: hosts, pathology, surveillance, and control. *Veterinary Pathology* 50(3), 488–499.

Gortazar, C., Diez-Delgado, I., Barasona, J.A., Vicente, J., De La Fuente, J. and Boadella, M. (2014) The wild side of disease control at the wildlife-livestock-human interface: a review. *Frontiers in Veterinary Science* 1, 27.

Knobler, S.L., Mack, A., Mahmoud, A. and Lemon, S.M. (eds) (2005) *The Threat of Pandemic Influenza: Are We Ready? Workshop Summary.* National Academies Press, Washington DC, USA.

OIE (1924) Organic Statutes of the Office International des Epizooties, 25 January 1924. Available at: http://www.oie.int/en/about-us/key-texts/basic-texts/organic-statutes/ (accessed 1 June 2016).

OIE (2011) Rinderpest eradication. *OIE Bulletin* 2. Available at: http://www.oie.int/fileadmin/Home/eng/Publications_%26_Documentation/docs/pdf/bulletin/Bull_2011-2-ENG.pdf (accessed 1 June 2016).

OIE (2015) *Terrestrial Animal Health Code*. Chapter 11.5. Bovine tuberculosis. Article 11.5.5. Available at: http://www.oie.int/index.php?id=169&L=0&htmfile=chapitre_bovine_tuberculosis.htm (accessed 1 June 2016).

OIE (2016a) WAHIS Portal: Animal Health Data. Available at http://www.oie.int/en/animal-health-in-the-world/wahis-portal-animal-health-data/ (accessed 1 June 2016).

OIE (2016b) *Manual of Diagnostic Tests and Vaccines for Terrestrial Animals. World Animal Health Organization. Paris, France.* Version adopted by the World Assembly of Delegates of the OIE in May 2009. Available at: http://www.oie.int/eng/normes/mmanual/A_summry.htm (accessed 1 June 2016).

Schiller, I., Oesch, B., Vordermeier, H.M., Palmer, M.V., Harris, B.N., Orloski, K.A., Buddle, B.M., Thacker, T.C., Lyashchenko, K.P. and Waters, W.R. (2010) Bovine tuberculosis: a review of current and emerging diagnostic techniques in view of their relevance for disease control and eradication. *Transboundary Emerging Diseases* 57(4), 205–220.

World Health Organization (WHO) (2015) *WHO Estimates of the Global burden of foodborne diseases: foodborne disease burden epidemiology reference group 2007–2015.* World Health Organization, Geneva, Switzerland, p. 268.

2 *Mycobacterium bovis* as the Causal Agent of Human Tuberculosis: Public Health Implications

Francisco Olea-Popelka,[1,*] **Anna S. Dean,**[2] **Adrian Muwonge,**[3] **Alejandro Perera,**[4] **Mario Raviglione**[2] **and Paula I. Fujiwara**[5]

[1]*College of Veterinary Medicine and Biomedical Sciences, Department of Clinical Sciences and Mycobacteria Research Laboratories, Colorado State University, Fort Collins, USA;* [2]*Global TB Programme, World Health Organization, Geneva, Switzerland;* [3]*Genetics and Genomics, Roslin Institute, Royal (Dick) School of Veterinary Studies, University of Edinburgh, Edinburgh, UK;* [4]*United States Embassy, Mexico City, US Department of Agriculture, Animal and Plant Health Inspection Service, Mexico City, Mexico;* [5]*International Union Against Tuberculosis and Lung Disease, Paris, France*

2.1 Introduction

Mycobacterium bovis, the causal agent of bovine tuberculosis (TB) can also infect and cause TB in a variety of domestic and wild animals (see Chapters 4, 6 and 7, this volume). Additionally, humans can become infected with *M. bovis* and progress to develop what is known as zoonotic TB (O'Reilly and Daborn, 1995; Cosivi *et al.*, 1998; de la Rua-Domenech, 2006). The link between bovine TB, milk consumption and TB in humans (especially in children) has been recognized for centuries (Michel *et al.*, 2009; Palmer and Water, 2011). In the USA in 1900, approximately 10% of human TB cases were due to exposure to TB-infected cattle or cattle products (Olmstead and Rhode, 2004). Most importantly, approximately 25% of TB cases in children were caused by *M. bovis* (Roswurm and Ranney, 1973). In the UK, a report published in 1947 showed that up to 2000 deaths from TB were due to *M. bovis* and approximately 30% of new TB infections in children under 5 years of age were due to *M. bovis* (O'Reilly and Daborn, 1995). The role of *M. bovis* as a source of human TB historically has been previously reviewed (Griffith, 1937, 1938; Grange and Collins, 1987; Cosivi *et al.*, 1998; Collins, 2000; Ayele *et al.*, 2004; Thoen and LoBue, 2007; Michel *et al.*, 2009, 2015; Thoen *et al.*, 2009; Katale *et al.*, 2012; De Garine-Wichatitsky *et al.*, 2013; Kaneene *et al.*, 2014).

Today, in 2017, the true annual incidence of zoonotic TB is unknown. Thus, its impact on the global burden of TB is poorly understood. This is due to the lack of systematic surveillance for *M. bovis* as a causal agent of human TB in low-income, high TB burden countries where bovine TB is also endemic. The most commonly used tests to diagnose human TB in many parts of the world, such as sputum smear microscopy or GeneXpert, do not differentiate *M. bovis* from *Mycobacterium tuberculosis* (Cosivi *et al.*, 1998; Drobniewski *et al.*, 2003; Thoen *et al.*, 2010;

*Email: folea@colostate.edu

Müller et al., 2013; Perez-Lago et al., 2014). Additionally, even where cultures are performed, culture on standard Löwenstein-Jensen medium cannot distinguish the two species (Afghani, 1998; Keating et al., 2005). Culture must be performed using either pyruvate-supplemented solid media or liquid culture systems. Thus, not only are true incidence and burden poorly understood, but there is also a general lack of awareness (Thoen et al., 2010) on the importance, challenges and public health implications posed by *M. bovis* as a causal agent of human TB (Perez-Lago et al., 2014). This has resulted in *M. bovis* being neglected and underestimated as relevant data are not routinely captured by the majority of national tuberculosis control programmes.

In recent years, there has been a growing number of publications highlighting the importance of *M. bovis* as a cause of TB in humans. For example, in 2014, two reviews concluded that effective diagnostic policies using existing (and new) molecular epidemiology tools with the integration of veterinary, human health and wildlife sectors are needed in order to better understand the true challenge posed by *M. bovis* (Pal et al., 2014; Perez-Lago et al., 2014). In 2016, El-Sayed et al. (2016) published a review highlighting the seriousness of *M. bovis* at the human–animal interface, focusing mostly on the importance of molecular epidemiological studies related to *M. bovis*. Olea-Popelka and colleagues 'called for action' to address the global challenges regarding the prevention, diagnosis, treatment and control of human TB caused by *M. bovis* (Olea-Popelka et al., 2017). All these publications emphasize the need to consider the microbiological, epidemiological and clinical characteristics of *M. bovis* in order to improve the prevention, diagnosis and treatment of zoonotic TB patients.

Initially, the impetus for action to control bovine TB came from evidence indicating that *M. bovis* was zoonotic in nature and as such, a threat both to the farming family caring for its infected cattle and the wider population consuming meat and unpasteurized dairy products. In high-income countries, the success of the early bovine TB control campaigns (Michel et al., 2009; Palmer and Waters, 2011), the introduction of universal meat inspection programmes and the implementation of milk pasteurization have shifted the emphasis away from the health and social relevance of the disease in cattle to the economic and trading implications of the disease for both the beef and dairy industries (Collins, 1999). Today, the number of humans becoming infected by *M. bovis* and suffering from zoonotic TB is relatively low (compared to the number of those infected by *M. tuberculosis*) in most high-income countries. However, the scenario is likely to be very different in low- and middle-income countries where bovine TB is endemic and uncontrolled, and where animal management practices, socio-economic and cultural factors facilitate *M. bovis* transmission to humans (Ayele et al., 2004; Michel et al., 2009).

From a public health perspective, it is imperative to understand, recognize and address the challenges faced by TB patients infected with *M. bovis* as patient treatment and care differ in comparison to the most common form of TB caused by *M. tuberculosis*. For example, *M. bovis* is naturally resistant to pyrazinamide (O'Donohue et al., 1985; Nieman et al., 2000), one of first-line medications in the standard treatment regimen of TB, and zoonotic TB caused by *M. bovis* in humans is more commonly associated with extra-pulmonary rather than pulmonary TB (Dürr et al., 2013). Furthermore, the epidemiology and most common transmission dynamics of *M. bovis* differ significantly from those of the airborne disease caused by *M. tuberculosis*. Furthermore, the risk for zoonotic TB increases in rural areas in developing regions of the world where bovine TB is endemic and/or people live in conditions that favour direct contact with infected animals or animal products, especially with consumption of unpasteurized milk and untreated animal products.

As we move from the era of the United Nation's Millennium Development Goals (United Nations, 2016) into the Sustainable Development Goals for the period 2016–2030, greater emphasis is being placed on the importance of adopting multidisciplinary approaches to improving health. This is particularly relevant for zoonotic diseases. In the context of the SDGs, the World Health Organization's (WHO) End TB Strategy (WHO, 2015a) seeks to end the global TB epidemic by 2035 and calls for diagnosis and treatment of every TB case regardless of the *Mycobacterium* species causing disease.

Furthermore, in support of WHO's End TB strategy, the Stop TB Partnership released the fourth edition of its 'Global Plan to End TB, 2016–2020: The Paradigm Shift' (Stop TB Partnership, 2015) identifying cattle herders, farmers, dairy workers and others as 'key affected populations' for the first time. The Global Research Alliance for Bovine TB (GRAbTB), working under the umbrella of One Health, is also a heartening sign of progress. Thus, the current policy environment is indeed favourable to pursue greater awareness and investments in the prevention and control of zoonotic TB. A One Health approach to *M. bovis* that integrates human, domestic and wild species, and environmental health is further described in Chapter 3, this volume.

In this chapter, we highlight the global public health implications still posed today by *M. bovis* as a source of human TB. Additionally, we discuss the implications of the well-known characteristics of *M. bovis* that must be considered when attempting to improve the prevention, diagnosis and treatment of human TB caused by *M. bovis*. Finally, we summarize data that have become available in the past three years and provide information regarding recent activities implemented at a global scale supporting the design and implementation of strategies aiming to address the major challenges remaining related to the prevention, diagnosis and treatment of human TB caused by *M. bovis*.

2.2 Estimates of the Global Burden of Human TB Caused by *M. bovis*

The available and historical data including estimates of TB caused by *M. bovis* in people globally, regionally and nationally have been previously published. In brief, Cosivi *et al.* (1998) conducted a comprehensive global review and summarized the available data on zoonotic TB due to *M. bovis* in developing countries. The author concluded that disease surveillance programmes for *M. bovis* in humans should be considered a priority and called for evaluation of the scale of the zoonotic TB problem, especially in rural communities and in the workplace. Fifteen years later, Müller *et al.* (2013) conducted a systematic review and meta-analysis of available zoonotic TB data with the purpose of estimating the global occurrence of zoonotic TB caused by *M. bovis*. This latter study concluded that the same challenges and concerns expressed 15 years previously by Cosivi *et al.* (1998) remain valid, including lack of surveillance and appropriate diagnostic tools to correctly identify *M. bovis* as the causal agent of human TB.

Historically, TB cases caused by *M. bovis* have most often been reported as a relative proportion of the total number of human TB cases, obscuring the fact that even a relatively small proportion of the approximately 10.4 million estimated TB cases per year globally (WHO, 2016) still represents a considerable absolute number of humans suffering from zoonotic TB, disproportionally affecting poor and marginalized communities. Furthermore, these available proportions are usually not based on nationally representative data, and instead they are often derived from studies involving only specific and selected groups of patients, such as those presenting to tertiary referral hospitals (Cosivi *et al.*, 1998; Müller *et al.*, 2013). In the past three decades, most published data on zoonotic TB in humans come from studies conducted within different epidemiological settings (i.e. some studies have come from areas where bovine TB is or is not endemic), without any standardization of study design, such as population demographics, patient inclusion criteria, sample size and laboratory methods used to isolate and differentiate *M. bovis* (Cosivi *et al.*, 1998; Drobniewski *et al.*, 2003; Thoen *et al.*, 2010; Müller *et al.*, 2013; Perez-Lago *et al.*, 2014). Because of the lack of accurate and representative data in developing regions, incorrect extrapolation of data from high-income, low TB burden countries has likely resulted in the misconception that globally only a small number of humans suffer from pulmonary and extra-pulmonary TB caused by *M. bovis*. Extrapolating available figures on zoonotic TB from high-income, low TB burden countries to the global context is not warranted (Thoen *et al.*, 2010). Additionally, areas where bovine TB is endemic sometimes overlap with areas where HIV prevalence is high (i.e. in some African countries). Consequently, it is not surprising to find a considerable amount of variability in the reported proportions of human TB cases caused by *M. bovis* in different studies. Without standardization of study design, the comparability of such studies is diminished; hence, the available estimates regarding the burden of zoonotic TB may not accurately represent the true incidence of this disease.

Despite the limitations with the quality and representativeness of currently available data regarding the global scenario for zoonotic TB, the estimated incident number of cases is concerning. The first comprehensive global estimates of the burden of zoonotic TB caused by *M. bovis* in people were published in 2015 by the WHO as part of the Global Burden of Foodborne Disease (Kirk *et al.*, 2015; WHO, 2015b). These estimates were derived from the systematic review conducted by Müller *et al.* (2013) of published data to estimate proportions of TB patients with zoonotic TB in different settings and identify countries endemic for bovine TB, which were then applied to WHO estimates of incidence and mortality of all forms of TB during 2010. The estimated global annual incidence of zoonotic TB was 121,268 (95% uncertainty interval: 99,852–150,239), with a median rate of 2 (95%UI: 1–4) new cases per 100,000 population per year. The highest population-level incidence was in the WHO African region, with an estimated median of 7 (95% UI: 4–9) new cases per 100,000 population. Additionally, 607,775 (95%UI: 458,364–826,115) disability-adjusted life-years (DALYs), representing healthy years of life lost due to illness, were estimated to be attributed to zoonotic TB globally. In the African region, this was estimated as 30 (95%UI: 19–42) DALYs per 100,000 population (WHO, 2015b). The annual estimated global mortality due to *M. bovis* during 2010 was 10,545 (95% UI: 7894–14,472). In 2016, for the first time, the annual WHO Global TB Report presented the incidence of human TB caused by *M. bovis*. For the year 2015, there were an estimated 149,000 new cases (95% uncertainty interval: 71,600–255,000) and 13,400 deaths (95% uncertainty interval: 5050–27,500). It is worth noting that the estimated number of people suffering annually from zoonotic TB largely exceeds the number of people affected by other diseases that receive greater attention, funding, and resources (WHO, 2012; von Philipsborn *et al.*, 2015). Despite these available estimates and likely widespread geographical distribution of associated zoonotic TB risk factors, *M. bovis* as a causal agent of human TB has remained largely ignored in the vast majority of low-income, high TB burden countries where bovine TB is also endemic.

The global incidence of zoonotic TB will continue to be updated annually by WHO based on the most recent estimation of the incidence of all forms of TB. However, there is a need for better quality national data in order to fully understand the true burden of disease, particularly in regions where bovine TB is endemic. It must also be remembered that the above estimates of disease only represent one component of the total impact of *M. bovis*. Reduced livestock productivity, economic losses and trade barriers due to infection in livestock must also be accounted for when considering the full scope of the disease. These aspects of zoonotic TB are covered in Chapters 1, 3 and 4 in this volume.

2.3 Socio-cultural and Demographic Factors Associated with Zoonotic TB Caused by *M. bovis*

The epidemiology and risk factors increasing the risk of human TB caused by *M. bovis* vary according to social, cultural and economic factors (Michel *et al.*, 2009; Ayele *et al.*, 2014). *M. bovis* infection in humans can be acquired both orally and via inhalation of aerosolized particles containing *M. bovis* from infected animals (Biet *et al.*, 2005) or rarely from person-to-person contact (LoBue *et al.*, 2003; Evans *et al.*, 2007).

2.3.1 Consumption of unpasteurized dairy products

The most common route of infection of *M. bovis* is through the oral route by consumption of contaminated milk or other dairy products (Acha and Szyfres, 1987). Thus, milk pasteurization plays a crucial role in preventing human infection (O'Reilly and Daborn, 1995; Collins, 2006). Pasteurization of milk, however, is often inaccessible in many low-income countries or in rural communities around the world. Although the boiling of milk at home provides sufficient pasteurization, this requires access to a fuel source. Ben *et al.* (2011) demonstrated the presence of *M. bovis* in raw milk samples obtained from cows in Tunisia, and warned that consumers of raw milk (or dairy products) are at high risk of zoonotic TB. Ereqat *et al.* (2013) for the first time isolated *M. bovis* from milk of apparently healthy animals (cattle and goats) in the West Bank in Palestine. In Brazil, Zarden *et al.* (2013), reported the isolation of *M. bovis* from milk samples from cows testing negative to the intradermal tuberculin test, the most commonly used test to identify cattle infected by *M. bovis*. Franco *et al.* (2013) concluded that in Brazil, consumption of raw bovine milk (or dairy products) may be regularly exposing human populations to mycobacteria. Roug *et al.* (2014) conducted a simulation model to evaluate strategies to reduce human exposure to *M. bovis* in pastoralist households of Tanzania. The authors concluded that heat treatment of milk may be an effective strategy to reduce human exposure to *M. bovis*-infected milk in settings where TB in cattle is endemic and a bovine TB control programme is not available. Michel *et al.* (2015) in a study conducted in agro-pastoral farming communities in South Africa, showed that *M. bovis* may survive in fresh and souring milk for periods of time that represent a risk for people consuming these products. Additionally, this study demonstrated an association between the temperature at which the milk was soured and stored and the survival time of *M. bovis*. All of the *M. bovis* concentrations inoculated into milk yielded viable *M. bovis* in milk at both temperatures (20°C and 33°C). *M. bovis* survived for at least 2 weeks at 20°C; however, at all different *M. bovis* concentrations tested at 33°C, *M. bovis* was absent within 3 days after inoculation. At higher temperatures (33°C), different *M. bovis* tested concentrations survived between 1 to 3 days. Thus, the public health implications of milk (and milk products) potentially containing *M. bovis* should not be underestimated.

On the other hand, there are areas in low-income countries where pasteurization is available but yet communities still consume unpasteurized milk. In Ethiopia, for example, unpasteurized milk was more consumed in urban and peri-urban areas where pasteurization is expected to be available and accessible (Desissa and Grace, 2012). In this study the observed significant difference in consumption behaviour was due to lack of awareness of the associated risk as well as engrained cultural consumption habits (Dessissa and Grace, 2012). Such findings emphasize the fact that socio-cultural aspects of communities, especially food consumption habits, are critical but challenging to change, hence can be barriers to defining and implementing risk mitigations strategies.

2.3.2 Consumption of raw meat

Consumption of meat (muscle mass) has not been documented as a concern regarding transmission of *M. bovis* to humans. In 2003, the UK Food Safety Agency reviewed the possible health risks to consumers of meat from cattle with evidence of *M. bovis* infection (Food Standards Agency, 2003). In this qualitative review, the authors concluded that: 'the risk, if any, from the consumption of meat sold as fresh meat for human consumption following assessment and action by the Meat Hygiene Service staff in UK abattoirs is very low' (Food Standards Agency, 2003). In New Zealand, a report concluded that there was no evidence that *M. bovis* infections in humans were caused by consumption of meat (Cressey *et al.*, 2006). In the Republic of Ireland, the Food Safety Authority indicated that the scientific information available did not permit a quantitative risk assessment regarding *M. bovis* in meat (Food Safety Authority of Ireland, 2008); however, this report indicated that 'on the basis of available evidence, it is reasonable to conclude that the occurrence of viable *M. bovis* in the muscle mass of cattle, and of other food-producing animals infected with *M. bovis*, is uncommon'. Additionally, it was concluded that the risk from the consumption of meat sold for human consumption following official inspection in abattoirs in Ireland was very low.

Most tuberculous lesions found in cattle at slaughter are confined to the lymph nodes associated with the head, thorax and, less commonly, abdomen. Other organs including the lungs, liver, spleen, kidneys and mammary gland along with the associated lymph nodes and related serous surfaces (pleura and peritoneum) are other less common sites of infection (Corner,

1994). It is uncommon that the muscle mass be affected by tuberculous lesions, and this has been documented only in the advanced stages of the disease (Drieux, 1957). In 1957, Drieux reviewed studies of the isolation of *M. bovis* from skeletal muscle in cattle with advanced TB. The majority (but not all) of the studies reviewed by Drieux failed to isolate *M. bovis* from muscle. However, two of the studies did recover *M. bovis* from muscle in a high proportion of cases tested. It should be noted that organs that do not display visible lesions of TB at post-mortem inspection may nevertheless carry *M. bovis* (Food Safety Authority of Ireland, 2008).

Although it is well recognized that meat consumption poses a considerably lower risk in the transmission of *M. bovis* when compared to the consumption of dairy products, it is nonetheless a risk that has been recognized in certain settings. For example, in Ethiopia, Ameni *et al.* (2003) showed that almost 99% of meat consumed in areas where bovine TB was endemic was either consumed raw or semi-cooked. Furthermore, the authors showed that there was a general lack of awareness of the risk associated with this behaviour. In West Africa, Hambolu *et al.* (2013) showed that 22% of meat handlers in Nigeria ate 'Fuku elegusi' (the practice of eating raw, visibly TB-infected parts of the lungs in order to convince customers to buy these parts) and only 28% of meat handlers were aware that eating 'Fuku elegusi' could be a source of *M. bovis* infection and zoonotic TB in humans. The magnitude of risk associated with such behaviour remains to be established and, thus, the role of meat products as a source of *M. bovis* for humans deserves further attention, particularly in geographical areas in which cultural and eating habits could facilitate transmission.

2.3.3 Occupational risk of contracting *M. bovis*

The risk for zoonotic TB disease increases in areas where bovine TB is endemic and people live in conditions that favour direct contact with infected animals. *M. bovis* poses an occupational risk throughout the world to farmers, pastoralists, veterinarians, zoo keepers, slaughterhouse workers, butchers and other types of workers with frequent direct contact with animal or animal products (Fanning and Edwards, 1991; Dalovisio *et al.*, 1992; Cosivi *et al.*, 1998; Adesokan *et al.*, 2012; Torres-Gonzalez *et al.*, 2013; Michel *et al.*, 2015; Khattak *et al.*, 2016). Aerosol infection has been suggested in farmers in contact with elk (Fanning and Edwards, 1991) and zoo keepers exposed to rhinoceroses infected with *M. bovis* (Dalovisio *et al.*, 1992). Cutaneous TB due to *M. bovis* infection has been documented in hunters handling infected wild animals (Wilkins *et al.*, 2008) and infected possums (Gallagher and Bannantine, 1998). In Ontario, Canada, veterinarians became infected while working in abattoirs as part of a depopulation campaign of infected deer and elk herds (Liss *et al.*, 1994). Adesokan *et al.* (2012) confirmed undetected pulmonary TB due to *M. bovis* among livestock traders in Nigeria. In Mexico, Torres-Gonzalez *et al.* (2013) reported a high prevalence of latent and pulmonary TB among people working with cattle infected with *M. bovis*, especially in people working in non-ventilated spaces. In these settings, the epidemiology and risk factors for zoonotic TB differ significantly from those for airborne disease caused by *M. tuberculosis*.

2.3.4 *M. bovis* human-to-human transmission

Although an uncommon route of transmission of *M. bovis*, person-to-person transmission has been reported (Yates and Grange, 1988; LoBue *et al.*, 2003; Smith *et al.*, 2004; Evans *et al.*, 2007; Sunder *et al.*, 2009; Adesokan *et al.*, 2012; Malama *et al.*, 2014; Sanou *et al.*, 2014; Buss *et al.*, 2016). In the US, the analysis of 8 years of data (2006–2013) by Scott *et al.* (2016) concluded that although the ingestion of unpasteurized dairy products was the main mode of transmission of *M. bovis* to humans, airborne transmission was suggested by their data. Pulmonary TB caused by *M. bovis* via airborne transmission among people therefore appears possible and deserves further investigation as a source of secondary transmission. As mentioned in section 2.3.3, there is also evidence for occupational airborne infection.

2.3.5 Children

In many regions of the world where bovine TB is endemic, children frequently consume unpasteurized milk. In the US, the predominance of *M. bovis* disease among children suggests recent infection, likely from contaminated food sources (Dankner and Davis, 2000; Hlavsa *et al.*, 2008). In the analysis conducted by Scott *et al.* (2016), children younger than 15 years of age born in Mexico or with at least one parent born there were more likely to have *M. bovis* infection compared to children born in the US. In children, severe forms of disease such as disseminated TB or meningitis are more common, exacerbated by a late diagnosis due to the fact that they are dependent on adults for accessing healthcare, do not easily produce sputum or may have extra-pulmonary disease.

Two recent paediatric case reports of gastrointestinal TB due to *M. bovis* published by Anantha *et al.* (2015) in Canada and Pemartín *et al.* (2015) in Spain further highlight the serious health consequences of *M. bovis* in children. The authors emphasized the need for increased awareness of abdominal TB caused by *M. bovis* that may mimic other conditions, resulting in delayed diagnosis and unnecessary surgery. This is of particular relevance for foreign-born individuals who travel periodically to TB-endemic regions. Another case report in the US by Hang *et al.* (2015) of an Hispanic girl with a submandibular mass caused by *M. bovis* further demonstrates the clinical challenges she faced, including failure of initial two-drug therapy, the need for surgery, followed by nine additional months of treatment.

2.3.6 Patient demographics

In the US, patients with TB caused by *M. bovis* are more likely to be Hispanic than patients with TB caused by *M. tuberculosis* (LoBue and Moser, 2005; Rodwell *et al.*, 2008; Scott *et al.*, 2016). In contrast, most zoonotic TB patients in the UK are white and older, born prior to the introduction of widespread milk pasteurization, suggesting re-activation of a latent infection acquired decades earlier (Mandal *et al.*, 2011). In African countries, several studies have identified risk factors for *M. bovis* transmission to humans, such as a lack of education including unawareness of zoonotic TB, consumption of unpasteurized milk products, and not using protective equipment in abattoirs. In Uganda, Kazoora *et al.* (2016) concluded that knowledge of interviewed cattle farmers regarding zoonotic TB caused by *M. bovis* in humans was poor. In Nigeria, two recent studies regarding knowledge, attitudes and practices conducted among abattoir workers concluded that there is an urgent need for public health authorities to intervene in controlling bovine TB (Sa'idu *et al.*, 2015) and that the knowledge on bovine TB among abattoir workers was low (Ismaila *et al.*, 2015). In Cameroon, Kelly *et al.* (2016) concluded that the control of bovine TB under the current cattle husbandry practices is challenging, particularly in mobile pastoralist herds, and that the prevention of *M. bovis* transmission in milk offers the best approach for human risk mitigation. However, this requires strategies that improve risk awareness among producers and consumers. In Ethiopia, Kidane *et al.* (2015) found that among high school students in Adis Ababa, a low proportion of students considered raw milk and yogurt as sources of *M. bovis* infection (47.3% and 15.8%, respectively). It was concluded that there was a much lower knowledge and awareness of bovine TB among students compared to human pulmonary TB.

Although extremely rare, transmission of *M. bovis* from pets to humans has been documented. In the UK, Shrikrishna *et al.* (2009) documented an owner and her pet dog having pulmonary TB caused by the same strain of *M. bovis*. In Texas, USA, Ramdas *et al.* (2015) documented two (indoor) cats suffering from pulmonary TB caused by *M. bovis* and discussed the potential association with at least one household member, who had died from pulmonary TB due to *M. bovis*. Although, the *M. bovis* strains did not exactly match, the authors concluded that the cat and human *M. bovis* strains were closely related, and highlighted the challenges of this unusual case of *M. bovis* infection. Due to the scarcity of data on this topic, the potential public health risk of *M. bovis* infection in pets deserves further attention.

2.3.7 HIV/AIDS

Human-to-human transmission of *M. bovis* has been shown to occur among HIV-positive patients (Bouvet *et al.*, 1993). Of particular concern is the transmission of *M. bovis* strains resistant to not only pyrazinamide, but other first-line anti-TB drugs such as isoniazid in HIV-positive persons (Dupon and Ragnaud, 1992; Bouvet *et al.*, 1993; Blázquez *et al.*, 1997; Samper *et al.*, 1997; Cosivi *et al.*, 1998; Fortún *et al.*, 2005) rendering the standard four-drug regimen of isoniazid, rifampicin, ethambutol and pyrazinamide much less effective. A study in the US identified that TB caused by *M. bovis* was common among persons living with HIV and was strongly associated with both Hispanic ethnicity and disseminated disease with abdominal involvement (Park *et al.*, 2010). In this study, as in others conducted previously in the US (Hlavsa *et al.*, 2008; Rodwell *et al.*, 2008), the authors concluded that unpasteurized dairy products were a likely source of acquisition and that HIV care providers should be aware of this risk and counsel patients appropriately. Again, while the resistance pattern is not unique to HIV-positive persons, their compromised immune systems increase the likelihood of recent infection progressing rapidly to severe clinical *M. bovis* disease and transmission to others. With 74% of HIV-related TB cases being in sub-Saharan Africa (WHO, 2016) as well as 70% of zoonotic TB cases caused by *M. bovis* estimated to occur in Africa (Müller *et al.*, 2013; WHO, 2015b), the potential overlap of HIV and *M. bovis* is concerning.

2.4 Clinical challenges posed by *M. bovis* as a causal agent of human TB

Data on the clinical impact of *M. bovis* as a cause of human TB are predominantly available from high-income countries where access to laboratory diagnostic tools allows speciation of the *M. tuberculosis* complex. It is important that clinicians, health workers and public health officials recognize the unique epidemiologic and clinical features of zoonotic TB.

2.4.1 Antimicrobial resistance

Inherent pyrazinamide (PZA) resistance

An additional complication that zoonotic TB patients face is that *M. bovis* is inherently resistant to pyrazinamide (O'Donohue *et al.*, 1985; Niemann *et al.*, 2000), a key medication in the standard first-line TB treatment regimen, thus presenting a special challenge for patient treatment and recovery. Unfortunately, most TB patients in the world begin TB treatment based on either clinical symptoms or sputum smear microscopy, without knowledge of drug susceptibility or identification of the causative *Mycobacterium* species, increasing the risk of inadequate treatment of patients with undiagnosed *M. bovis*. As a result, patients with TB due to *M. bovis* may receive sub-optimal treatment, which could select for further resistance and explain higher mortality rates in *M. bovis*-infected patients (de la Rua-Domenech, 2006; Rodwell *et al.*, 2008). Globally in 2014, only 12% of the 2.7 million new bacteriologically-confirmed TB cases were tested for drug resistance (WHO, 2015a).

In Belgium, Allix-Beguec *et al.* (2010) concluded that the absence of prompt identification of *M. bovis* in an adult case had adverse consequences for clinical management. Specifically, the authors indicated that due to the lack of speciation of the *Mycobacterium*, 'pyrazinamide was inadequately administered in the 2 months of induction chemotherapy and, worst, was inappropriately used to replace isoniazid in the follow-up treatment because of toxic hepatitis'. In addition, this case constitutes an additional example of the persistent significance of *M. bovis* as a zoonotic pathogen, even in countries such as Belgium which has been declared officially free of cattle TB since 2003. In the US, the recommendation for 9 months of antimicrobial therapy utilizing isoniazid and rifampicin for TB patients infected with *M. bovis* instead of the standard four-drug 6-month regimen for *M. tuberculosis* (CDC, 2003; LoBue and Moser, 2005) presents additional challenges due to decreased patient adherence and increased costs associated with prolonged treatment.

Other resistance patterns

Strains of *M. bovis* have been shown to be resistant to isoniazid. McLaughlin *et al.* (2012) reported that 28.5% of *M. bovis* isolates evaluated in their study in the US were resistant to both pyrazinamide and isoniazid. Other reports (LoBue *et al.*, 2003; CDC, 2005) have also identified *M. bovis* with resistance to isoniazid, further complicating the treatment of these patients. Cases of *M. bovis* multidrug-resistant strains (displaying resistance to both isoniazid and rifampicin, the two most powerful first-line drugs) have been reported in Scotland (Armstrong and Christie, 1998), in Spain among HIV-positive patients (Guerrero *et al.*, 1997) and in an immunocompetent patient (Palenque *et al.*, 1998), and in Mexico (Vazquez-Chacon *et al.*, 2015). Multidrug-resistant TB (regardless of the causative agent) poses a serious public health challenge, with only 50% of patients being successfully treated globally in 2014 (WHO, 2015a). Hence, it is important to quantify and evaluate not only the impact of the inherent pyrazinamide-resistance of *M. bovis* but also the potential acquired resistance to other anti-TB drugs on treatment outcomes. Understandably, the success of treatment may be considerably worse for TB patients with *M. bovis* strains resistant to multiple anti-TB drugs.

2.4.2 Extra-pulmonary tuberculosis

Despite the fact that TB disease caused by *M. bovis* is clinically, radiographically and pathologically indistinguishable from TB caused by *M. tuberculosis* (Cosivi *et al.*, 1998; Grange, 2001; Wedlock *et al.*, 2002; Michel *et al.*, 2009), there is nonetheless an association between *M. bovis* infection and extra-pulmonary sites (de Kantor *et al.*, 2010; Dürr *et al.*, 2013). In Europe and the US, one-half to three-quarters of zoonotic TB patients are affected by extra-pulmonary disease, including lymph nodes, the gastrointestinal tract and urogenital tract. In regions where bovine TB is endemic, foodborne infection (milk) is the principal cause of cervical lymphadenopathy and abdominal and other forms of non-pulmonary TB (Cosivi *et al.*, 1998). The predilection of *M. bovis* for extra-pulmonary sites raises the risk of misdiagnosis or late diagnosis (Sunnetcioglu *et al.*, 2015), therefore delaying the initiation of treatment. In India, Shah *et al.* (2006) reported the results of a study aiming to detect *M. tuberculosis* and *M. bovis* in human cerebrospinal fluid (CSF) from TB patients including patients with tuberculous meningitis. The study evaluated 212 CSF samples including 100 from children. This study showed that in 17% (36 out of 212) of CSF samples, *M. bovis* was detected (versus only 2.8% containing *M. tuberculosis*). The authors concluded that appropriate molecular diagnostic techniques would allow the correct identification of *M. bovis* and could aid and improve the prevention of human TB. Although most TB caused by *M. tuberculosis* in Europe and the US affects the lungs, approximately one-quarter presents as extra-pulmonary disease (Dürr *et al.*, 2013). Extra-pulmonary TB cannot therefore be assumed to be caused by *M. bovis*. In Ethiopia, where rates of extra-pulmonary TB are relatively high, an association with *M. bovis* infection could not be demonstrated. This may be due to an overall low prevalence of *M. bovis* infection in livestock (Berg *et al.*, 2015). Unfortunately, in most parts of the world, the ability to diagnose extra-pulmonary TB is limited.

2.5 Conclusion

In light of the considerable number of people estimated to contract zoonotic TB annually, and the important epidemiologic and clinical differences of *M. bovis* compared to the more common causal agent of human TB (*M. tuberculosis*), it is important to recognize the implications for prevention, diagnosis and treatment of human TB caused by *M. bovis*. It is clear that there is a need to strengthen the identification and prevention of *M. bovis* as a causal agent of human TB, in light of the aligned policy agendas of the End TB Strategy of WHO, the UN Sustainable Development Goals and the Stop TB Partnership's Global Plan to End TB.

Considering the public health implications and challenges associated with zoonotic TB, it is crucial to, first, obtain an accurate picture of the burden both at national and global levels. For this, comprehensive surveillance approaches and laboratory methods must be implemented.

This will improve our ability to diagnose TB cases caused by *M. bovis*, particularly in poor or rural communities who are unaware of the risks of contracting zoonotic TB from unpasteurized dairy products and contaminated meat.

Given the available evidence, *M. bovis* cannot continue to be neglected as a cause of zoonotic TB. The key first steps in addressing zoonotic TB are: (i) governments must acknowledge *M. bovis* in official national policies as a source of TB warranting attention; (ii) knowledge, attitudes and practices of both healthcare providers and communities at risk must be better understood in order to identify gaps and develop appropriate interventions; and (iii) existing laboratory methods that differentiate *M. bovis* from *M. tuberculosis* should be more widely implemented. With these first steps, the world will be closer to the goal of ending suffering from TB, no matter what its source. Ultimately, the prevention and control of *M. bovis* infection and bovine TB in cattle (and other animal species) by the veterinary sector is crucial to prevent the spread of *M. bovis* to humans.

References

Acha, P.N. and Szyfres, B. (1987) Zoonotic tuberculosis. In: *Zoonoses and Communicable Diseases Common to Man and Animals* 2nd edn. Pan American Health Organization/World Health Organization: Scientific Publication No. 503, Washington DC, USA.

Adesokan, H.K., Jenkins, A.O., van Soolingen, D. and Cadmus, S.I. (2012) *Mycobacterium bovis* infection in livestock workers in Ibadan, Nigeria: evidence of occupational exposure. *International Journal of Tuberculosis and Lung Disease* 16(10), 1388–1392.

Afghani, B. (1998) Rapid differentiation of *Mycobacterium tuberculosis* and *Mycobacterium bovis* using glycerol susceptibility and quantitative polymerase chain reaction. *Journal of Investigative Medicine* 46(2), 73–75.

Allix-Beguec, C., Fauville-Dufaux, M., Stoffels, K., Ommeslag, D., Walravens, K., et al. (2010) Importance of identifying *Mycobacterium bovis* as a causative agent of human tuberculosis. *The European Respiratory Journal* 35, 692–694.

Ameni, G., Amenu, K. and Tibbo, M. (2003) Bovine tuberculosis: prevalence and risk factor assessment in cattle and cattle owners in Wuchale-Jida District, Central Ethiopia. *The International Journal of Applied Research in Veterinary Medicine* 1(1), 17–26.

Anantha, R.V., Salvadori, M.I., Hussein, M.H. and Merritt, N. (2015) Abdominal cocoon syndrome caused by *Mycobacterium bovis* from consumption of unpasteurised cow's milk. *The Lancet Infectious Diseases* 15, 1498.

Armstrong, J. and Christie, P. (1998) Two cases of multidrug resistant *Mycobacterium bovis* infection in Scotland. *Euro Surveillance 1998*, 2(37), pii=1159. Available at: http://www.eurosurveillance.org/ViewArticle.aspx?ArticleId=1159 (accessed 1 July 2017).

Ayele, W.Y., Neill, S.D., Zinsstag, J., Weiss, M.G. and Pavlik, I. (2004) Bovine tuberculosis: an old disease but a new threat to Africa. *International Journal of Tuberculosis and Lung Disease* 8(8), 924–937.

Ben, K.I., Boschiroli, M.L., Souissi, F., Cherif, N., Benzarti, M., et al. (2011) Isolation and molecular characterisation of *Mycobacterium bovis* from raw milk in Tunisia. *African Health Sciences* 11(Suppl 1), S2–S5.

Berg, S., Schelling, E., Hailu, E., Firdessa, R., Gumi, B., et al. (2015) Investigation of the high rates of extrapulmonary tuberculosis in Ethiopia reveals no single driving factor and minimal evidence for zoonotic transmission of *Mycobacterium bovis* infection. *BMC Infectious Diseases* 15, 112.

Biet, F., Boschiroli, M.L., Thorel, M.F. and Guilloteau, L.A. (2005) Zoonotic aspects of *Mycobacterium bovis* and *Mycobacterium avium*-intracellulare complex (MAC). *Veterinary Research* 36(3), 411–436.

Blázquez, J., Espinosa de Los Monteros, L.E., Samper, S., Martín, C., Guerrero, A., et al. (1997) Genetic characterization of multidrug-resistant *Mycobacterium bovis* strains from a hospital outbreak involving human immunodeficiency virus-positive patients. *Journal of Clinical Microbiology* 35(6), 1390–1393.

Bouvet, E., Casalino, E., Mendoza-Sassi, G., Lariven, S., Vallee, E. and Pernet, M. (1993) A nosocomial outbreak of multidrug-resistant *Mycobacterium bovis* among HIV-infected patients. A case-control study. *AIDS* 7, 1453–1460.

Buss, B.F., Keyser-Metobo, A., Rother, J., Holtz, L., Gall, K., *et al.* (2016) Possible Airborne Person-to-Person Transmission of *Mycobacterium bovis* – Nebraska 2014–2015. *Morbidity and Mortality Weekly Report (MMWR)* 65(8), 197–201.

CDC (2003) Centers for Disease Control and Prevention Treatment of Tuberculosis. *Morbidity and Mortality Weekly Report (MMWR)*. 2003; 52 (No. RR–11). Available at: http://www.cdc.gov/mmwr/PDF/rr/rr5211.pdf. (accessed May 2016).

CDC (2005) Centers for Disease Control and Prevention. Human tuberculosis caused by *Mycobacterium bovis*—New York City, 2001–2004. *Morbidity and Mortality Weekly Report (MMWR)* 54, 605–608.

Collins, C.H. (2000) The bovine tubercle bacillus. *British Journal of Biomedical Science* 57(3), 234–240.

Collins, J.D. (1999) Tuberculosis in cattle: reducing the risk of herd exposure. *UK Vet* 5, 35–39.

Collins, J.D. (2006) Tuberculosis in cattle: strategic planning for the future. *Veterinary Microbiology* 25; 112(2–4), 369–381.

Corner, L.A. (1994) Post-mortem diagnosis of *Mycobacterium bovis* infection in cattle. *Veterinary Microbiology* 40, 53–63.

Cosivi, O., Grange, J.M., Daborn, C.J., Raviglione, M.C., Fujikura, T., *et al.* (1998) Zoonotic tuberculosis due to *Mycobacterium bovis* in developing countries. *Emerging Infectious Diseases* 4, 59–70.

Cressey, P., Lake, R. and Hudson, A. (2006) Risk Profile: *Mycobacterium bovis* in Red Meat. New Zealand Food Safety Authority, Ministry for Primary Industries, Wellington, New Zealand.

Dalovisio, J.R., Stetter, M. and Mikota-Wells, S. (1992) Rhinoceros' rhinorrhea: cause of an outbreak of infection due to airborne *Mycobacterium bovis* in zookeepers. *Clinical Infectious Diseases* 15(4), 598–600.

Dankner, W.M. and Davis, C.E. (2000) *Mycobacterium bovis* as a significant cause of tuberculosis in children residing along the United States–Mexico border in the Baja California region. *Pediatrics* 105(6), E79.

De Garine-Wichatitsky, M., Caron, A., Kock, R., Tschopp, R., Munyeme, M., *et al.* (2013) A review of bovine tuberculosis at the wildlife-livestock-human interface in sub-Saharan Africa. *Epidemiology and Infection* 141(7), 1342–1356.

de Kantor, I.N., LoBue, P.A. and Thoen, C.O. (2010) Human tuberculosis caused by *Mycobacterium bovis* in the United States, Latin America and the Caribbean. *The International Journal of Tuberculosis and Lung Disease* 14(11), 1369–1373.

de la Rua-Domenech (2006) Human *Mycobacterium bovis* infection in the United Kingdom: Incidence, risks, control measures and review of the zoonotic aspects of bovine tuberculosis. *Tuberculosis* 86(2), 77–109.

Desissa, F. and Grace, D. (2012) Raw milk consumption behaviour and assessment of its risk factors among dairy producers in urban and peri-urban areas of Debre-Zeit, Ethiopia: Implication for public health. Paper presented at the Tropentag 2012, Göttingen, Germany, 19–21 September 2012.

Drieux, H. (1957) Post-mortem inspection and judgement of tuberculous carcasses. In: *Meat Hygiene*. Food and Agriculture Organisation of the United Nations, Geneva, Switzerland, pp. 195–215.

Drobniewski, F.M., Strutt, G., Smith, R., Magee, J. and Flanagan, P. (2003) Audit of scope and culture techniques applied to samples for the diagnosis of *Mycobacterium bovis* by hospital laboratories in England and Wales. *Epidemiology and Infection* 130, 235–237.

Dupon, M. and Ragnaud, J.M. (1992) Tuberculosis in patients infected with human immunodeficiency virus 1. A retrospective multicentre study of 123 cases in France. *Quarterly Journal of Medicine* [New Series 85], 306, 719–730.

Dürr, S., Müller, B., Alonso, S., Hattendorf, J., Laisse, C.J., *et al.* (2013) Differences in primary sites of infection between zoonotic and human tuberculosis: results from a worldwide systematic review. *PLOS Neglected Tropical Diseases* 7, e2399.

El-Sayed, A., El-Shannat, S., Kamel, M., Castañeda-Vazquez, M.A. and Castañeda-Vazquez, H. (2016) Molecular epidemiology of *Mycobacterium bovis* in humans and cattle. *Zoonoses Public Health* 63, 251–264.

Ereqat, S., Nasereddin, A., Levine, H., Azmi, K., Al-Jawabreh, A., *et al.* (2013) First-time detection of *Mycobacterium bovis* in livestock tissues and milk in the West Bank, Palestinian Territories. *PlosOne Neglected Tropical Diseases* 7(9), e2417.

Evans, J.T., Smith, E.G., Banerjee, A., Smith, R.M., Dale, J., Innes, J.A., Hunt, D., Tweddell, A., Wood, A., Anderson, C., Hewinson, R.G., Smith, N.H., Hawkey, P.M. and Sonnenberg, P. (2007) Cluster of human tuberculosis caused by *Mycobacterium bovis*: evidence for person-to-person transmission in the UK. *The Lancet* 369, 1270–1276.

Fanning, A. and Edwards, S. (1991) *Mycobacterium bovis* infection in human beings in contact with elk (*Cervus elaphus*) in Alberta, Canada. *The Lancet* 338(8777), 1253–1255.

Food Safety Authority of Ireland (2008) *Zoonotic Tuberculosis and Food Safety*, 2nd edn. Food Safety Authority of Ireland, Dublin, Ireland.

Fortún, J., Martín-Dávila, P., Navas, E., Pérez-Elías, M.J., Cobo, J., *et al.* (2005) Linezolid for the treatment of multidrug-resistant tuberculosis. *Journal of Antimicrobial Chemotherapy* 56(1), 180–185.

Franco, M.M., Paes, A.C., Ribeiro, M.G., de Figueiredo Pantoja, J.C., Santos, A.C., *et al.* (2013) Occurrence of mycobacteria in bovine milk samples from both individual and collective bulk tanks at farms and informal markets in the southeast region of Sao Paulo, Brazil. *BMC Veterinary Research* 9, 85.

Gallagher, J. and Bannantine, J.P. (1998) *Mycobacterial Diseases*. Oxford University Press, New York, USA.

Grange, J.M. (2001) *Mycobacterium bovis* infection in human beings. *Tuberculosis* 81, 71–77.

Grange, J.M. and Collins, C.H. (1987) Bovine tubercle bacilli and disease in animals and man. *Epidemiology and Infection* 99(2), 221–234.

Griffith, A.S. (1937) Bovine tuberculosis in man. *Tuberculosis* 18(12), 529–543.

Griffith, A.S. (1938) Bovine tuberculosis in the human subject. *Proceedings of the Royal Society of Medicine* 31(10), 1208–1212.

Guerrero, A., Cobo, J., Fortun, J., Navas, E., Quereda, C., *et al.* (1997) Nosocomial transmission of *Mycobacterium bovis* resistant to 11 drugs in people with advanced HIV-1 infection. *Lancet* 350, 1738–1742.

Hambolu, D., Freeman, J. and Taddese, H.B. (2013) Predictors of bovine TB risk behaviour amongst meat handlers in Nigeria: a cross-sectional study guided by the health belief model. *PLOSOne* 8(2), e56091.

Hang, N.T., Maeda, S., Keicho, N., Thuong, P.H. and Endo, H. (2015) Sublineages of *Mycobacterium tuberculosis* Beijing genotype strains and unfavorable outcomes of anti-tuberculosis treatment. *Tuberculosis* 95(3), 336–342.

Hlavsa, M.C., Moonan, P.K., Cowan, L.S., Navin, T.R., Kammerer, J.S., *et al.* (2008) Human tuberculosis due to *Mycobacterium bovis* in the United States, 1995–2005. *Clinical Infectious Diseases* 47, 168–175.

Ismaila, U.G., Rahman, H.A. and Saliluddin, S.M. (2015) Knowledge on Bovine Tuberculosis among Abattoir Workers in Gusau, Zamfara State, Nigeria. *International Journal of Public Health and Clinical Sciences* 2(3), 45–58.

Kaneene, J.B., Miller, R., Steele, J.H. and Thoen, C.O. (2014) Preventing and controlling zoonotic tuberculosis: a One Health approach. *Veterinaria Italiana* 50(1), 7–22.

Katale, B., Mbugi, E., Kendal, S., Fyumagwa, R., Kibiki, G., *et al.* (2012) Bovine tuberculosis at the human-livestock-wildlife interface: Is it a public health problem in Tanzania? A review. *Onderstepoort Journal of Veterinary Research* 79(2), 8.

Kazoora, H.B., Majalija, S., Kiwanuka, N. and Kaneene, J.B. (2016) Knowledge, attitudes and practices regarding risk to human infection due to *Mycobacterium bovis* among cattle farming communities in western Uganda. *Zoonoses and Public Health* 63(8), 616–623.

Keating, L.A., Wheeler, P.R., Mansoor, H., Inwald, J.K., Dale, J., *et al.* (2005) The pyruvate requirement of some members of the *Mycobacterium tuberculosis* complex is due to an inactive pyruvate kinase: implications for in vivo growth. *Molecular Microbiology* 56(1), 163–174.

Kelly, R.F., Hamman, S.M., Morgan, K.L., Nkongho, E.F., Ngwa, V.N., *et al.* (2016) Knowledge of bovine tuberculosis, cattle husbandry and dairy practices amongst pastoralists and small-scale dairy farmers in cameroon. *PLoS ONE* 11(1), e0146538.

Khattak, I., Mushtaq, M.H., Ahmad, M.U.D., Khan, M.S. and Haider, J. (2016) Zoonotic tuberculosis in occupationally exposed groups in Pakistan. *Occupational Medicine* 66(5), 371–376.

Kidane, A.H., Sifer, D., Aklilu, M. and Pal, M. (2015) Knowledge, attitude and practice towards human and bovine tuberculosis among high school students in Addis Ababa, Ethiopia. *International Journal of Livestock Research* 5(1), 1–11.

Kirk, M.D., Pires, S.M., Black, R.E., Caipo, M., Crump, J.A., *et al.* (2015) World Health Organization Estimates of the Global and Regional Disease Burden of 22 Foodborne Bacterial, Protozoal, and Viral Diseases: A Data Synthesis. 2015. *PLOS Medicine* 12(12), e1001940.

Liss, G.M., Wong, L., Kittle, D.C., Simor, A., Naus, M., *et al.* (1994) Occupational exposure to *Mycobacterium bovis* infection in deer and elk in Ontario. *Canadian Journal of Public Health* 85, 326–329.

LoBue, P.A. and Moser, K.S. (2005) Treatment of *Mycobacterium bovis* infected tuberculosis patients: San Diego County, California, United States, 1994–2003. *Tubercle and Lung Disease* 9, 333–338.

LoBue, P.A., Betacourt, W., Peter, C. and Moser, K.S. (2003) Epidemiology of *Mycobacterium bovis* disease in San Diego County, 1994–2000. *International Journal of Tuberculosis and Lung Disease* 7(2), 180–185.

Malama, S., Johansen, T.B., Muma, J.B., Munyeme, M., Mbulo, G., *et al.* (2014) Characterization of *Mycobacterium bovis* from humans and cattle in Namwala District, Zambia. *Veterinary Medicine International*, Article ID 187842.

Mandal, S., Bradshaw, L., Anderson, L.F., Brown, T., Evans, J.T., *et al.* (2011) Investigating transmission of *Mycobacterium bovis* in the United Kingdom in 2005 to 2008. *Journal of Clinical Microbiology* 49, 1943–1950.

McLaughlin, A.M., Gibbons, N., Fitzgibbon, M., Power, J.T., Foley, S.C., *et al.* (2012) Primary isoniazid resistance in *Mycobacterium bovis* disease: a prospect of concern. *American Journal of Respiratory and Critical Care Medicine* 186(1), 110–111.

Michel, A.L., Müller, B. and van Helden, P.D. (2009) *Mycobacterium bovis* at the animal-human interface: a problem, or not? *Veterinary Microbiology* 140, 371–381.

Michel, A.L., Geoghegan, C., Hlokwe, T., Raseleka, K., Getz, W.M. and Marcotty, T. (2015) Longevity of *Mycobacterium bovis* in raw and traditional souring milk as a function of storage temperature and dose. *PLoS ONE* 10(6), e0129926.

Müller, B., Dürr, S., Alonso, S., Hattendorf, J., Laisse, C.J., *et al.* (2013) Zoonotic *Mycobacterium bovis*-induced tuberculosis in humans. *Emerging Infectious Diseases* 19, 899–908.

Niemann, S., Harmsen, D., Rüsch-Gerdes, S. and Richter, E. (2000) Differentiation of clinical *Mycobacterium tuberculosis* complex isolates by gyrB DNA sequence polymorphism analysis. *Journal of Clinical Microbiology* 38(9), 3231–3234.

O'Donohue, W.J. Jr., Bedi, S., Bittner, M.J. and Preheim, L.C. (1985) Short-course chemotherapy for pulmonary infection due to *Mycobacterium bovis*. *Archives of Internal Medicine* 145, 703–705.

Olea-Popelka, F., Muwonge, A., Perera, A., Dean, A.S., Mumford, E., *et al.* (2017) Zoonotic tuberculosis in human beings caused by *Mycobacterium bovis*—a call for action. *The Lancet Infectious Diseases* 17(1), e21–e25.

Olmstead, A.L. and Rhode, P.W. (2004) An impossible undertaking: the eradication of bovine tuberculosis in the United States. *Journal of Economic History* 64(3), 734–772.

O'Reilly, L.M. and Daborn, C.J. (1995) The epidemiology of *Mycobacterium bovis* infections in animals and man: a review. *Tubercle and Lung Disease* 76 (Suppl 1), 1–46.

Pal, M., Zenebe, N. and Rahman, M.T. (2014) Growing significance of *Mycobacterium bovis* in human health. *Microbes and Health* 3(1), 29–34.

Palenque, E., Villena, V., Rebollo, M.J., Jiminez, M.S. and Samper, S. (1998) Transmission of multidrug-resistant *Mycobacterium bovis* to an immunocompetent patient. *Clinical Infectious Diseases* 26, 995–996.

Palmer, M.V. and Waters, W.R. (2011) Bovine tuberculosis and the establishment of an eradication program in the United States: role of veterinarians. *Veterinary Medicine International*, Volume 2011, Article ID 816345.

Park, D., Qin, H., Jain, S., Preziosi, M., Minuto, J.J., *et al.* (2010) Tuberculosis due to *Mycobacterium bovis* in patients coinfected with human immunodeficiency virus. *Clinical Infectious Diseases* 51(11), 1343–1346.

Pemartín, B., Portolés Morales, M., Elena Carazo, M., Marco Macián, A. and Isabel Piqueras, A. (2015) *Mycobacterium bovis* abdominal tuberculosis in a young child. *The Pediatric Infectious Disease Journal* 34(10), 1133–1135.

Perez-Lago, L., Navarro, Y. and Garcia-de-Viedma, D. (2014) Current knowledge and pending challenges in zoonosis caused by *Mycobacterium bovis*: A review. *Research in Veterinary Science* 97, S94–S100.

Ramdas, K.E.F., Lyashchenko, K.P., Greenwald, R., Robbe-Austerman, S., McManis, C. and Waters, W.R. (2015) *Mycobacterium bovis* infection in humans and cats in same household, Texas, USA, 2012. *Emerging Infectious Diseases* 21(3), 480–483.

Rodwell, T.C., Moore, M., Moser, K.S., Brodine, S.K. and Strathdee, S.A. (2008) Tuberculosis from *Mycobacterium bovis* in binational communities, United States. *Emerging Infectious Diseases* 14(6), 909–916.

Roswurm, J.D. and Ranney, A.F. (1973) Sharpening the attack on bovine tuberculosis. *American Journal of Public Health* 63(10), 884–886.

Roug, A., Perez, A., Mazet, J.A.K., Clifford, D.L., VanWormera, E., *et al.* (2014) Comparison of intervention methods for reducing human exposure to *Mycobacterium bovis* through milk in pastoralist households of Tanzania. *Preventive Veterinary Medicine* 115(3–4), 157–165.

Sa'idu, A.S., Okolocha, E.C., Dzikwi, A.A., *et al.* (2015) Public health implications and risk factors assessment of *Mycobacterium bovis* infections among abattoir personnel in Bauchi State, Nigeria. *Journal of Veterinary Medicine* vol. 2015, Article ID 718193.

Samper, S., Martín, C., Pinedo, A., Rivero, A., Blázquez, J., *et al.* (1997) Transmission between HIV-infected patients of multidrug-resistant tuberculosis caused by *Mycobacterium bovis*. *AIDS* 11(10), 1237–1242.

Sanou, A., Tarnagda, Z., Kanyala, E., Zingué, D., Nouctara, M., *et al.* (2014) *Mycobacterium bovis* in Burkina Faso: epidemiologic and genetic links between human and cattle isolates. *PLOS Neglected Tropical Diseases* 8(10), e3142.

Scott, C., Cavanaugh, J.S., Pratt, R., Silk, B.J., LoBue, P. and Moonan, P.K. (2016) Human tuberculosis caused by *Mycobacterium bovis* in the United States, 2006–2013. *Clinical Infectious Diseases* 63(5), 594–601.

Shah, N.P., Singhal, A., Jain, A., Kumar, P., Uppal, S.S., *et al.* (2006) Occurrence of overlooked zoonotic tuberculosis: detection of *Mycobacterium bovis* in human cerebrospinal fluid. *Journal of Clinical Microbiology* 44(4), 1352–1358.

Shrikrishna, D., de la Rua-Domenech, R., Smith, N.H., *et al.* (2009) Human and canine pulmonary *Mycobacterium bovis* infection in the same household: re-emergence of an old zoonotic threat? *Thorax* 64, 89–91.

Smith, R., Drobniewski, F., Gibson, A., Colloff, A. and Coutts, I. (2004) *Mycobacterium bovis* infection, United Kingdom. *Emerging Infectious Diseases* 10, 539–541.

Stop TB Partnership (2015) Global Plan to End TB 2016–2020 – The Paradigm Shift. Available at: http://www.stoptb.org/assets/documents/global/plan/GlobalPlanToEndTB_TheParadigmShift_2016-2020_StopTBPartnership.pdf (accessed 29 May 2016).

Sunder, S., Lanotte, P., Godreuil, S., Martin, C., Boschiroli, M.L. and Besnier, J.M. (2009) Human-to-human transmission of tuberculosis caused by *Mycobacterium bovis* in immunocompetent patients. *Journal of Clinical Microbiology* 47, 1249–1251.

Sunnetcioglu, A., Sunnetcioglu, M., Binici, I., Baran, A.I., Karahocagil, M.K. and Saydan, M.R. (2015) Comparative analysis of pulmonary and extrapulmonary tuberculosis of 411 cases. *Annals of Clinical Microbiology and Antimicrobials* 14, 34.

Thoen, C.O. and LoBue, P.A. (2007) *Mycobacterium bovis* tuberculosis: forgotten, but not gone. *Lancet* 369(9569), 1236–1238.

Thoen, C.O., Lobue, P.A., Enarson, D.A., Kaneene, J.B. and de Kantor, I.N. (2009) Tuberculosis: a re-emerging disease in animals and humans. *Veterinaria Italiana* 45(1), 135–181.

Thoen, C.O., LoBue, P.A. and de Kantor, I. (2010) Why has zoonotic tuberculosis not received much attention? *Tubercle and Lung Disease* 14, 1073–1074.

Torres-Gonzalez, P., Soberanis-Ramos, O., Martinez-Gamboa, A., Chavez-Mazari, B., Barrios-Herrera, M.T., *et al.* (2013) Prevalence of latent and active tuberculosis among dairy farm workers exposed to cattle infected by *Mycobacterium bovis*. *PLOS Neglected Tropical Diseases* 7(4), e2177.

United Nations Sustainable Development Goals (2016) Available at: http://www.un.org/sustainabledevelopment/sustainable-development-goals/ (accessed May 2016).

United Kingdom Food Standards Agency (2003) Available at: https://www.food.gov.uk/sites/default/files/multimedia/pdfs/committee/acm981a_mbovis.pdf (accessed May 2016).

Vazquez-Chacon, C.A., Martínez-Guarneros, A., Couvin, D., González-Y-Merchand, J.A., Rivera-Gutierrez, S., *et al.* (2015) Human multidrug-resistant *Mycobacterium bovis* infection in Mexico. *Tuberculosis* 95, 802–809.

von Philipsborn, P., Steinbeis, F., Bender, M.E., Regmi, S. and Tinnemann, P. (2015) Poverty-related and neglected diseases – an economic and epidemiological analysis of poverty relatedness and neglect in research and development. *Global Health Action* 8, 25818.

Wedlock, D.N., Skinner, M.A., de Lisle, G.W. and Buddle, B.M. (2002) Control of *Mycobacterium bovis* infections and the risk to human populations. *Microbes and Infection* 4, 471–480.

Wilkins, M.J., Meyerson, J., Bartlett, P.C., Spieldenner, S.L., Berry, D.E., *et al.* (2008) Human *Mycobacterium bovis* infection and bovine tuberculosis outbreak, Michigan, 1994–2007. *Emerging Infectious Diseases* 14(4), 657–660.

WHO (2012) Global report for research on infectious diseases of poverty. 2012. http://whqlibdoc.who.int/publications/2012/9789241564489_eng. pdf?ua=1 (accessed 6 June 2015).
WHO (2015a) World Health Organization Gear up to End TB- Introducing the WHO End TB Strategy. 2015. Available at: http://www.who.int/tb/EndTBadvocacy_brochure/en/ (accessed 10 May 2015).
WHO (2015b) World Health Organization: Estimates of the global burden of foodborne diseases 2015. Available at: http://www.who.int/foodsafety/publications/foodborne_disease/fergreport/en/ (accessed 1 March 2016).
WHO (2016) Global Tuberculosis Report. Available at: http://www.who.int/tb/publications/global_report/en/ (accessed 1 February 2017).
Yates, M.D. and Grange, J.M. (1988) Incidence and nature of human tuberculosis due to bovine tubercle bacilli in South-East England: 1977–1987. *Epidemiology and Infection* 101, 225–229.
Zarden, C.F.O., Marassi, C.D., Figueiredo, E.E.S. and Lilenbaum, W. (2013) *Mycobacterium bovis* detection from milk of negative skin test cows. *Veterinary Record* 172(5). DOI: 10.1136/vr.101054.

3 Economics of Bovine Tuberculosis: A One Health Issue

Hind Yahyaoui Azami[1,2,3] and Jakob Zinsstag[2,3],*

[1]Institut Agronomique et Vétérinaire Hassan II, Rabat, Morocco; [2]Swiss Tropical and Public Health Institute, Basel, Switzerland; [3]University of Basel, Basel, Switzerland

---

This chapter is focused on the economics of bovine tuberculosis (TB), taking into consideration the burden of this disease for livestock and also for human health, with a strong emphasis on One Health (OH) as a control approach. The current chapter starts with an overview of One Health, followed by a review of the economics of bovine TB as an OH issue, through a summary of One Health and its added value for bovine TB and human TB control.

3.1 One Health

OH can be defined as the added value of closer cooperation between human and animal health in terms of better health of humans and animals, financial savings and improved ecosystem services (Zinsstag et al., 2015). OH is part of the broader consideration of ecology and health. It contributes to improving health by engaging different institutions and disciplines in a closer way by improved communication, closer collaboration and better information sharing based on the recognition that human and animal health are mutually dependent.

Obstacles of the broad acceptance of the benefits gained from an OH approach are mostly economic. In fact, it is critical for the establishment of an OH approach to demonstrate that public and private stakeholders may save money from a closer cooperation (Zinsstag et al., 2012).

Veterinary attention should be drawn to many sectors related directly or indirectly to animal health, such as international trade and travel, global climate changes, habitat destruction, overpopulation, ecotourism and food safety, and all those sectors should be aware of the positive impact of the collaboration with other disciplines. However, the establishment of an OH initiative and setup of its principles should be performed at the academic level; in addition to the creation of specialized Masters' in OH (Osburn et al., 2009), the academic training of OH should be adapted to different countries and contexts in order to be most efficient. Still, the OH approach should be embraced also by several institutions and organizations outside academia, such as industrial firms, especially those that will benefit from addressing the challenges posed by bovine TB using an OH approach (e.g. the milk and meat industries).

Public health schools remain among the biggest institutions that deploy considerable efforts to educate global health experts and prepare them to confront the global burden diseases. One of the strengths of public health schools is their multidisciplinary orientation and their aspiration to develop, test and validate new approaches, technologies and systems in order to reach the global health needs, especially

---

* Email: jakob.zinsstag@swisstph.ch

© CAB International 2018. Bovine Tuberculosis
(eds M. Chambers, S. Gordon, F. Olea-Popelka, P. Barrow)

in developing countries (Fried *et al.*, 2010). Moreover, OH courses are available in many universities, non-governmental organizations and government agencies, for example, the University of Edinburgh, London School of Hygiene and Tropical Medicine, Swiss Tropical and Public Health Institute, and many other universities and institutes.

Examples of OH approaches include a vaccination campaign in Chad for both pastoralists (vaccination against diphtheria, whooping cough, tetanus and against polio) and their livestock (vaccination against anthrax, pasteurellosis, blackleg and contagious bovine pleuropneumonia), in addition to the delivery of healthcare. This was a successful intervention integrating human and animal health workers, where this joint action allowed a reduction of costs by 15% compared to a separate campaign (Bechir *et al.*, 2003; Schelling *et al.*, 2007).

Moreover, it has been validated in a prevalence study performed in Chad for brucellosis and Q-fever that using an OH approach in prevalence investigations of a zoonosis could decrease the detection time when sampling humans and animals in parallel (Schelling *et al.*, 2003). However, this joint investigation should be justified with a higher incremental knowledge, and more importantly, no concessions should be made in the quality of the methods (Narrod *et al.*, 2012).

Zinsstag *et al.* (2007) demonstrated, using brucellosis, rabies and avian influenza examples, that interventions against zoonoses become cost saving when considered from a societal perspective. An intervention may become highly cost effective when costs are shared between different sectors in proportion to their benefits (Roth *et al.*, 2003). In contrast to developed countries, many zoonoses are still endemic in many developing countries, as financial and organizational resources cannot be focused on the animal reservoir (Zinsstag *et al.*, 2005).

3.2 Human Tuberculosis: The International Epidemiological Situation and Control Strategy

According to the World Health Organization (WHO), in 2015, TB caused 1.8 million deaths worldwide, which puts human TB as a leading cause of death. In addition, 12% of all TB cases are co-infected with HIV. The estimated number of new cases of human TB in the world for 2015 was 10.4 million. The incidence of TB is variable from one region to another; Southeast Asia and the Western Pacific accounts for 58% of all TB cases. Africa has 28% of worldwide TB cases, but has the most severe burden relative to population (WHO, 2016).

On the other hand, Western Europe and North America showed a low incidence of human TB compared to the most populous countries of Asia, where human TB is very prevalent (e.g. Bangladesh, India, China, Indonesia, and Pakistan) (Lawn and Zumla, 2011). In addition, in some developing countries, an increase in new TB cases has been observed within the last 20 years, and this could be explained, among other reasons, by better data management and diagnostic rates (WHO, 2016).

In May 2014, the End TB strategy was established with the goals of reducing the number of TB deaths by 90% by 2030 (compared to 2015 rates) and reducing the number of new TB cases by 80% (WHO, 2016).

3.3 The Economic and Public Health Burden of Bovine Tuberculosis

Bovine TB affects the national economy of the countries where this disease is endemic by causing a decrease in productivity, condemnation of meat in the abattoirs and an influence on the international trade of animal products (Michel *et al.*, 2010). Ongoing bovine TB transmission also has important effects on ecosystems by affecting wildlife (Caron *et al.*, 2003). Bovine TB is more difficult to eliminate from wildlife than from cattle. This is currently an obstacle for the eradication of bovine TB in some developed countries, for example, badgers in the UK and Ireland (Mathews *et al.*, 2006; Gormley and Corner, 2013), the brushtail possum in New Zealand (Barron *et al.*, 2015), wild boar (*Sus scrofa*) in the Iberian Peninsula (Palmer, 2013) and white-tailed deer (*Odocoileus virginianus*) in Michigan, USA (O'Brien *et al.*, 2009).

The public health burden of zoonotic TB in industrialized countries is low because of the pasteurization of milk and/or its effective elimination in cattle. Rare cases are contracted abroad (de la Rua-Domenech, 2006). For example, in Australia *Mycobacterium bovis* represented 0.2% of all human TB cases in 2010, and *M. bovis* infection is linked with employment in the livestock industry and immigration from countries in which bovine TB is endemic (Ingram *et al.*, 2010). In the USA, between 1995 and 2005, the majority of human *M. bovis* patients were born outside of the USA and could have contracted zoonotic TB abroad. In addition, the consumption of fresh cheese ('queso fresco') produced from unpasteurized milk in Mexico has been described to be a potential source of *M. bovis* in the USA (Hlavsa *et al.*, 2008). Mexico is a country where bovine TB has a high prevalence in cattle, and studies have found high prevalence in humans (Sreevatsan *et al.*, 2000; LoBue *et al.*, 2003; de Kantor and Ritacco, 2006). A recent study described a prevalence of 26.2% of *M. bovis* among human TB patients ($n=1165$) in Mexico. However, this high proportion of *M. bovis* among human TB patients has been explained by the authors as potentially linked to immunosuppressed patients; in addition, isolates obtained from HIV-infected patients accounted for 19.2% of the local samples in the same study (Bobadilla-del Valle *et al.*, 2015).

Bovine TB has been previously classified by the WHO to be a neglected zoonosis in developing countries, where the public health burden of bovine TB is high and many risk factors linked to the transmission and persistence of *M. bovis* are present, for example, consumption of unpasteurized milk (Ayele *et al.*, 2004). Moreover, neglected zoonoses such as bovine TB in developing countries are associated with poverty (Maudlin *et al.*, 2009). The quantified burden of zoonotic TB on public health is still not well known in developing countries. A recent review of *M. bovis* among humans in Africa reported a mean prevalence of 2.8% of *M. bovis* among human TB patients. Considering an incidence rate of 264/100,000 population/year, this review resulted in a crude estimate of 7 zoonotic TB cases/100,000 population per year (Müller *et al.*, 2013); however, more studies are needed to better investigate the public health burden of bovine TB in developing countries. In June 2016, the WHO included zoonotic TB as a priority and it is now endorsed by the Strategic and Technical Advisory Group. In order to follow this development, OH approaches are needed to continue to improve the situation.

3.3.1 Livestock

Bovine TB causes economic losses to the livestock industry, as it increases mortality and reduces milk and meat production. It also results in condemnation of organs and carcasses in the slaughterhouses when animals show gross visible lesions suggestive of bovine TB infection (Michel *et al.*, 2010). To date no study has been performed in Africa to estimate the productivity losses in terms of meat and milk caused by bovine TB.

In Ireland, a study showed that bovine TB infection caused a decrease of milk production by 0.5% to 14.6%; however, decreased milk production has been shown to be a risk factor for bovine TB (Boland *et al.*, 2010). These findings are in line with earlier estimates of milk production losses of 10% among tuberculin-positive animals in the former East Germany (Meisinger, 1970). In Bangladesh, a study showed bovine TB to be responsible for 18% of milk losses (Rahman and Samad, 2008). In addition, annual calving rates are reduced by 5% among bovine TB-positive animals, thus affecting the fertility and demographic composition of the herd (Bernues *et al.*, 1997). Overall, the cost of bovine TB to the Ethiopian livestock production systems was estimated at 1% of the net present value in the rural and 4% to 6% in urban areas (Tschopp *et al.*, 2012).

3.3.2 Human health

The emergence of drug-resistant *M. bovis* is an important public health problem that affects the success of TB control programmes in many developing countries, for instance in Mexico (Vazquez-Chacon *et al.*, 2015). Consequently, it causes an increased illness burden and financial losses due to relapses considering the resistance of *M. bovis* to a first-line drug (pyrazinamide) used in human TB treatment (Scorpio and Zhang, 1996; McLaughlin, 2012; Bobadilla-del Valle et al., 2015).

In most developing countries, no microbiological identification of TB causative agents is made before the administration of treatment. Considering the natural resistance of *M. bovis* to pyrazinamide, in addition to the re-emerging mutations in *M. bovis* genome, which cause resistance to other TB drugs (McLaughlin, 2012), a human infection with *M. bovis* could be considered as one of the causes contributing to the relapse of TB patients. Consequently, there is an urgent need to quantify the exact burden of zoonotic TB among human TB patients in developing countries and, more importantly, among the groups that are the most at risk of contracting *M. bovis* from cattle.

3.4 Bovine Tuberculosis: Transmission and Risk Factors for Cattle and Humans

Bovine TB is a zoonosis caused by *M. bovis*, a Gram-positive bacteria belonging to the *Mycobacterium tuberculosis* complex. The most important host for *M. bovis* is cattle (Amanfu, 2006); however, this species infects a wide range of domestic and wild animals as well as humans (Palmer, 2013; Pesciaroli et al., 2014).

A brief description of factors impacting transmission of *M. bovis* among cattle and to and between humans is presented in this section to highlight the need of an OH approach to control bovine and zoonotic TB. For more details regarding *M. bovis* transmission between cattle see Chapter 4 and for *M. bovis* public health implications see Chapter 2.

Several risk factors are linked with bovine TB infection in cattle. The risk of bovine TB infection has been described to increase with age (Brooks-Pollock et al., 2013), while local breeds have been linked with lower prevalence of bovine TB (Moiane et al., 2014). The risk of bovine TB infection regarding gender has been observed to be linked to livestock management practices and cultural behavioural habits related to each country (Humblet et al., 2009). In developing African countries, imported cattle are usually kept under intensive conditions, a factor that has been previously described as a risk factor for bovine TB infection (Elias et al., 2008). In addition, intensive breeding is usually practiced in larger herds, a factor that has been shown to increase the risk of bovine TB infection (Humblet et al., 2009). The type of production could also be a risk factor for bovine TB, as described in a cohort study in New Zealand from 1980 to 2004, where dairy herds were observed to have a higher risk of infection compared to fattening schemes (Porphyre et al., 2008).

Two routes of transmission have been described in humans: for adult and older patients, airborne transmission is the most common route causing pulmonary TB, while in younger patients, foodborne transmission occurs more often, which may lead to extrapulmonary tuberculosis (Hlavsa et al., 2008). Consumption of unpasteurized milk has been recognized as a major risk factor (Cosivi et al., 1998). However, the transmission of *M. bovis* to humans can be enhanced by other factors, such as HIV co-infection (Grange, 2001; Hlavsa et al., 2008). Person-to-person transmission of *M. bovis* has been previously reported in immune-deficient patients (Roring et al., 2002; Evans et al., 2007), as well as in immune-competent patients as described in France in 2009 (Sunder et al., 2009). The transmission of *M. bovis* between animals and humans depends on many risk factors, which vary from one epidemiological context to another. In developing countries, the livestock management system is a very important risk factor for bovine TB transmission. As the economy of a country grows, the livestock keepers tend to move from more extensive pastoral systems to more intensive livestock management for dairy production. In such systems, animals are closer together in less ventilated spaces and with less sunlight. Such intensified production systems provide a more favourable environment for the persistence of the disease, as *M. bovis* is more easily transmitted (Shitaye et al., 2007; Elias et al., 2008).

Moreover, human TB due to *M. bovis* has been suggested as an occupational hazard after the isolation of *M. bovis* from 5 abattoir workers among 3000 abattoir workers during a 2-year period in Australia (Robinson et al., 1988). In Pakistan, human TB caused by *M. bovis* was found in livestock keepers and abattoir workers.

Almost all of these workers do not work safely and they do not protect themselves (Khattak et al., 2016). These facts suggest that biosafety measures should be applied for workers in direct contact with *M. bovis* hazards from livestock to abattoirs, and strict routine surveillance for bovine TB gross visible lesions should be applied in order to protect workers and, in turn, the consumer from *M. bovis* exposure.

3.5 The Cost of Bovine Tuberculosis

The economics of bovine TB have been summarized by Zinsstag et al. (2006). The authors emphasized the multifaceted and multi-sector nature of bovine TB with costs to livestock production and animal health, in addition to wildlife and human health. However most of the time economic analyses of bovine TB focused only in one sector: the cost to livestock production. In areas where cattle are the only reservoir host, the control of bovine TB is possible with a test-and-slaughter policy, whereas in countries with wildlife reservoirs it is more difficult and increases the cost of efforts to control bovine TB. The cost for the control of bovine TB in the UK decreased from an average of £92 million annually from 2003 to 2005 (Bovine TB Info, 2016) to £74 million in 2006 (Mathews et al., 2006) and increased again to £99 million pounds in 2013 (Department for Environment, Food and Rural Affairs, 2014). A total of £66 million has been directed for operational, policy and lab work performed by the animal health services and the veterinary laboratories agency; in addition to the payment for private veterinarians for TB testing, £23.5 million of the total amount is for cattle compensation costs (Department for Environment, Food and Rural Affairs, 2013). In Turkey, the annual socio-economic impact of bovine TB to the agriculture and health sectors is estimated to range from US$15 to US$59 million (Barwinek and Taylor, 1996), while in Argentina, the losses due to bovine TB has been estimated to be US$63 million as reported by Cosivi et al. (1998).

Very few cost estimates are available for bovine TB in developing countries. As one of the first, in Ethiopia the cost of this disease was estimated using a livestock demographic model (LDPS2, Food and Agriculture Organization) with some modifications to allow the stochastic simulation of parameters. It was shown that the cost of bovine TB in the peri-urban dairy production system in areas of Addis Ababa (where the disease has a higher prevalence) was found to range from US$0.5 to US$4.9 million in 2005 and in 2011, respectively, whereas in the rural areas, where bovine TB has a lower prevalence, the cost of bovine TB ranged from US$75.2 million in 2005 to US$358 million in 2011 (Tschopp et al., 2012). This cost analysis in Ethiopia concluded that intervention to control bovine TB in the country would not be cost effective and was not possible within the current economic situation of Ethiopia (Tschopp et al., 2012).

In addition, a recent review in Ethiopia identified the test-and-slaughter control strategy to be financially and logistically unfeasible for bovine TB. This review also highlighted the need to explore alternative control options such as milk pasteurization, meat condemnation in the abattoirs and animal movement control (Tschopp and Aseffa, 2016).

The above analysis was not multi-sectorial in the sense that it considered that the estimation of the full societal cost of bovine TB should take into account the social and private sectors, direct and indirect losses to livestock production, and animal and human health.

Table 3.1 summarizes the different losses triggered by bovine TB in the human and animal sectors. The human health sector losses could be estimated considering the burden of *M. bovis* on human TB cases.

Bovine TB is not a disease that receives the most attention in developing countries, as many other infectious diseases in animal health are given higher prioritization (e.g. foot and mouth disease and peste des petits ruminants). In addition, as the burden of bovine TB has not yet been estimated in most of the countries, the stakeholders are not aware of the real burden of this disease, especially for human health. In many developing countries, physicians are not convinced of the added value of working closer with the animal health sector in order to control this disease, as they assume the proportion of *M. bovis* among human TB patients to be very low, although this is not yet estimated in many developing countries (e.g. Morocco), and that

Table 3.1. Direct and indirect economic losses associated with bovine tuberculosis in human and animal sectors.

	Animal	Human
Direct	Condemned meat in slaughterhouses Diminution of the animal value	Diagnostic and hospitalization (ministry of health) Out-of-pocket expenses for healthcare (contribution of the patient)
Indirect	Diminution of milk production Diminution of fertility Change of herd demographic composition	DALY's lost Transport costs (travel expenses) Expenses related to the patient visitors and accompanying person Jobs lost (change in the household income)

M. bovis has not been officially considered or investigated as the causal agent of human TB. In countries where bovine TB has a high prevalence in cattle, and where no prevention control measures are applied (e.g. mandatory milk pasteurization), the proportion of *M. bovis* infections among human patients could potentially be higher than expected.

3.6 One Health Economics of Bovine Tuberculosis

OH approaches to control zoonoses have been applied in developing countries, mainly in epidemiological investigations. Examples include human and animal seroprevalence studies performed in Kyrgyzstan (Zinsstag *et al.*, 2009; Kasymbekov *et al.*, 2013) and in Mongolia (Tsend *et al.*, 2014). Moreover, OH showed a great potential in the contribution to rabies elimination in Africa as explained by Léchenne *et al.* (2015).

To apply an OH approach to bovine TB, the first step to be undertaken is to investigate the burden of *M. bovis* among human TB patients. This information could be used in order to start a dialogue between the human and animal health sectors. Before an integrated approach to control human TB and bovine TB can be developed, an economic study assessing the cost of the control of human TB using an OH approach should be performed, in addition to the evaluation of the added value of this approach. Potential savings achievable through the implementation of OH concept in 139 World Bank client countries have been estimated to range from 0% to 40% depending on the task considered (World Bank, 2010).

The adequate resources needed to achieve this collaboration should be available; in addition, the persons involved in OH interventions should be trained in order to have the necessary skills needed for a better management of the intervention (WHO *et al.*, 2012).

Decision makers are a key stakeholder in bovine TB control strategy, and they should be involved in the process from the beginning. The economic and societal impact of each approach suggested must be communicated to the decision makers, in addition to a time line for intervention and a cost-effectiveness analysis (WHO *et al.*, 2012). Interventions to control a zoonosis should be performed in parallel with a health education campaign, as this will contribute to a better acceptance of the control programme by the local population and its sustainability (Ducrotoy *et al.*, 2015).

3.7 Bovine Tuberculosis as a One Health Issue

The burden of *M. bovis* for public health is very low for developed countries, where the disease in cattle has a low prevalence or has been eradicated. In developing countries, the burden of *M. bovis* in humans is known for only a few countries. In a systematic review and meta-analysis, Müller *et al.* (2013) reported an average prevalence of *M. bovis* among humans of about 2.8% (7 zoonotic TB cases/100,000 population per year) in Africa, based on information from African countries for which data is available. However, no data are available for quantifying the number of human TB patients infected with *M. bovis* in many developing countries in Africa and elsewhere. This could be due to a weak communication between human and veterinary health systems, which calls for an OH approach. In addition to a lack of awareness of a potential high burden of *M. bovis* among humans, in settings where bovine TB has a high prevalence among cattle and several risk factors for transmission of bovine TB to humans are present (e.g. consumption of unpasteurized milk, close contact between humans and cattle), the burden of *M. bovis* should be urgently considered.

Morocco is a developing country where the prevalence of bovine TB among cattle is 18% (FAO, 2011), and 40% of the population live in rural areas (La Banque Mondiale, 2014) in close contact with cattle. The burden of *M. bovis* among human TB cases should be investigated, as the risk factors for zoonotic TB transmission from animals to humans are present. In this context, an OH approach should be introduced where the human health and veterinary efforts are integrated in order to investigate the real burden of *M. bovis* in humans in such settings, but such collaboration needs an improved communication between both sectors.

A recent transmission model (Fig. 3.1) of bovine TB in Morocco showed that the disease could be controlled within 20 years, if 60% of Moroccan cattle were tested annually and infected animals were slaughtered. This 20-year campaign is projected to cost €1.53 billion (Abakar *et al.*, 2017). Further analyses on the profitability and cost effectiveness are ongoing. The transmission model used to estimate the cost of bovine TB elimination in Morocco considered three categories for cattle (susceptible, exposed with latent TB, and infected with active TB). The human population was divided into four categories (susceptible, exposed with latent zoonotic TB, infected with active TB, and recovered from TB). In order to represent the human burden of bovine TB, a transmission from infected cattle to exposed humans was considered in the model (Abakar *et al.*, 2017).

3.8 Towards the Control and Elimination of Bovine Tuberculosis in Developing Countries

In Japan, the tuberculin skin test was introduced in 1948, and the test-and-slaughter strategy was applied, followed by an annual examination. Consequently, bovine TB prevalence dropped quickly and the disease was nearly eliminated from cattle in Japan (Shimao, 2010). Several developed countries were able to eliminate bovine TB using the test-and-slaughter strategy, and the success of this strategy was supported by the absence of a wildlife reservoir (Wedlock *et al.*, 2002). Switzerland is one of the success stories of bovine TB eradication, where

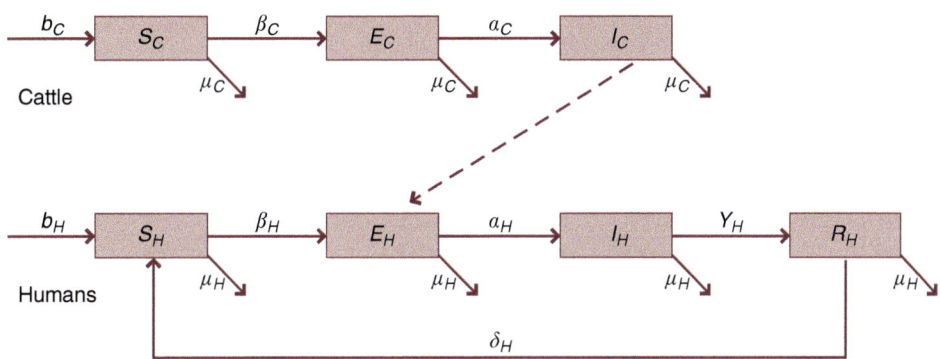

Fig. 3.1. Schematic diagram of the bovine TB cattle–human transmission model for Morocco (Abakar *et al.*, 2017).

the test-and-slaughter strategy was applied for 10 years followed by 20 years of surveillance campaign (Schiller et al., 2011). Australia also successfully controlled bovine TB using a mandatory test-and-slaughter strategy (Cousins and Roberts, 2001). Test-and-slaughter is the only control strategy that shows success for the control and elimination of bovine TB; however, this strategy remains unaffordable for developing countries, primarily because of the compensation needed for the slaughtered cattle (Ayele et al., 2004).

In order to control a particular disease, a clear understanding of the biology and epidemiology of the causal agent is an important starting point that allows for the identification of all the realistic intervention points and the design of control strategies that are in line with the economic situation of the country. The implementation of a control strategy should be done in a way that allows progressive adjustments. Epidemiological surveillance procedures and tools should be used to monitor the progress of the control strategy and adjust it if necessary (Morris, 2015). According to Morris (2015), the most problematic point in dealing with the control of a disease is the fact that the previously explained points are marginalized. Disease control could be achieved in a more efficient way by integrating suitable management tools by the appropriate stakeholders (Cowie et al., 2015). Bovine TB control should be motivated by both the public health implications of *M. bovis* and the economic losses triggered (Amanfu, 2006). Transdisciplinary research using participatory stakeholder involvement could be used in order to contribute to the control of bovine TB from developing countries, like Morocco, where there is very little or almost no dialogue between the different stakeholders (veterinarians, medical doctors, decision makers and farmers).

The importance of an OH-integrated approach including livestock, wildlife and public health sectors was identified as a key element in bovine TB control in Ethiopia (Tschopp and Aseffa, 2016). In developing countries, the control of bovine TB must begin with many transdisciplinary workshops in order to set a dialogue between the different stakeholders, as well as create a trust environment between these sectors. In this process, farmers and decision makers will be informed by the scientists about the economic losses caused by bovine TB and about the different ways or actions that could be undertaken in order to control this disease. The needs of all the stakeholders involved in controlling bovine TB should be considered, as this will ensure their engagement in the application of control strategies and contribute to its sustainability.

In developing countries, bovine TB control strategy should be focused on many levels. Good management of the resources that will be involved in the campaign is required, in addition to training the teams that will participate in the intervention. In parallel, an awareness campaign should be launched in order to make the local population aware of the effectiveness of the control strategy and its positive effect on the long term. Sustainability of the control strategy is essential for the success in controlling bovine TB and its elimination in the long term. The integration of all the stakeholders in all the processes from the formulation to the application of the control strategy and including the monitoring is crucial to ensure the achievement of the interventions.

References

Abakar, F., Yahyaoui Azami, H., Justus Bless, P., Crump, L., Lohmann, P., et al. (2017) Transmission dynamics and elimination potential of zoonotic tuberculosis in Morocco. *PLOS Neglected Tropical Diseases* 11(2), e0005214.

Amanfu, W. (2006) The situation of tuberculosis and tuberculosis control in animals of economic interest. *Tuberculosis* 86(3–4), 330–335.

Ayele, W.Y., Neill, S.D., Zinsstag, J., Weiss, M.G. and Pavlik, I. (2004) Bovine Tuberculosis: an old disease but a new threat to Africa. *The International Journal of Tuberculosis and Lung Disease* 8(8), 924–937.

Barron, M.C., Tompkins, D.M., Ramsey, D.S.L. and Bosson, M.A.J. (2015) The role of multiple wildlife hosts in the persistence and spread of bovine Tuberculosis in New Zealand. *New Zealand Veterinary Journal* 63 Suppl 1(June), 68–76.

Barwinek, F. and Taylor, N.M. (1996) *Assessment of the Socio-Economic Importance of Bovine Tuberculosis in Turkey and Possible Strategies for Control or Eradication: Turkish-German Animal Health Information Project General Direktorate of Protection and Control.* GTZ, Ankara, Turkey.

Bechir, M., Schelling, E., Wyss, K., Daugla, D.M., Daoud, S., *et al.* (2003) An innovative approach combining human and animal vaccination campaigns in nomadic settings of Chad: experiences and costs. *Medecine tropicale: revue du Corps de sante colonial* 64(5), 497–502.

Bernues, A., Manrique, E. and Maza, M.T. (1997) Economic evaluation of bovine Brucellosis and Tuberculosis eradication programmes in a mountain area of Spain. *Preventive Veterinary Medicine* 30(2), 137–149.

Bobadilla-del Valle, M., Torres-González, P., Cervera-Hernández, M.E., Martínez-Gamboa, A., Crabtree-Ramirez, B., *et al.* (2015) Trends of *Mycobacterium bovis* isolation and first-line anti-tuberculosis drug susceptibility profile: a fifteen-year laboratory-based surveillance. *PLoS Neglected Tropical Diseases* 9(9) e0004124.

Boland, F., Kelly, G.E., Good, M. and More, S.J. (2010) Bovine tuberculosis and milk production in infected dairy herds in Ireland. *Preventive Veterinary Medicine* 93(2), 153–161.

Bovine TB Info (2016) Bovine TB in the UK, England, Ireland, Wales and New Zealand. Available at: http://www.bovinetb.info/ (accessed 29 June 2016).

Brooks-Pollock, E., Conlan, A.J.K., Mitchell, A.P., Blackwell, R., Trevelyan, J., *et al.* (2013) Age-dependent patterns of bovine tuberculosis in cattle. *Veterinary Research* 44, 97.

Caron, A., Cross, P.C. and du Toit, J.T. (2003) Ecological implications of bovine tuberculosis in African buffalo herds. *Ecological Applications* 13(5), 1338–1345.

Cosivi, O., Grange, J.M., Daborn, C.J., Raviglione, M.C., Fujikura, T., *et al.* (1998) Zoonotic tuberculosis due to *Mycobacterium bovis* in developing countries. *Emerging Infectious Diseases* 4(1), 59–70.

Cousins, D.V. and Roberts, J.L. (2001) Australia's campaign to eradicate bovine tuberculosis: the battle for freedom and beyond. *Tuberculosis* 81(1–2), 5–15.

Cowie, C.E., Gortázar, C., White, P.C.L., Hutchings, M.R. and Vicente, J. (2015) Stakeholder opinions on the practicality of management interventions to control bovine tuberculosis. *The Veterinary Journal* 204(2), 179–185.

de Kantor, I.N. and Ritacco, V. (2006) An update on bovine tuberculosis programmes in Latin American and Caribbean countries. *Veterinary Microbiology*, 4th International Conference on *Mycobacterium bovis* 112(2–4), 111–118.

de la Rua-Domenech, R. (2006) Human *Mycobacterium bovis* infection in the United Kingdom: incidence, risks, control measures and review of the zoonotic aspects of bovine tuberculosis. *Tuberculosis* 86(2), 77–109.

Department for Environment, Food and Rural Affairs (2013) Various Bovine TB Costs (2008 to 2013). Available at: https://www.gov.uk/government/publications/various-bovine-tb-costs-2008-to-2013. (accessed 22 May 2008 to 2013).

Department for Environment, Food and Rural Affairs (2014) Bovine TB Control Costs in 2013. Available at: https://www.gov.uk/government/publications/bovine-tb-control-costs-in-2013 (accessed 22 May 2013).

Ducrotoy, M.J., Yahyaoui Azami, H., El Berbri, I., Bouslikhane, M., Fassi Fihri, O., *et al.* (2015) Integrated health messaging for multiple neglected zoonoses: approaches, challenges and opportunities in Morocco. *Acta Tropica* 152(December), 17–25.

Elias, K., Hussein, D., Asseged, B., Wondwossen, T. and Gebeyehu, M. (2008) Status of bovine tuberculosis in Addis Ababa dairy farms. *Revue Scientifique et Technique (International Office of Epizootics)* 27(3), 915–923.

Evans, J.T., Smith, E.G., Banerjee, A., Smith, R.M., Dale, J., *et al.* (2007) Cluster of human tuberculosis caused by *Mycobacterium bovis*: evidence for person-to-person transmission in the UK. *The Lancet* 369(9569), 1270–1276.

FAO (2011) Principales Réalisations Depuis L'ouverture de La Représentation de La FAO À Rabat En 1982. Available at: www.fao.org/3/a-ba0008f.pdf (accessed 12 December 2017).

Fried, L.P., Bentley, M.E., Buekens, P., Burke, D.S., Frenk, J.J., *et al.* (2010) Global health is public health. *The Lancet* 375(9714), 535–537.

Gormley, E. and Corner, L.A.L. (2013) Control strategies for wildlife tuberculosis in Ireland. *Transboundary and Emerging Diseases* 60 Suppl 1(November), 128–135.

Grange, J.M. (2001) *Mycobacterium bovis* infection in human beings. *Tuberculosis* 81(1–2), 71–77.

Hlavsa, M.C., Moonan, P.K., Cowan, L.S., Navin, T.R., Kammerer, J.S., et al. (2008) Human tuberculosis due to *Mycobacterium bovis* in the United States, 1995–2005. *Clinical Infectious Diseases* 47(2), 168–175.

Humblet, M.-F., Boschiroli, M.L. and Saegerman, C. (2009) Classification of worldwide bovine tuberculosis risk factors in cattle: a stratified approach. *Veterinary Research* 40(5), 1–24.

Ingram, P.R., Bremner, P., Inglis, T.J., Murray, R.J. and Cousins, D.V. (2010) Zoonotic tuberculosis: on the decline. *Communicable Diseases Intelligence Quarterly Report* 34(3), 339.

Kasymbekov, J., Imanseitov, J., Ballif, M., Schürch, N., Paniga, S., et al. (2013) Molecular epidemiology and antibiotic susceptibility of livestock *Brucella melitensis* isolates from Naryn Oblast, Kyrgyzstan. *PLOS Neglected Tropical Diseases* 7(2), e2047.

Khattak, I., Mushtaq, M.H., Ahmad, M.U.D., Khan, M.S. and Haider, J. (2016) Zoonotic tuberculosis in occupationally exposed groups in Pakistan. *Occupational Medicine* 66(5), 371–376.

La banque mondiale (2014) Population rural (% de La Population Totale). Available at: http://donnees.banquemondiale.org/indicateur/SP.RUR.TOTL.ZS (accessed 12 December 2017).

Lawn, S.D. and Zumla, A.I. (2011) Tuberculosis. *The Lancet* 378(9785), 57–72.

Léchenne, M., Miranda, M.E. and Zinsstag, J. (2015) *Integrated Rabies Control in One Health: The Theory and Practice of Integrated Health Approaches*. CAB International, Wallingford, UK.

LoBue, P., Betacourt, W., Peter, C. and Moser, K. (2003) Epidemiology of *Mycobacterium bovis* disease in San Diego county, 1994–2000. *The International Journal of Tuberculosis and Lung Disease* 7(2), 180–185.

Mathews, F., Macdonald, D.W., Taylor, G.M., Gelling, M., Norman, R.A., et al. (2006) Bovine tuberculosis (*Mycobacterium bovis*) in British farmland wildlife: the importance to agriculture. *Proceedings of the Royal Society of London B: Biological Sciences* 273(1584), 357–365.

Maudlin, I., Eisler, M.C. and Welburn, S.C. (2009) Neglected and endemic zoonoses. *Philosophical Transactions of the Royal Society of London B: Biological Sciences* 364(1530), 2777–2787.

McLaughlin, A.M. and Gibbons, N. (2012) Primary isoniazid resistance in *Mycobacterium bovis* disease: a prospect of concern. *American Journal of Respiratory and Critical Care Medicine* 186(1), 110–111.

Meisinger, G. (1970) Economic effects of the elimination of bovine tuberculosis on the productivity of cattle herds. 2. Effect on meat production. *Monatshefte Für Veterinärmedizin* 25(1), 7.

Michel, A.L., Müller, B. and van Helden, P.D. (2010) *Mycobacterium bovis* at the animal–human interface: a problem, or not? *Veterinary Microbiology, Zoonoses: Advances and Perspectives* 140(3–4), 371–381.

Moiane, I., Machado, A., Santos, N., Nhambir, A., Inlamea, O., et al. (2014) Prevalence of bovine tuberculosis and risk factor assessment in cattle in rural livestock areas of Govuro district in the Southeast of Mozambique. *PLoS One* 9(3), e91527.

Morris, R.S. (2015) Diseases, dilemmas, decisions: converting epidemiological dilemmas into successful disease control decisions. *Preventive Veterinary Medicine* 122(1–2), 242–252.

Müller, B., Dürr, S., Alonso, S., Hattendorf, J., Laisse, C.J., et al. (2013) Zoonotic *Mycobacterium bovis*-induced tuberculosis in humans. *Emerging Infectious Diseases* 19(6), 899–908.

Narrod, C., Zinsstag, J. and Tiongco, M. (2012) A one health framework for estimating the economic costs of zoonotic diseases on society. *EcoHealth* 9(2), 150–162.

O'Brien, D.J., Schmitt, S.M., Lyashchenko, K.P., Waters, W.R., Berry, D.E., et al. (2009) Evaluation of blood assays for detection of *Mycobacterium bovis* in white-tailed deer (*Odocoileus virginianus*) in Michigan. *Journal of Wildlife Diseases* 45(1), 153–164.

Osburn, B., Scott, C. and Gibbs, P. (2009) One world—one medicine—one health: emerging veterinary challenges and opportunities. *Revue Scientifique et Technique* 28(2), 481.

Palmer, M.V. (2013) *Mycobacterium bovis*: characteristics of wildlife reservoir hosts. *Transboundary and Emerging Diseases* 60(Suppl. 1), 1–13.

Pesciaroli, M., Alvarez, J., Boniotti, M.B., Cagiola, M., Di Marco, V., et al. (2014) Tuberculosis in domestic animal species. *Research in Veterinary Science* 97(Suppl. Oct), S78–85.

Porphyre, T., Stevenson, M.A. and McKenzie, J. (2008) Risk factors for bovine tuberculosis in New Zealand cattle farms and their relationship with possum control strategies. *Preventive Veterinary Medicine* 86(1), 93–106.

Rahman, M.A. and Samad, M.A. (2008) Prevalence of bovine tuberculosis and its effects on milk production in red chittagong cattle. *Bangladesh Journal of Veterinary Medicine* 6(2), 175–178.

Robinson, P., Morris, D. and Antic, R. (1988) *Mycobacterium bovis* as an occupational hazard in abattoir workers. *Australian and New Zealand Journal of Medicine* 18(5), 701–703.

Roring, S., Scott, A., Brittain, D., Walker, I., Hewinson, G., et al. (2002) Development of variable-number tandem repeat typing of *Mycobacterium bovis*: comparison of results with those obtained by using existing exact tandem repeats and spoligotyping. *Journal of Clinical Microbiology* 40(6), 2126–2133.

Roth, F., Zinsstag, J., Orkhon, D., Chimed-Ochir, G., Hutton, G., et al. (2003) Human Health Benefits from Livestock Vaccination for Brucellosis: Case Study. *Bulletin of the World Health Organization* 81(12), 867–876.

Schelling, E., Diguimbaye, C., Daoud, S., Nicolet, J., Boerlin, P., et al. (2003) Brucellosis and Q-fever seroprevalences of nomadic pastoralists and their livestock in Chad. *Preventive Veterinary Medicine* 61(4), 279–293.

Schelling, E., Bechir, M., Ahmed, M.A., Wyss, K., Randolph, T.F. and Zinsstag, J. (2007) Human and animal vaccination delivery to remote nomadic families, Chad. *Emerging Infectious Diseases* 13(3), 373–379.

Schiller, I., Waters, W.R., Vordermeier, H.M., Jemmi, T., Welsh, M., et al. (2011) Bovine tuberculosis in Europe from the perspective of an officially tuberculosis free country: trade, surveillance and diagnostics. *Veterinary Microbiology* 151(1–2), 153–159.

Scorpio, A. and Zhang, Y. (1996) Mutations in pncA, a gene encoding pyrazinamidase/nicotinamidase, cause resistance to the antituberculous drug pyrazinamide in tubercle bacillus. *Nature Medicine* 2(6), 662–667.

Shimao, T. (2010) Control of cattle TB in Japan. *Kekkaku: [Tuberculosis]* 85(8), 661–666.

Shitaye, J.E., Tsegaye, W. and Pavlik, I. (2007) Bovine tuberculosis infection in animal and human populations in Ethiopia: a review. *Veterinarni Medicina-Praha-* 52(8), 317.

Sreevatsan, S., Bookout, J.B., Ringpis, F., Perumaalla, V.S., Ficht, T.A., et al. (2000) A multiplex approach to molecular detection of *Brucella abortus* and/or *Mycobacterium bovis* infection in cattle. *Journal of Clinical Microbiology* 38(7), 2602–2610.

Sunder, S., Lanotte, P., Godreuil, S., Martin, C., Boschiroli, M.L. and Besnier, J.M. (2009) Human-to-human transmission of tuberculosis caused by *Mycobacterium bovis* in immunocompetent patients. *Journal of Clinical Microbiology* 47(4), 1249–1251.

Tschopp, R. and Aseffa, A. (2016) Bovine tuberculosis and other Mycobacteria in animals in Ethiopia: a systematic review. *Jacobs Journal of Epidemiology and Preventive Medicine* 2(2), 26.

Tschopp, R., Hattendorf, J., Roth, F., Choudhoury, A., Shaw, A., et al. (2012) Cost estimate of bovine tuberculosis to Ethiopia. *One Health: The Human-Animal-Environment Interfaces in Emerging Infectious Diseases*, Springer, Berlin, Germany, pp. 249–268.

Tsend, S., Baljinnyam, Z., Suuri, B., Dashbal, E., Oidov, B., et al. (2014) Seroprevalence survey of brucellosis among rural people in Mongolia. *Western Pacific Surveillance and Response* 5(4).

Vazquez-Chacon, C.A., Martínez-Guarneros, A., Couvin, D., González-Y-Merchand, J.A., Rivera-Gutierrez, S., et al. (2015) Human multidrug-resistant *Mycobacterium bovis* infection in Mexico. *Tuberculosis* 95(6), 802–809.

Wedlock, D.N., Skinner, M.A., de Lisle, G.W. and Buddle, B.M. (2002) Control of *Mycobacterium bovis* infections and the risk to human populations. *Microbes and Infection/Institut Pasteur* 4(4), 471–480.

World Bank (2010) People, Pathogens, and Our Planet. Volume 2: The Economics of One Health. Available at: https://openknowledge.worldbank.org/handle/10986/11892 (accessed December 12, 2017).

WHO, FAO, UN, and OIE (2012) High-Level Technical Meeting to Address Health Risks at the Human-Animal Ecosystems Interfaces: Mexico City, Mexico 15–17 November 2011. Available at: http://www.who.int/iris/handle/10665/78100 (accessed 7 December 2017).

WHO (2016) Global Tuberculosis Report 2015. Available at: http://www.who.int/tb/publications/global_report/en/ (accessed 12 January 2015).

Zinsstag, J., Schelling, E., Wyss, K. and Mahamat, M.B. (2005) Potential of cooperation between human and animal health to strengthen health systems. *The Lancet* 366 (9503), 2142–2145.

Zinsstag, J., Schelling, E., Roth, F., Kazwala, R., Thoen, C.O., et al. (2006) Economics of bovine tuberculosis. *Mycobacterium bovis Infection in Animals and Humans*. Blackwell Publishing Ltd, pp. 68–83.

Zinsstag, J., Schelling, E., Roth, F., Bonfoh, B., de Savigny, D. and Tanner, M. (2007) Human benefits of animal interventions for zoonosis control. *Emerging Infectious Diseases* 13(4), 527–531.

Zinsstag, J., Schelling, E., Bonfoh, B., Fooks, A.R., Kasymbekov, J., *et al.* (2009) Towards a 'One Health' research and application tool box. *Veterinaria Italiana* 45(1), 121–133.

Zinsstag, J., Mackenzie, J.S., Jeggo, M., Heymann, D.L., Patz, J.A. and Daszak, P. (2012) Mainstreaming one health. *EcoHealth* 9(2), 107–110.

Zinsstag, J., Schelling, E., Waltner-Toews, D., Whittaker, M. and Tanner, M. (2015) *One Health: The Theory and Practice of Integrated Health Approaches*. CAB International, Wallingford, UK.

4 The Epidemiology of *Mycobacterium bovis* Infection in Cattle

Andrew J.K. Conlan* and James L.N. Wood
Disease Dynamics Unit, Department of Veterinary Medicine, University of Cambridge, Cambridge, UK

The epidemiology of bovine tuberculosis is, by its very nature, inconsistent. *Mycobacterium bovis* is poorly transmissible between cattle, but has a high potential for spread due to the chronic nature of infection. The risk of infection, susceptibility and progression of disease in individual animals is highly variable but it does vary systematically with age (Brooks-Pollock *et al.*, 2013; Downs *et al.*, 2016), breed (Ameni *et al.*, 2007), host genetics (Allen *et al.*, 2010; Bermingham *et al.*, 2014) and production type (Broughan *et al.*, 2016), which in themselves will vary in different epidemiological contexts. Resolving the impact of these biological factors on transmission is difficult as transmission rates, the duration of latency and the immunological response of infected animals to diagnostic tests all compete on timescales comparable to the life expectancy of the host. As a consequence, despite rich detailed surveillance data and a history of study stretching over a century, the epidemiology of bovine tuberculosis (TB) is still characterized as much by what we do not know as it is by what we do.

In this chapter, we critically assess some of the historic epidemiological data that shaped many of our views on the epidemiology of *M. bovis* in cattle. With reference to simple, and less simple, epidemiological models, we consider the strength of different pieces of evidence, the uncertainty that remains and the implications for control of *M. bovis* in different contexts.

We begin by reviewing the life history of infection and routes of transmission of *M. bovis* within herds. We then revisit the data from unmanaged herds endemically infected with bovine tuberculosis (Francis, 1947) and consider the implications of these data for the likely patterns of transmission of infection within herds. We compare these insights to more recent analyses of transmission in managed herds – in particular from Great Britain where detailed surveillance and demographic data sets have led to the development and estimation of several new models of bovine TB transmission both within and between herds. Finally, we consider the role that infection in sympatric wildlife populations has for both the inference of patterns of transmission within cattle populations and the prospects for control.

4.1 Life History of Infection and Transmission

Comstock, Levesay and Woolpert described human tuberculosis as an infectious disease where 'the incubation period . . . ranges from a few weeks to a lifetime' (Comstock *et al.*, 1974).

---

* Email: ajkc2@cam.ac.uk

© CAB International 2018. *Bovine Tuberculosis*
(eds M. Chambers, S. Gordon, F. Olea-Popelka, P. Barrow)

This sentiment could equally well apply to bovine tuberculosis, but there are important contrasts in the progression of disease in humans and cattle. In human tuberculosis, only a small fraction (~10%) of infected individuals that react positively to a tuberculin skin test will ever develop symptomatic disease. The rate of progression of tuberculosis in humans depends on the age at infection, with children more likely to develop active tuberculosis (Comstock et al., 1974). However, older people may also develop disease due to endogenous reactivation of infection that was acquired decades earlier in life (Comstock, 1982). This dichotomy is reflected in mathematical models of the transmission of *Mycobacterium tuberculosis* by explicitly modelling these two groups as separate model compartments relating to 'fast' and 'slow' progressors (Blower et al., 1995).

Such distinct heterogeneity in progression is assumed not to be important for *M. bovis* infection in cattle (Francis, 1947) and this is reflected in the structure of mathematical models for the transmission of *M. bovis*, which focus rather on the relationship between immunological status with respect to diagnostic tests and infectiousness. Our understanding of the progression and routes of transmission of *M. bovis* between cattle is underpinned by a long history of experimental and field studies. The commonalities and inconstancies of this body of work have been reviewed extensively by previous authors (Francis, 1947; Menzies and Neill, 2000; Goodchild and Clifton-Hadley, 2001) and are also challenged by recent work on the distribution of lesions in reactor animals (Brooks-Pollock et al., 2013; Downs et al., 2016). Here, we review the key findings of these studies within a conceptual model of disease progression (Fig. 4.1) that synthesizes the assumptions commonly used to develop mechanistic transmission models for *M. bovis* in cattle.

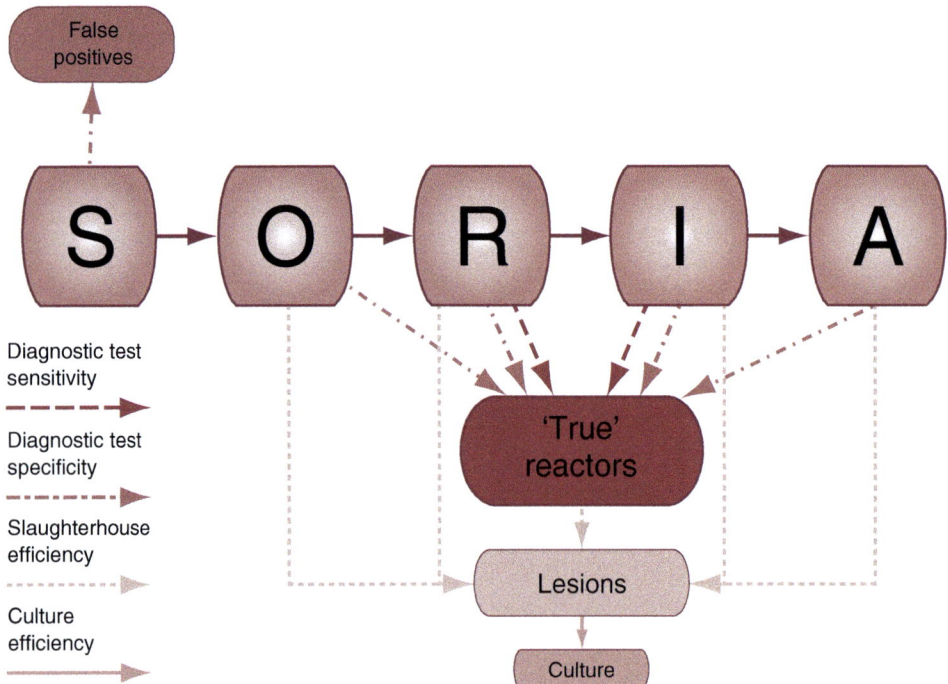

Fig. 4.1. Conceptual model of progression of bovine tuberculosis infection and relationship of model compartments to surveillance and control measures. S, susceptible; O, occult/unreactive; R, reactive; I, infectious; A, anergic.

4.1.1 A conceptual model of bovine tuberculosis progression

After infection, susceptible animals (S) enter an occult (O), or unreactive, period where they are infected, but do not react in diagnostic tests. Early experimental and field studies established an occult period between inoculation and cattle reacting to tuberculin. Francis (1947) concluded that this occult period had a duration of 20 to 30 days but could range between 8 and 50 days. These early insights are consistent with more modern data suggesting that artificially challenged animals are detectable within 3 weeks of infection (Thom et al., 2006).

The duration of latency in infectious diseases, including murine *M. tuberculosis* infection, can, at least theoretically, vary with infectious dose (Meynell and Meynell, 1958). This raises the possibility that experimental estimates may underestimate the occult period due to the (comparatively) large doses used in challenge studies. However, animals given as low a dose as one colony forming unit have also been demonstrated to become test positive within the same 3-week timescale (Dean et al., 2005). Epidemiological data from Great Britain provides further evidence that the occult period must be relatively short. Although latency periods in general are poorly identified by transmission models (Conlan et al., 2012, 2015; Bekara et al., 2014; Brooks-Pollock et al., 2014; O'Hare et al., 2014), occult periods greatly in excess of the experimentally derived range of 8 to 50 days would generate unrealistically high rates of recurrence in low incidence areas based on estimates of cattle-to-cattle transmission rates (Conlan et al., 2012).

There is marked confusion in the literature in the use of the term 'latency', which is assumed to mean clinical latency for much of the human literature, but usually refers to epidemiological latency for most studies of the cattle disease.

Despite over a century of study, the relationship between infection, diagnostic status, shedding of live bacteria and infectiousness of animals are still poorly characterized. Shedding of bacteria by naturally infected animals is intermittent and unpredictable, which along with culture times of up to 3 months devalues efforts to isolate *M. bovis* from live animals in the field. Experimentally challenged animals have been shown to shed bacteria within the first 10 to 60 days after intranasal challenge (Neill et al., 1988, 1989; Kao et al., 2007). Subsequently, shedding is intermittent and unpredictable, with the frequency of shedding held to increase with the progression of visible signs of disease and pathology.

This intermittency in shedding makes quantifying a period of epidemiological latency for bovine tuberculosis particularly difficult. This interval between infection and infectiousness is of critical importance for transmission as it sets the natural timescale over which changes in transmission, and therefore the impacts of control, are expected to be manifest. Some mathematical models of bovine TB assume that there is an additional 'reactive' latent period (R) where animals are reactive to the skin test but are not yet infectious (I). Barlow's original model of bovine TB in New Zealand herds assumed a range of epidemiological latency (the period spent in O and R states combined) of 180 to 600 days, while acknowledging a likely shorter range of 87 to 226 days in experimentally infected calves (Neill et al., 1992). Subsequent attempts to estimate this timescale rigorously from test-and-slaughter surveillance data sets have only served to increase this uncertainty (Conlan et al., 2012, 2015; Bekara et al., 2014; Brooks-Pollock et al., 2014; O'Hare et al., 2014).

Brooks-Pollock et al. (2014) estimated a much longer average (epidemiological) latent period of 11.1 years (95% credible interval of 3.29–25.7 years) from their national level models of bovine TB spread within Great Britain. Estimates from herd-level models fitted to the same British data aggregated at the herd level vary considerably (Conlan et al., 2012, 2015; O'Hare et al., 2014). However, this variability can be attributed to the very different prior assumptions made by authors in different studies, with vague assumptions on latency (Conlan et al., 2015) leading to longer estimated periods of latency consistent with Brooks-Pollock et al. (2014). A further apparent inconsistency in these recent modelling studies is that more parsimonious models, where animals are assumed to be infectious immediately on meeting infection, but at a lower overall rate of infectiousness, fit the British data equally well as models that include a latent period (Conlan et al., 2012, 2015).

Taken together, these inconsistencies suggest that the period of epidemiological latency is poorly identifiable from testing data. Models can fit the patterns of transmission within, and likely between, herds equally well with very short or long average periods of latency by trading off against other unknown parameters such as the average rate of transmission and test characteristics. Extreme estimates of latency, longer than the average lifetime of an animal within this population, may seem unrealistic at first sight, but in fact point to inadequacies in our conceptual model of infection (Fig. 4.1). The standard compartmental model we have outlined assumes all animals progress through the compartments of the model at fixed (average) rates. With no heterogeneity between individuals, estimating a low rate of progression to infectiousness is the only mechanism through which the model can capture the variability observed between outbreaks. O'Hare et al. (2014) found evidence that the inclusion of such heterogeneity in the form of a few 'super-spreading' cattle can improve the fit of herd level models, but this could also be generated by seasonal differences in contact rates (Bekara et al., 2014) or by a difference in individuals' rates of progression as previously discussed for models of human tuberculosis infection (Blower et al., 1995).

The final compartment of our conceptual model, accounts for severely infected animals with extensive lesions which nonetheless exhibit no reaction to tuberculin (Francis, 1947; Monaghan et al., 1994). Such 'anergic' animals (A) were thought to be relatively rare even in endemically infected herds, and have thus been considered to be unlikely to play a significant role in the transmission of bovine TB in regularly tested herds (Barlow et al., 1997). This assumption is supported by the relatively small numbers of animals presenting at slaughterhouses with lesions from regularly tested herds (Frankena et al., 2007; Olea-Popelka et al., 2012; Shittu et al., 2013) – and are more the inevitable consequence of gaps in surveillance, not least with an imperfect test (Mitchell et al., 2006), rather than necessarily a failure of testing. However, in uncontrolled populations where bovine tuberculosis is endemic or emerging, anergic animals may well be masking an even higher burden of infection within herds (Thakur et al., 2010; Firdessa et al., 2012).

4.1.2 The hidden burden of infection

The structure of epidemic models for bovine TB reflects the importance of diagnostic test performance in both controlling and estimating the rate of transmission. Tuberculin testing remains the imperfect gold standard for quantifying the prevalence of infection and demonstrating freedom from infection for herds and animals (Monaghan et al., 1994; de la Rua-Domenech et al., 2006; Nuñez-Garcia et al., 2017). The sensitivity and specificity of tuberculin testing are well known to vary with respect to the format of the test (e.g. single intradermal, comparative), potency of tuberculin (Downs et al., 2013) and even the compliance of veterinarians to protocol (Humblet et al., 2011). Variability in compliance is in some sense understandable given the considerable health and safety challenges, for both veterinarians and farmers, of administering the test. Conscious and unconscious decisions concerning the time spent per animal and the handling of borderline reactions will also be influenced by the epidemiological context of the herd being tested. This veterinary discretion, although a complicating factor for the interpretation of epidemiological data, has been argued to be a strength of the statutory system allowing the impacts of disease, if not the disease itself, to be more appropriately managed (Enticott, 2012).

Less appreciated, however, is the dynamic relationship between transmission, test sensitivity and the hidden burden of infection missed by testing. Transmission models for bovine tuberculosis are structured to account for the systematic reduction in test sensitivity for early and late infections. Within our conceptual framework, 'true' reactor animals that are actually infected are detected from the R and I compartments (Fig. 4.1) with an efficiency determined by the diagnostic test sensitivity. Exposure to other environmental sources of *Mycobacterium* is likely to be an important contributory factor to false positive reactions to the skin test. To account for this, models allow false positive animals to be detected from any compartment with a risk determined by the test specificity parameter. However, post-mortem inspection and culture, which can itself be considered as an insensitive but perfectly specific diagnostic test, can in principle identify animals at any stage of progression (i.e. from infected compartments O, R, I, A).

Empirical estimates of the sensitivity and specificity of tuberculin tests rely on post-mortem comparison to culture of *M. bovis* from test-positive and -negative animals, respectively. The discrepancy between these relative measures of diagnostic test performance and the true sensitivity and specificity (with respect to disease status) will depend on the extent of misclassification of test-negative animals. In turn, this hidden burden of infection due to test-insensitive animals will vary with the prevalence of infection and past history of transmission. Herds with a recent high rate of transmission will have a disproportionately high proportion of occult animals, whereas a herd that has been heavily infected for a long period of time may have a greater proportion of anergic animals.

Quantifying the burden of infection missed by testing therefore requires dynamic models of transmission that track the history of infection and removal of animals (Conlan *et al.*, 2012). From the modeller's perspective, this relationship means that the parameters governing test characteristics in mathematical models of transmission, where we know the true infection status of animals, cannot be simply equated to relative measures from visible lesions. More fundamentally, alternative diagnostic tests for bovine tuberculosis have different windows of sensitivities with gamma-interferon tests more likely to pick up earlier infection (de la Rua-Domenech *et al.*, 2006) and antibody tests more likely to pick up later infection (Whelan *et al.*, 2010). Simple comparison of the performance of bovine TB tests with respect to lesions could therefore be highly misleading, a concern reinforced by recent latent class analysis (Nuñez-Garcia *et al.*, 2017) that suggests that the true sensitivity of the single intradermal comparative cervical tuberculin skin (SICCT) test may be as low as 50% (26–78%, 95% credible intervals) compared to the commonly accepted median estimate of relative sensitivity of 80% (range of estimates from 50–100%; de la Rua-Domenech *et al.*, 2006). However, as we discuss in Section 4.3, the way we use testing is just as important – if not more so – than the performance of the test in individual animals.

4.1.3 Routes and mechanisms of transmission between cattle

Bovine tuberculosis in cattle is primarily a pulmonary infection (Francis, 1947; Liebana *et al.*, 2008), which suggests that respiratory transmission is the primary route of cattle-to-cattle transmission (Menzies and Neill, 2000; Goodchild *et al.*, 2015). However, pseudo-vertical transmission through milk – the main historic zoonotic risk for humans – is also a likely alternative route of infection for calves. Although only a relatively small proportion of infected animals in an uncontrolled situation (1–2%) develop infection within the udders, bulk milk feeding practices may pose a high risk. Alimentary infection is rarely detected, particularly in managed populations, although bacteria have also been recovered from faeces from experimentally challenged animals (Neill *et al.*, 1988).

Pathology can suggest the likely routes of infection, and is often appealed to justify the importance of a particular route of transmission. However compelling these narratives may be, the reality is that no study to date has successfully quantified the relative importance of direct contact, aerosol spread and indirect environmental spread through fomites to the risk of acquiring infection. Historical studies in the south of England found that *M. bovis* could remain alive and virulent on pasture for at least 49 days during the summer (Maddock, 1933). Environmental factors are likely to affect this viability with more recent studies in New Zealand (Jackson *et al.*, 1995) and Michigan, USA (Fine *et al.*, 2011) finding considerable variability in the viability of bacteria between seasons. For chronic, relatively poorly transmissible pathogens such as *M. bovis*, the duration of exposure is as important a component as the dose. While the exposure from direct contact might be orders of magnitude greater than contamination on pasture, the frequency of exposure through grazing may amplify the overall risk of acquiring infection.

Environmental transmission was largely ruled out in the 1930s based on experimental infection studies, which demonstrated that transmission to calves was possible from pastures sprayed with artificially high concentrations of *M. bovis* (Maddock, 1933), but transmission was not observed on pasture contaminated by artificially inoculated animals (Maddock, 1934). However, animals in this second study were only exposed to pasture for 3 weeks after the infected animals were removed to eliminate the risk of direct transmission. This is a very short period of exposure given the low rates of direct transmission that have been observed between susceptible and test-positive animals held in direct contact over far longer exposure times of 12 months (Khatri et al., 2012). Environmentally mediated exposure cannot therefore be ruled out completely, particularly for extensively managed farms in developing countries (Ameni et al., 2007), but also as a mechanism for within-farm persistence of infection. The lower risk of recurrence of bovine TB incidence in Scotland and low-risk areas of England compared to high-risk areas in England is most often attributed to a reduced prevalence of disease within wildlife (Karolemeas et al., 2011). However, the reduced viability of environmental M. bovis in Scotland due to climatic factors could also be a contributory factor. Climate has been reported as a risk factor for TB incidence (Wint et al., 2002); however, several confounding factors could explain this association including the density of cattle, badgers and liver fluke which is known to interfere with the action of the diagnostic skin test (Flynn et al., 2007).

4.2 Patterns of Transmission Within Unmanaged Herds

Regardless of the route of exposure, what is clear is that bovine tuberculosis is a relatively poorly transmissible pathogen that nonetheless has a considerable potential for transmission within herds due to the chronic and progressive nature of infection. The potential for transmission of an infectious disease can be characterized by the basic reproduction number (R_0), defined as the expected number of new infections when a single infectious individual is introduced into a fully susceptible population. Heuristically, the basic reproduction ratio can be thought of as depending on two factors: the duration of time they are infectious and the probability of transmission per unit time (β'),

itself a function of the rate of contact between susceptible and infected animals and the relative infectiousness and susceptibility of different hosts. For a chronic infection such as bovine tuberculosis, the duration of infection is, to a first approximation, the life expectancy of the animal. Thus:

$$R_0 = \beta L$$

In an unmanaged population R_0 will be closely related to the proportion of the population free from disease (s) when the population is infected endemically (Keeling and Rohani, 2008):

$$R_0 \approx 1/s$$

Setting aside the likely presence of hidden infection, the fraction of endemically infected herds unreactive to tuberculin can therefore provide a 'first-estimate' of the basic reproductive ratio of bovine tuberculosis. Early prevalence studies in Europe, collated by Francis (1947), reported herd level prevalence from Denmark (1896) and Great Britain (1945) of between 4% and 60% corresponding to a range for the within herd R_0 of between 1.04 and 1.67.

Variations between regions, animal husbandry, breed and format of the tuberculin test is responsible for some of this variability, but two systematic aspects were highlighted by Francis in his seminal book that have important implications for how epidemiological modellers would come to describe cattle-to-cattle transmission.

4.2.1 Density-dependent transmission

Francis noted that the proportion of cattle testing positive to tuberculin increased with herd size (Fig. 4.2a): 'For every addition of ten cattle to a herd the incidence of tuberculosis increases by about 4 per cent'.

This observation, together with a more general association of the risk of tuberculosis infection or breakdowns with herd size, is perhaps the most consistently reported aspect of bovine tuberculosis epidemiology in cattle (Skuce et al., 2012). The implication of this observation is that the potential for transmission of bovine tuberculosis, as measured by R_0, is increasing along with the size of the herd (Fig. 4.2b).

Such a so-called density-dependent, but really a herd size-dependent, relationship for

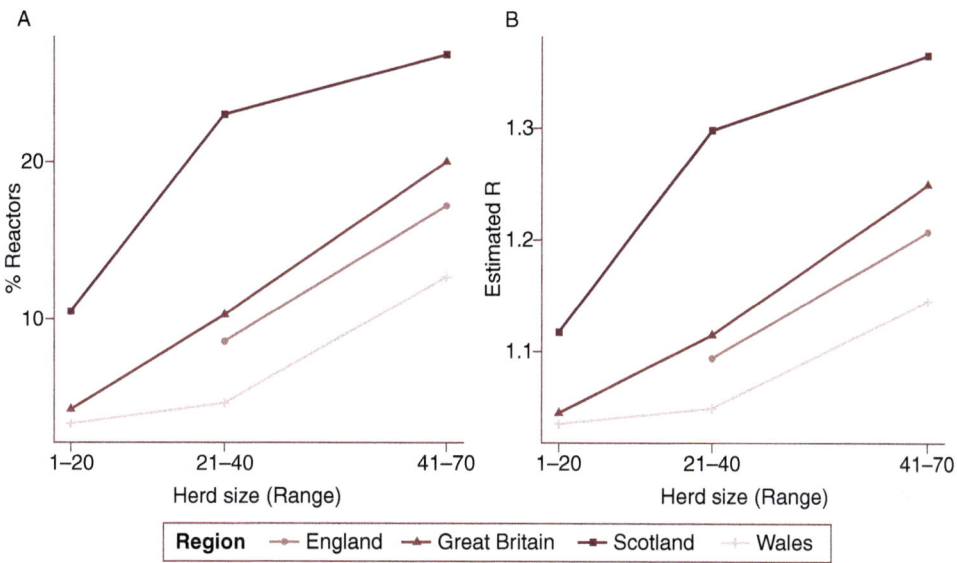

Fig. 4.2. (a) Average percentage of animals reacting to the tuberculin skin test with increasing herd size. (b) Estimated reproduction ratio based upon the apparent average prevalence of tuberculin reactors within these coarse herd size ranges. Adapted from Francis, J. (1947) *Bovine Tuberculosis*, Table XI.

transmission is a common (McCallum et al., 2001), but controversial (Begon et al., 2002), assumption for epidemic models in animal populations. The controversy comes from the fundamental assumption at the heart of most epidemic models that the rate of transmission is mediated by the direct contact, or interaction of susceptible and infectious individuals. Given this assumption, at least for a well-mixed, homogenous population, we would expect the rate of encounters between individuals to scale with the number of susceptible individuals and the proportion of infective animals. In this situation, so-called frequency-dependent transmission, the value of R_0 scales independently of herd size:

$$R_0 = \beta L$$

Following Francis's observation, epidemic models for bovine tuberculosis typically assume density-dependent transmission where the rate of infection depends on both the numbers of susceptible and infectives and R_0 increases linearly with herd size (H):

$$R_0 = \beta L H$$

While this assumption is more consistent with the empirical patterns of prevalence for bovine tuberculosis, it raises technical concerns not the least of which is that R_0 potentially increases without bound with the size of the population. It is also unclear what a herd size dependence on rate of transmission means mechanistically as the empirical association could be confounded by differences in husbandry, demography or even the balance of direct and indirect transmission acting upon herds.

This distinction in how transmission is modelled is not just a technical matter, but has fundamental consequences for the likely efficacy of controls. If transmission is density dependent, then we would expect controls, in particular vaccination, to become increasingly less effective with the size of the herd. Different authors have chosen to use either density-dependent transmission (Barlow et al., 1997; Kao et al., 1997; O'Hare et al., 2014) or frequency-dependent transmission (Fischer et al., 2005; van Asseldonk et al., 2005) with potentially profound implications for their conclusions of the relative merits of alternative control interventions.

Conlan and colleagues attempted to resolve this controversy by introducing a non-linearly density-dependent term where R_0 scales with an additional parameter q, that measures the strength of density dependence:

$R_0 = \beta L H^{1-q}$

with $q = 0$ corresponding to density dependence and $q = 1$ frequency dependence (Conlan et al., 2012). Unfortunately, at least from herd level models, the density-dependent parameter is poorly identified, with a suggestion that transmission is closer to density rather than frequency dependence for a range of alternative models (Conlan et al., 2012, 2015). However, the additional flexibility of the non-linear density-dependent term provides the opportunity to fit the empirical increase phenomenologically while ensuring that transmission rates are bounded as herd sizes increase.

4.2.2 Age-dependent patterns of incidence and transmission

The first estimate of R_0 from the overall within-herd prevalence, considered above, depends on an implicit assumption that the risk of transmission within the herd is constant with respect to age. We can test the validity of this assumption by calculating the force of infection – or the rate at which test-negative animals become test-positive – with respect to age. Data from the 19th and early 20th centuries, once again tabulated by Francis, demonstrates the increasing risk of becoming test-positive with respect to age that we would expect given the progressive nature of bovine TB infection (Fig 4.3a). However, at least from these historical data, the rate at which animals became test-positive decreases with age (Fig. 4.3b) with a peak in the very youngest age group considered by Francis (0–0.5 years old). This pattern is perhaps suggestive of pseudo-vertical transmission, but it should also be noted that tuberculin testing is no longer carried out in calves under the age of 6 weeks. Interpreting such historic data is fraught with difficulty with many potential confounding factors. While this general pattern remains true in contemporary managed populations for infected animals detected through meat inspection (Frankena et al., 2007; Shittu et al., 2013), it is not the case for the rates of culture confirmation of reactor animals in managed herds (Brooks-Pollock et al., 2013) and contemporary unmanaged herds in Ethiopia (Firdessa et al., 2012) and India (Thakur et al., 2010) where the proportion of

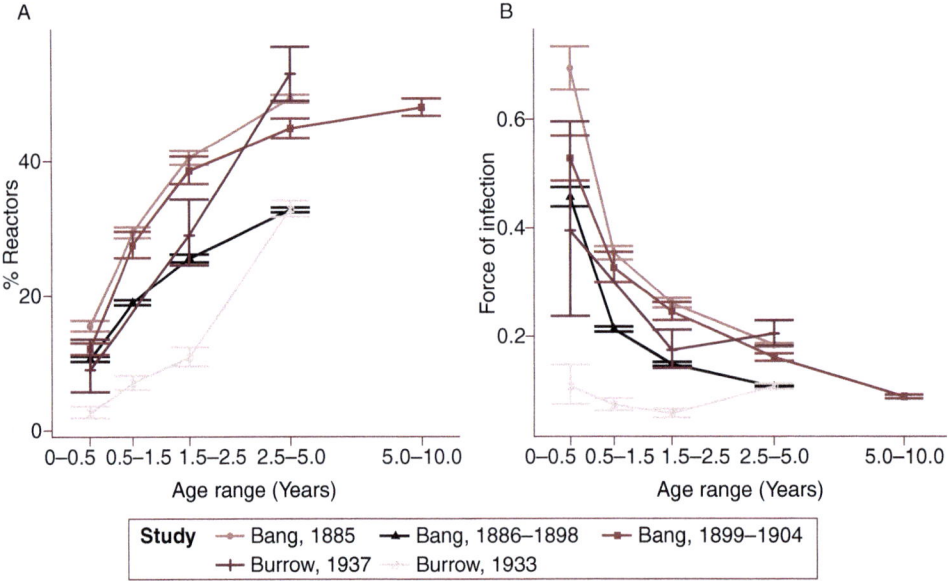

Fig. 4.3. (a) Percentage of animals reacting to skin test within coarse age groups (b) Estimated force of infection within the same age groups. Adapted from Francis, J. (1947) *Bovine Tuberculosis*, Table I.

cattle testing positive to tuberculin peaks with middle-age cattle.

4.3 Patterns of Transmission in Managed Populations: The Confounding Impact of Control

Control programmes for the management of bovine tuberculosis in industrial countries provide perhaps the richest sources of epidemiological data on bovine TB. However, the dynamic and context-sensitive nature of control programmes for bovine TB confounds the patterns of disease within herds that may be expected from studying the disease in unmanaged populations. The frequency of testing and removal of animals occurs on a timescale far shorter than the natural timescales of transmission which is reflected in the epidemiological patterns we see in these populations.

In this section, we concentrate on the epidemiology of bovine tuberculosis in the UK and the Republic of Ireland. The relatively high prevalence of infection in the face of national control programmes (Abernethy et al., 2013) combined with detailed demographic and cattle movement data (Mitchell et al., 2005) has facilitated highly sophisticated analyses and modelling of transmission. These analyses attempt to unpick the mechanisms of transmission, local persistence and efficiency of tuberculin testing that are responsible for the successes, and failures, of control in these populations.

4.3.1 Patterns of within-herd incidence

Control of bovine tuberculosis, particularly in Europe, is targeted at the herd level. Herds are tuberculin tested to demonstrate their freedom from infection at an interval that depends on their risk of infection. Detection of test-positive animals triggers a so-called herd 'breakdown', the lifting of officially TB-free status and the imposition of movement restrictions onto the affected herd. After the initial successes of the attestation era (1935–1960) (Pritchard, 1988) and before the introduction of annual testing for the whole of Wales in 2008, the frequency of routine testing in Great Britain was determined by the historical incidence within a herd's parish (the Parish Testing Interval, or PTI). This translated to herds in high-risk areas being expected to be tested annually, while lower-risk areas were required to test at progressively longer intervals of 2, 3 and 4 years.

Taken in itself, this temporal structuring of testing in Great Britain might have been expected to result in a greater number of reactor animals being found in breakdowns that started in low-risk areas. PTI 4 herds potentially had up to four times longer for disease to transmit before it could be disclosed by testing. However, the distribution of reactor animals removed from herds at their disclosing test was in fact remarkably consistent between testing areas – with the most frequent result being a single reactor animal triggering a breakdown (Fig. 4.4). This apparent incongruity is resolved when we note that the second most frequent situation was for a breakdown to start with no reactor animals – the consequence of an animal with lesions consistent with *M. bovis* infection being detected at slaughter and triggering a whole herd test earlier than the routine schedule would have required.

This single statistic is a powerful illustration of the dynamic link between the frequency of testing and potential for transmission within managed populations. The consistency of the within-herd distribution of reactors is a measure of the degree to which the second principle arm of surveillance, meat inspection or slaughterhouse surveillance, has worked to limit the potential transmission of bTB within herds. The proportion of breakdowns triggered at the slaughterhouse was considerably higher in low-risk areas (Conlan et al., 2012), effectively limiting the duration of time that infection could remain hidden within herds in low-risk areas before herd-level measures could be imposed. The power of slaughterhouse surveillance comes from the sheer number of animals that are inspected, such that even with a relatively poor sensitivity at the individual animal level, which can vary considerably between slaughterhouses (Frankena et al., 2007; Olea-Popelka et al., 2012; Shittu et al., 2013), there can be a significant benefit at the population level.

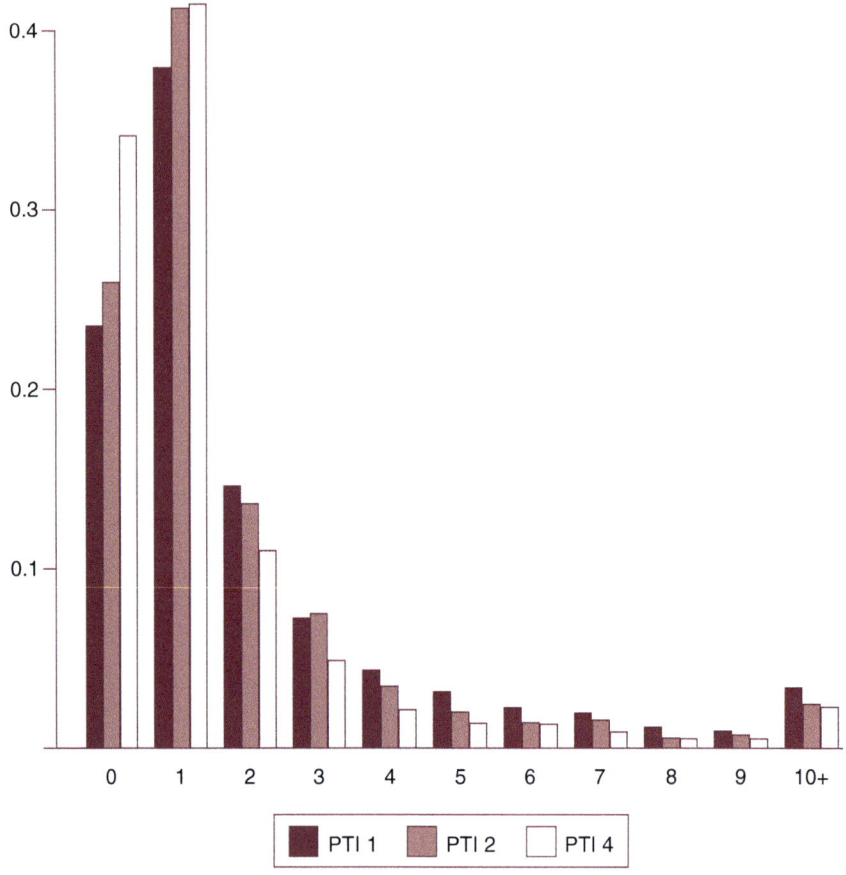

Fig. 4.4. Distribution of reactor animals disclosed at the beginning of a herd breakdown in PTI 1, 2 and 4 historical testing areas in Great Britain (2003–2005).

4.3.2 Persistence of infection within herds

The dynamic link between testing and the potential for transmission is increased further by the intensification of testing that results from disclosure within a herd. Herds are repeatedly tested at short intervals of at least 60 days until they test clear. The duration of breakdowns is incredibly heterogeneous. Although the majority of breakdowns resolve within 240 days (a maximum of four short interval tests), approximately 30% breakdowns will be prolonged, with some herds remaining under movement restrictions for years (Karolemeas et al., 2010). While the intrinsic dynamics of transmission of bovine TB no doubt contribute to this variability, the strongest risk factor for breakdowns in Great Britain to become prolonged is the confirmation of a reactor animal by visible lesions and culture. Such laboratory confirmation has a systematic effect of increasing the number of clear tests required to clear restrictions and demanding the use of a 'severe' interpretation of the SICCT test where an increase in sensitivity is traded for a reduction in specificity (i.e. the expected number of false positive tests).

The effectiveness of testing also plays a role in understanding the high rate of recurrence, which is another important measure of within-herd persistence. By far the greatest, and most consistent, risk factor for a herd having a breakdown of bovine TB is a past history of infection (Skuce et al., 2012; Broughan et al., 2016). In Great Britain between 2003 and 2005, approximately 38% of breakdowns recurred within

24 months of clearing restrictions (Karolemeas et al., 2011). Heuristically, recurrence can be explained either by the presence of infection missed by testing during the original breakdown or the re-introduction of infection through cattle movements, residual infection within the farm's environment or cross-species transmission from wildlife.

We used herd-level models with a structure similar to our conceptual model (see Fig. 4.1) to estimate the extent to which these patterns of persistence were consistent with re-introduction of infection or a hidden burden of infection missed by testing (Conlan et al., 2012). Our results suggested that at most 21% (12–33%) of breakdowns harbour a median of one infected animal (95% CI: 1–4) and at most 50% (95% CI: 33–67) of recurrent breakdowns could be explained by infection missed by testing.

4.3.3 Between-herd transmission of bovine tuberculosis and the role of cryptic infection in wildlife

The introduction of statutory reporting of cattle movements in the wake of the bovine spongiform encephalopathy epidemic has provided exquisite cattle movement data for the UK (Mitchell et al., 2005), Ireland and other European countries. In the UK, the so-called cattle tracing system has allowed sophisticated network analyses to be carried out that attempt to quantify the contribution of cattle movements to between-herd transmission.

Second only to a past history of infection, cattle movements from high-risk herds are perhaps the greatest, and most consistent, risk factor for bovine TB breakdowns outperforming environmental and other geographic factors (Gilbert et al., 2005). The importance of cattle movements to transmission was most dramatically demonstrated by the geographic expansion of disease that followed re-stocking of farms after the 2001 Foot and Mouth Epidemic (Carrique-Mas et al., 2008). However, the combination of insensitive cattle tests and slow transmission means that the relative contribution of environmental sources and cattle movements to between-herd transmission of bovine tuberculosis is surprisingly hard to quantify. The situation in Scotland is perhaps the exception to this, where all, or nearly all, recent breakdowns have been attributed to cattle movement (Bessell et al., 2013), even though at least one was detected late after substantial within-herd transmission that cattle movement allowed to be seeded into several other herds.

The low prevalence of infection in Scotland limits the utility in estimating rates of between-herd transmission. In order to progress, national level network models have had to make relatively strong assumptions about the role of wildlife in transmission that colour their findings. Green et al. (2008) developed a relatively simple framework for weighting the contribution of cattle movements to other sources where the risk of infection from environmental sources was modelled as a constant risk.

This pragmatic assumption, necessary due to our lack of systematic surveillance of wildlife populations, neglects the feedback loop that exists when a disease is freely transmitted between two host populations. Amid all of the controversy over the role of badgers, and culling efforts on the epidemiology of M. bovis in cattle, what is clear is that the disease can be transmitted between both species and interference with one host affects the prevalence of disease in the other (Godfray et al., 2013). This is most clearly demonstrated by the close geographical association in the genotypes of M. bovis isolated from cattle and badgers (Goodchild et al., 2012), but the relative rates of transmission between populations are not identifiable given available methods and data, with considerable uncertainty in estimates even with strong assumptions about directionality (Donnelly and Nouvellet, 2013).

The importance of considering the full dynamics of this two-host ecological system was highlighted by Brooks-Pollock and Wood (2015), who demonstrated how even relatively low levels of between-species infection can allow infection to persist in one host, be it cattle or badger, even when the inherent within-species reproductive ratio is below the threshold value of 1. In this situation, which on the balance of evidence is likely in Great Britain, marginal gains from intervention measures could be sufficient to tip the two-host system below threshold – particularly if the measures target interspecific spread.

Brooks-Pollock and colleague's national level network model from 2014 provided an important mid-way ground between assuming a constant risk from wildlife and a fully specified two-host model (Brooks-Pollock *et al.*, 2014). In this model the environmental reservoir is dynamic, increasing proportionally to the local prevalence of disease in cattle and decaying at a constant rate. This does not quite amount to an implicit assumption that disease will not persist within the environment in the absence of cattle infection – the estimated rate of decay may in principle be small enough that persistence is ensured over any reasonable timescale of interest. The mechanism is therefore likely to be able to account statistically for the background risk of infection, but lacks the detail necessary to make predictions about the impact of interventions that target transmission between badgers and cattle, or on the badger population itself.

The major contributions of the Brooks-Pollock model are a framework within which alternative transmission models may be systematically estimated from data (using approximate Bayesian computation) and a more robust quantification of the risks of cattle movements between herds to spread of the disease than was previously possible. Brooks-Pollock found that the herd reproduction ratio – the number of expected new breakdowns resulting from a given breakdown – was highly skewed. The majority of breakdowns lead to no transmission to other herds, but there is a fat tail of super-spreading herds responsible for multiple new incidents. This variability, driven by the trading practices and demographic structure of herds complements the variation seen in the within-herd R_0 and numbers of disclosed reactors at the herd level (Fig. 4.4). Herds that trade frequently are at a lower risk of within-herd transmission due to the relatively short duration of time individual animals remain within the herd – but these same herds may well pose a greater risk of transmission between herds.

4.4 Conclusion

Control of bovine TB in cattle is difficult, but in situations without sympatric host species tuberculin testing-based slaughter programs have been successful in eliminating disease. Control in populations with multiple host species involved will always be more challenging.

References

Abernethy, D.A., Upton, P., Higgins, I.M., McGrath, G., Goodchild, A.V., *et al.* (2013) Bovine tuberculosis trends in the UK and the Republic of Ireland, 1995–2010. *Veterinary Record* 172(12), 312.

Allen, A.R., Minozzi, G., Glass, E.J., Skuce, R.A., McDowell, S.W.J., *et al.* (2010) Bovine tuberculosis: the genetic basis of host susceptibility. *Proceedings of the Royal Society of London B: Biological Sciences*, 277(1695), 2737–2745.

Ameni, G., Aseffa, A., Engers, H., Young, D., Gordon, S., *et al.* (2007) High prevalence and increased severity of pathology of bovine tuberculosis in holsteins compared to zebu breeds under field cattle husbandry in central Ethiopia. *Clinical and Vaccine Immunology* 14(10), 1356–1361.

Barlow, N.D., Kean, J.M., Hickling, G., Livingstone, P.G. and Robson, A.B. (1997) A simulation model for the spread of bovine tuberculosis within New Zealand cattle herds. *Preventive Veterinary Medicine* 32(1), 57–75.

Begon, M., Bennett, M., Bowers, R.G., French, N.P., Hazel, S.M. and Turner, J. (2002) A clarification of transmission terms in host-microparasite models: numbers, densities and areas. *Epidemiology and Infection* 129(1), 147–153.

Bekara, M.E.A., Courcoul, A., Bénet, J.J. and Durand, B. (2014) Modeling tuberculosis dynamics, detection and control in cattle herds. *PLoS One* 9(9), e108584.

Bermingham, M.L., Bishop, S.C., Woolliams, J.A., Pong-Wong, R., Allen, A.R., *et al.* (2014) Genome-wide association study identifies novel loci associated with resistance to bovine tuberculosis. *Heredity* 112(5), 543–551.

Bessell, P.R., Orton, R., O'Hare, A., Mellor, D.J., Logue, D. and Kao, R.R. (2013) Developing a framework for risk-based surveillance of tuberculosis in cattle: a case study of its application in Scotland. *Epidemiology & Infection* 141(2), 314–323.

Blower, S.M., McLean, A.R., Porco, T.C., Small, P.M., Hopewell, P.C., et al. (1995) The intrinsic transmission dynamics of tuberculosis epidemics. *Nature Medicine* 1(8), 815–821.

Brooks-Pollock, E. and Wood, J.L.N. (2015) Eliminating bovine tuberculosis in cattle and badgers: insight from a dynamic model. *Proceedings of the Royal Society B* 282(1808), 20150374.

Brooks-Pollock, E., Conlan, A.J.K., Mitchell, A.P., Blackwell, R., McKinley, T.J. and Wood, J.L.N. (2013) Age-dependent patterns of bovine tuberculosis in cattle. *Veterinary Research* 44, 97.

Brooks-Pollock, E., Roberts, G.O. and Keeling, M.J. (2014) A dynamic model of bovine tuberculosis spread and control in Great Britain. *Nature* 511(7508), 228–231.

Broughan, J.M., Judge, J., Ely, E., Delahay, R.J., Wilson, G., et al. (2016) A review of risk factors for bovine tuberculosis infection in cattle in the UK and Ireland. *Epidemiology & Infection* 144(14), 2899–2926.

Carrique-Mas, J.J., Medley, G.F. and Green, L.E. (2008) Risks for bovine tuberculosis in british cattle farms restocked after the foot and mouth disease epidemic of 2001. *Preventive Veterinary Medicine* 84(1–2), 85–93.

Comstock, G.W. (1982) Epidemiology of tuberculosis. *American Review of Respiratory Disease* 125(3P2), 8–15.

Comstock, G.W., Livesay, V.T. and Woolpert, S.F. (1974) The prognosis of a positive tuberculin reaction in childhood and adolescence. *American Journal of Epidemiology* 99(2), 131–138.

Conlan, A.J.K., McKinley, T.J., Karolemeas, K., Brooks Pollock, E., Goodchild, A.V., et al. (2012) Estimating the hidden burden of bovine tuberculosis in Great Britain. *PLoS Computational Biology* 8(10), e1002730.

Conlan, A.J.K., Brooks Pollock, E., McKinley, T.J., Mitchell, A.P., Jones, G.J., et al. (2015) Potential benefits of cattle vaccination as a supplementary control for bovine tuberculosis. *PLoS Computational Biology* 11(2), e1004038.

Dean, G.S., Rhodes, S.G., Coad, M., Whelan, A.O., Cockle, P.J., et al. (2005) Minimum infective dose of *Mycobacterium bovis* in cattle. *Infection and Immunity* 73(10), 6467–6471.

de la Rua-Domenech, R., Goodchild, A.T., Vordermeier, H.M., Hewinson, R.G., Christiansen, K.H. and Clifton-Hadley, R.S. (2006) Ante mortem diagnosis of tuberculosis in cattle: a review of the tuberculin tests, γ-interferon assay and other ancillary diagnostic techniques. *Research in Veterinary Science* 81(2), 190–210.

Donnelly, C.A. and Nouvellet, P. (2013) The contribution of badgers to confirmed tuberculosis in cattle in high-incidence areas in England. *PLOS Currents Outbreaks* October 10, Edition 1.

Downs, S.H., Clifton-Hadley, R.S., Upton, P.A., Milne, I.C., Ely, E.R., et al. (2013) Tuberculin manufacturing source and breakdown incidence rate of bovine tuberculosis in british cattle, 2005–2009. *Veterinary Record* 172(4), 98–98.

Downs, S.H., Broughan, J.M., Goodchild, A.V., Upton, P.A. and Durr, P.A. (2016) Responses to diagnostic tests for bovine tuberculosis in dairy and non-dairy cattle naturally exposed to *Mycobacterium bovis* in Great Britain. *The Veterinary Journal* 216 (October), 8–17.

Enticott, G. (2012) The local universality of veterinary expertise and the geography of animal disease. *Transactions of the Institute of British Geographers* 37(1), 75–88.

Fine, A.E., Bolin, C.A., Gardiner, J.C. and Kaneene, J.B. (2011) A study of the persistence of *Mycobacterium bovis* in the environment under natural weather conditions in Michigan, USA. *Veterinary Medicine International* 2011 (April), e765430.

Firdessa, R., Tschopp, R., Wubete, A., Sombo, M., Hailu, E., et al. (2012) High prevalence of bovine tuberculosis in dairy cattle in central Ethiopia: implications for the dairy industry and public health. *PLoS One* 7(12), e52851.

Fischer, E.A.J., van Roermund, H.J.W., Hemerik, L., van Asseldonk, M.A.P.M. and de Jong, M.C.M. (2005) Evaluation of surveillance strategies for bovine tuberculosis (*Mycobacterium bovis*) using an individual based epidemiological model. *Preventive Veterinary Medicine* 67(4), 283–301.

Flynn, R.J., Mannion, C., Golden, O., Hacariz, O. and Mulcahy, G. (2007) Experimental *Fasciola hepatica* infection alters responses to tests used for diagnosis of bovine tuberculosis. *Infection and Immunity* 75(3), 1373–1381.

Francis, J. (1947) *Bovine Tuberculosis*. Staples Press Limited, London, UK.

Frankena, K., White, P.W., O'Keeffe, J., Costello, E., Martin, S.W., et al. (2007) Quantification of the relative efficiency of factory surveillance in the disclosure of tuberculosis lesions in attested Irish cattle. *Veterinary Record* 161(20), 679–684.

Gilbert, M., Mitchell, A., Bourn, D., Mawdsley, J., Clifton-Hadley, R. and Wint, W. (2005) Cattle movements and bovine tuberculosis in Great Britain. *Nature* 435(7041), 491–496.

Godfray, H.C.J., Donnelly, C.A., Kao, R.R., Macdonald, D.W., McDonald, R.A., *et al.* (2013) A restatement of the natural science evidence base relevant to the control of bovine tuberculosis in Great Britain. *Proceedings of the Royal Society B* 280(1768), 20131634.

Goodchild, A.V. and Clifton-Hadley, R.S. (2001) Cattle-to-cattle transmission of *Mycobacterium bovis*. *Tuberculosis* 81(1), 23–41.

Goodchild, A.V., Watkins, G.H., Sayers, A.R., Jones, J.R. and Clifton-Hadley, R.S. (2012) Geographical association between the genotype of bovine tuberculosis in found dead badgers and in cattle herds. *Veterinary Record* 170(10), 259–259.

Goodchild, A.V., Downs, S.H., Upton, P., Wood, J.L.N. and de la Rua-Domenech, R. (2015) Specificity of the comparative skin test for bovine tuberculosis in Great Britain. *The Veterinary Record* 177(10), 258.

Green, D.M., Kiss, I.Z., Mitchell, A.P. and Kao, R.R. (2008) Estimates for local and movement-based transmission of bovine tuberculosis in British cattle. *Proceedings of the Royal Society of London B: Biological Sciences* 275(1638), 1001–1005.

Humblet, M.-F., Walravens, K., Salandre, O., Boschiroli, M.L., Gilbert, M., Berkvens, D., *et al.* (2011) Monitoring of the intra-dermal tuberculosis skin test performed by Belgian field practitioners. *Research in Veterinary Science* 91(2), 199–207.

Jackson, R., de Lisle, G.W. and Morris, R.S. (1995) A study of the environmental survival of *Mycobacterium bovis* on a farm in New Zealand. *New Zealand Veterinary Journal* 43(7), 346–352.

Kao, R.R., Gravenor, M.B., Charleston, B., Hope, J.C., Martin, M. and Howard, C.J. (2007) *Mycobacterium bovis* shedding patterns from experimentally infected calves and the effect of concurrent infection with bovine viral diarrhoea virus. *Journal of The Royal Society Interface* 4(14), 545–551.

Kao, R.R., Roberts, M.G. and Ryan, T.J. (1997) A model of bovine tuberculosis control in domesticated cattle herds. *Proceedings of the Royal Society of London B: Biological Sciences* 264(1384), 1069–1076.

Karolemeas, K., McKinley, T.J., Clifton-Hadley, R.S., Goodchild, A.V., Mitchell, A., *et al.* (2010) Predicting prolonged bovine tuberculosis breakdowns in Great Britain as an aid to control. *Preventive Veterinary Medicine*, Special section: Calvin W. Schwabe Symposium 2009 Methodologies in Epidemiological Research 97(3–4),183–190.

Karolemeas, K., McKinley, T.J., Clifton-Hadley, R.S., Goodchild, A.V., Mitchell, A., *et al.* (2011) Recurrence of bovine tuberculosis breakdowns in Great Britain: risk factors and prediction. *Preventive Veterinary Medicine* 102(1), 22–29.

Keeling, M.J. and Rohani, P. (2008) *Modeling Infectious Diseases in Humans and Animals*. Princeton University Press, Princeton, USA.

Khatri, B.L., Coad, M., Clifford, D.J., Hewinson, R.G., Whelan, A.O. and Vordermeier, H.M. (2012) A natural-transmission model of bovine tuberculosis provides novel disease insights. *Veterinary Record* 171(18), 448.

Liebana, E., Johnson, L., Gough, J., Durr, P., Jahans, K., *et al.* (2008) Pathology of naturally occurring bovine tuberculosis in England and Wales. *The Veterinary Journal* 176(3), 354–360.

Maddock, E.C.G. (1933) Studies on the survival time of the bovine tubercle bacillus in soil, soil and dung, in dung and on grass, with experiments on the preliminary treatment of infected organic matter and the cultivation of the organism. *Epidemiology & Infection* 33(1), 103–117.

Maddock, E.C.G. (1934) Further studies on the survival time of the bovine tubercle bacillus in soil, soil and dung, in dung and on grass, with experiments on feeding guinea-pigs and calves on grass artificially infected with bovine tubercle bacilli. *The Journal of Hygiene* 34(3), 372–379.

McCallum, H., Barlow, N. and Hone, J. (2001) How should pathogen transmission be modelled? *Trends in Ecology & Evolution* 16(6), 295–300.

Menzies, F.D. and Neill, S.D. (2000) Cattle-to-cattle transmission of bovine tuberculosis. *The Veterinary Journal* 160(2), 92–106.

Meynell, G.G. and Meynell, E.W. (1958) The growth of micro-organisms in vivo with particular reference to the relation between dose and latent period. *The Journal of Hygiene* 56(3), 323–346.

Mitchell, A., Bourn, D., Mawdsley, J., Wint, W., Clifton-Hadley, R. and Gilbert, M. (2005) Characteristics of cattle movements in Britain – an analysis of records from the cattle tracing system. *Animal Science* 80(3), 265–273.

Mitchell, A.P., Green, L.E., Clifton-Hadley, R., Mawdsley, J., Sayers, R. and Medley, G.F. (2006) Analysis of single intradermal comparative cervical test (SICCT) coverage in the GB cattle population. In: Mellor, D.J. and Russell, A.M. (eds) *Proceedings of Society of Veterinary Epidemiology and Preventative Medicine*, SVEPM, Nottingham, UK, 70–86.

Monaghan, M.L., Doherty, M.L., Collins, J.D., Kazda, J.F. and Quinn, P.J. (1994) The tuberculin test. *Veterinary Microbiology* 40(1), 111–124.

Neill, S.D., Hanna, J., Mackie, D.P. and Bryson, T.G. (1992) Isolation of *Mycobacterium bovis* from the respiratory tracts of skin test-negative cattle. *Veterinary Record* 131(3), 45–47.

Neill, S.D., Hanna, J., O'Brien, J.J. and McCracken, R.M. (1988) Excretion of *Mycobacterium bovis* by experimentally infected cattle. *Veterinary Record* 123(13), 340–343.

Neill, S.D., Hanna, J., O'Brien, J.J. and McCracken, R.M. (1989) Transmission of tuberculosis from experimentally infected cattle to in-contact calves. *Veterinary Record* 124(11), 269–271.

Nuñez-Garcia, J., Downs, S.H., Parry, J.E., Abernethy, D.A., Broughan, J.M., et al. (2017) Meta-analyses of the sensitivity and specificity of ante-mortem and post-mortem diagnostic tests for bovine tuberculosis in the UK and Ireland. *Preventive Veterinary Medicine* doi: 10.1016/j.prevetmed.2017.02.017.

O'Hare, A., Orton, R.J., Bessell, P.R. and Kao, R.R. (2014) Estimating epidemiological parameters for bovine tuberculosis in british cattle using a bayesian partial-likelihood approach. *Proceedings of the Royal Society of London B: Biological Sciences* 281(1783), 20140248.

Olea-Popelka, F., Freeman, Z., White, P., Costello, E., O'Keeffe, J., et al. (2012) Relative effectiveness of Irish factories in the surveillance of slaughtered cattle for visible lesions of tuberculosis, 2005–2007. *Irish Veterinary Journal* 65, 2.

Pritchard, D.G. (1988) A century of bovine tuberculosis 1888–1988: conquest and controversy. *Journal of Comparative Pathology* 99(4), 357–399.

Shittu, A., Clifton-Hadley, R.S., Ely, E.R., Upton, P.U. and Downs, S.H. (2013) Factors associated with bovine tuberculosis confirmation rates in suspect lesions found in cattle at routine slaughter in Great Britain, 2003–2008. *Preventive Veterinary Medicine* 110(3–4), 395–404.

Skuce, R.A., Allen, A.R. and McDowell, S.W.J. (2012) Herd-level risk factors for bovine tuberculosis: a literature review. *Veterinary Medicine International* 2012(June), e621210.

Thakur, A., Sharma, M., Katoch, V.C., Dhar, P. and Katoch, R.C. (2010) A study on the prevalence of bovine tuberculosis in farmed dairy cattle in Himachal Pradesh. *Veterinary World* 3(9), 408–413.

Thom, M.L., Hope, J.C., McAulay, M., Villarreal-Ramos, B., Coffey, T.J., et al. (2006) The effect of tuberculin testing on the development of cell-mediated immune responses during *Mycobacterium bovis* infection. *Veterinary Immunology and Immunopathology* 114(1–2), 25–36.

van Asseldonk, M.A.P.M., van Roermund, H.J.W., Fischer, E.A.J., de Jong, M.C.M. and Huirne, R.B.M. (2005) Stochastic efficiency analysis of bovine tuberculosis-surveillance programs in the Netherlands. *Preventive Veterinary Medicine* 69(1–2), 39–52.

Whelan, C., Whelan, A.O., Shuralev, E., Kwok, H.F., Hewinson, G., et al. (2010) Performance of the Enferplex TB assay with cattle in Great Britain and assessment of its suitability as a test to distinguish infected and vaccinated animals. *Clinical and Vaccine Immunology* 17(5), 813–817.

Wint, G.R.W., Robinson, T.P., Bourn, D.M., Durr, P.A., Hay, S.I., et al. (2002) Mapping bovine tuberculosis in Great Britain using environmental data. *Trends in Microbiology* 10(10), 441–444.

5 *Mycobacterium bovis* Molecular Typing and Surveillance

Robin A. Skuce,[1,2,]* Andrew W. Byrne,[1,2] Angela Lahuerta-Marin[1] and Adrian Allen[1]

[1]*Veterinary Sciences Division, Agri-Food and Biosciences Institute, Belfast, UK;*
[2]*School of Biological Sciences, Queens University Belfast, Belfast, UK*

5.1 Bovine Tuberculosis

Mycobacterium bovis is a highly 'successful' pathogen with a worldwide distribution (Bezos *et al.*, 2014). In several countries, bovine tuberculosis (TB) remains a major and costly infectious disease of cattle and other domesticated, feral and wild animals (Pollock and Neill, 2002; Mathews *et al.*, 2006; Carslake *et al.*, 2011). It is considered the most complex and costly multispecies endemic disease currently facing the government, veterinary profession and farming industry in the UK and Ireland at least (Reynolds, 2006; Sheridan, 2011), where it impacts negatively on-farm profitability, trade and the welfare of affected farming families. It can also decimate years of livestock genetic improvement.

5.2 Rationale

In order to improve bovine TB control, it remains fundamental to describe and explain the basic biological processes of maintenance and transmission. However, despite substantial research, surprisingly little is known about transmission routes. Consequently, there is a continuing need to better understand bovine TB epidemiology and the interaction within and between cattle, wildlife and other potential environmental reservoirs. The ability to take advantage of structured surveillance and reproducibly discriminate *M. bovis* isolates into different molecular types has the potential to clarify sources of infection, major routes of transmission and potentially their relative importance. The methods, practices and data have essentially two applications: (i) to investigate important aspects of bovine TB ecology, evolution and epidemiology using descriptive, analytical and disease mathematical modelling studies; and (ii) to inform TB outbreak investigations and contact tracings (Benton *et al.*, 2014). There is substantial spend on components of current bovine TB control programmes, such as disease tracing and contiguous testing, and analysis of local molecular typing data has the potential to assess their efficacy, to monitor control and future interventions.

5.3 The Bacteria that Cause Tuberculosis

M. bovis is a member of the closely related *M. tuberculosis* complex (MTC) mycobacteria (Brosch *et al.*, 2002; Coll *et al.*, 2014a, b). On a global scale, the MTC can be subdivided using genome-enabled tests into discrete lineages that show strong phylogeographical localization to

---

* Email: robin.skuce@afbini.gov.uk

geographical regions (Hershberg et al., 2008; Wirth et al., 2008). This consistent observation has significant implications for control (Gagneux and Small, 2007) and despite sharing >99.95% nucleotide identity the MTC resolves into a series of 'ecotypes', each with its own non-absolute host-preference (Smith et al., 2006a; Whelan et al., 2010). It is biologically untenable that genetic variation in both the host and the pathogen does not influence the outcome of exposure, infection, disease and infectivity (Allen et al., 2010). Phylogenetic analysis of the MTC shows that the animal-adapted strains are found in a single major lineage marked by the deletion of chromosomal region of difference 9 (RD9-deleted) (Brosch et al., 2002). This important work has since been extended (Smith et al., 2006a, 2006b; Smith and Upton, 2012) to predict the most likely genotype in a series of inferred ancestors for modern animal-adapted MTC bacteria.

5.4 Epidemiology

Classical epidemiology attempts to identify those factors that determine disease distribution in time and space within and across populations. Furthermore, epidemiology is concerned with the mechanism(s) that determine disease transmission, manifestation and progression. The epidemiology of bovine TB worldwide is notoriously complex (Drewe et al., 2014), with current evidence indicating both cattle and wildlife infection sources in a number of ecosystems, the relative significance of which is uncertain and will vary amongst species, across regions and over time. Factors such as the adequacy of cattle control measures, the infection pressure in wildlife populations and the interaction between cattle and wildlife species are important (Skuce et al., 2012).

5.4.1 Molecular epidemiology

As a sub-specialism of epidemiology and driven by rapid advances in genome analyses and comparative genomics (Loman and Pallen, 2015), molecular epidemiology is the application of molecular taxonomy, phylogeny or population genetics techniques to epidemiologic problems. Molecular techniques further stratify data for epidemiologic activities, including disease surveillance, outbreak investigations, identifying transmission patterns and risk factors amongst apparently unconnected cases, characterizing host-pathogen interactions and assessing relative pathogen virulence.

Rapid improvements in the performance and scalability of pathogen molecular typing and access to meta-data are revolutionizing and modernizing disease control and surveillance in human health (Aarestrup et al., 2012). They are predicted to have a similarly transforming impact on animal health. This relatively new discipline provides an opportunity to revisit the received wisdom about infectious disease dynamics and has become an essential component of most modern infectious disease investigations (Muellner et al., 2011, 2015). Here we discuss how M. bovis molecular epidemiology has already improved our limited understanding of bovine TB ecology, evolution and epidemiology and the opportunities and limitations presented by the impending pathogen genomics revolution (Kwong et al., 2015). Molecular typing should not be seen as an end in itself; it should add value to, and is no replacement for, sound epidemiological design and implementation. The benefits of deployment should flow from the policy decisions that are informed by the evidence and estimates provided by rational molecular epidemiology studies.

The development and application of molecular epidemiology to more fully understand disease ecology and epidemiology is particularly well demonstrated in the highly related pathogen *M. tuberculosis* (Schurch and van Soolingen, 2012; Jagielski et al., 2016). While there have been significant methodological and data advances over recent years, these methods have been used effectively to monitor and investigate TB transmission dynamics, to detect laboratory cross-contamination, to differentiate relapse from re-infection, to evaluate those risk factors that place TB cases in a cluster of the same molecular type and to investigate emerging drug resistance. These methods have also revolutionized our understanding of the evolution and phylogeography of this important human pathogen (Comas and Gagneux, 2011; Pepperell et al., 2011). Molecular surveillance (Muellner et al., 2015) of *M. tuberculosis* to support outbreak analysis and contact tracing is now valued and well established in several countries, notably the USA (Centers for Disease Control and Prevention, 2012) and the Netherlands (Borgdorff and Soolingen, 2013), although the cost versus benefit of some systems has been questioned recently (Mears *et al.*, 2015).

5.4.2 Data sources and surveillance

In countries with advanced test and control programmes, animal-level testing, at prescribed intervals, is well established and confirmation by specialist bacterial culture provides an opportunity for structured *M. bovis* molecular type surveillance. In order to understand the diversity in the local *M. bovis* population it is important that representative sampling, whether retrospective or prospective, be achieved (Skuce *et al.*, 2010). Comprehensive herd-level, and in some cases animal-level, surveillance of *M. bovis* types in confirmed outbreaks has become established, most notably in the UK, where very large datasets have been assembled and are being analysed (Skuce *et al.*, 2010; Broughan *et al.*, 2015), and also in the USA, France, Spain, New Zealand etc., as discussed later. In order to effectively index the genetic diversity in a particular region it remains important to configure molecular epidemiology tests at a resolution that matches the epidemiological questions being addressed.

Until relatively recently, the bovine TB molecular epidemiology literature was dominated by method development and validation studies, rather than applications of mature technologies. While the bovine TB molecular type data are apparently 'simple' on a superficial level, it is important that such data are interpreted with caution and only in the context of other relevant epidemiological and genetic data, particularly retrospective data gathered over several years. Outbreak investigators find the data useful in the outbreak setting where it can support, or challenge, a hypothesis. Stakeholders expect competent authorities to deploy all available data and tools in a cost-effective manner to investigate local bovine TB breakdowns. Relations between all parties should improve where this is seen to be the case.

The epidemiology of bovine TB is highly complex and many of the processes driving the current epidemic are not fully recorded or observed (O'Hare *et al.*, 2014; Trewby *et al.*, 2016). An important example of such a process is animal movements between herds and via markets, which can act as a means of disseminating infection (Gilbert *et al.*, 2005). In addition, herds and animals also tend to be geo-referenced to the centre of the main farm holding. In reality the location attributed to cattle may be a systematic error, although the trend will be evident (Durr and Froggatt, 2002; Enright and Kao, 2016). Farm fragmentation and unrecorded cattle movements have the potential to significantly increase the size of epidemics driven by livestock movements and undermine the value of cattle tracing systems (Enright and Kao, 2016). Even in countries with exceptionally well-recorded animal test and movement data there may still be significant deficiencies in terms of data resolution in both space and time. An important challenge in understanding how, when and where bovine TB transmits to, from and between cattle, wildlife and the environment is that infections are not immediately apparent. The ante and post mortem cattle tests used in official schemes have high specificity but only moderate sensitivity (Nuñez-Garcia *et al.*, 2017; Lahuerta-Marin *et al.*, 2015), and countries differ significantly in the extent of culture confirmation undertaken (de la Rua-Domenech *et al.*, 2006; Clegg *et al.*, 2011; Abernethy *et al.*, 2013; Bermingham *et al.*, 2015). This impacts the representativeness of subsequent molecular surveillance of confirmed cases where epidemiologists will only ever see a reduced part of the transmission tree and have to make at least some assumptions (Biek and Real, 2010; Biek *et al.*, 2015).

Due to the slow growth of the organism, molecular typing data are often only available well after the disease control decisions need to be made. However, while real-time data are most useful, inference of trends in the data can inform on ways to modify and enhance approaches to disease control. As increasingly sophisticated mapping and database solutions are implemented to help exploit these data (Rodriguez-Campos *et al.*, 2012a), novel insights are being gained. Advances in bacterial physiology (O'Connor *et al.*, 2015), direct detection and metagenomics (Doughty *et al.*, 2014; Votintseva *et al.*, 2015) may further improve the prospects for real-time molecular surveillance.

5.4.3 Molecular typing methodology

Prior to the DNA-based studies, much of what was known about mycobacterial ecology, pathogenesis and epidemiology came from early methods used to identify these challenging bacteria. Such methods relied on strain phenotypic characteristics, including colony morphology, susceptibility to antimicrobials, biochemical and serological reactivity and mycobacterial phage typing. While some are still of value, such phenotypic methods have largely been superseded by methods that index structural genetic diversity in mycobacterial genomes (Jagielski *et al.*, 2016). Due to the high degree of genetic similarity and extreme clonality in modern MTC bacteria and the consequent co-linearity of their genomes, these methods are applicable and remarkably congruent across the ecotypes that comprise the MTC. The methods do vary in some performance characteristics, for example their discriminatory power, and they do have various strengths and weaknesses (Schurch and van Soolingen, 2012). Structural genetic markers that tend to evolve unidirectionally (e.g. SNPs and deletions) are well suited to phylogenetic and evolutionary studies, whereas markers that evolve more quickly and bi-directionally (e.g. mini-satellites and repeat variations) are prone to convergent evolution (homoplasy) but are better suited to outbreak investigations.

Prior to DNA amplification technologies, molecular epidemiology was based on gel electrophoretic analysis of bacterial whole-genome restriction enzyme analysis (REA) or the subsequent restriction fragment length polymorphism (RFLP) analysis, which probed REA profiles with repetitive DNA sequences. REA (Collins, 1999) and RFLP typing (van Soolingen, 2001) were standardized and became routine procedures in several public health and some veterinary research laboratories. While considered discriminating at the time, these techniques were technically demanding, requiring expensive software for archiving complex banding patterns and inter-laboratory reproducibility was not trivial (Heersma *et al.*, 1998). Most *M. bovis* isolates sampled worldwide turned out to belong to the same clonal complex and tended to have only one copy of the IS*6110* RFLP target (Smith, 2012).

Due to the landmark achievements of the first genome sequences for *M. tuberculosis* (Cole *et al.*, 1998) and *M. bovis* (Cole, 2002; Garnier *et al.*, 2003), the mycobacterial diagnostics and research community now has a tool box of molecular genetic tests that discriminate the MTC at different geographic and evolutionary scales (Pepperell *et al.*, 2011, 2013; O'Neill *et al.*, 2015). The first of the more portable PCR-enabled methods was spoligotyping (Kamerbeek *et al.*, 1997). This technique indexes unidirectional possession of short repeat sequences at a locus since shown to be a clustered regularly interspersed polymorphic repeat (CRISPR), a locus now finding game-changing applications in gene-drive and genome-editing technologies (Carlson *et al.*, 2016; Wright *et al.*, 2016). Spoligotyping methodology, including nomenclature, is internationally accepted (Mbovis.org, SITVIT2) and provides a moderate level of discrimination between isolates.

Significantly higher discrimination was achieved by configuring molecular typing tests based on multi-locus tandem repeat variation in mycobacterial interspersed repetitive units (MIRUs) and variable number of tandem repeats (VNTRs), the so-called MIRU-VNTR or multi-locus VNTR analysis (MLVA) techniques. Methodology and applications are reviewed elsewhere (Drewe and Smith, 2014; Robbe-Austerman and Turcotte, 2014) and will not be repeated in detail here. Unfortunately, nomenclature for naming *M. bovis* molecular types using these tests has not been settled internationally.

5.5 International Findings of *M. bovis* Molecular Typing

Here we summarize some general findings from deployment of genome-enabled molecular typing tests internationally. Systematic analysis of *M. bovis* sampled worldwide has disclosed striking region-to-region difference in the *M. bovis* clonal complexes that dominate within regions (Rodriguez-Campos *et al.*, 2012a; Smith, 2012; Allen *et al.*, 2013).

5.5.1 Europe

The European 1 clonal complex, which dominates and is virtually fixed in the UK and Ireland, is marked by a specific genomic deletion (RDEu1). It can be inferred that the UK and Ireland *M. bovis* population is largely different to that which dominates the rest of Europe. European 1 also dominates in many other countries (Canada, USA, Australia, New Zealand, Argentina, Chile, South Africa, etc.), which are former trading colonies of Britain. There is now genetic evidence that European 1 most likely originated in the British Isles and was exported to many countries worldwide and founded their now dominant populations (Smith *et al.*, 2011). Brazil is dominated by the European 2 clonal complex, which is also concentrated in Portugal, reflecting the historical connection between those countries (Rodriguez-Campos *et al.*, 2012b).

The fact that European 1 *M. bovis* has now been completely eradicated (e.g. in Australia) or largely eradicated in some countries (e.g. New Zealand) by test-and-slaughter policies, implies that European 1 can be eradicated with current tools, albeit over lengthy time periods. There seems nothing 'special' about European 1 that should make it impossible to eradicate. Also, European 1 has been isolated from a wide range of animal species; this implies that it is no more, or no less, capable of establishing in wildlife, depending on whether they are classified as dead-end or maintenance hosts. It seems plausible that intensive application of a test-and-slaughter policy based on tuberculin testing would have applied a strong selective pressure on the pathogen population and selected what might be described as 'escape mutants' of the tuberculin test. Whether European 1 has such a selective advantage that allowed it to reach high frequency within the UK and Ireland and beyond seems unlikely since European 1 was present before and after the dramatic reduction in bovine TB due to full implementation of the UK and Ireland control programmes. It is not clear if the RDEu1 deletion confers such a fitness advantage, and just because a clonal complex is common does not necessarily mean that it has a fitness advantage. However, one potential selective advantage has been proposed: control over insertion sequence copy number, which could impact gene expression and may have allowed these bacteria to become a globally distributed and important group (Smith *et al.*, 2011; Smith, 2012).

To investigate the evolutionary history of *M. bovis* within the UK and Ireland, rational population samples were typed at a range of informative mutations. Due to the clonal nature of modern TB bacteria, where mutations pass to all progeny, it is possible to propose the evolutionary events leading to the dominance of current clones. It is likely that the UK and Ireland, historically the British Isles, were founded by an *M. bovis* that was already deleted at RDEu1, potentially alongside other lineages that are now extinct. Regardless of the exact colonization history, the Eu1 lineage is now predominant in Britain and Ireland (Allen *et al.*, 2013). The British and Irish *M. bovis* populations are remarkably similar (Allen *et al.*, 2013). As well as sharing the RDEu1 deletion, they have the same basic linear phylogeny, providing further evidence that a single introduction into these islands occurred, potentially at a time when cattle populations were more homogenized prior to movement controls. Diversification within each territory has since occurred, with shared and region-specific genotypes identified. These locally evolved variants are useful in attributing source to imported cases and this facilitates a crude estimate of the impact of imports from other regions on outbreak and reactor numbers in each region.

Surveillance of *M. bovis* by spoligotyping and MLVA is an ongoing part of the strategy for TB control in Britain. Spoligotyping data have been used to infer the occurrence and clonal expansion of a common molecular type in Britain, possibly due to a selective advantage or invasion of a new ecological niche or host (Smith *et al.*, 2003). Spoligotyping and MLVA data have also been used to identify instances of human *M. bovis* infection (Gibson *et al.*, 2004; Stone *et al.*, 2011) and onward transmission to other humans (Evans *et al.*, 2007). Similarly, MLVA data have been used to identify incidents of disease in cattle caused by import from distant sources (Gopal *et al.*, 2006). The genetic structure evident in the MLVA, spoligotype and SNP-based molecular data has led to novel research hypotheses on diagnostics and vaccines (Smith *et al.*, 2006a, 2011; Allen *et al.*, 2013) and helped understand the population structure and evolutionary history of the pathogen across the British Isles, Western Europe and beyond. MLVA and spoligotyping confirmed that *M. bovis* recovered from European badgers (*Meles meles*) exhibits a strong geographic association with cattle herds sharing the same molecular type (Goodchild *et al.*, 2012).

Irish efforts began in concert with Northern Ireland, specifically with regard to spoligotyping and RFLP technologies (Roring *et al.*, 1998) applied to bovine, cervine, ovine, caprine, porcine and meline samples (Costello *et al.*, 1999). Distribution of most common molecular types was seen across all species and indicated that transmission between multiple hosts was a feature of *M. bovis* epidemiology (Costello *et al.*, 1999). RFLP techniques were subsequently deployed in the analysis of *M. bovis* isolates from badgers and cattle in four areas subjected to badger culling (Olea-Popelka *et al.*, 2005). Despite good evidence of cattle and badgers sharing the same molecular type, badger isolates exhibited low spatial clustering that may constitute evidence of increased badger mobility over time (Olea-Popelka *et al.*, 2005). Surveillance data indicated that combined spoligotype and MLVA methods had enhanced resolution (McLernon *et al.*, 2010), and when applied to badgers with differing disease prevalence across a wide geographic area (Furphy *et al.*, 2012), indicated that two distinct MLVA types were associated with high and low prevalence populations and that multiple strain types could be found in the same host (Furphy *et al.*, 2012).

IS*6110* RFLP was used by Spanish researchers to investigate *M. bovis* isolates from cattle and goat hosts (Gutierrez *et al.*, 1995) but lacked resolution. Subsequently, spoligotyping provided superior resolution (Aranaz *et al.*, 1996), proving useful in ruling out epidemiological association between cattle and human cases of *M. bovis* (Romero and Aranaz, 2006). Combined MLVA and spoligotyping has since been used to infer *M. bovis* transmission between wild boar and domestic pigs (Parra *et al.*, 2003), to survey *M. bovis* diversity in wildlife including deer and wild boar (Parra *et al.*, 2005; Mentaberre *et al.*, 2014), to confirm a role for wildlife in transmission to domestic animals and vice versa (Romero *et al.*, 2008) and to investigate *M. bovis* diversity in widely distributed bovine hosts (Rodriguez-Campos *et al.*, 2013). With the advent of MLVA (Navarro *et al.*, 2014), the ease with which molecular epidemiological information could be gathered has increased the utility of these data and a MLVA and spoligotype database has been developed to aid epidemiological surveillance in Spain (Rodriguez-Campos *et al.*, 2012a). More recent application of MLVA and spoligotyping in a high prevalence area indicated that persistence of the same molecular types within small spatial localities was a driver of ongoing infection rather than re-introduction from external sources (de la Cruz *et al.*, 2014), and that multiple molecular types were found in single hosts as a result of super-infection (Navarro *et al.*, 2015).

Italian researchers have applied spoligo-, MLVA and IS*6110* RFLP typing to human *M. bovis* isolates (Lari *et al.*, 2006, 2011). A study in Tuscany identified that 2.3% of 829 cases were caused by *M. bovis* infection (Lari *et al.*, 2007). Subsequently, optimization of an MLVA panel for the Italian *M. bovis* population was undertaken using isolates collected from cattle between 2000 and 2006 in northern Italy (Boniotti *et al.*, 2009). In a recent specific epidemiological application, MLVA and spoligotyping data helped identify a stable source of *M. bovis* infection in a joint enterprise cattle and goat farm (Zanardi *et al.*, 2013) where the presence of a strain identical to that isolated in a previous breakdown suggested on-farm persistence, potentially in goats, which were not being tested under the statutory TB eradication scheme (Zanardi *et al.*, 2013).

Some of the earliest work on characterization and standardization of MLVA methodologies to the MTC was undertaken in France in the mid-2000s (Le Fleche *et al.*, 2006). Application of these techniques to human patients confirmed that *M. bovis* was responsible for 2% of human TB cases during a 5-year retrospective study (Mignard *et al.*, 2006). The lack of clonal evolution and relatedness between these human cases was useful in excluding transmission between human cases (Mignard *et al.*, 2006). More recently, large-scale spoligotyping and MLVA of 4654 cattle and wildlife isolates collected since 1978 has increased the knowledge of the local *M. bovis* population structure, which consists of several clonal groups, some exhibiting geographic restriction (Hauer *et al.*, 2015).

Longitudinal typing data were observed to track reduction in pathogen diversity as France's eradication scheme gathered momentum in the preceding decade (Hauer *et al.*, 2015). MLVA has been applied to cattle *M. bovis* isolates in order to better understand the population structure and epidemiology of the pathogen in Belgium (Allix *et al.*, 2006). Human and deer isolates from Sweden have been genotyped using IS*6110* RFLP (Szewzyk *et al.*, 1995). The genetic differences observed confirmed that both hosts were affected by distinct bacterial lineages, thereby ruling out disease transmission (Szewzyk *et al.*, 1995).

5.5.2 Africa

Spoligotype and MLVA analysis of *M. bovis* isolates from cattle slaughtered in Algeria confirmed the presence of molecular types associated with previously documented European strains (Sahraoui *et al.*, 2009). In Tunisia, initial development of spoligotyping and an MLVA panel has taken place and revealed the widespread distribution of molecular types associated with European cattle (Lamine-Khemiri *et al.*, 2013). Both studies presented data consistent with the legacy of European colonialism in North Africa. Initial efforts to characterize the *M. bovis* population of Cameroon relied on RFLP and pulsed field gel electrophoresis (PFGE) methods (Njanpop-Lafourcade *et al.*, 2001). Subsequent application of spoligotyping and MLVA to 180 Cameroonian cattle samples detected greater diversity and molecular types associated with neighbouring Nigeria (Cadmus *et al.*, 2011). More recently, comparative genomics and genotyping of a large sequence polymorphism has enabled the detection of a dominant *M. bovis* clonal complex, named Af1, in Saharan West Africa encompassing the cattle populations of Mali, Nigeria, Chad and Cameroon (Müller *et al.*, 2009). MLVA of cattle isolates from all territories indicated very limited sharing of molecular types indicating recent mixing via cattle movement (Müller *et al.*, 2009). Similar work in neighbouring Burkina Faso revealed the same clonal complex dominance and sharing of spoligotypes, with MLVA, suggesting country-specific evolution of molecular types (Sanou *et al.*, 2014).

In Ethiopia early application of MLVA and spoligotyping revealed novel molecular types in the Addis Ababa area (Ameni *et al.*, 2007). Further application of spoligotyping in northern Ethiopia revealed clustering of six molecular types, three of which were novel (Ameni *et al.*, 2010). MLVA and spoligotyping have been used in central Ethiopia (Firdessa *et al.*, 2012), while further optimization of the techniques has been published (Biffa *et al.*, 2014). In Uganda, spoligotyping and RFLP typing confirmed *M. bovis* infection and distinguished members of the MTC (Oloya *et al.*, 2007). In Tanzania, MLVA and spoligotyping have been applied to *M. bovis* isolates from multiple hosts, including humans, livestock and wildlife, where ongoing transmission was occurring, but transmission to humans was not occurring (Katale *et al.*, 2015). Comparative genomics revealed a chromosomal deletion/large sequence polymorphism unique to *M. bovis* isolates from the East African countries of Ethiopia, Uganda, Burundi and Tanzania, marking a further clonal complex named as Af2 (Berg *et al.*, 2012).

In South Africa, IS*6110* RFLP was used to investigate the epidemiology of *M. bovis* transmission between buffalo and other wildlife species in the Kruger National Park (Michel *et al.*, 2009). Molecular typing confirmed that buffalo interacting with cattle was the source of *M. bovis* entering the park (Michel *et al.*, 2009). Local optimization of an MLVA panel for the Kruger National Park facilitated distinction of related and unrelated cases (Hlokwe *et al.*, 2013), and subsequently MLVA and spoligotyping were used to detect spillover from wildlife hosts in the greater Kruger National Park area to bordering regions with livestock (Musoke *et al.*, 2015). Further north in Zambia, spoligotyping has revealed shared molecular types of *M. bovis* in cattle and humans affected by tuberculosis suggesting zoonotic transmission (Malama *et al.*, 2014).

5.5.3 The Americas

In the USA, RFLP methods were applied initially to isolates from cattle, captive elk and other wildlife species (Whipple *et al.*, 1997). In general, the same *M. bovis* molecular type was observed for multiple animals from the same cattle herd, with distinct types seen in separate herds, consistent with the independent evolution of regional variants (Whipple et al., 1997). Molecular types in many wildlife species were indistinguishable from those in captive elk populations, indicating an epidemiological link (Whipple et al., 1997). More recently, spoligotyping data have confirmed that most sources of *M. bovis* infection in humans and cattle in California were Mexican cattle (Rodwell et al., 2010). A discriminating MLVA test was configured and showed remarkable congruence with epidemiological data when tested on selected USA isolates (Martinez et al., 2008). Molecular typing data were exploited to assess the extent of, and risk factors for, *M. bovis* infections in humans in the USA 2006–2013 (Scott et al., 2016).

Early application of molecular epidemiology to *M. bovis* in South America used the RFLP technique (Fisanotti, 1998) and suggested that regional variants were associated with Argentina, Paraguay and Brazil (Fisanotti, 1998). Spoligo- and RFLP typing confirmed these original observations (Zumarraga et al., 1999). Spoligotyping, RFLP and MLVA have subsequently been applied to human and cattle populations in Argentina, confirming that the most common molecular type in cattle was also observed in 2% of human pulmonary tuberculosis cases (Etchechoury et al., 2010). Several human cases exhibited identical molecular types that were distinct from cattle isolates, perhaps indicative of human to human transmission (Etchechoury et al., 2010). More recently, MLVA and IS*6110* RFLP typing confirmed *M. bovis/M. avium hominissuis* co-infection in pigs (Barandiaran et al., 2014). In Brazil, an optimized MLVA panel alongside spoligotyping increased the discrimination of *M. bovis* (Parreiras et al., 2012), and has been used to infer multiple introductions into single herds (Figueiredo et al., 2012).

5.5.4 Oceania

In Australia, REA and RFLP produced informative molecular epidemiological data in the early 1990s (Cousins et al., 1993). PFGE was used to differentiate strains from different regions and to infer transmission within different hosts and between farms (Feizabadi et al., 1996). However, Australia's declaration of Officially Bovine Tuberculosis Free (Lamoureux et al., 2012) status in December 1997 (More et al., 2015) predated much of the more recent development of molecular epidemiological tools.

Des Collins from New Zealand is quite rightly recognized as having pioneered the molecular epidemiology of *M. bovis* (Collins and De Lisle, 1984), initially with the REA technique. Molecular epidemiology has remained a valued and cost-effective tool in the country's bovine TB eradication scheme (Livingstone et al., 2015a, b), helping to direct potentially costly control interventions by determining whether new breakdowns are more likely the result of transmission from domestic livestock or wildlife (Ryan et al., 2006; Price-Carter et al., 2011; Buddle et al., 2015).

5.6 Local Findings from Northern Ireland and Lessons Learned

Here we discuss findings from Northern Ireland in a little more detail. While *M. bovis* molecular typing provides useful information in the outbreak investigation setting, its optimal use is likely to be in describing population-level epidemiological effects (cattle movements, cattle–cattle transmission, wildlife–cattle transmission, relative virulence, etc.).

Northern Ireland has implemented herd-level MLVA surveillance since 2003 (Skuce et al., 2010) and animal-level MLVA surveillance since 2010. Significantly, the spatial distribution of *M. bovis* MLVA types sampled was not random; highly significant geographical localization of *M. bovis* genotypes was clearly evident and suggested that sources tended to be local and that TB was a locally driven epidemic. Each MLVA type could be considered as responsible for its own micro-epidemic and the observed geographical localization implies that the epidemic comprises a group of local micro-epidemics (Smith et al., 2003).

MLVA types in purchased cattle were slightly more dispersed (less clustered) than those from home-bred cattle. However, on occasions MLVA types were clearly translocated significant distances from their normal geographical 'home range', often confirmed by cattle movement tracings. Due to the striking biogeography and geographical localization of molecular types, isolates have a genetic signature characteristic of their geographic origin. This is now an important, consistent and exploitable finding in several countries (Smith *et al.*, 2003; Skuce *et al.*, 2010; Robbe-Austerman and Turcotte, 2014). When deployed in the outbreak investigation setting, and in conjunction with cattle movement databases and wildlife surveillance, this is a powerful means of investigating source, maintenance and spread of bovine TB. Depending on their movement history, infected cattle either 'qualified' or were 'excluded' from particular outbreaks or clusters (Skuce *et al.*, 2010). Where *M. bovis* molecular types were recovered at some distance from even a coarse definition of their normal home range, this demonstrated a role for cattle movement in dispersal of bovine TB. Hence, it will be important to investigate the extent to which recorded local and longer-range cattle movements and cattle social (contact/movement) networks could explain the observed geographical localization of *M. bovis* molecular types. TB molecular types were also found outside their normal home range in home-bred cattle, indicating previous contact and transmission involving cattle from a distant home range.

The existence of home ranges for molecular types from molecular surveillance provides for a distinction between 'purchased' infection and infection 'acquired on arrival' in most cases, i.e. local versus non-local source(s). In Northern Ireland, significant numbers of specific MLVA types were found outside their normal home range. Many such animals had ear tags that linked them directly with their proposed MLVA type home range. The remainder may have had more complex links (secondary, tertiary, etc.) to the home range (Skuce and others, unpublished data).

Whether geographical localization of *M. bovis* molecular types in cattle reflects the underlying spatial segregation of the disease in wildlife remains to be determined in Northern Ireland. Considering the detailed livestock, landscape and wildlife data sources that are now being collected in various ecological studies, there is an opportunity to investigate the extent to which the geographical localization of *M. bovis* molecular types in cattle reflects variables such as cattle contact and movement networks, landscape features, badger genetic structure, etc. (Biek and Real, 2010).

Several local studies confirm that the number of reactors by herd is highly skewed and consequently a relatively small number of herds provide a disproportionate number of reactors. In Northern Ireland, herd- and animal-level molecular surveillance has identified >300 *M. bovis* MLVA types in >50,000 isolates (Skuce *et al.*, 2010; Trewby *et al.*, 2016). Herd-level MLVA surveillance disclosed on average 73 MLVA types each year, with 29 MLVA types present in all years sampled, implying that a relatively small number of MLVA types provides a disproportionate number of culture-confirmed cases. In human TB epidemiology, such data are consistent with the presence of the 'super-spreader' phenotype (Ypma *et al.*, 2013), TB cases that contribute disproportionately to transmission. For *M. bovis* in Northern Ireland, such 'super-spreaders' could reside at herd and animal levels. For example, certain herds may act as key nodes and may be highly connected in transmission networks underpinned by animal movement through trade. For *M. bovis*, such data are also consistent with the clonal expansion of molecular types identified in British data (Smith *et al.*, 2003).

The most parsimonious explanation for observing the same, or very similar, genotypes in large multi-reactor herds would tend to be that extensive cattle–cattle transmission (amplification, regardless of initial source) is occurring. Smaller herds with multiple reactors tended to contain multiple MLVA types, the most plausible explanation being multiple introductions from several external sources. However, it remains important to index and understand microevolutionary events within-herd (Navarro *et al.*, 2016). *M. bovis* MLVA types were observed to expand and contract, at least in their frequency (Skuce *et al.*, 2010). Hence, the local population seems to have remained largely, but not entirely static, which probably reflects the expansion and contraction of molecular types in different locations (Smith *et al.*, 2003) in response to the efficacy of local control measures, the transmission dynamics of the various genotypes and other undefined factors, such as potential competition between types and constraints imposed by host and environmental features. The phylogenetic relatedness of MLVA types can be determined and used to elucidate the evolutionary history of various molecular types and clusters. Such approaches clearly show the ongoing generation of new variants, a substantial number of which are identified each year, comprising ~50% of the total MLVA types (not isolates) recovered.

M. bovis genotyping in conjunction with comprehensive cattle movement databases and structured wildlife surveillance offers a powerful tool for investigating bovine TB source, maintenance and spread (Skuce *et al.*, 2010). The population structure of *M. bovis* and the performance characteristics of molecular typing support its use to answer detailed epidemiological questions of direct policy relevance.

5.7 Pathogen Genotype–Phenotype Associations

The striking phylogeography disclosed recently for the major lineages of the MTC has important implications for lineage–lineage phenotypic differences (Caws *et al.*, 2008; Hershberg *et al.*, 2008). However, these observed inter-strain differences are more convincing in experimental studies than they are at the population scale (Coscolla and Gagneux, 2010). Whether *M. bovis* molecular types also display different detectable, reproducible and relevant phenotypes is being investigated.

In a Northern Ireland study, two proxy measures for skin test detectability by pathogen molecular type (MLVA) were developed: (i) whether tuberculin test results differed significantly by MLVA type; and (ii) whether the distribution of MLVA types was significantly different between TB reactors and tuberculin-negative abattoir cases. Subtle, but ultimately non-significant, differences were detected in the relative detectability by MLVA type. In addition, no significant difference was detected in the disclosure rate of non-reactor abattoirs (Wright *et al.*, 2013a). In a further statistical analysis, an MLVA type effect was detected on virulence and pathogenesis but not on outbreak size (Wright *et al.*, 2013b). The *M. bovis* population in Northern Ireland is comprised exclusively of the European 1 clonal complex and shows very limited diversity at that scale, so it is not unexpected that no significant differences were detected in the phenotypes investigated. Recent studies in North America (Waters *et al.*, 2014) did not detect a significant genotype–phenotype difference in the isolates tested. However, differences at the spoligotype scale were reported in Argentina (Garbaccio *et al.*, 2014). It remains to be determined whether phenotypic differences, if detectable, are expressed between different clonal complexes, or within them. Additionally, phenotype may be influenced by RNA regulation and differences in epigenetic profile may be seen in *M. bovis* lineages (Drewe and Smith, 2014). Genomics has been used to investigate phenotypic differences between *M. bovis* and *M. caprae* and between *M. bovis* isolates of the same spoligotype and provides evidence for potential correlates of bacterial viability and virulence (de la Fuente *et al.*, 2015).

Northern Ireland has also investigated the extent of *M. bovis* infection in road-kill badgers. Where *M. bovis* was confirmed, isolates were also MLVA typed. In all cases the MLVA types identified in badgers were also found in local cattle. *M. bovis* MLVA types in badgers also showed strong geographical clustering to regions and this pattern was very similar to that disclosed in cattle herds. *M. bovis* MLVA types in both cattle and badgers were mostly clustered to the same geographical regions. This is indirect evidence of an 'association' between TB infections in cattle and badgers. However, this association does not indicate the direction of transmission, or the relative importance of badger-driven versus cattle-driven transmission in generating this association whether on an individual animal/herd, regional or province-wide basis. Similar findings and interpretations have been reported from studies in other countries, including Ireland, England and Wales (Olea-Popelka *et al.*, 2005; Goodchild *et al.*, 2012).

5.8 Whole-Genome Sequencing and Genomic Epidemiology

Although there remain significant blind spots and missing data, molecular epidemiology studies have improved the understanding of bovine TB epidemiology, ecology and evolution. Here we consider the opportunities and limitations presented by the game-changing revolution in pathogen genomic epidemiology (Kwong et al., 2015).

Technology does not stand still for long and the revolution in whole-genome sequencing (WGS) is transforming pathogen molecular epidemiology and will ultimately provide portable, high-performance tests for outbreak investigation and epidemiological research. Increasingly sophisticated analytical tools that combine the whole-genome sequences of large samples of pathogen isolates with geospatial and temporal data are leading to unprecedented improvements in understanding of the origins, evolution, pathogenicity and epidemiology of infectious diseases, with the prospect of greatly improved real-time surveillance of disease outbreaks (Bentley and Parkhill, 2015; Croucher and Didelot, 2015). Following rapid developments in bacterial WGS, it is now cost effective to read and compare the complete genome of bacteria; this provides the highest possible discrimination between isolates and enhanced resolution of complex epi-systems (Luheshi et al., 2015; Lee and Behr, 2016). Mutations which accrue as bacteria spread between hosts allow scientists to produce and compare detailed pathogen family trees and to compare these to the geographical distribution of the bacteria.

Several recent studies on human TB genomic epidemiology illustrate particularly well the power and, indeed, some of the limitations of this phylodynamic approach to investigating TB transmission dynamics (Gardy et al., 2011; Walker et al., 2013a, 2013b, 2014; Didelot et al., 2014; Tang and Gardy, 2014; Guthrie and Gardy, 2015; Nikolayevskyy et al., 2016). To some extent, such studies are confounded by missing data and the exceptionally slow mutation rate characteristic of this pathogen (Ford et al., 2013; Lillebaek et al., 2016). It has proven important to estimate the mutation rate of the M. tuberculosis lineage(s) under study, to more fully understand within-host diversity (Thacker et al., 2015; Didelot et al., 2016) and, uniquely, to calibrate and date-stamp the transmission trees derived (Ford et al., 2013; Colijn and Gardy, 2014; Didelot et al., 2014; Thacker et al., 2015) when attempting to investigate transmission dynamics using genomic epidemiology. Increasingly advanced statistical and epidemiological modelling approaches are required to more fully exploit TB phylodynamics (Didelot, 2013; Coll et al., 2014b; Didelot et al., 2014; Jombart et al., 2014a, 2014b). However, bacterial WGS is increasingly being seen as an enabling technology for the high-resolution microbial forensic analysis of pathogens and mycobacterial molecular surveillance systems are being implemented (Pankhurst et al., 2016).

A pilot study in Northern Ireland investigated the potential of molecular typing, bacterial WGS and mathematical modelling to investigate how bovine TB might spread between and within cattle herds and local wildlife (Biek et al., 2012). Previous MLVA surveillance had shown that cattle and badgers were associated at a regional scale, but lacked genetic evidence linking cattle and badgers at the farm scale. The pilot investigated a local TB 'micro-epidemic' comprising five cattle herds with a 10-year history of repeated TB breakdowns (due to a novel molecular type, MLVA010) and four TB-positive road traffic accident (RTA) badgers. Bacterial whole-genomes were sequenced from a sample of the TB-positive cattle ($n = 26$) and the four RTA badgers. The study showed the following: (i) most breakdowns involved genetically distinct bacteria; and (ii) cattle and local badger bacteria were very highly related and often indistinguishable, implying that transmission between cattle and badgers occurred frequently, recently and at a very local (farm-level) scale. This study produced the first direct genetic evidence of ongoing bovine TB transmission between cattle and badgers at the individual farm level. However, the number of isolates examined was too low to draw robust conclusions about the direction of transmission between cattle and badgers at that stage. Results were also consistent with some ongoing cattle–cattle transmission (amplification) occurring in some study herds. Recorded cattle movements, between the five study herds, did not seem to be significant in determining the geographical distribution of the pathogen. However, since sampling was localized, movement effects may have been underestimated.

Further isolates were recovered from the expanding micro-epidemic of MLVA010 (Trewby et al., 2016). As before, this micro-epidemic was locally driven and recorded cattle movements were not a strong predictor of the distribution of the bacteria, which do spread in the landscape over time. It remains plausible that the mechanism of spread is not adequately captured in official records. The number of badger-derived isolates examined was again too low to draw robust conclusions about the direction of transmission between cattle and badgers within the home range of MLVA010.

This extended study illustrates the potential and some of the limitations inherent in this phylodynamics approach. The exceptionally slow mutation rate imposes some limitations on what can be achieved, even from bacterial WGS data. For example, it may not be possible to determine the underlying transmission tree, the 'who infected whom?' question, as similarly concluded in human TB studies. This study illustrated the increased precision and discrimination provided by bacterial WGS and was able to detect some MLVA switching events that would otherwise have been undetected. More widespread application of bacterial WGS to *M. bovis* genomic epidemiology should provide novel and important insights into the dynamics of *M. bovis* persistence and spread. The most relevant control questions may be better addressed using approaches that integrate more directly bacterial WGS with additional epidemiological data. However, if sampling of hosts has been sufficiently dense and over sufficient time, it may be possible to identify 'transitions' between hosts and to provide some estimate of the extent to which local prevalence is cattle-driven versus wildlife-driven.

In Michigan, USA, *M. bovis* from experimentally infected white tail deer populations has been subjected to pathogen WGS, revealing within-host evolution and diversification of the pathogen in different tissues (Thacker *et al.*, 2015). More recently, genomic epidemiological approaches have revealed potential airborne transmission of *M. bovis* between human hosts in Nebraska (Buss *et al.*, 2016) and introduction of infection into Minnesota with possible links to Mexico and south-western states of the USA (Glaser *et al.*, 2016). In the latter case, phylogenetic techniques were used to confirm the breakdown was a result of a very recent, single introduction (Glaser *et al.*, 2016).

Bacterial WGS looks set to revolutionize the way we do veterinary bacteriology, much as it is doing for human medical microbiology (Loman *et al.*, 2012; Loman and Pallen, 2015; Arnold, 2016). It is likely that pathogen WGS will replace many traditional methods for detection, identification, antimicrobial resistance (AMR) testing and epidemiological typing where the resolution of WGS can be scaled to provide the desired resolution, including the highest possible resolution of disease transmission dynamics. When integrated with dense epidemiological, ecological and population genetics data and advanced mathematical modelling, including Bayesian inferences (Kao *et al.*, 2014, 2016; Biek *et al.*, 2015; Trewby *et al.*, 2016), this powerful approach, once the sole preserve of studies on fast evolving RNA viruses (du Plessis and Stadler, 2015), is providing unprecedented insight into disease maintenance and spread in the landscape in epi-systems involving complex host, pathogen and environment interactions (Blanchong *et al.*, 2016). An elegant recent approach of genomic epidemiology to study *Brucella abortus* illustrates the power of this new approach. Using animal location and movement data, mathematical modelling and Bayesian inferences they detected transmission events (transitions) between domestic and wildlife host species (Kamath *et al.*, 2016).

These phylodynamic approaches have their limitations with pathogens that exhibit low mutation rates such as *M. bovis* (Biek *et al.*, 2015). However, the unprecedented level of resolution that genomic data provides, especially when applied over densely sampled bacterial populations from multiple hosts and collected over long time frames, promises to be a game changer (Sintchenko and Holmes, 2015). It is consequently a time of upheaval in bacterial molecular epidemiology as researchers adapt to new tools that are opening up new opportunities (Gaiarsa *et al.*, 2015). A major challenge in the near future will be how to better implement bacterial WGS for disease forensics. It will become necessary for laboratories to agree a nomenclature scheme for naming *M. bovis* genomes that facilitates inter-laboratory comparisons and the inclusion of extant whole-genome sequences that have been deposited in open-access databases. It is already feasible to generate a spoligotype pattern from raw sequence reads (Coll *et al.*, 2012). Provided sequencing costs continue to fall and issues around incorporation of existing typing data, standardization of nomenclature and methodologies can be resolved, whole-genome approaches are likely to become the new standard for molecular epidemiology (Didelot *et al.*, 2012).

5.9 Conclusions

The population structure of *M. bovis* and the performance characteristics of molecular and genomic epidemiology support their use in molecular surveillance and to answer detailed epidemiological questions of direct policy relevance. They should offer powerful and practical 'decision-support' tools for investigating the maintenance and spread of bovine TB. These approaches should more accurately identify clusters and unsuspected transmission events, particularly where the breakdown index case can be identified as an 'out of home range' cattle movement. This provides a unique opportunity to monitor and quantify the extent, if any, of secondary (cattle–cattle) spread within and between herds, and any spillover/spillback involving local wildlife.

The *M. bovis* population structure is particularly, maybe even uniquely, amenable to this approach. Molecular and genomic epidemiology has the performance characteristics to support its use as a surveillance and investigative tool, to monitor the efficacy of current control programmes and future interventions. It has the potential to refine the modelling and analysis of detailed epidemiological questions. The application to epidemiological and evolutionary studies provides unique and valuable insights into the current bovine TB epidemic.

There remain opportunities to investigate, in a structured manner, what molecular and genomic epidemiology data tell us about TB in sporadic, multi-reactor, persistent, recurrent and restocked herds, etc. It is predictable that this technology will become more useful as the epidemic (hopefully) declines. One reason why human TB genomic epidemiology can currently make stronger inferences about transmission dynamics is that the epi-system is significantly less complex. For bovine TB, there are multiple exposed hosts (cattle and wildlife) and the potential for the environment to be contaminated. Consequently, it is currently very challenging to disaggregate these, especially at a local scale. However, should TB in cattle be substantially reduced, it will become relatively more straightforward to assess spillover and which wildlife hosts/populations are spilling over. Pathogen genotyping continues to unravel the biology of mycobacteria and offers significant promise in the fight against and prevention of the diseases caused by these troublesome pathogens (Wlodarska *et al.*, 2015).

References

Aarestrup, F.M., Brown, E.W., Detter, C., Gerner-Smidt, P., Gilmour, M.W., *et al.* (2012) Integrating genome-based informatics to modernize global disease monitoring, information sharing, and response. *Emerging Infectious Diseases* 18(11), e1.

Abernethy, D.A., Upton, P., Higgins, I.M., McGrath, G., Goodchild, A.V., *et al.* (2013) Bovine tuberculosis trends in the UK and the Republic of Ireland, 1995–2010. *Veterinary Record* 172(12), 312.

Allen, A.R., Minozzi, G., Glass, E.J., Skuce, R.A., McDowell, S.W., *et al.* (2010) Bovine tuberculosis: the genetic basis of host susceptibility. *Proceedings Biological Sciences* 277(1695), 2737–2745.

Allen, A.R., Dale, J., McCormick, C., Mallon, T.R., Costello, E., *et al.* (2013) The phylogeny and population structure of *Mycobacterium bovis* in the British Isles. *Infection, Genetics and Evolution* 20, 8–15.

Allix, C., Walravens, K., Saegerman, C., Godfroid, J., Supply, P. and Fauville-Dufaux, M. (2006) Evaluation of the epidemiological relevance of variable-number tandem-repeat genotyping of *Mycobacterium bovis* and comparison of the method with IS6110 restriction fragment length polymorphism analysis and spoligotyping. *Journal of Clinical Microbiology* 44(6), 1951–1962.

Ameni, G., Aseffa, A., Sirak, A., Engers, H., Young, D.B., *et al.* (2007) Effect of skin testing and segregation on the prevalence of bovine tuberculosis, and molecular typing of *Mycobacterium bovis*, in Ethiopia. *Veterinary Record* 161(23), 782–786.

Ameni, G., Desta, F. and Firdessa, R. (2010) Molecular typing of *Mycobacterium bovis* isolated from tuberculosis lesions of cattle in north eastern Ethiopia. *Veterinary Record* 167(4), 138–141.

Aranaz, A., Liebana, E., Mateos, A., Dominguez, L., Vidal, D., et al. (1996) Spacer oligonucleotide typing of *Mycobacterium bovis* strains from cattle and other animals: a tool for studying epidemiology of tuberculosis. *Journal of Clinical Microbiology* 34(11), 2734–2740.

Arnold, C. (2016) Considerations in centralizing whole genome sequencing for microbiology in a public health setting. *Expert Review of Molecular Diagnostics* 16(6), 619–621.

Barandiaran, S., Perez, A.M., Gioffre, A.K., Martinez Vivot, M., Cataldi, A.A. and Zumarraga, M.J. (2014) Tuberculosis in swine co-infected with *Mycobacterium avium* subsp. *hominissuis* and *Mycobacterium bovis* in a cluster from Argentina. *Epidemiology and Infection* 143(05), 966–974.

Bentley, S.D. and Parkhill, J. (2015) Genomic perspectives on the evolution and spread of bacterial pathogens. *Proceedings Biological Sciences* 282(1821), 20150488.

Benton, C., Delahay, R., Trewby, H. and Hodgson, D.J. (2014) What has molecular epidemiology ever done for wildlife disease research? Past contributions and future directions. *European Journal of Wildlife Research* 61(1).

Berg, S., Garcia-Pelayo, M.C., Muller, B., Hailu, E., Asiimwe, B., et al. (2012) African 2, a clonal complex of *Mycobacterium bovis* epidemiologically important in East Africa. *Journal of Bacteriology* 194(6), 1641.

Bermingham, M.L., Handel, I.G., Glass, E.J., Woolliams, J.A., de Clare Bronsvoort, B.M., et al. (2015) Hui and Walter's latent-class model extended to estimate diagnostic test properties from surveillance data: a latent model for latent data. *Scientific Reports* 5, 11861.

Bezos, J., Alvarez, J., Romero, B., de Juan, L. and Dominguez, L. (2014) Bovine tuberculosis: historical perspective. *Research in Veterinary Science* 97 Suppl, S3–4.

Biek, R. and Real, L.A. (2010) The landscape genetics of infectious disease emergence and spread. *Molecular Ecology* 19(17), 3515–3531.

Biek, R., O'Hare, A., Wright, D., Mallon, T., McCormick, C., et al. (2012) Whole genome sequencing reveals local transmission patterns of *Mycobacterium bovis* in sympatric cattle and badger populations. *PLoS Pathogens* 8(11), e1003008.

Biek, R., Pybus, O.G., Lloyd-Smith, J.O. and Didelot, X. (2015) Measurably evolving pathogens in the genomic era. *Trends in Ecology & Evolution* 30(6), 306–313.

Biffa, D., Johansen, T.B., Godfroid, J., Muwonge, A., Skjerve, E. and Djonne, B. (2014) Multi-locus variable-number tandem repeat analysis (MLVA) reveals heterogeneity of *Mycobacterium bovis* strains and multiple genotype infections of cattle in Ethiopia. *Infection, Genetics and Evolution* 23, 13–19.

Blanchong, J.A., Robinson, S.J., Samuel, M.D. and Foster, J.T. (2016) Application of genetics and genomics to wildlife epidemiology. *The Journal of Wildlife Management* 80(4).

Boniotti, M.B., Goria, M., Loda, D., Garrone, A., Benedetto, A., et al. (2009) Molecular typing of *Mycobacterium bovis* strains isolated in Italy from 2000 to 2006 and evaluation of variable-number tandem repeats for geographically optimized genotyping. *Journal of Clinical Microbiology* 47(3), 636–644.

Borgdorff, M.W. and van Soolingen, D. (2013) The re-emergence of tuberculosis: what have we learnt from molecular epidemiology? *Clinical Microbiology and Infection* 19(10), 889–901.

Brosch, R., Gordon, S.V., Marmiesse, M., Brodin, P., Buchrieser, C., et al. (2002) A new evolutionary scenario for the *Mycobacterium tuberculosis* complex. *Proceedings of the National Academy of Sciences of the United States of America* 99(6), 3684–3689.

Broughan, J.M., Harris, K.A., Brouwer, A., Downs, S.H., Goodchild, A.V., et al. (2015) Bovine TB infection status in cattle in Great Britain in 2013. *Veterinary Record* 176(13), 326–330.

Buddle, B.M., de Lisle, G.W., Griffin, J.F.T. and Hutchings, S.A. (2015) Epidemiology, diagnostics, and management of tuberculosis in domestic cattle and deer in New Zealand in the face of a wildlife reservoir. *New Zealand Veterinary Journal* 63(sup1), 19–27.

Buss, B.F., Keyser-Metobo, A., Rother, J., Holtz, L., Gall, K., et al. (2016) Possible airborne person-to-person transmission of *Mycobacterium bovis* – Nebraska 2014–2015. MMWR *Morbidity and Mortality Weekly Report* 65(8), 197–201.

Cadmus, S.I.B., Gordon, S.V., Hewinson, R.G. and Smith, N.H. (2011) Exploring the use of molecular epidemiology to track bovine tuberculosis in Nigeria: An overview from 2002 to 2004. *Veterinary Microbiology* 151(1–2), 133–138.

Carlson, D.F., Lancto, C.A., Zang, B., Kim, E.S., Walton, M., et al. (2016) Production of hornless dairy cattle from genome-edited cell lines. *Nature Biotechnology* 34(5), 479–481.

Carslake, D., Grant, W., Green, L.E., Cave, J., Greaves, J., et al. (2011) Endemic cattle diseases: comparative epidemiology and governance. *Philosophical Transactions of the Royal Society of London. Series B, Biological Sciences* 366(1573), 1975–1986.

Caws, M., Thwaites, G., Dunstan, S., Hawn, T.R., Lan, N.T., *et al.* (2008) The influence of host and bacterial genotype on the development of disseminated disease with *Mycobacterium tuberculosis*. *PLoS Pathogens* 4(3), e1000034.

Centers for Disease Control and Prevention (2012) Tuberculosis genotyping–United States, 2004–2010. MMWR *Morbidity and Mortality Weekly Report* 61(36), 723–725.

Clegg, T.A., Duignan, A., Whelan, C., Gormley, E., Good, M., *et al.* (2011) Using latent class analysis to estimate the test characteristics of the gamma-interferon test, the single intradermal comparative tuberculin test and a multiplex immunoassay under Irish conditions. *Veterinary Microbiology* 151(1–2), 68–76.

Cole, S.T. (2002) Comparative and functional genomics of the *Mycobacterium tuberculosis* complex. *Microbiology* 148(Pt 10), 2919–2928.

Cole, S.T., Brosch, R., Parkhill, J., Garnier, T., Churcher, C., *et al.* (1998) Deciphering the biology of *Mycobacterium tuberculosis* from the complete genome sequence. *Nature* 393(6685), 537–544.

Colijn, C. and Gardy, J. (2014) Phylogenetic tree shapes resolve disease transmission patterns. *Evolution, Medicine, and Public Health* 2014(1), 96–108.

Coll, F., Mallard, K., Preston, M.D., Bentley, S., Parkhill, J., *et al.* (2012) SpolPred: rapid and accurate prediction of *Mycobacterium tuberculosis* spoligotypes from short genomic sequences. *Bioinformatics* 28(22), 2991–2993.

Coll, F., McNerney, R., Guerra-Assuncao, J.A., Glynn, J.R., Perdigao, J., *et al.* (2014a) A robust SNP barcode for typing *Mycobacterium tuberculosis* complex strains. *Nature Communications* 5, 4812.

Coll, F., Preston, M., Guerra-Assuncao, J.A., Hill-Cawthorn, G., Harris, D., *et al.* (2014b) PolyTB: a genomic variation map for *Mycobacterium tuberculosis*. *Tuberculosis (Edinb)* 94(3), 346–354.

Collins, D.M. (1999) DNA typing of *Mycobacterium bovis* strains from the Castlepoint area of the Wairarapa. *The New Zealand Veterinary Journal* 47(6), 207–209.

Collins, D.M. and De Lisle, G.W. (1984) DNA restriction endonuclease analysis of *Mycobacterium tuberculosis* and *Mycobacterium bovis* BCG. *Microbiology* (Reading, England). 130(4), 1019–1021.

Comas, I. and Gagneux, S. (2011) A role for systems epidemiology in tuberculosis research. *Trends in Microbiolology* 19(10), 492–500.

Coscolla, M. and Gagneux, S. (2010) Does *M. tuberculosis* genomic diversity explain disease diversity? *Drug Discovery Today: Disease Mechanisms* 7(1), e43–e59.

Costello, E., O'Grady, D., Flynn, O., O'Brien, R., Rogers, M., *et al.* (1999) Study of restriction fragment length polymorphism analysis and spoligotyping for epidemiological investigation of *Mycobacterium bovis* infection. *Journal of Clinical Microbiology* 37(10), 3217–3222.

Cousins, D.V., Williams, S.N., Ross, B.C. and Ellis, T.M. (1993) Use of a repetitive element isolated from *Mycobacterium tuberculosis* in hybridization studies with *Mycobacterium bovis*: a new tool for epidemiological studies of bovine tuberculosis. *Veterinary Microbiology* 37(1–2), 1–17.

Croucher, N.J. and Didelot, X. (2015) The application of genomics to tracing bacterial pathogen transmission. *Current Opinion in Microbiology* 23, 62–67.

de la Cruz, M.L., Perez, A., Bezos, J., Pages, E., Casal, C., *et al.* (2014) Spatial dynamics of bovine tuberculosis in the autonomous community of Madrid, Spain (2010–2012). *PLoS ONE* 9(12), e115632.

de la Fuente, J., Diez-Delgado, I., Contreras, M., Vicente, J., Cabezas-Cruz, A., *et al.* (2015) Comparative genomics of field isolates of *Mycobacterium bovis* and *M. caprae* provides evidence for possible correlates with bacterial viability and virulence. *PLoS Neglected Tropical Diseases* 9(11), e0004232.

de la Rua-Domenech, R., Goodchild, A.T., Vordermeier, H.M., Hewinson, R.G., Christiansen, K.H. and Clifton-Hadley, R.S. (2006) Ante mortem diagnosis of tuberculosis in cattle: a review of the tuberculin tests, gamma-interferon assay and other ancillary diagnostic techniques. *Research in Veterinary Science* 81(2), 190–210.

Didelot, X. (2013) Genomic analysis to improve the management of outbreaks of bacterial infection. *Expert Review of Anti-infective Therapy* 11(4), 335–337.

Didelot, X., Bowden, R., Wilson, D.J., Peto, T.E.A. and Crook, D.W. (2012) Transforming clinical microbiology with bacterial genome sequencing. *Nature Reviews Genetics* 13(9), 601–612.

Didelot, X., Gardy, J. and Colijn, C. (2014) Bayesian inference of infectious disease transmission from whole-genome sequence data. *Molecular Biology and Evolution* 31(7), 1869–1879.

Didelot, X., Walker, A.S., Peto, T.E., Crook, D.W. and Wilson, D.J. (2016) Within-host evolution of bacterial pathogens. *Nature Reviews Microbiology* 14(3), 150–162.

Doughty, E.L., Sergeant, M.J., Adetifa, I., Antonio, M. and Pallen, M.J. (2014) Culture-independent detection and characterisation of *Mycobacterium tuberculosis* and *M. africanum* in sputum samples using shotgun metagenomics on a benchtop sequencer. *PeerJ* 2, e585.

Drewe, J.A. and Smith, N.H. (2014) Molecular epidemiology of *Mycobacterium bovis*. In: Thoen, C.O., Steele, J.H., Kaneene, J.B. (eds) *Zoonotic Tuberculosis:* Mycobacterium bovis *and Other Pathogenic Mycobacteria*, 3rd edn. Wiley, Hoboken, USA.

Drewe, J.A., Pfeiffer, D.U. and Kaneene, J.B. (2014) Epidemiology of *Mycobacterium bovis*. In: Thoen, C.O., Steele, J.H., Kaneene, J.B. (eds) *Zoonotic Tuberculosis:* Mycobacterium bovis *and Other Pathogenic Mycobacteria*, 3rd edn. Wiley, Hoboken, USA.

Durr, P.A. and Froggatt, A.E. (2002) How best to geo-reference farms? A case study from Cornwall, England. *Preventive Veterinary Medicine* 56(1), 51–62.

Enright, J. and Kao, R.R. (2016) A descriptive analysis of the growth of unrecorded interactions amongst cattle-raising premises in Scotland and their implications for disease spread. *BMC Veterinary Research* 12, 37.

Etchechoury, I., Valencia, G.E., Morcillo, N., Sequeira, M.D., Imperiale, B., *et al.* (2010) Molecular typing of *Mycobacterium bovis* isolates in Argentina: first description of a person-to-person transmission case. *Zoonoses and Public Health* 57(6), 375–381.

Evans, J.T., Smith, E.G., Banerjee, A., Smith, R.M.M., Dale, J., *et al.* (2007) Cluster of human tuberculosis caused by *Mycobacterium bovis*: evidence for person-to-person transmission in the UK. *The Lancet* 369(9569), 1270–1276.

Feizabadi, M.M., Robertson, I.D., Cousins, D.V. and Hampson, D.J. (1996) Genomic analysis of *Mycobacterium bovis* and other members of the *Mycobacterium tuberculosis* complex by isoenzyme analysis and pulsed-field gel electrophoresis. *Journal of Clinical Microbiology* 34(5), 1136–1142.

Firdessa, R., Tschopp, R., Wubete, A., Sombo, M., Hailu, E., *et al.* (2012) High prevalence of bovine tuberculosis in dairy cattle in central Ethiopia: implications for the dairy industry and public health. *PLoS ONE* 7(12), e52851.

Figueiredo, E.E., Ramos, D.F., Medeiros, L., Silvestre, F.G., Lilenbaum, W., *et al.* (2012) Multiple strains of *Mycobacterium bovis* revealed by molecular typing in a herd of cattle. *The Veterinary Journal* 193(1), 296–298.

Fisanotti, J. (1998) Molecular epidemiology of *Mycobacterium bovis* isolates from South America. *Veterinary Microbiology* 60(2–4), 251–257.

Ford, C.B., Shah, R.R., Maeda, M.K., Gagneux, S., Murray, M.B., *et al.* (2013) *Mycobacterium tuberculosis* mutation rate estimates from different lineages predict substantial differences in the emergence of drug-resistant tuberculosis. *Nature Genetics* 45(7), 784–790.

Furphy, C., Costello, E., Murphy, D., Corner, L.A.L. and Gormley, E. (2012) DNA typing of *Mycobacterium bovis* isolates from badgers (*Meles meles*) culled from areas in Ireland with different levels of tuberculosis prevalence. *Veterinary Medicine International* 2012, 1–6.

Gagneux, S. and Small, P.M. (2007) Global phylogeography of *Mycobacterium tuberculosis* and implications for tuberculosis product development. *The Lancet Infectious Diseases* 7(5), 328–337.

Gaiarsa, S., De Marco, L., Comandatore, F., Marone, P., Bandi, C. and Sassera, D. (2015) Bacterial genomic epidemiology, from local outbreak characterization to species-history reconstruction. *Pathogens and Global Health* 109(7), 319–327.

Garbaccio, S., Macias, A., Shimizu, E., Paolicchi, F., Pezzone, N., *et al.* (2014) Association between spoligotype-VNTR types and virulence of *Mycobacterium bovis* in cattle. *Virulence* 5(2), 297–302.

Gardy, J.L., Johnston, J.C., Ho Sui, S.J., Cook, V.J., Shah, L., *et al.* (2011) Whole-genome sequencing and social-network analysis of a tuberculosis outbreak. *The New England Journal of Medicine* 364(8), 730–739.

Garnier, T., Eiglmeier, K., Camus, J.C., Medina, N., Mansoor, H., *et al.* (2003) The complete genome sequence of *Mycobacterium bovis*. *Proceedings of the National Academy of Sciences of the United States of America* 100(13), 7877–7882.

Gibson, A.L., Hewinson, G., Goodchild, T., Watt, B., Story, A., *et al.* (2004) Molecular epidemiology of disease due to *Mycobacterium bovis* in humans in the United Kingdom. *Journal of Clinical Microbiology* 42(1), 431–434.

Gilbert, M., Mitchell, A., Bourn, D., Mawdsley, J., Clifton-Hadley, R. and Wint, W. (2005) Cattle movements and bovine tuberculosis in Great Britain. *Nature* 435(7041), 491–496.

Glaser, L., Carstensen, M., Shaw, S., Robbe-Austerman, S., Wunschmann, A., *et al.* (2016) Descriptive epidemiology and whole genome sequencing analysis for an outbreak of bovine tuberculosis in beef cattle and white-tailed deer in Northwestern Minnesota. *PLOS ONE* 11(1), e0145735.

Goodchild, A.V., Watkins, G.H., Sayers, A.R., Jones, J.R. and Clifton-Hadley, R.S. (2012) Geographical association between the genotype of bovine tuberculosis in found dead badgers and in cattle herds. *Veterinary Record* 170(10), 259.

Gopal, R., Goodchild, A., Hewinson, G., de la Rua Domenech, R. and Clifton-Hadley, R. (2006) Introduction of bovine tuberculosis to north-east England by bought-in cattle. *Veterinary Record* 159(9), 265–271.

Guthrie, J.L. and Gardy, J.L. (2015) Accelerating tuberculosis elimination in low-incidence settings: the role of genomics. *European Respiratory Journal* 46(6), 1840–1841.

Gutierrez, M., Samper, S., Gavigan, J.A., García Marín, J.F. and Martin, C. (1995) Differentiation by molecular typing of *Mycobacterium bovis* strains causing tuberculosis in cattle and goats. *Journal of Clinical Microbiology* 33(11), 2953–2956.

Hauer, A., De Cruz, K., Cochard, T., Godreuil, S., Karoui, C., *et al.* (2015) Genetic evolution of *Mycobacterium bovis* causing tuberculosis in livestock and wildlife in France since 1978. *PLOS ONE* 10(2), e0117103.

Heersma, H.F., Kremer, K. and van Embden, J.D. (1998) Computer analysis of IS6110 RFLP patterns of *Mycobacterium tuberculosis*. *Methods in Molecular Biology* 101, 395–422.

Hershberg, R., Lipatov, M., Small, P.M., Sheffer, H., Niemann, S., *et al.* (2008) High functional diversity in *Mycobacterium tuberculosis* driven by genetic drift and human demography. *PLoS Biology* 6(12), e311.

Hlokwe, T.M., van Helden, P. and Michel, A. (2013) Evaluation of the discriminatory power of variable number of tandem repeat typing of *Mycobacterium bovis* isolates from Southern Africa. *Transboundary and Emerging Diseases* 60, 111–120.

Jagielski, T., Minias, A., van Ingen, J., Rastogi, N., Brzostek, A., *et al.* (2016) Methodological and clinical aspects of the molecular epidemiology of *Mycobacterium tuberculosis* and other mycobacteria. *Clinical Microbiology Reviews* 29(2), 239–290.

Jombart, T., Cori, A., Didelot, X., Cauchemez, S., Fraser, C. and Ferguson, N. (2014a) Bayesian reconstruction of disease outbreaks by combining epidemiologic and genomic data. *PLoS Computational Biology* 10(1), e1003457.

Jombart, T., Aanensen, D.M., Baguelin, M., Birrell, P., Cauchemez, S., *et al.* (2014b) OutbreakTools: a new platform for disease outbreak analysis using the R software. *Epidemics* 7, 28–34.

Kamath, P.L., Foster, J.T., Drees, K.P., Luikart, G., Quance, C., *et al.* (2016) Genomics reveals historic and contemporary transmission dynamics of a bacterial disease among wildlife and livestock. *Nature Communications* 7, 11448.

Kamerbeek, J., Schouls, L., Kolk, A., van Agterveld, M., van Soolingen, D., *et al.* (1997) Simultaneous detection and strain differentiation of *Mycobacterium tuberculosis* for diagnosis and epidemiology. *Journal of Clinical Microbiology* 35(4), 907–914.

Kao, R.R., Haydon, D.T., Lycett, S.J. and Murcia, P.R. (2014) Supersize me: how whole-genome sequencing and big data are transforming epidemiology. *Trends in Microbiology* 22(5), 282–291.

Kao, R.R., Price-Carter, M. and Robbe-Austerman, S. (2016) Use of genomics to track bovine tuberculosis transmission. *Revue Scientifique Et Technique* 35(1), 241–268.

Katale, B.Z., Mbugi, E.V., Siame, K.K., Keyyu, J.D., Kendall, S., *et al.* (2015) Isolation and potential for transmission of *Mycobacterium bovis* at Human-livestock-wildlife interface of the Serengeti ecosystem, Northern Tanzania. *Transboundary and Emerging Diseases* 64(3), 815–825.

Kwong, J.C., McCallum, N., Sintchenko, V. and Howden, B.P. (2015) Whole genome sequencing in clinical and public health microbiology. *Pathology* 47(3), 199–210.

Lahuerta-Marin A., Gallagher M., McBride S., Skuce R., Menzies F. *et al.*(2015) Should they stay, or should they go? Relative future risk of bovine tuberculosis for interferon-gamma test-positive cattle left on farms. *Vet Research* 46(90).

Lamine-Khemiri, H., Martinez, R., Garcia-Jimenez, W.L., Benitez-Medina, J.M., Cortes, M., *et al.* (2013) Genotypic characterization by spoligotyping and VNTR typing of *Mycobacterium bovis* and *Mycobacterium caprae* isolates from cattle of Tunisia. *Tropical Animal Health and Production* 46(2), 305–311.

Lamoureux, B.E., Palmieri, P.A., Jackson, A.P. and Hobfoll, S.E. (2012) Child sexual abuse and adulthood interpersonal outcomes: examining pathways for intervention. *Psychological Trauma* 4(6), 605–613.

Lari, N., Rindi, L., Bonanni, D., Tortoli, E. and Garzelli, C. (2006) Molecular analysis of clinical isolates of *Mycobacterium bovis* recovered from humans in Italy. *Journal of Clinical Microbiology* 44(11), 4218–4221.

Lari, N., Rindi, L., Bonanni, D., Rastogi, N., Sola, C., *et al.* (2007) Three-year longitudinal study of genotypes of *Mycobacterium tuberculosis* isolates in Tuscany, Italy. *Journal of Clinical Microbiology* 45(6), 1851–1857.

Lari, N., Bimbi, N., Rindi, L., Tortoli, E. and Garzelli, C. (2011) Genetic diversity of human isolates of *Mycobacterium bovis* assessed by spoligotyping and variable number tandem repeat genotyping. *Infection, Genetics and Evolution* 11(1), 175–180.

Lee, R.S. and Behr, M.A. (2016) The implications of whole-genome sequencing in the control of tuberculosis. *Therapeutic Advances in Infectious Disease* 3(2), 47–62.

Le Fleche, P., Jacques, I., Grayon, M., Al Dahouk, S., Bouchon, P., *et al.* (2006) Evaluation and selection of tandem repeat loci for a *Brucella* MLVA typing assay. *BMC Microbiology* 6(1), 9.

Lillebaek, T., Norman, A., Rasmussen, E.M., Marvig, R.L., Folkvardsen, D.B., *et al.* (2016) Substantial molecular evolution and mutation rates in prolonged latent *Mycobacterium tuberculosis* infection in humans. *International Journal of Medical Microbiology* 306(7), 580–585.

Livingstone, P.G., Hancox, N., Nugent, G., Mackereth, G. and Hutchings, S.A. (2015a) Development of the New Zealand strategy for local eradication of tuberculosis from wildlife and livestock. *The New Zealand Veterinary Journal* 63(Suppl 1), 98–107.

Livingstone, P.G., Hancox, N., Nugent, G. and de Lisle, G.W. (2015b) Toward eradication: the effect of *Mycobacterium bovis* infection in wildlife on the evolution and future direction of bovine tuberculosis management in New Zealand. *The New Zealand Veterinary Journal* 63(Suppl 1), 4–18.

Loman, N.J. and Pallen, M.J. (2015) Twenty years of bacterial genome sequencing. *Nature Reviews Microbiology* 13(12), 787–794.

Loman, N.J., Constantinidou, C., Chan, J.Z., Halachev, M., Sergeant, M., *et al.* (2012) High-throughput bacterial genome sequencing: an embarrassment of choice, a world of opportunity. *Nature Reviews Microbiology* 10(9), 599–606.

Luheshi, L.M., Raza, S. and Peacock, S.J. (2015) Moving pathogen genomics out of the lab and into the clinic: what will it take? *Genome Medicine* 7(1), 132.

Malama, S., Muma, J., Munyeme, M., Mbulo, G., Muwonge, A., *et al.* (2014) Isolation and molecular characterization of *Mycobacterium tuberculosis* from humans and cattle in Namwala district, Zambia. *EcoHealth* 11(4), 564–570.

Martinez, L.R., Harris, B., Black, W.C., Meyer, R.M., Brennan, P.J., *et al.* (2008) Genotyping North American animal *Mycobacterium bovis* isolates using multilocus variable number tandem repeat analysis. *Journal of Veterinary Diagnostic Investigation* 20(6), 707–715.

Mathews, F., Macdonald, D.W., Taylor, G.M., Gelling, M., Norman, R.A., *et al.* (2006) Bovine tuberculosis (*Mycobacterium bovis*) in British farmland wildlife: the importance to agriculture. *Proceedings Biological Sciences* 273(1584), 357–365.

McLernon, J., Costello, E., Flynn, O., Madigan, G. and Ryan, F. (2010) Evaluation of mycobacterial interspersed repetitive-unit-variable-number tandem-repeat analysis and spoligotyping for genotyping of *Mycobacterium bovis* isolates and a comparison with restriction fragment length polymorphism typing. *Journal of Clinical Microbiology* 48(12), 4541–4545.

Mears, J., Vynnycky, E., Lord, J., Borgdorff, M.W., Cohen, T., *et al.* (2015) The prospective evaluation of the TB strain typing service in England: a mixed methods study. *Thorax* 71(8), 734–741.

Mentaberre, G., Romero, B., de Juan, L., Navarro-Gonzalez, N., Velarde, R., *et al.* (2014) Long-term assessment of wild boar harvesting and cattle removal for bovine tuberculosis control in free ranging populations. *PLoS ONE* 9(2), e88824.

Michel, A.L., Coetzee, M.L., Keet, D.F., Mare, L., Warren, R., *et al.* (2009) Molecular epidemiology of *Mycobacterium bovis* isolates from free-ranging wildlife in South African game reserves. *Veterinary Microbiology* 133(4), 335–343.

Mignard, S., Pichat, C. and Carret, G. (2006) *Mycobacterium bovis* infection, Lyon, France. *Emerging Infectious Diseases* 12(7), 1431–1433.

More, S.J., Radunz, B. and Glanville, R.J. (2015) Lessons learned during the successful eradication of bovine tuberculosis from Australia. *Veterinary Record* 177(9), 224–232.

Muellner, P., Zadoks, R.N., Perez, A.M., Spencer, S.E., Schukken, Y.H. and French, N.P. (2011) The integration of molecular tools into veterinary and spatial epidemiology. *Spatial and Spatio-temporal Epidemiology* 2(3), 159–171.

Muellner, P., Stark, K.D., Dufour, S. and Zadoks, R.N. (2015) 'Next-Generation' surveillance: An epidemiologists' perspective on the use of molecular information in food safety and animal health decision-making. *Zoonoses Public Health* 63(5), 351–357.

Müller, B., Hilty, M., Berg, S., Garcia-Pelayo, M.C., Dale, J., et al. (2009) African 1, an epidemiologically important clonal complex of *Mycobacterium bovis* dominant in Mali, Nigeria, Cameroon, and Chad. *Journal of Bacteriology* 191(6), 1951–1960.

Musoke, J., Hlokwe, T., Marcotty, T., du Plessis, B.J.A. and Michel, A.L. (2015) Spillover of *Mycobacterium bovis* from wildlife to livestock, South Africa. *Emerging Infectious Diseases* 21(3), 448–451.

Navarro, Y., Herranz, M., Romero, B., Bouza, E., Dominguez, L., et al. (2014) High-throughput multiplex MIRU-VNTR typing of *Mycobacterium bovis*. *Research in Veterinary Science* 96(3), 422–425.

Navarro, Y., Romero, B., Copano, M.F., Bouza, E., Dominguez, L., et al. (2015) Multiple sampling and discriminatory fingerprinting reveals clonally complex and compartmentalized infections by *M. bovis* in cattle. *Veterinary Microbiology* 175(1), 99–104.

Navarro, Y., Romero, B., Bouza, E., Dominguez, L., de Juan, L. and Garcia-de-Viedma, D. (2016) Detailed chronological analysis of microevolution events in herds infected persistently by *Mycobacterium bovis*. *Veterinary Microbiology* 183, 97–102.

Nikolayevskyy, V., Kranzer, K., Niemann, S. and Drobniewski, F. (2016) Whole genome sequencing of *Mycobacterium tuberculosis* for detection of recent transmission and tracing outbreaks: A systematic review. *Tuberculosis (Edinb)* 98, 77–85.

Njanpop-Lafourcade, B.M., Inwald, J., Ostyn, A., Durand, B., Hughes, S., et al. (2001) Molecular typing of *Mycobacterium bovis* Isolates from Cameroon. *Journal of Clinical Microbiology* 39(1), 222–227.

Nuñez-Garcia, J., Downs, S.H., Parry, J.E., Abernethy, D.A., Broughan, J.M., et al. (2017) Meta-analyses of the sensitivity and specificity of ante-mortem and post-mortem diagnostic tests for bovine tuberculosis in the UK and Ireland. *Preventive Veterinary Medicine* Mar 6, doi: 10.1016/j.prevetmed.2017.02.017.

O'Connor, B.D., Woltmann, G., Patel, H., Turapov, O., Haldar, P. and Mukamolova, G.V. (2015) Can resuscitation-promoting factors be used to improve culture rates of extra-pulmonary tuberculosis? *International Journal of Tuberculosis and Lung Disease* 19(12), 1556–1557.

O'Hare, A., Orton, R.J., Bessell, P.R. and Kao, R.R. (2014) Estimating epidemiological parameters for bovine tuberculosis in British cattle using a Bayesian partial-likelihood approach. *Proceedings Biological Sciences* 281(1783), 20140248.

Olea-Popelka, F.J., Flynn, O., Costello, E., McGrath, G., Collins, J.D., et al. (2005) Spatial relationship between *Mycobacterium bovis* strains in cattle and badgers in four areas in Ireland. *Preventive Veterinary Medicine* 71(1–2), 57–70.

Oloya, J., Kazwala, R., Lund, A., Opuda-Asibo, J., Demelash, B., et al. (2007) Characterisation of mycobacteria isolated from slaughter cattle in pastoral regions of Uganda. *BMC Microbiology* 7(1), 95.

O'Neill, M.B., Mortimer, T.D. and Pepperell, C.S. (2015) Diversity of *Mycobacterium tuberculosis* across evolutionary scales. *PLoS Pathogens* 11(11), e1005257.

Pankhurst, L.J., Del Ojo Elias, C., Votintseva, A.A., Walker, T.M., Cole, K., et al. (2016) Rapid, comprehensive, and affordable mycobacterial diagnosis with whole-genome sequencing: a prospective study. *The Lancet Respiratory Medicine* 4(1), 49–58.

Parra, A., Fernandez-Llario, P., Tato, A., Larrasa, J., Garcia, A., et al. (2003) Epidemiology of *Mycobacterium bovis* infections of pigs and wild boars using a molecular approach. *Veterinary Microbiology* 97(1–2), 123–133.

Parra, A., Larrasa, J., Garcia, A., Alonso, J. and Mendoza, J. (2005) Molecular epidemiology of bovine tuberculosis in wild animals in Spain: A first approach to risk factor analysis. *Veterinary Microbiology* 110(3–4), 293–300.

Parreiras, P.M., Andrade, G.I., Nascimento, T.F., Oelemann, M.C., Gomes, H.M., et al. (2012) Spoligotyping and variable number tandem repeat analysis of *Mycobacterium bovis* isolates from cattle in Brazil. *Memórias do Instituto Oswaldo Cruz* 107(1), 64–73.

Pepperell, C.S., Granka, J.M., Alexander, D.C., Behr, M.A., Chui, L., et al. (2011) Dispersal of *Mycobacterium tuberculosis* via the Canadian fur trade. *Proceedings of the National Academy of Sciences of the United States of America* 108(16), 6526–6531.

Pepperell, C.S., Casto, A.M., Kitchen, A., Granka, J.M., Cornejo, O.E, et al. (2013) The role of selection in shaping diversity of natural *M. tuberculosis* populations. *PLoS Pathogens* 9(8), e1003543.

du Plessis, L. and Stadler, T. (2015) Getting to the root of epidemic spread with phylodynamic analysis of genomic data. *Trends in Microbiology* 23(7), 383–386.

Pollock, J.M. and Neill, S.D. (2002) *Mycobacterium bovis* infection and tuberculosis in cattle. *Veterinary Journal* 163(2), 115–127.

Price-Carter, M., Rooker, S. and Collins, D.M. (2011) Comparison of 45 variable number tandem repeat (VNTR) and two direct repeat (DR) assays to restriction endonuclease analysis for typing isolates of *Mycobacterium bovis*. *Veterinary Microbiology* 150(1–2), 107–114.

Reynolds, D. (2006) A review of tuberculosis science and policy in Great Britain. *Veterinary Microbiology* 112(2–4), 119–126.

Robbe-Austerman, S. and Turcotte, C. (2014) New and current approaches for isolation, identification, and genotyping of *Mycobacterium bovis*. In: Thoen, C.O., Steele, J.H., Kaneene, J.B. (eds) *Zoonotic Tuberculosis:* Mycobacterium bovis *and Other Pathogenic Mycobacteria*, 3rd edn. Wiley, Hoboken, USA.

Rodriguez-Campos, S., Gonzalez, S., de Juan, L., Romero, B., Bezos, J., *et al.* (2012a) A database for animal tuberculosis (mycoDB.es) within the context of the Spanish national programme for eradication of bovine tuberculosis. *Infection, Genetics and Evolution* 12(4), 877–882.

Rodriguez-Campos, S., Schurch, A.C., Dale, J., Lohan, A.J., Cunha, M.V., *et al.* (2012b) European 2 – a clonal complex of *Mycobacterium bovis* dominant in the Iberian Peninsula. *Infection, Genetics and Evolution* 12(4), 866–872.

Rodriguez-Campos, S., Navarro, Y., Romero, B., de Juan, L., Bezos, J., *et al.* (2013) Splitting of a prevalent *Mycobacterium bovis* spoligotype by variable-number tandem-repeat typing reveals high heterogeneity in an evolving clonal group. *Journal of Clinical Microbiology* 51(11), 3658–3665.

Rodwell, T.C., Kapasi, A.J., Moore, M., Milian-Suazo, F., Harris, B., *et al.* (2010) Tracing the origins of *Mycobacterium bovis* tuberculosis in humans in the USA to cattle in Mexico using spoligotyping. *International Journal of Infectious Diseases* 14, e129–e35.

Romero, B., Aranaz, A., Juan, L., Alvarez, J., Bezos, J., *et al.* (2006) Molecular epidemiology of multidrug-resistant *Mycobacterium bovis* Isolates with the same spoligotyping profile as isolates from animals. *Journal of Clinical Microbiology* 44(9), 3405–3408.

Romero, B., Aranaz, A., Sandoval, Å., Ålvarez, J., de Juan, L., *et al.* (2008) Persistence and molecular evolution of Mycobacterium bovis population from cattle and wildlife in Donana National Park revealed by genotype variation. *Veterinary Microbiology* 132(1–2), 87–95.

Roring, S., Brittain, D., Bunschoten, A.E., Hughes, M.S., Skuce, R.A., *et al.* (1998) Spacer oligotyping of *Mycobacterium bovis* isolates compared to typing by restriction fragment length polymorphism using PGRS, DR and IS6110 probes. *Veterinary Microbiology* 61(1–2), 111–120.

Ryan, T.J., Livingstone, P.G., Ramsey, D.S., de Lisle, G.W., Nugent, G., *et al.* (2006) Advances in understanding disease epidemiology and implications for control and eradication of tuberculosis in livestock: the experience from New Zealand. *Veterinary Microbiology* 112(2–4), 211–219.

Sahraoui, N., Muller, B., Guetarni, D., Boulahbal, F., Yala, D., *et al.* (2009) Molecular characterization of *Mycobacterium bovis* strains isolated from cattle slaughtered at two abattoirs in Algeria. *BMC Veterinary Research* 5(1), 4.

Sanou, A., Tarnagda, Z., Kanyala, E., Zingue, D., Nouctara, M., *et al.* (2014) *Mycobacterium bovis* in Burkina Faso: Epidemiologic and genetic links between human and cattle isolates. *PLoS Neglected Tropical Diseases* 8(10), e3142.

Schurch, A.C. and van Soolingen, D. (2012) DNA fingerprinting of *Mycobacterium tuberculosis*: from phage typing to whole-genome sequencing. *Infection, Genetics and Evolution* 12(4), 602–609.

Scott, C., Cavanaugh, J.S., Pratt, R., Silk, B.J., LoBue, P. and Moonan, P.K. (2016) Human tuberculosis caused by *Mycobacterium bovis* in the United States, 2006–2013. *Clinical Infectious Diseases* 63(5), 594–601.

Sheridan, M. (2011) Progress in tuberculosis eradication in Ireland. *Veterinary Microbiology* 151(1–2), 160–169.

Sintchenko, V. and Holmes, E.C. (2015) The role of pathogen genomics in assessing disease transmission. *BMJ* 350, h1314.

Skuce, R.A., Mallon, T.R., McCormick, C.M., McBride, S.H., Clarke, G., *et al.* (2010) *Mycobacterium bovis* genotypes in Northern Ireland: herd-level surveillance (2003 to 2008). *Veterinary Record* 167(18), 684–689.

Skuce, R.A., Allen, A.R. and McDowell, S.W. (2012) Herd-level risk factors for bovine tuberculosis: a literature review. *Veterinary Medicine International* 2012, 621210.

Smith, N.H. (2012) The global distribution and phylogeography of *Mycobacterium bovis* clonal complexes. *Infection, Genetics and Evolution* 12(4), 857–865.

Smith, N.H. and Upton, P. (2012) Naming spoligotype patterns for the RD9-deleted lineage of the *Mycobacterium tuberculosis* complex; www.Mbovis.org. *Infection, Genetics and Evolution* 12(4), 873–876.

Smith, N.H., Dale, J., Inwald, J., Palmer, S., Gordon, S.V., *et al.* (2003) The population structure of *Mycobacterium bovis* in Great Britain: clonal expansion. *Proceedings of the National Academy of Sciences of the United States of America* 100(25), 15271–15275.

Smith, N.H., Kremer, K., Inwald, J., Dale, J., Driscoll, J.R., *et al.* (2006a) Ecotypes of the *Mycobacterium tuberculosis* complex. *Journal of Theoretical Biology* 239(2), 220–225.

Smith, N.H., Gordon, S.V., de la Rua-Domenech, R., Clifton-Hadley, R.S. and Hewinson, R.G. (2006b) Bottlenecks and broomsticks: the molecular evolution of *Mycobacterium bovis*. *Nature Reviews Microbiology* 4(9), 670–681.

Smith, N.H., Berg, S., Dale, J., Allen, A., Rodriguez, S., *et al.* (2011) European 1: a globally important clonal complex of *Mycobacterium bovis*. *Infection, Genetics and Evolution* 11(6), 1340–1351.

Stone, M.J., Brown, T.J. and Drobniewski, F.A. (2011) Human *Mycobacterium bovis* infections in London and southeast England: Table 1. *Journal of Clinical Microbiology* 50(1), 164–165.

Szewzyk, R., Svenson, S.B., Hoffner, S.E., Bolske, G., Wahlstrom, H., *et al.* (1995) Molecular epidemiological studies of *Mycobacterium bovis* infections in humans and animals in Sweden. *Journal of Clinical Microbiology* 33(12), 3183–3185.

Tang, P. and Gardy, J.L. (2014) Stopping outbreaks with real-time genomic epidemiology. *Genome Medicine* 6(11), 104.

Thacker, T.C., Palmer, M.V., Robbe-Austerman, S., Stuber, T.P. and Waters, W.R. (2015) Anatomical distribution of *Mycobacterium bovis* genotypes in experimentally infected white-tailed deer. *Veterinary Microbiology* 180(1–2), 75–81.

Trewby, H., Wright, D., Breadon, E.L., Lycett, S.J., Mallon, T.R., *et al.* (2016) Use of bacterial whole-genome sequencing to investigate local persistence and spread in bovine tuberculosis. *Epidemics* 14, 26–35.

Van Soolingen, D. (2001) Molecular epidemiology of tuberculosis and other mycobacterial infections: main methodologies and achievements. *Journal of Internal Medicine* 249(1), 1–26.

Votintseva, A.A., Pankhurst, L.J., Anson, L.W., Morgan, M.R., Gascoyne-Binzi, D., *et al.* (2015) Mycobacterial DNA extraction for whole-genome sequencing from early positive liquid (MGIT) cultures. *Journal of Clinical Microbiology* 53(4), 1137–1143.

Walker, T.M., Monk, P., Smith, E.G. and Peto, T.E. (2013a) Contact investigations for outbreaks of *Mycobacterium tuberculosis*: advances through whole genome sequencing. *Clinical Microbiology and Infection* 19(9), 796–802.

Walker, T.M., Ip, C.L., Harrell, R.H., Evans, J.T., Kapatai, G., *et al.* (2013b) Whole-genome sequencing to delineate *Mycobacterium tuberculosis* outbreaks: a retrospective observational study. *Lancet Infectious Diseases* 13(2), 137–146.

Walker, T.M., Lalor, M.K., Broda, A., Saldana Ortega, L., Morgan, M., *et al.* (2014) Assessment of *Mycobacterium tuberculosis* transmission in Oxfordshire, UK, 2007–12, with whole pathogen genome sequences: an observational study. *The Lancet Respiratory Medicine* 2(4), 285–292.

Waters, W.R., Thacker, T.C., Nelson, J.T., DiCarlo, D.M., Maggioli, M.F., *et al.* (2014) Virulence of two strains of *Mycobacterium bovis* in cattle following aerosol infection. *Journal of Comparative Pathology* 151(4), 410–419.

Whelan, A.O., Coad, M., Cockle, P.J., Hewinson, G., Vordermeier, M. and Gordon, S.V. (2010) Revisiting host preference in the *Mycobacterium tuberculosis* complex: experimental infection shows *M. tuberculosis* H37Rv to be avirulent in cattle. *PLoS One* 5(1), e8527.

Whipple, D.L., Clarke, P.R., Jarnagin, J.L. and Payeur, J.B. (1997) Restriction fragment length polymorphism analysis of *Mycobacterium bovis* isolates from captive and free-ranging animals. *Journal of Veterinary Diagnostic Investigation* 9(4), 381–386.

Wirth, T., Hildebrand, F., Allix-Beguec, C., Wolbeling, F., Kubica, T., *et al.* (2008) Origin, spread and demography of the *Mycobacterium tuberculosis* complex. *PLoS Pathogens* 4(9), e1000160.

Wlodarska, M., Johnston, J.C., Gardy, J.L. and Tang, P. (2015) A microbiological revolution meets an ancient disease: improving the management of tuberculosis with genomics. *Clinical Microbiology Reviews* 28(2), 523–539.

Wright, D.M., Allen, A.R., Mallon, T.R., McDowell, S.W., Bishop, S.C., *et al.* (2013a) Detectability of bovine TB using the tuberculin skin test does not vary significantly according to pathogen genotype within Northern Ireland. *Infection, Genetics and Evolution* 19, 15–22.

Wright, D.M., Allen, A.R., Mallon, T.R., McDowell, S.W., Bishop, S.C., et al. (2013b) Field-isolated genotypes of *Mycobacterium bovis* vary in virulence and influence case pathology but do not affect outbreak size. *PLoS One* 8(9), e74503.

Wright, A.V., Nunez, J.K. and Doudna, J.A. (2016) Biology and applications of CRISPR systems: Harnessing nature's toolbox for genome engineering. *Cell* 164(1–2), 29–44.

Ypma, R.J., Altes, H.K., van Soolingen, D., Wallinga, J. and van Ballegooijen, W.M. (2013) A sign of superspreading in tuberculosis: highly skewed distribution of genotypic cluster sizes. *Epidemiology* 24(3), 395–400.

Zanardi, G., Boniotti, M.B., Gaffuri, A., Casto, B., Zanoni, M. and Pacciarini, M.L. (2013) Tuberculosis transmission by *Mycobacterium bovis* in a mixed cattle and goat herd. *Research in Veterinary Science* 95(2), 430–433.

Zumarraga, M.J., Martin, C., Samper, S., Alito, A., Latini, O., et al. (1999) Usefulness of spoligotyping in molecular epidemiology of *Mycobacterium bovis*-related infections in South America. *Journal of Clinical Microbiology* 37(2), 296–303.

6 Bovine Tuberculosis in Other Domestic Species

Anita L. Michel*

Department Veterinary Tropical Diseases, Bovine Tuberculosis and Brucellosis Research Programme, Faculty of Veterinary Science, University of Pretoria, Onderstepoort, South Africa

6.1 Introduction

The ability of *Mycobacterium bovis* to cause disease in a wide range of domestic and wild mammal species classifies this pathogen among the globally most widespread infectious causes of livestock production losses across many, highly diverse animal production systems (Buhr *et al.*, 2009; Humblet *et al.*, 2009; Schiller *et al.*, 2011; Food and Agriculture Organisation, 2012). In the World Organisation for Animal Health (OIE) Terrestrial Animal Health Code, bovine tuberculosis (TB) is currently listed within the categories of diseases of cattle and those of farmed Cervidae, which indicates a recognition by the OIE of the rising importance of *M. bovis* infections in production animals other than domestic cattle in terms of global trade (OIE, 2016).

The public health importance of *M. bovis* stems from the effective transmission to humans through consumption of infected cow's milk or, alternatively and less frequently, via aerosol in occupational risk groups such as farmers, veterinarians and abattoir workers (Michel *et al.*, 2010). The risk of contracting zoonotic tuberculosis from consumption of meat is considered low in countries with effective meat inspection. However, in developing countries where livestock is largely slaughtered informally and without veterinary inspection, consumption of high-risk parts such as lymph nodes and internal organs is common (Dlamini, 2013; Hambolu *et al.*, 2013) and presents an additional mode of transmission (see Chapter 2 for public health details and Chapter 3 for a discussion of One Health).

In production animals other than cattle, the risk profile for zoonotic transmission should, in principle, be regarded the same because it is based primarily on utilization of milk and meat and to a smaller extent on close contact. The species-specific pathogenesis of *M. bovis* in other food-producing animals needs to be visited in more detail to establish and manage the associated human health risk.

This chapter presents the current body of knowledge of *M. bovis* infection and disease is reviewed with regard to the following species: sheep, goats, pigs, water buffalo and camel.

6.2 *M. bovis* Infection in Sheep and Goats

Domestic small ruminants, like other mammals, are susceptible to *M. bovis* infection despite the scarcity of the disease for most of the 20th century (Cordes *et al.*, 1981; Bezos *et al.*, 2015).

---

* Email: anita.michel@up.ac.za

Before the introduction of national bovine tuberculosis control and eradication programmes when large proportions of the European cattle herds were infected with *M. bovis*, the prevalence of goats with tuberculosis slaughtered did not exceed 1% (Myers and Steele, 1969; Huitema, 1988) and tuberculosis in sheep was barely known. In North and South America, Asia and Australia the disease also seemed to be very rare and associated with the occurrence of widespread tuberculosis in cattle (Myers and Steele, 1969; Nanda & Gopal Singh, cited in Lall, 1969; O'Reilly and Daborn, 1995).

In recent decades, a broader geographical distribution of *M. bovis* infection in goats and sheep has been reported including Africa (van den Heever, 1984; Cadmus *et al.*, 2009; Hiko and Agga, 2011; Naima *et al.*, 2011; Boukary *et al.*, 2012), South America (Higino *et al.*, 2011), New Zealand (Cordes *et al.*, 1981; Davidson *et al.*, 1981), Sudan (Tag el Din and el Nour Gamaan, 1982), Pakistan (Javed *et al.*, 2010) and Europe (Shanahan *et al.*, 2011; Van Der Burgt *et al.*, 2013) with an emphasis on Mediterranean countries (Muñoz Mendoza *et al.*, 2012; Zanardi *et al.*, 2013).

Apart from *M. bovis*, *M. caprae* is the main causative agent of tuberculosis in goats and sheep (Bezos *et al.*, 2014). Since its discovery in Spain (Aranaz *et al.*, 1999) and elevation to species level as an independent member of the *M. tuberculosis* complex (MTBC) (Aranaz *et al.*, 2003) it has also been reported to infect other domestic and wild animal species as well as humans mainly in Europe (Pate *et al.*, 2006; Cvetnić *et al.*, 2007; Rodriguez *et al.*, 2011). In Spain it is responsible for 7.4% of MTBC isolates whereby the epidemiology is driven by caprine infections (Rodriguez *et al.*, 2011).

It was generally accepted that outbreaks in sheep or goats were the result of spillover from bovine TB reservoir species, whether domestic or wild (Cordes *et al.*, 1981; Malone *et al.*, 2003). While this route of transmission is probably a reality in many cases, it should not distract from the potential of both sheep and goats to act as reservoir hosts under certain conditions (Napp *et al.*, 2013). Intensification of dairy goat production has led to large herd sizes often housed all year and resulting in high animal densities facilitating rapid spread of infection among goats. As a result, high within-herd prevalences and mortality rates of up to 50% are not uncommon and cause severe economic losses to producers (Crawshaw *et al.*, 2008; Quintas *et al.*, 2010; Bezos *et al.*, 2014; Harwood, 2014).

In contrast, sheep are mostly managed extensively, and while their species-specific behaviour is usually a limiting factor to incidental *M. bovis* exposure from other infected hosts, infections do occur where sheep share their environment with cattle herds infected with high *M. bovis* prevalence (Cordes *et al.*, 1981; Malone *et al.*, 2003). Under these circumstances, *M. bovis* is transmitted either by aerosol or by ingestion and results in encapsulated granulomatous lesions, occasionally with mineralized foci, in the respiratory tract and mesenteric lymph nodes.

Clinical signs in goats include dry cough and progressive emaciation, whereas tuberculosis in sheep remains generally unnoticed. The lesions are mostly located in the lungs and their draining lymph nodes where they present as caseous lymphadenitis with nodules of various sizes with a yellowish–white, moist appearance. Several reports have described liquifactive necrosis and cavitary lung lesions filled with exudate as typical features of tuberculosis in goats (Daniel *et al.*, 2009; Domingo *et al.*, 2014) which, according to Sanchez (2011) is similar to human tuberculosis and contributes to a high transmissibility of the disease. The occasional occurrence of mammary tuberculosis raises a public health concern for consumers of goat milk (Huitema, 1988).

On rare occasions, *M. tuberculosis* infection has been reported in goats in the UK (Crawshaw *et al.*, 2008) and Africa (Cadmus *et al.*, 2009; Hiko and Agga, 2011; Kassa *et al.*, 2012). In an experimental infection study, Bezos and coworkers challenged goats with *M. bovis*, *M. caprae* and *M. tuberculosis* and showed that although *M. tuberculosis* induced specific pathology, the lesion scores were lowest for *M. tuberculosis* (Bezos *et al.*, 2015). This may suggest that goats contract *M. tuberculosis* from close contact with infected humans, but they are a dead-end or spillover host and have no significant role to play in the epidemiology of *M. tuberculosis*. In the zoonotic context, goats have been implied to serve as source of human infection with *M. bovis* (Gutierrez *et al.*, 1997) and *M. caprae* (Nebreda *et al.*, 2016). However, little is known about the zoonotic risk to consumers in rural areas of Sudan where it is customary to eat raw sheep liver, lung, rumen reticulum and omasum (Tag el Din and el Nour Gamaan, 1982).

As far as other members of the MTBC are concerned few have been associated with lesions resembling tuberculosis in goats. Recently, *M. microti* was isolated from a dairy goat in France that was most likely infected from a badger carrying the same spoligotype (Michelet et al., 2016).

Even though the disease is considered to be endemic in goats in Spain, prevalence data are limited to targeted studies in specific areas. This is because tuberculosis in goats is not covered by national control strategies and eradication programmes (Shanahan et al., 2011; Kassa et al., 2012; Napp et al., 2013; Harwood, 2014). For this reason, there is no compulsory testing of small ruminants for *M. bovis* and no internationally recognized test exists today. As long as the control of tuberculosis in small ruminants remains voluntary, the disease can be expected to spread and the prevalence to increase.

The relative higher frequency of outbreaks observed in goats compared to sheep is attributed to husbandry factors rather than a difference in susceptibility. The previously held belief that goats and sheep are purely spillover species has been challenged and the maintenance potential of goat and sheep flocks has been reported (Malone et al., 2003; Muñoz Mendoza et al., 2012; Napp et al., 2013).

6.3 *M. bovis* Infection in Domestic Pigs

From all mycobacterial infections, pigs are most susceptible to *M. avium* complex (MAC), especially *M. avium* subsp. *hominisuis* (Mah) and occasionally *M. avium* subsp. *avium* (Maa) (Mijs et al., 2002; Cvetnić et al., 2007; Agdestein et al., 2014; Pérez de Val et al., 2014). Within the MTBC, *M. bovis* is most frequently associated with tuberculosis in pigs. The historical significance of *M. bovis* infections in pig herds globally is difficult to establish from a review of the published literature because earlier reports classified all cases caused by *M. bovis* and by MAC as swine tuberculosis (Myers and Steele, 1969).

Despite the similarity of clinical and pathological characteristics associated with either MAC or MTBC in pigs, it is of utmost importance to distinguish between these causative agents as they play a different role in the epidemiology and control of tuberculosis-like lesions. Infection of pigs with *M. avium* or *M. bovis* results in localized indistinguishable granulomatous lesions mostly located in the mandibular and mesenteric lymph nodes without prior manifestation of clinical signs (Matlova et al., 2004; Cvetnić et al., 2007). Therefore, their detection is limited to observation of tuberculosis-like lesions in slaughter pigs at the abattoir. Country- and setting-specific predominance of either *Mycobacterium* organism is observed and depends on the epidemiological situation of bovine TB in cattle and wildlife as well as on pig husbandry factors. Mah is a ubiquitous environmental organism and Maa is distributed by birds. Therefore, infection in pigs can have a wide geographical distribution given exposure of pig herds to the environment in outdoor production systems (Lahiri et al., 2014), or through the use of untreated feed and bedding materials containing Mah (Matlova et al., 2004; Johansen et al., 2014). Mah causes opportunistic infections in swine resulting in condemnations at the abattoir with economic losses, but there is also growing concern about possible zoonotic transmission to humans (Tirkkonen et al., 2007; Leão et al., 2014) where it can cause pulmonary disease (Lahiri et al., 2014) and lymphadenitis (Despierres et al., 2012). In some studies, co-infection of *M. bovis* and *M. avium* strains has been observed and may be underdiagnosed in others due to the competition of these bacteria in culture and the paucibacillary nature of lesions (Santos et al., 2010; Barandiaran et al., 2015).

Infection of pigs with *M. bovis* occurs in countries where bovine tuberculosis is endemic in cattle or wildlife, while successful control and the prevalence in pigs is likely to reflect the local situation in the reservoir (Corner et al., 1981; Bernard et al., 2005; Barandiaran et al., 2011; Muwonge et al., 2012; Bailey et al., 2013; Broughan et al., 2013). Elimination of bovine TB in the reservoir leads to a decline and later the disappearance of *M. bovis* from pigs and to a relative increase of *M. avium*-derived mycobacterial disease in swine (Lesslie et al., 1968; Schliesser, 1985; Möbius et al., 2006).

M. bovis infection in pigs is the result of exposure from contaminated pastures, feeding of contaminated milk or contact with wildlife including carrion (O'Reilly and Daborn, 1995; Cousins, 2001; Bailey *et al.*, 2013; Nugent *et al.*, 2015). The presence of such a source of infection in combination with opportunities of exposure has become scarce in many developed countries as they have eradicated bovine TB from their cattle population and contact with infected feed or wildlife is practically impossible under the strict biosecurity measures applicable to commercial intensive pig productions. The bulk of recent knowledge of the epidemiology of *M. bovis* in domestic pigs therefore relies on reports from free-ranging and feral pig populations in Spain and New Zealand. In western Spain, extensively bred Iberian race pigs were found to be infected with *M. bovis* in the absence of cattle but in contact with a large population of wild boar that are maintenance hosts of *M. bovis* (Naranjo *et al.*, 2008). The lesions in both domestic pigs and wild boar were mainly located in the respiratory tract and included open lesions, indicating a respiratory route of infection between them (Parra *et al.*, 2003). Under specific conditions like those described here, which are characterized by a high pig population density and frequent contact with a sympatric reservoir of *M. bovis* exhibiting the same species-specific behaviour, it appears possible that certain populations of domestic pigs are capable of transmitting *M. bovis*.

In pigs experimentally challenged with high infective doses of up to 10^8 colony forming units, expansive lesions with liquefied necrotic centres and large numbers of extracellular bacilli as well as macrophages containing *M. bovis* in the airways were observed (Bolin *et al.*, 1997). If under similar natural conditions live pigs may transmit *M. bovis* in their respiratory secretions, there is currently no evidence that the rate of intra-species transmission is sufficient to establish infection in the pig population. Therefore, the presence of respiratory lesions alone may not prove a maintenance status but it classifies such populations as spillover hosts with amplifier potential.

Similarly, generalized tuberculosis was observed in the majority of semi free-ranging Sicilian domestic black pigs sampled from infected herds (Di Marco *et al.*, 2012). Like in other domestic pigs, the *M. bovis* prevalence increased with age and the most common site for macroscopic lesions was the head but the appearance and dissemination of lesions differed. The lesions in black pigs mostly lacked the fibrous layer of encapsulated lesions found in other pigs, suggesting that these pigs may be able to effectively excrete mycobacteria via aerosol or in their faeces (Di Marco *et al.*, 2012).

A contrasting situation has been reported from New Zealand where strong evidence exists that feral pigs easily contract *M. bovis* from infected possums through scavenging. Possums are the main wildlife reservoir of bovine tuberculosis in New Zealand (Nugent, 2011). A series of well-documented investigations have been conducted on pig-related factors in the transmission cycle of bovine tuberculosis. The release of 15 domestic pigs as sentinels in an area where wildlife tuberculosis was widespread demonstrated that pigs are very susceptible to *M. bovis* as infection was confirmed in all pigs, and in some as early as 2 months after release. Visible lesions in the mandibular lymph nodes were common to all pigs, whereas only a few animals showed involvement of thoracic lymph nodes, suggesting oral rather than a respiratory route of infection (Nugent *et al.*, 2002). This is in line with other studies involving farmed slaughter pigs that found a similar distribution of lesions with a predilection for the head lymph nodes (Cousins *et al.*, 2004; Bailey *et al.*, 2013). In pigs experimentally infected with moderate to low doses of *M. bovis*, the earliest lesions were detectable approximately 3 weeks after inoculation and contained large numbers of bacilli which gradually decreased over time. At 2 months most lesions had developed into well-circumscribed often encapsulated granulomas containing few bacilli and with a potential to heal (Francis, 1958; Bolin *et al.*, 1997; Bailey *et al.*, 2013). The white–yellow caseocalcerous tubercles are similar to those found in cattle but generally do not exceed 40 mm in diameter (Cousins *et al.*, 2004; Bailey *et al.*, 2013). Occasionally, generalized cases with dissemination of lesions to the liver, spleen and lungs and associated lymph nodes have been reported. Affected lungs may present with caseous bronchopneumonia but in other organs lesions appear fibrotic and less calcified.

These findings gave rise to the view that feral pigs in New Zealand are foremost spillover and dead-end hosts with no significant risk of intra- or inter-species transmission (Nugent and Whitford, 2003). Compelling evidence was provided by various studies. In areas where possums were controlled by poisoning, tuberculosis levels in resident feral pigs declined quickly and fell to near zero within a few years as opposed to areas without possum control (Nugent and Whitford, 2008; Nugent et al., 2012). In the final phase of the Australian tuberculosis eradication campaign directed at feral buffalo and cattle in the Northern Territory, the *M. bovis* prevalence had not only declined sharply in the target species but also in sympatric feral pigs, in which previously infection rates had reached up to 100% (McInerney et al., 1995). The use of pigs as sentinels in a surveillance programme in high-risk areas for *M. bovis* along international borders has been reported from the USA (Campbell et al., 2011).

Although pig-to-pig transmission probably exists in New Zealand, it may be very limited and due to cannibalism rather than to other forms of horizontal, vertical or pseudovertical transmission in feral pigs. No evidence of *M. bovis* excretion via urine, faeces or the nasal cavity could be found (Lugton, 1997, cited in Nugent and Whitford, 2003), and no piglets under the age of 2 months have been found infected. A case of a sow and her piglets being infected turned out to be genetically unrelated outbreaks, suggesting scavenging as the underlying source of the infections (Nugent and Whitford, 2003). The explanation may be similar where multiple cases of *M. bovis* in pigs were encountered on the same farm in Great Britain (Bailey et al., 2013).

M. tuberculosis infection is a sporadic infection in swine and an indication of transmission between humans and pigs. Due to the nature of the localized lesions in the head lymph nodes, the infection occurs most likely as the result of spillover from the human reservoir with little potential for spillback. Following the same principles as *M. bovis*, the prevalence reflects the epidemiological situation in humans and cases have been reported from countries with a high tuberculosis burden in humans including Nigeria (Jenkins et al., 2011), Ethiopia (Arega et al., 2013) and South Africa (Michel, unpublished data).

Other incidental infections of pigs with members of the *Mycobacterium tuberculosis* complex have been described for *M. microti* (Taylor et al., 2006) and *M. caprae* (Cvetnić et al., 2006; Rodriguez et al., 2011).

6.4 *M. bovis* Infection in Domestic Asian Water Buffalo

Asian water buffalo (*Bubalo bubalis*) were domesticated approximately 5000 years ago. Their natural distribution includes the Indian subcontinent and southeast Asia from where they have been introduced to Europe, the Americas and some parts of Africa, mostly Egypt. The susceptibility of water buffalo to *M. bovis* as well as the pathogenesis was found to be comparable to domestic cattle, leading to the assumption that water buffalo can serve as a reservoir and source of zoonotic infection to humans (Lall, 1969; Barbosa et al., 2014; Khattak et al., 2016). The largest buffalo population in the West is found in Brazil where *M. bovis* infection at an animal level of between 1.4% and 20.4% has been reported (Barbosa et al., 2014; Minharro et al., 2016), classifying bovine tuberculosis as cause of significant economic losses in Brazil.

In India, tuberculosis was historically widely distributed in water buffalo. A survey conducted in the 1950s in four states among 40,000 water buffalo revealed a reactor rate of 13.8%. Where cattle and buffalo were kept on the same farm, infection rates were higher in buffalo than in cattle (Lall, 1969). In Nepal, corresponding infection rates of 16% were found in water buffalo and cattle with both species sporadically excreting *M. bovis* in milk and faeces (Jha et al., 2007). Skin testing of water buffalo in Pakistan revealed a reactor prevalence of 5.7% (Khattak et al., 2016). Within Europe, water buffalo play a locally isolated but important role in the production of 'mozzarella di bufala' cheese in southern Italy, and the eradication of bovine tuberculosis from both cattle and buffalo populations is threatened by a renewed increase in case incidence of 0.65% (Alfano et al., 2014).

6.5 *M. bovis* Infection in Old World Camelids

Bactrian and dromedary camels are domesticated Old World camelid species. There are today about 27 million camels globally, 80% of which are dromedary and 20% are Bactrian camels (Food and Agriculture Organization, 2012). The latter exclusively occupy the cold deserts of Asia. Camels are working animals that are used as pack animals or for riding, and to contribute milk, fibre, hides, draught power and meat to the livelihoods of agro-pastoral communities in Africa and Asia (Wardeh, 2004). The dromedary camel is also bred for camel racing and there is a growing feral population of about one million dromedary camels in Australia (Schwartz, 2013). In Africa, especially in Sahel countries and East Africa, camel populations make a significant contribution to national economies and bear an unutilized economic potential (Farah, 2004). In sub-Saharan Africa, camels contribute 7% of total milk production while the highest numbers of dairy cattle are found in Somalia, Mali, Ethiopia and Niger where they contribute to food security (Food and Agriculture Organization, 2017).

Camels are susceptible to members of the MTBC, of which *M. bovis* is the most frequently reported causative agent of camel tuberculosis. The disease has long been recognized and can be fatal, but appears to have a rare occurrence in nomadic camels (Fassi-Fehri, 1987; Kinne *et al.*, 2006; Wernery *et al.*, 2014). In a review of tuberculosis in camels Mason (1917) described its sporadic occurrence in India, Sudan and Algeria, and a much more widespread distribution of the disease in Egypt since the late 19th century (Littlewood, 1888, cited in Mason, 1917). In 1987, Mustafa briefly reviewed the literature and concluded that tuberculosis in camels may be exacerbated under intensive farming conditions and when farmed and housed in close contact with cattle (Mustafa, 1987). Under these circumstances isolation of *M. bovis* from bulk camel milk was reported in Russia (Donchenko *et al.*, 1975, cited in Mustafa, 1987). In 2008, Manal and Gobran investigated a total of 704 camels slaughtered at different abattoirs in Egypt. The animals originated from farms with and without cattle, and tuberculosis was only confirmed in camels at a prevalence of 0.7% from farms co-inhabited by cattle (Manal and Gobran, 2008).

Although tuberculosis is today considered of increasing socio-economic and public health importance (see Chapter 2 for details), there is a large paucity of prevalence and epidemiological data from most camel-breeding countries. It is unknown whether this is due to a lack of reporting or to the absence of the disease. Somalia has the largest camel population in Africa, followed by Mali, yet less than half a dozen reports, which only marginally mention tuberculosis in Somalia, could be traced (Abdurahman and Bornstein, 1991). Sporadic studies reported the presence of *M. bovis* in camels in Niger (Boukary *et al.*, 2012), Nigeria (Bala *et al.*, 2011; Abubakar *et al.*, 2012), Mauritania (Chartier *et al.*, 1991), Egypt, Ethiopia, India and Pakistan. In Eritrea, tuberculosis in camels is infrequently encountered, but in a recent survey among 198 dromedary camels using the single comparative intradermal tuberculin test (SCITT) a prevalence of 1.5% was observed (Ghebremariam, M.K., personal communication). When a lower cut-off was applied, as previously suggested for cattle, the prevalence increased almost eightfold to 11.6%. As shown by other investigators, the SCITT appears to be prone to false positive reactions and of doubtful diagnostic value in camels, possibly due the high rate of infections with non-tuberculous mycobacteria. The lower SCITT cut-off may therefore have to be used with caution (Bush *et al.*, 1990; Wernery *et al.*, 2007; Alvarez *et al.*, 2012). The few detailed reports on diagnostic assays in Old Word camelids were reviewed by Alvarez who cited the findings by Schillinger (1987) according to which between 10% and 20% false positive skin test reactions were observed in Australian dromedaries with a tuberculosis free status (Alvarez *et al.*, 2012). Bush *et al.* (1990), on the other hand, found that the SCITT also failed to detect *M. bovis* infection in two Bactrian camels, one of which exhibited localized and the other one generalized tuberculosis (Bush *et al.*, 1990). The SCITT forms the basis for tuberculosis testing in many animal species but appears unsuitable for screening or control in camels (Wernery *et al.*, 2014).

Infectious conditions of the lungs were reported in 10% of slaughter camels (Zubair *et al.*, 2004). Tuberculosis-like lesions in the respiratory tract of camels can, apart from *M. bovis*, be associated with non-tuberculous mycobacteria including *M. kansasii*, *M. fortuitum*, *M. smegmatis* or *Rhodococcus equi* (Elmossalami *et al.*, 1971; Kinne *et al.*, 2011). As a consequence, prevalence data based on the observation of gross lesions alone may be an overestimate of *M. bovis*-associated camel tuberculosis. In Ethiopia, the prevalence of tuberculosis-like lesions in two studies was 10% and 4.5%; of these, only 22% and 21%, respectively, were caused by *M. bovis*, corresponding to a final bovine tuberculosis prevalence of less than 1% (Mamo *et al.*, 2011; Kasaye *et al.*, 2013).

As established for small ruminants and pigs, there is agreement between various studies in different countries that age was found to be positively associated with the prevalence of tuberculosis in camels (Mamo *et al.*, 2011; Narnaware *et al.*, 2015). In view of their life expectancy, which ranges from 22 to 35 years, the cumulative risk of old camels to be infected with and to transmit *M. bovis* is significantly higher than in other domestic animals (Wosene, 1991).

Clinical signs of tuberculosis in camels may be absent in early stages, but later on generally include anorexia and progressive but often rapid emaciation (Narnaware *et al.*, 2015). Pathological changes caused by *M. bovis* present as granulomatous, caseous-necrotizing lesions that are macroscopically comparable to those in cattle. Microscopically, the only marked difference is the scarcity of giant cells in the lesions. Calcification and fibroplastic reactions may be observed (Elmossalami *et al.*, 1971; Bush *et al.*, 1990). The lesions are predominantly found in the lungs and mediastinal lymph nodes, retropharyngeal and mesenteric lymph nodes with occasional cases of dissemination to the kidneys, liver, spleen, heart and pericardium, mesentery, trachea, pancreas and peripheral lymph nodes (Bush *et al.*, 1990; Chartier *et al.*, 1991; Kasaye *et al.*, 2013; Narnaware *et al.*, 2015). Acid-fast organisms are either absent or scant.

The exact route of *M. bovis* transmission between camels is unknown, but the lung-centred pathology strongly suggests that camels contract the pathogen via aerosols either during close contact or through dust particles (Wernery and Rüger-Kaaden, 2002). In exceptional cases of generalized tuberculosis with kidney involvement, shedding of bacilli in the urine has been reported (Dekker *et al.*, 1962). There are no reports on possible vertical or pseudovertical transmission of *M. bovis* in camels, neither has tuberculous mastitis been described. This may suggest that *M. bovis* excretion in milk is an unlikely event reserved for generalized cases under intensive husbandry conditions. There is reason to believe that the arid climate and the traditional nomadic, semi free-ranging husbandry system prevailing in most camel-owning communities neither facilitate close, prolonged contact nor the confined conditions that are conducive to high transmission rates by aerosol. Their current status as spillover host may therefore be seen as a function of the incapacitating circumstances for *M. bovis* transmission rather than a low degree of susceptibility, similar to the varying roles of wild boar as hosts of *M. bovis* in Mediterranean Europe. However, with the increasing global demand for camel milk the production in intensive camel farms in East Africa has tripled in the past 50 years and presently contributes 7% of the milk produced in sub-Saharan Africa (Schwartz, 2013). Further intensification of camel production in the absence of tuberculosis surveillance and control programmes may certainly pave the way for a changing role of *M. bovis* in camel health and production.

Tuberculosis is a serious disease concern and cause of death in zoological collections. While *M. tuberculosis* is the more common cause of tuberculosis in this setting, both localized and generalized cases have been described which were caused by *M. bovis* (Bush *et al.*, 1990) but also by *M. caprae* (Erler *et al.*, 2004; Pate *et al.*, 2006), *M. pinnipedii* and *M. orygis* in a camel in the UAE (Kinne *et al.*, 2006; Wernery *et al.*, 2007; Wernery and Kinne, 2012).

6.6 Conclusion

Domestic animals are susceptible to *M. bovis* resulting in an extensive host spectrum. Where differences in the frequency of outbreaks are observed, those have been attributed to species-specific behaviour or husbandry practices rather than to differences in host susceptibility. Overall, tuberculosis in domestic animals other than cattle is a sporadic event and, with the exception of small ruminants and water buffalo, strongly associated with spillover of infection from cattle or wildlife. Therefore, in regions where bovine tuberculosis has been successfully eradicated from cattle or where contact between reservoir species (cattle or wildlife) and spillover species is uncommon, tuberculosis in other species is believed to be very rare.

There is a general paucity of information on the true prevalence and distribution of *M. bovis* infection in domestic species other than cattle, especially where they are farmed extensively or live under semi free-roaming conditions. Water buffalo and small ruminants have maintenance host potential and, given the high risk for economic losses and zoonotic *M. bovis* transmission, there is a need to integrate those species in the national bovine tuberculosis control programmes.

References

Abdurahman, O.S. and Bornstein, S. (1991) Diseases of camels (*Camelus dromedarius*) in Somalia and prospects for better health. *Nomadic Peoples* 104–112.

Abubakar, U.B., Kudi, A.C., Abdulkadri, I.A., Okaiyeto, S.O. and Ibrahim, S. (2012) Prevalence of tuberculosis in slaughtered camels (*Camelus dromedarius*) based on post-mortem meat inspection and Zeihl-Neelsen Stain in Nigeria. *Journal of Camel Practice and Research* 19, 29–32.

Agdestein, A., Olsen, I., Jørgensen, A., Djønne, B. and Johansen, T.B. (2014) Novel insights into transmission routes of *Mycobacterium avium* in pigs and possible implications for human health. *Veterinary Research* 45, 46.

Alfano, F., Peletto, S., Lucibelli, M.G., Borriello, G., Urciuolo, G., et al., (2014) Identification of single nucleotide polymorphisms in toll-like receptor candidate genes associated with tuberculosis infection in water buffalo (*Bubalus bubalis*). *BMC Genetics* 15, 139.

Alvarez, J., Bezos, J., Juan, L., Vordermeier, M., Rodriguez, S., et al. (2012) Diagnosis of tuberculosis in camelids: old problems, current solutions and future challenges. *Transboundary & Emerging Diseases* 59, 1–10.

Aranaz, A., Liebana, E., Gomez-Mampaso, E., Galan, J.C., Cousins, D., et al., (1999) *Mycobacterium tuberculosis* subsp. *caprae* subsp. nov.: a taxonomic study of a new member of the Mycobacterium tuberculosis complex isolated from goats in Spain. *International Journal of Systematic Bacteriology* 49(3), 1263–1273.

Aranaz, A., Cousins, D., Mateos, A. and Dominguez, L. (2003) Elevation of *Mycobacterium tuberculosis* subsp. *caprae* Aranaz et al., 1999 to species rank as *Mycobacterium caprae* comb. nov., sp. nov. *International Journal of Systematic & Evolutionary Microbiology* 53, 1785–1789.

Arega, S.M., Conraths, F.J. and Ameni, G. (2013) Prevalence of tuberculosis in pigs slaughtered at two abattoirs in Ethiopia and molecular characterization of *Mycobacterium tuberculosis* isolated from tuberculous-like lesions in pigs. *BMC Veterinary Research* 9, 97.

Bailey, S.S., Crawshaw, T.R., Smith, N.H. and Palgrave, C.J. (2013) *Mycobacterium bovis* infection in domestic pigs in Great Britain. *Veterinary Journal* 198, 391–397.

Bala, A.N., Garba, A.E. and Yazah, A.J. (2011) Bacterial and parasitic zoonoses encountered at slaughter in Maiduguri abattoir, Northeastern Nigeria. *Veterinary World* 4, 437–443.

Barandiaran, S., Martinez Vivot, M., Moras, E.V., Cataldi, A.A. and Zumarraga, M.J. (2011) *Mycobacterium bovis* in swine: spoligotyping of isolates from Argentina. *Veterinary Medicine International* 2011, 979647.

Barandiaran, S., Pérez, A.M., Gioffré, A.K., Martínez Vivot, M., Cataldi, A.A. and Zumárraga, M.J. (2015) Tuberculosis in swine co-infected with *Mycobacterium avium* subsp. *hominissuis* and *Mycobacterium bovis* in a cluster from Argentina. *Epidemiology and Infection* 143, 966–974.

Barbosa, J.D., da Silva, J.B., Rangel, C.P., da Fonseca, A.H., Silva, N.S., et al. (2014) Tuberculosis prevalence and risk factors for water buffalo in Pará, Brazil. *Tropical Animal Health and Production* 46, 513–517.

Bernard, F., Vincent, C., Matthieu, L., David, R. and James, D. (2005) Tuberculosis and brucellosis prevalence survey on dairy cattle in Mbarara milk basin. *Preventive Veterinary Medicine* 15, 267–281.

Bezos, J., Marqués, S., Álvarez, J., Casal, C., Romero, B., et al. (2014) Evaluation of single and comparative intradermal tuberculin tests for tuberculosis eradication in caprine flocks in Castilla y León (Spain). *Research in Veterinary Science* 96, 39–46.

Bezos, J., Casal, C., Díez-Delgado, I., Romero, B., Liandris, E., *et al.* (2015) Goats challenged with different members of the *Mycobacterium tuberculosis* complex display different clinical pictures. *Veterinary Immunology and Immunopathology* 167, 185–189.

Bolin, C.A., Whipple, D.L., Khanna, K.V., Risdahl, J.M., Peterson, P.K. and Molitor, T.W. (1997) Infection of swine with *Mycobacterium bovis* as a model of human tuberculosis. *Journal of Infectious Diseases* 176, 1559–1566.

Boukary, A.R., Thys, E., Rigouts, L., Matthys, F., Berkvens, D., *et al.* (2012) Risk factors associated with bovine tuberculosis and molecular characterization of *Mycobacterium bovis* strains in urban settings in Niger. *Transboundary and Emerging Diseases* 59, 490–502.

Broughan, J.M., Downs, S.H., Crawshaw, T.R., Upton, P.A., Brewer, J. and Clifton-Hadley, R.S. (2013) *Mycobacterium bovis* infections in domesticated non-bovine mammalian species. Part 1: review of epidemiology and laboratory submissions in Great Britain 2004–2010. *Veterinary Journal* 198, 339–345.

Buhr, B., McKeever, K. and Adachi, K. (2009) *Economic Impact of Bovine Tuberculosis on Minnesota's Cattle and Beef Sector*. University of Nebraska – Lincoln, Michigan Bovine Tuberculosis Bibliography and Database. Paper 20. Available at: http://digitalcommons.unl.edu/michbovinetb/20 (accessed 24 July 2016).

Bush, M., Montali, R.J., Phillips L.J. Jr and Holobaugh, P.A. (1990) Bovine tuberculosis in a bactrian camel herd: clinical, therapeutic, and pathologic findings. *Journal of Zoo and Wildlife Medicine* 21, 171–179.

Cadmus, S.I., Adesokan, H.K., Jenkins, A.O. and van Soolingen, D. (2009) *Mycobacterium bovis* and *M. tuberculosis* in goats, Nigeria. *Emerging Infectious Diseases* 15, 2066–2067.

Campbell, T.A., Long, D.B., Bazan, L.R., Thomsen, B.V., Robbe-Austerman, S., *et al.* (2011) Absence of *Mycobacterium bovis* in feral swine (*Sus scrofa*) from the southern Texas border region. *Journal of Wildlife Diseases* 47, 974–978.

Chartier, F., Chartier, C., Thorel, M.F. and Crespeau, F. (1991) A new case of *Mycobacterium bovis* pulmonary tuberculosis in the dromedary (*Camelus dromedarius*) in Mauritania. *Revue d'elevage et de medecine veterinaire des pays tropicaux* 44, 43–47.

Cordes, D.O., Bullians, J.A., Lake, D.E. and Carter, M.E. (1981) Observations on tuberculosis caused by *Mycobacterium bovis* in sheep. *New Zealand Veterinary Journal* 29, 60–62.

Corner, L.A., Barrett, R.H., Lepper, A.W., Lewis, V. and Pearson, C.W. (1981) A survey of mycobacteriosis of feral pigs in the Northern Territory. *Australian Veterinary Journal* 57, 537–542.

Cousins, D.V. (2001) *Mycobacterium bovis* infection and control in domestic livestock. *Revue Scientifique et Technique* 20, 71–85.

Cousins, D.V., Huchzermeyer, H.F., Griffin, J.F., Brueckner, G.K., van Rensburg, I.B.J. and Kriek, N.P.J. (2004) Tuberculosis. In: *Infectious Diseases of Livestock*. Oxford University Press, Cape Town, South Africa.

Crawshaw, T., Daniel, R., Clifton-Hadley, R., Clark, J., Evans, H., *et al.* (2008) TB in goats caused by *Mycobacterium bovis*. *Veterinary Record* 163, 127.

Cvetnić, Ž., Špišić, S., Katalinić-Janković, V., Marjanovic, S., Obrovac, M., *et al.* (2006) *Mycobacterium caprae* infection in cattle and pigs on one family farm in Croatia: a case report. *Veterinarni Medicina* 51, 523–531.

Cvetnić, Ž., Katalinić-Janković, V., Sostaric, B., Špišić, S., Obrovac, M., *et al.* (2007) *Mycobacterium caprae* in cattle and humans in Croatia. *International Journal of Tuberculosis & Lung Disease* 11, 652–658.

Cvetnić, Ž., Špišić, S., Benić, M., Katalinić-Janković, V., Pate, M., *et al.* (2007) Mycobacterial infection of pigs in Croatia. *Acta Veterinaria Hungarica* 55, 1–9.

Daniel, R., Evans, H., Rolfe, S., De La Rua-Domenech, R., Crawshaw, T., *et al.* (2009) Papers: outbreak of tuberculosis caused by *Mycobacterium bovis* in golden Guernsey goats in Great Britain. *Veterinary Record* 165, 335–342.

Davidson, R.M., Alley, M.R. and Beatson, N.S. (1981) Tuberculosis in a flock of sheep. *New Zealand Veterinary Journal* 29, 1–2.

Dekker, N.D.M. and van der Schaaf, A. (1962) Open tuberculosis in a camel. *Tijschrift voor Diergeneeskunde* 87, 1133–1140.

Despierres, L., Cohen-Bacrie, S., Richet, H. and Drancourt, M. (2012) Diversity of *Mycobacterium avium* subsp. *hominissuis* mycobacteria causing lymphadenitis, France. *European Journal of Clinical Microbiology and Infectious Diseases* 31, 1373–1379.

Di Marco, V., Mazzone, P., Capucchio, M.T., Boniotti, M.B., Aronica, V., *et al.*, (2012) Epidemiological significance of the domestic black pig (*Sus scrofa*) in maintenance of bovine tuberculosis in Sicily. *Journal of Clinical Microbiology* 50, 1209–1218.

Dlamini, M. (2013) *A Study on Bovine Tuberculosis and Associated Risk Factors for Humans in Swaziland*. MSc dissertation, University of Pretoria, Pretoria, South Africa.

Domingo, M., Vidal, E. and Marco, A. (2014) Pathology of bovine tuberculosis. *Research in Veterinary Science* 97, S20–S29.

Elmossalami, E., Siam, M.A. and Sergany, M.E. (1971) Studies on tuberculous-like lesions in slaughtered camels. *Zentralblatt für Veterinärmedizin Reihe B* 18, 253–261.

Erler, W., Martin, G., Sachse, K., Naumann, L., Kahlau, D., *et al*., (2004) Molecular fingerprinting of *Mycobacterium bovis* subsp. *caprae* isolates from Central Europe. *Journal of Clinical Microbiology* 42, 2234–2238.

Farah, Z. (2004) An introduction to the camel. In: Farah, Z. and A. Fischer (eds): *Milk and meat from the camel – Handbook on products and processing.* Vdf Hochschulverlag, Zűrich, Switzerland, pp. 15–28.

Fassi-Fehri, M.M. (1987) Diseases of camels. *Revue Scientifique Technique OIE* 6, 337–354.

Food and Agriculture Organization (2012) Tuberculosis, *EMPRES Transboundary Animal Diseases Bulletin,* (Online), vol. 40. Available at: http://www.fao.org/docrep/015/i2811e/i2811e.pdf. (accessed 17 December 2015).

Food and Agriculture Organization (2017) *Dairy production and products.* Available at: http://www.fao.org/agriculture/dairy-gateway/milk-production/dairy-animals/camels/en/#.V54oZfl9600) (accessed 5 June 2017).

Francis, J. (1958) *Tuberculosis in Animals and Man: A Study in Comparative Pathology.* Cassell, Bristol, UK.

Gutierrez, M., Samper, S., Jimenez, M.S., van Embden, J.D., Marin, J.F. and Martin, C. (1997) Identification by spoligotyping of a caprine genotype in *Mycobacterium bovis* strains causing human tuberculosis. *Journal of Clinical Microbiology* 35, 3328–3330.

Hambolu, D., Freeman, J. and Taddese, H.B. (2013) Predictors of bovine TB risk behaviour amongst meat handlers in Nigeria: a cross-sectional study guided by the health belief model. *PLoS One* 8, e56091.

Harwood, D. (2014) Bovine TB in goats. *Veterinary Record* 174, 456.

Higino, S.S.S., Pinheiro, S.R., de Souza, G.O., Dib, C.C., do Rosário, T.R., *et al*. (2011) *Mycobacterium bovis* infection in goats from the Northeast region of Brazil. *Brazilian Journal of Microbiology* 42, 1437–1439.

Hiko, A. and Agga, G.E. (2011) First-time detection of mycobacterium species from goats in Ethiopia. *Tropical Animal Health and Production* 43, 133–139.

Huitema, H. (1988) *Tuberculosis in Animals and Man.* Royal Netherlands Tuberculosis Association, The Hague, Netherlands.

Humblet, M.F., Boschiroli, M.L. and Saegerman, C. (2009) Classification of worldwide bovine tuberculosis risk factors in cattle: a stratified approach. *Veterinary Research* 40, 50.

Javed, M.T., Munir, A., Shahid, M., Severi, G., Irfan, M., *et al*. (2010) Percentage of reactor animals to single comparative cervical intradermal tuberculin (SCCIT) in small ruminants in Punjab Pakistan. *Acta Tropica* 113, 88–91.

Jenkins, A.O., Cadmus, S.I.B., Venter, E.H., Pourcel, C., Hauk, Y., *et al*. (2011) Molecular epidemiology of human and animal tuberculosis in Ibadan, Southwestern Nigeria. *Veterinary Microbiology* 151, 139–147.

Jha, V.C., Morita, Y., Dhakal, M., Besnet, B., Sato, T., *et al*. (2007) Isolation of *Mycobacterium* spp. from milking buffaloes and cattle in Nepal. *Journal Veterinary Medical Science* 69, 819–825.

Johansen, T.B., Agdestein, A., Lium, B., Jørgensen, A. and Djønne, B. (2014) *Mycobacterium avium* subsp. *hominissuis* infection in swine associated with peat used for bedding. *BioMed Research International* 2014, 189649.

Kasaye, S., Molla, W. and Amini, G. (2013) Prevalence of camel tuberculosis at Akaki abattoir at Addis Ababa in Ethiopia. *African Journal of Microbiology Research* 7, 2184–2189.

Kassa, G.M., Abebe, F., Worku, Y., Legesse, M., Medhin, G., *et al*. (2012) Tuberculosis in goats and sheep in Afar Pastoral Region of Ethiopia and isolation of mycobacterium tuberculosis from goat. *Veterinary Medicine International* 2012, 869146.

Khattak, I., Mushtaq, M.H., Ahmad, M.D., Khan, M.S., Chaudhry, M. and Sadique, U. (2016) Risk factors associated with *Mycobacterium bovis* skin positivity in cattle and buffalo in Peshawar, Pakistan. *Tropical Animal Health and Production* 48, 479–485.

Kinne, J., Johnson, B., Jahans, K.L., Smith, N.H., Ul-Haq, A. and Wernery, U. (2006) Camel tuberculosis: a case report. *Tropical Animal Health & Production* 38, 207–213.

Kinne, J., Madarame, H., Takai, S., Jose, S. and Wernery, U. (2011) Disseminated *Rhodococcus equi* infection in dromedary camels (*Camelus dromedarius*). *Veterinary Microbiology* 149, 269–272.

Lahiri, A., Kneisel, J., Kloster, I., Kamal, E. and Lewin, A. (2014) Abundance of *Mycobacterium avium* ssp. *hominissuis* in soil and dust in Germany – implications for the infection route. *Letters in Applied Microbiology* 59, 65–70.

Lall, J.M. (1969) Tuberculosis among animals in India. *Veterinary Bulletin* 39, 385–390.

Leão, C., Canto, A., Machado, D., Sanches, I.S., Couto, I., *et al.* (2014) Relatedness of *Mycobacterium avium* subspecies *hominissuis* clinical isolates of human and porcine origins assessed by MLVA. *Veterinary Microbiology* 173, 92–100.

Lesslie, I.W., Birn, K.J., Stuart, P., O'Neill, P.A. and Smith, J. (1968) Tuberculosis in the pig and the tuberculin test. *Veterinary Record* 83, 647–651.

Malone, F.E., Wilson, E.C., Pollock, J.M. and Skuce, R.A. (2003) Investigations into an outbreak of tuberculosis in a flock of sheep in contact with tuberculous cattle. *Journal of Veterinary Medicine Series B: Infectious Diseases and Veterinary Public Health* 50, 500–504.

Mamo, G., Bayleyegn, G., Tessema, T.S., Legesse, M., Medhin, G., *et al.* (2011) Pathology of camel tuberculosis and molecular characterization of its causative agents in pastoral regions of Ethiopia. *PLoS One* 6(1), e15862.

Manal, M.Y. and Gobran, R.A. (2008) Some studies on tuberculosis in camel. *Egyptian Journal of Comparative Pathology and Clinical Pathology* 21, 58–74.

Mason, F.E. (1917) Tuberculosis in camels. *Journal of Comparative Pathology and Therapeutics* 30, 80–84.

Matlova, L., Dvorska, L., Palecek, K., Maurenc, L., Bartos, M. and Pavlik, I. (2004) Impact of sawdust and wood shavings in bedding on pig tuberculous lesions in lymph nodes, and IS1245 RFLP analysis of *Mycobacterium avium* subsp. *hominissuis* of serotypes 6 and 8 isolated from pigs and environment. *Veterinary Microbiology* 102, 227–236.

McInerney, J., Small, K.J. and Caley, P. (1995) Prevalence of *Mycobacterium bovis* infection in feral pigs in the Northern Territory. *Australian Veterinary Journal* 72, 448–451.

Michel, A.L., Müller, B. and Helden, P.D. (2010) *Mycobacterium bovis* at the animal-human interface: a problem, or not? *Veterinary Microbiology* 140, 371–381.

Michelet, L., de Cruz, K., Phalente, Y., Karoui, C., Hénault, S., *et al.* (2016) *Mycobacterium microti* infection in dairy goats, France. *Emerging Infectious Diseases* 22, 569–570.

Mijs, W., de Haas, P., Rossau, R., Van Der Laan, T., Rigouts, L., *et al.* (2002) Molecular evidence to support a proposal to reserve the designation *Mycobacterium avium* subsp. *avium* for bird-type isolates and *M. avium* subsp. *hominissuis* for the human/porcine type of *M. avium*. *International Journal of Systematic and Evolutionary Microbiology* 52, 1505–1518.

Minharro, S., de Morais Alves, C., Mota, P.M.P.C., Dorneles, E.M.S., de Alencar, A.P., *et al.* (2016) Tuberculosis in water buffalo (*Bubalis bubalis*) in the Baixo Araguari Region, Amapá, Brazil. *Semina: Ciências Agrárias* 37, 885–890.

Möbius, P., Lentzsch, P., Moser, I., Naumann, L., Martin, G. and Köhler, H. (2006) Comparative macrorestriction and RFLP analysis of *Mycobacterium avium* subsp. *avium* and *Mycobacterium avium* subsp. *hominissuis* isolates from man, pig, and cattle. *Veterinary Microbiology* 117, 284–291.

Muñoz Mendoza, M., Juan, L.D., Menéndez, S., Ocampo, A., Mourelo, J., *et al.* (2012) Tuberculosis due to *Mycobacterium bovis* and *Mycobacterium caprae* in sheep. *Veterinary Journal* 191, 267–269.

Mustafa, I.E. (1987) Bacterial diseases of dromedaries and Bactrian camels. *Revue Scientifique Technique Office International Epizootics* 6, 391–405.

Muwonge, A., Johansen, T.B., Vigdis, E., Godfroid, J., Olea-Popelka, F., *et al.* (2012) *Mycobacterium bovis* infections in slaughter pigs in Mubende district, Uganda: a public health concern. *BMC Veterinary Research* 8, 168.

Myers, J.A. and Steele, J.H. (eds) (1969) *Bovine Tuberculosis Control in Man and Animals*. Warren H Green, St. Louis, USA.

Naima, S., Borna, M., Bakir, M., Djamel, Y., Fadila, B., *et al.* (2011) Tuberculosis in cattle and goats in the North of Algeria. *Veterinary Research* 4, 100–103.

Napp, S., Allepuz, A., Mercader, I., Nofrarias, M., Lopez-Soria, S., *et al.* (2013) Evidence of goats acting as domestic reservoirs of bovine tuberculosis. *Veterinary Record* 172, 663.

Naranjo, V., Gortazar, C., Vicente, J. and de la Fuente, J. (2008) Evidence of the role of European wild boar as a reservoir of *Mycobacterium tuberculosis* complex. *Veterinary Microbiology* 127, 1–9.

Narnaware, S.D., Dahiya, S.S., Tuteja, F.C., Nagarajan, G., Nath, K. and Patil, N.V. (2015) Pathology and diagnosis of *Mycobacterium bovis* in naturally infected dromedary camels (*Camelus dromedarius*) in India. *Tropical Animal Health and Production* 47, 1633–1636.

Nebreda, T., Álvarez-Prida, E., Blanco, B., Remacha, M.A., Samper, S. and Jiménez, M.S. (2016) Peritoneal tuberculosis due to *Mycobacterium caprae*. *IDCases* 4, 50–52.

Nugent, G. (2011) Maintenance, spillover and spillback transmission of bovine tuberculosis in multi-host wildlife complexes: a New Zealand case study. *Veterinary Microbiology* 151, 34–42.

Nugent, G. and Whitford, J. (2003) *Pigs as Hosts of Bovine Tuberculosis in New Zealand – a review. R-10577: part 1 of a two-part project*, Animal Health Board. Available at: http://www.tbfree.org.nz/Portals/0/2014AugResearchPapers/Nugent%20G,%20Reddiex%20B,%20Whitford%20J,%20Yockney%20I.%20Pig%20as%20hosts%20of%20bovine%20tuberculosis%20in%20New%20Zealand%20_%20a%20review.pdf (accessed 26 June 2016).

Nugent, G. and Whitford, J. (2008) *Confirmation of the Spatial Scale and Duration of Spillback Risk from Tb infected Pigs. Project No. R-10688*, Animal Health Board. Available at: http://www.tbfree.org.nz/Portals/0/2014AugResearchPapers/Nugent%20G,%20Whitford%20EJ.%20Confirmation%20of%20the%20Spatial%20Scale%20and%20Duration%20of%20Spillback%20Risk%20from%20Tb-infected%20Pigs.pdf (accessed 26 June 2016).

Nugent, G., Whitford, J. and Young, N. (2002) Use of released pigs as sentinels for *Mycobacterium bovis*. *Journal of Wildlife Diseases* 38, 665–677.

Nugent, G., Whitford, J., Yockney, I.J. and Cross, M.L. (2012) Reduced spillover transmission of *Mycobacterium bovis* to feral pigs (*Sus scofa*) following population control of brushtail possums (*Trichosurus vulpecula*). *Epidemiology and Infection* 140, 1036–1047.

Nugent, G., Gortazar, C. and Knowles, G. (2015) The epidemiology of *Mycobacterium bovis* in wild deer and feral pigs and their roles in the establishment and spread of bovine tuberculosis in New Zealand wildlife. *New Zealand Veterinary Journal* 63, 54–67.

OIE (2016) *2016 Terrestrial Animal Health Code.* Chapter 1.3. *Diseases, infections and infestations.* Available at: www.oie.org (accessed 28 February 2017).

O'Reilly, L.M. and Daborn, C.J. (1995) The epidemiology of *Mycobacterium bovis* infections in animals and man: a review. *Tubercle and Lung Disease* 76, 1–46.

Parra, A., Fernandez-Llario, P., Tato, A., Larrasa, J., Garcia, A., *et al.* (2003) Epidemiology of *Mycobacterium bovis* infections of pigs and wild boars using a molecular approach. *Veterinary Microbiology* 97, 123–133.

Pate, M., Svara, T., Gombac, M., Paller, T., Zolnir-Dovc, M., *et al.*, (2006) Outbreak of tuberculosis caused by *Mycobacterium caprae* in a zoological garden. *Journal of Veterinary Medicine Series B* 53, 387–392.

Pérez de Val, B., Grau-Roma, L., Segalés, J., Domingo, M. and Vidal, E. (2014) Mycobacteriosis outbreak caused by *Mycobacterium avium* subsp. *avium* detected through meat inspection in five porcine fattening farms. *Veterinary Record* 174, 96.

Quintas, H., Reis, J., Pires, I. and Alegria, N. (2010) Tuberculosis in goats. *Veterinary Record* 166, 437–438.

Rodriguez, S., Bezos, J., Romero, B., de Juan, L., Alvarez, J., *et al.*, (2011) *Mycobacterium caprae* infection in livestock and wildlife, Spain. *Emerging Infectious Diseases* 17, 532–535.

Sanchez, J., Tomás, L., Ortega, N., Buendía, A.J., del Rio, L., *et al.* (2011) Microscopical and immunological features of tuberculoid granulomata and cavitary pulmonary tuberculosis in naturally infected goats. *Journal of Comparative Pathology* 145, 107–117.

Santos, N., Geraldes, M., Afonso, A., Almeida, V. and Correia-Neves, M. (2010) Diagnosis of tuberculosis in the wild boar (*Sus scrofa*): a comparison of methods applicable to hunter-harvested animals. *PLoS One* 5(9), e12663.

Schiller, I., RayWaters, W., Vordermeier, H.M., Jemmi, T., Welsh, M., *et al.*, (2011) Bovine tuberculosis in Europe from the perspective of an officially tuberculosis free country: trade, surveillance and diagnostics. *Veterinary Microbiology* 151, 153–159.

Schillinger, D. (1987) Kamel (*Camelus dromedarius*). *Sem. Sonderdruck Vet. Labhard Verlag Konstanz*, Germany, 9, 50–53.

Schliesser, T. (1985) Mycobacterium. In: Blobel, H. and Schliesser, T. (eds) *Handbuch der bakteriellen Infektionen bei Tieren*. Gutstav Fischer Verlag, Stuttgart, Germany, pp. 155–313.

Schwartz, H.J. (2013) *Global Development of Camel Populations, Production Systems, and Systems Productivity.* International Camel Conference Bahawalpur, Pakistan. Available at http://amor.cms.hu-berlin.de/~h1981d0z/ (accessed 14 December 2017).

Shanahan, A., Good, M., Duignan, A., Curtin, T. and More, S.J. (2011) Tuberculosis in goats on a farm in Ireland: epidemiological investigation and control. *Veterinary Record* 168, 485.

Tag el Din, M.H. and el Nour Gamaan, I. (1982) Tuberculosis in sheep in the Sudan. *Tropical Animal Health and Production* 14, 26.

Taylor, C., Jahans, K., Palmer, S., Okker, M., Brown, J. and Steer, K. (2006) *Mycobacterium microti* isolated from two pigs. *Veterinary Record* 159, 59–60.

Tirkkonen, T., Pakarinen, J., Moisander, A.-M., Mäkinen, J., Soini, H. and Ali-Vehmas, T. (2007) High genetic relatedness among *Mycobacterium avium* strains isolated from pigs and humans revealed by comparative IS1245 RFLP analysis. *Veterinary Microbiology* 125, 175–181.

van den Heever, L.W. (1984) Tuberculosis in milch goats. *Journal of the South African Veterinary Association* 55, 219–220.

Van Der Burgt, G.M., Drummond, F., Crawshaw, T. and Morris, S. (2013) An outbreak of tuberculosis in Lleyn sheep in the UK associated with clinical signs. *Veterinary Record* 172, 69.

Wardeh, M.F. (2004) Classification of the camel. *Journal of Camel Science* 1, 1–7.

Wernery, U. and Kinne, J. (2012) Tuberculosis in camelids: a review. *Revue Scientifique et Technique (International Office of Epizootics)* 31, 899–906.

Wernery, U. and Rüger-Kaaden, O. (2002) Tuberculosis. *Infectious Diseases in Camelids,* 2nd edn, Blackwell Science, Berlin, Germany, pp. 91–97.

Wernery, U., Kinne, J., Jahans, K.L., Vordermeier, H.M., Esfandiari, J., *et al.* (2007) Tuberculosis outbreak in a dromedary racing herd and rapid serological detection of infected camels. *Veterinary Microbiology* 122, 108–115.

Wernery, U., Kinne, J. and Schuster, R.K. (2014) *Camelid Infectious Disorders.* OIE, Paris.

Wosene, A. (1991) Traditional husbandry practices and major health problems of camels in the Ogaden (Ethiopia). *Nomadic Peoples* 21–30.

Zanardi, G., Boniotti, M.B., Gaffuri, A., Casto, B., Zanoni, M. and Pacciarini, M.L. (2013) Tuberculosis transmission by *Mycobacterium bovis* in a mixed cattle and goat herd. *Research in Veterinary Science* 95, 430–433.

Zubair, R., Khan, A.M.Z. and Sabri, M.A. (2004) Pathology of camel lungs. *Journal of Camel Science* 1, 103–106.

7 Role of Wildlife in the Epidemiology of *Mycobacterium bovis*

Naomi J. Fox,[1] Paul A. Barrow[2] and Michael R. Hutchings[1,]*

[1]SRUC, Edinburgh, UK; [2]The University of Nottingham, Nottingham, UK

Although *Mycobacterium bovis* is classically thought of as a cattle disease, this name belies its diverse range of hosts. *M. bovis* has one of the widest known host ranges of any zoonotic pathogen, and has been isolated from multiple members of a majority of mammal orders, from rodents and insectivores, to primates and carnivores (O'Reilly and Daborn, 1995; Coleman and Cooke, 2001; Delahay *et al.*, 2002).

The presence of wildlife hosts may hinder attempts to eradicate *M. bovis* in livestock. However, the isolation of *M. bovis* from an animal population does not necessarily implicate that species as important in disease outbreaks. A host's role in disease dynamics is dependent on a plethora of interacting factors, including the structure and location of lesions determining levels and routes of excretion, host behaviour, and likelihood of contact (direct and indirect) between infectious and susceptible individuals. Through understanding how these factors vary within and between host species, their potential role in disease maintenance and transmission can be elucidated.

7.1 *M. bovis* Infection in Key Wildlife Hosts

Given the breadth of the known host range of *M. bovis*, we summarize infection in host species thought to play a role in the epidemiology of livestock disease. There is a vast literature on *M. bovis* in these hosts and so here we focus on the sites of infection that result in excretion, which when combined with behaviour, provides potential routes of intra- and inter-specific transmission that drive infection prevalence and persistence. The detailed pathological picture observed in some of these species is covered in Chapter 8.

7.1.1 Possums

Brushtail possums (*Trichosurus vulpecula*) are a key wildlife maintenance host for *M. bovis* in New Zealand. Although prevalence of *M. bovis* in possums is generally low with an average of 5%, they are considered highly susceptible and locally prevalence can reach 60% (Coleman and Cooke, 2001). The average density of brushtail possums in New Zealand is around 1 possum/ha (Nugent *et al.*, 2015a), although uncontrolled populations in diverse forests can exceed 20 possums/ha (Coleman *et al.*, 1980), providing potential for large numbers of infected animals. Disease progression in individuals is rapid with minimal encapsulation, and extensive necrosis within lesions is concomitant with downregulation of macrophage activity, suggesting a failure of innate

---

* Email: Mike.Hutchings@sruc.ac.uk

© CAB International 2018. *Bovine Tuberculosis*
(eds M. Chambers, S. Gordon, F. Olea-Popelka, P. Barrow)

immunity. Possum susceptibility has been demonstrated in experimental infections, where aerosol or intra-tracheal administration of 10–100 colony forming units (CFU) leads to rapid disease progression and death in 8–10 weeks (Aldwell *et al.*, 2003).

In infected possums, lesions are predominantly found in the lungs and peripheral superficial lymph nodes, with bacterial counts reaching 10^7 CFU/g of lung tissue (Nugent *et al.*, 2015a). Fulminating *M. bovis* in naturally infected possums is rapidly lethal, with possums showing clinical signs of tuberculosis dying within an average of 4.7 months (Ramsey and Cowan, 2003). In cachectic individuals in the terminal stage, infections are often generalized, with lesions in the liver, spleen, lungs or kidneys (Jackson *et al.*, 1995). At this stage, purulent material can be discharged from suppurating lesions in superficial lymph nodes (Gortazar *et al.*, 2015).

The mechanisms of infection are unclear, and transmission experiments have shone little light on the process (Corner *et al.*, 2002). However, potential routes can be gleaned from lesion distributions. In possums with tuberculosis, lesions are common in the lungs (Jackson *et al.*, 1995) which, in non-ruminants, is indicative of respiratory transmission. Evidence of respiratory transmission is further compounded by the presence of *M. bovis* from tracheal washings and the discharging fistula of superficial lymph nodes, whereas bacterial isolation from urine and faecal samples from infected possums is rare. Lesions are also common in the peripheral lymph nodes (e.g. the axillary and inguinal) (Jackson *et al.*, 1995), suggestive of percutaneous infection from scratches received during fighting or mating. The presence of tuberculosis lesions in possum mammary glands suggests that pseudovertical transmission via milk may occur (Jackson *et al.*, 1995). It has been suggested that initial infections in possums were from spillover from wild deer, as the first outbreaks in possums coincided with the beginning of commercial deer hunting (circa 1960). It was common practice to leave the heads and offal from hunted deer in the field, leaving possums to scavenge on potentially infected material (Nugent, 2011).

7.1.2 Badgers

Badgers (*Meles meles*) are considered the most important wildlife host of *M. bovis* in the UK and Ireland (Delahay *et al.*, 2002; Phillips *et al.*, 2003), and infected animals have occasionally been isolated from other countries (Bouvier *et al.*, 1962). Badgers are highly social animals and at high densities form social groups that defend distinct territories (Roper *et al.*, 1986). There is wide variation in estimates of *M. bovis* prevalence in badgers, with infections showing high spatial aggregation (Delahay *et al.*, 2000; Woodroffe *et al.*, 2005). At the local population level, there is no consistent correlation between badger density and TB prevalence (Vicente *et al.*, 2007a; Delahay *et al.*, 2013), although the incidence of new cases does correlate with the frequency of intergroup movements (Vicente *et al.*, 2007a).

The principal site of infection in badgers is the lower respiratory tract, with a high frequency of lung infections and high prevalence of pulmonary lesions (Gallagher and Nelson, 1979; Gallagher and Clifton-Hadley, 2000; Gavier-Widen *et al.*, 2001; Jenkins *et al.*, 2007a). This suggests that inhalation of infectious aerosol particles and infection by the respiratory route is the most likely route of transmission (Gavier-Widen *et al.*, 2001; Jenkins *et al.*, 2007a). In contrast, infection via the gastrointestinal tract is rare, possibly due to the highly acidic conditions (Vandal *et al.*, 2009). Bacilli excreted in badger urine, sputum, faeces and abscess pus are thought to contaminate the environment (Gallagher *et al.*, 1976; Gallagher and Clifton-Hadley, 2000). Of the excreta, urine from animals with infected kidneys has the highest numbers of bacilli at 250×10^3 CFU/ml urine (Gallagher and Clifton-Hadley, 2000).

As competent hosts, the majority of infections in badgers are latent, lesions are often resolved, and even complete elimination of *M. bovis* infection has been observed (Gallagher *et al.*, 1998). Consequently, badgers can survive infection for several years, excreting bacteria while maintaining social interactions (Cheeseman *et al.*, 1989). Badgers of all ages are susceptible; however, infection risk increases with age (Jenkins *et al.*, 2007a). Males have a higher prevalence than females, which is attributed to behavioural differences, with the males involved in aggressive behaviour associated with territorial defence (Gallagher and Clifton-Hadley, 2000). Following detection of bacterial excretion, males succumb to infection sooner than infected females (Graham et al., 2013; Tomlinson et al., 2013).

Badgers live in social groups typically comprised of three to ten individuals (Vicente et al., 2007a), and their behaviour strongly influences M. bovis transmission. Aerosol transmission is proximity dependent, and groups living with communal use of underground chambers (within setts) provides the opportunity for disease spread. Scent plays a key role in badger communication and all adult badgers scent mark territories, by defaecation, urination and anal and sub-caudal excretion, including at latrine sites (Neal, 1986). Bite wounds are commonly obtained during territorial defence and mating behaviours, especially in males (Gallagher and Nelson, 1979; Cheeseman et al., 1989). Environmental contamination from latrine use and inoculation from biting behaviours provide potential intra-specific transmission routes. To further complicate the relationship between badger behaviour and transmission, M. bovis culture-positive badgers show increased ranging behaviour compared to test-negative individuals (Garnett et al., 2005), are more socially isolated within their own groups, and display an increase in intergroup contacts (Weber et al., 2013).

7.1.3 Wild boar and feral pigs

High prevalences of M. bovis infection have been recorded in wild suid populations. In Spain, for example, where wild boar populations densities can reach 90 individuals per km^2 (Acevedo et al., 2007), M. bovis prevalence up to 100% has been recorded ($n=14$) (Vicente et al., 2006). There is geographic variation in M. bovis levels, for example prevalence values of 0–40% have been recorded in Australia, where densities are typically below 11 individuals per km^2 (Naranjo et al., 2008).

No sex differences in prevalence have been found, but the probability of infection does increase with age (Vicente et al., 2013) and roles in transmission are likely to be age dependent. Martín-Hernando et al. (2007) found a high proportion of juveniles had severe lesions in multiple anatomical areas, and the potential to excrete mycobacteria by several routes. As these are the age groups when dispersion is at a maximum, they have the potential to contribute to spatial spread. In contrast, piglets are thought to play a limited role in transmission, as in experimental studies transmission between infected and uninfected piglets is rare (Gortazar et al., 2015). Piglets have the potential to acquire infection by pseudovertical transmission, as tuberculous lesions have been found in the mammary glands of sows (Martín-Hernando et al., 2007). The distribution of tuberculous lesions vary across boar populations with high M. bovis prevalence; it is likely that individuals with generalized infection and high lesion scores play a disproportionate role in initiating new infections (Martín-Hernando et al., 2007).

It is possible that infections occur through both respiratory and food-borne routes, as wild boar have been found with tuberculous lesions only in the thoracic region (usually bronchial lymph nodes) or with only abdominal lesions (usually mesenteric lymph nodes) (Martín-Hernando et al., 2007). In addition to the geographical variation in disease prevalence, there is also spatial variation in disease progression. For example, lesions in the thoracic region are displayed in almost 50% of M. bovis-infected wild boar in Mediterranean Spain (Martín-Hernando et al., 2007), while fewer than 10% of infected wild boar in Atlantic Spain consistently present thoracic lesions (Muñoz-Mendoza et al., 2013). In contrast, the tuberculous lesions in feral pigs in New Zealand are mainly found in the head, in association with the lymph nodes (Nugent, 2011). Such variation in pathogenesis is indicative of differing infection sources.

Suids are implicated as spreaders of M. bovis (Martín-Hernando et al., 2007; Naranjo et al., 2008). There is potential for mycobacteria to be excreted in the saliva as wild boar have a high proportion of tuberculous lesions in mandibular lymph nodes and tonsils, and mycobacteria have been identified in the excretory ducts of the mandibular salivary glands of wild boar (Martín-Hernando et al., 2007). Given the distribution of lesions, respiratory infection from direct social contacts is possible as social family groups roam and forage together (Vicente et al., 2013). In contrast, transmission through urine is unlikely, as neither lesions nor mycobacteria have been found in wild boar kidneys (Naranjo et al., 2008). Numerous suid behaviours promote ingestion and inhalation of M. bovis bacilli, including their broad dietary spectrum (Dondo et al., 2007) and penchant for rooting and wallowing in muddy water, where M. bovis can survive outside the host (Young et al., 2005). Wild boar also have a predilection for carrion consumption, and it is likely that scavenging carrion and hunted animal remains left in the field plays an important role in transmission (Vicente et al., 2007b).

7.1.4 Deer

Consistent with the broad host range, M. bovis infection has been reported in at least 14 species of deer, including red deer (Cervus elaphus), North American elk (Cervus elaphus nelsoni), tule elk (Cervus elaphus nannodes), sika deer (Cervus nippon), sambar deer (Cervus unicolor swinhoei), fallow deer (Dama dama), white-tailed deer (Odocoileus virginianus), mule deer (Odocoileus hemionus), black-tailed deer (Odocoileus hemionus columbianus), axis deer (Axis axis), roe deer (Capreolus capreolus), Chinese muntjac deer (Muntiacus reevesi), reindeer (Rangifer tarandus) and moose (Alces alces) (Palmer et al., 2015). Severe outbreaks in wild deer are uncommon, and less frequent than in captive deer (Griffin and Buchan, 1994; Hunter, 1996).

The majority of data on wild deer hosts are from white-tailed deer in North America as they are believed to play an important role in disease maintenance, especially in areas of Michigan where M. bovis is endemic in the white-tailed deer population (Conner et al., 2008). M. bovis infection in deer has also been studied widely in other regions, including the UK (Delahay et al., 2007), Spain (Vicente et al., 2006; Martín-Hernando et al., 2010) and New Zealand (Griffin and Buchan, 1994; Lugton et al., 1998).

Prevalence in endemic deer populations can remain low (Delahay et al., 2007; O'Brien et al., 2011) and is often highly clustered with likelihood of infection increasing with age (O'Brien et al., 2006). Infections are often subacute and chronic, with infected hosts able to survive for over a decade (Nugent, 2011). However, some die soon after contracting the infection with those showing clinical signs (e.g. weight loss, rough coat, poor body condition) harbouring a grave prognosis (Griffin and Buchan, 1994). When tuberculous lesions are present, the most common sites are the lungs, the retropharyngeal lymph nodes and thoracic lymph nodes (Delahay et al., 2002). These lesion locations suggest the respiratory route is the primary route of infection, although cutaneous infection through open wounds is also possible. While lymphadenitis is often exhibited in infected deer, with the involvement of at least one of the lymph nodes, generalized disease in other organs can also occur (Griffin and Buchan, 1994; Lugton et al., 1998; Griffin and Mackintosh, 2000). For example, in parts of Spain generalized disease has been observed in over 50% of cases in some M. bovis outbreaks in red and fallow deer (Vicente et al., 2006; Martín-Hernando et al., 2010), and around one-third of naturally infected white-tailed deer display lesions in the head and thorax (Fitzgerald and Kaneene, 2013). In New Zealand's wild deer population, generalized M. bovis is relatively uncommon, with no visible lesions in 25% of culture-positive deer (Lugton et al., 1998). There is potential for onward transmission to other hosts as deer have been found with large, numerous and poorly encapsulated granulomas containing high concentrations of bacilli, and formation of discharging abscesses associated with the enlargement of superficial lymph nodes (Johnson et al., 2008). This is supported by evidence that naïve deer kept in direct contact with experimentally infected deer can contract M. bovis (Palmer et al., 2001). There remains a potential for transmission between wild and farmed deer although contact between the two is thought to be a rare event.

Disease distribution can be affected by cervid social structures. In white-tailed deer, M. bovis has a heterogeneous distribution as females are segregated in matrilineal groups with high site fidelity, and infection levels are high in some groups and low in others. Higher *M. bovis* prevalence is found in males, which have larger home ranges and make contact with more unrelated deer (Cosgrove *et al.*, 2012). There is a positive correlation between deer density and disease prevalence (Hickling, 2002), with a decrease in disease prevalence in both white-tailed deer and elk following population reductions (Shury and Bergeson, 2011). As transmission is density dependent it is affected by population management measures, with supplemental feeding leading to an overall increase in *M. bovis* transmission and more spatially homogenous disease distribution. The transmission implications of supplemental feeding have been highlighted by Palmer *et al.* (2004a), who demonstrated indirect experimental *M. bovis* infection in deer through the sharing of feed.

7.2 Multi-Host Complexes and the Ecology of *M. bovis* Dynamics and Persistence

The previous section discussed *M. bovis* infection in key host species. For each species, transmission is dependent on the pathology of infection, excretion potential, the minimum infective dose and interactions between infected and susceptible individuals. However, numerous host species often co-exist, and maintenance of *M. bovis* at the system level is dependent on multi-species complexes. On a simplistic level, hosts are often described as either maintenance hosts or spillover hosts. Maintenance hosts can maintain infection in a given area via intra-specific routes of transmission, without any inter-specific transmission (domestic or wild). In contrast, persistence of infection in spillover hosts requires continuous inter-specific transmission. Although both maintenance and spillover hosts can act as disease vectors, it is generally considered that the *M. bovis* hosts with greatest implications for disease control are maintenance hosts with high potential to transmit to other species. However, it is at least theoretically possible for host communities comprised of only spillover species to maintain infection. In such cases, control applied to any single species is likely to exaggerate their perceived role in maintaining the infection.

The role of maintenance hosts is typified in New Zealand's brushtail possums, where *M. bovis* can persist in possum populations that are completely isolated from infected livestock (Morris and Pfeiffer, 1995). In these areas, epidemiology suggests that pigs, ferrets and deer are spillover hosts (Morris and Pfeiffer, 1995; Ragg *et al.*, 1995; Jackson, 2002). The predominance of tuberculous lesions in the head and gastrointestinal tract of sympatric scavengers in New Zealand (e.g. wild pigs and ferrets) suggests that such wildlife are infected through scavenging carcasses of infected possums (Ragg *et al.*, 1995; Coleman and Cooke, 2001). The role of deer as spillover hosts is supported by evidence that *M. bovis* in deer was eradicated in areas where possum population control was carried out, but levels in deer were maintained in corresponding areas where possum numbers were not reduced (Palmer *et al.*, 2015). Captive deer have been observed licking and biting moribund *M. bovis*-infected possums (Sauter and Morris, 1995), demonstrating a potential transmission route.

The role of sympatric wildlife species in disease transmission and maintenance varies geographically with land use, ecology and habitat, and consequent host behaviours and population densities. While deer are considered spillover hosts in New Zealand, where hunting pressure is high and population densities are low, in Michigan, USA, self-sustaining outbreaks in wild cervid populations have been reported (O'Brien *et al.*, 2002). Their role in maintenance and transmission is partly due to their high population density, with concentrations of deer at artificial feeding sites that can facilitate transmission (O'Brien *et al.*, 2011). As a consequence of density dependent transmission, control efforts focus on population reduction.

The status of suids as hosts of *M. bovis* also varies dramatically, and is dependent on density, levels of infection in sympatric species, dispersion and ecological factors. The highest prevalences of *M. bovis* in wild boar are found in regions with highest population densities, which are usually artificially maintained through intensive game management (i.e. supplementary feeding and watering, translocating and fencing). In areas of high suid population density, intra-specific transmission can be sufficient for *M. bovis* to be independently maintained without spillover from other species (Naranjo et al., 2008). This is supported by evidence from estates fenced off from other domestic livestock for over two decades, where *M. bovis* has been found circulating in wild ungulates (Gortazar et al., 2005). Areas where wild boar are believed to act as maintenance hosts include the Mediterranean regions of south-western Spain and south-eastern Portugal. In such regions, reductions in numbers of wild boar have led to declines in *M. bovis* levels in sympatric cattle and deer (Boadella et al., 2012; García-Jiménez et al., 2013). In contrast, intra-specific transmission is low in areas with low pig population densities, and outside of the afore-mentioned Mediterranean regions feral pigs are considered to be dead-end hosts. However, spillover from other host species can be frequent. In areas with low pig population densities but high levels of infection in sympatric wildlife, prevalence in feral pigs can reach 100%, yet prevalence in these pigs rapidly declines following implementation of intensive lethal control targeted at other host species (e.g. brushtail possums in New Zealand [Nugent et al., 2015b] and bovids in Australia [McInerney et al., 1995; Corner, 2006]). In such regions, suids are useful sentinel hosts for determining *M. bovis* presence in target areas, due to their large home range size and omnivorous proclivity for scavenging carcasses of infected hosts (Nugent et al., 2002). This example highlights the importance of understanding the role of different host species in infection maintenance, rather than merely targeting those showing high disease prevalence.

The role of individual species in multi-host systems is complex, and not simply density dependent. Although high density maintenance hosts play a driving role in disease dynamics, low-density spillover hosts are an important component of host communities. Spillover species with large home ranges and long-lived, sub-clinical infections can act as spatial and temporal vectors, spilling back *M. bovis* to true maintenance hosts as their expansive ranges overlap with naïve populations, or as maintenance host densities recover following population reduction. Wild deer provide an example of this phenomenon. Outside of the US, the main role of deer in disease maintenance is attributed to their longevity and large home ranges (Nugent et al., 2015a). After *M. bovis* has been eliminated in its true maintenance hosts through control of short-lived carriers (e.g. possums), subclinically infected deer can act as temporal vectors surviving for many years and carrying *M. bovis*. They can then spill infection back to more susceptible yet short-lived host species as populations of these hosts recover rapidly after culling efforts. The large home ranges of wild deer also provide a mechanism for *M. bovis* to be translocated to new areas, prior to spillback into more common host species. If this phenomenon is known to be present, it is straightforward to take into account in the development of control strategies.

In multi-host systems it is often difficult to isolate the role of individual species. Such complexity is epitomized in the species-rich reserves of Southern Africa. *M. bovis* has been found in 16 different species in Southern Africa, with evidence of inter- and intra-species transmission (Hlokwe et al., 2014). There is evidence that *M. bovis* distribution is increasing, and the number of known host species is on the rise (Hlokwe et al., 2014). Thought to be first introduced into the national parks by cattle in nearby farms, African buffalo are now thought to be the primary maintenance hosts of *M. bovis*, capable of retaining it in ecosystems in the absence of domestic cattle (Michel et al., 2006). However, other species (e.g. greater kudu and lechwe) have also been shown to act as maintenance hosts (Michel et al., 2006; Mwacalimba et al., 2013). *M. bovis* is also found in predator species, and high prevalences are found in lion prides (Keet et al., 2010). As predators preferentially target weak and debilitated prey, wild ungulates succumbing to clinical infection are clear targets for predation, and large predators and scavenging omnivores are exposed to high quantities of infectious tissue. Due to the high species richness and inter-species exposure levels it has not been possible to determine whether such species (e.g. lions) can be maintenance hosts, and the true role of individual species in the multi-faceted, multi-host complex is not fully understood.

As has been demonstrated in New Zealand, culling of wildlife hosts can be an effective way of controlling *M. bovis*. However, possums are an alien species in New Zealand and a similar control approach is not feasible if culling could threaten the survival of protected and endangered indigenous species. Southern African national parks have a responsibility to protect a number of the species that host *M. bovis*, complicating control options. Due to the deleterious impact of culling, control strategies have focused on preventing the movement of infected wildlife to curtail further spread. However, if *M. bovis* diagnosis in wildlife increases movement restrictions, endemic areas (e.g. Kruger National Park) can become conservation islands. As movement of endangered species between national parks becomes restricted, conservation efforts can suffer from the limited exchange of genetic resources (Michel *et al.*, 2006). Such dilemmas in how to control *M. bovis* in species-rich ecosystems of high conservation importance are further complicated by the paucity of understanding on the true roles that each host species play. However, control in Southern Africa remains critical as *M. bovis* threatens the survival of endangered species (Michel *et al.*, 2006) and poses a zoonotic risk, especially in HIV-endemic communities surrounding conservation areas (Hlokwe *et al.*, 2014).

7.3 Transmission at the Livestock–Wildlife Interface

Given the diversity in host species and transmission routes, transmission of *M. bovis* at the livestock–wildlife interface is perhaps unsurprising. However, the role of wildlife in the epidemiology of livestock disease can be controversial. There are many studies that quantify wildlife–livestock interactions, both direct (e.g. Bohm *et al.*, 2009) and indirect (e.g. Hutchings and Harris, 1997), that may represent routes of *M. bovis* transmission. However, there is often little if any direct evidence of transmission, let alone quantification of the rates of transmission. The best evidence supporting the role of wildlife in the epidemiology of *M. bovis* in livestock comes from the results of disease control actions.

Local eradication of *M. bovis* in cattle and national TB-free status has been achieved following the implementation of disease control methods applied to livestock species alone (More *et al.*, 2015; and see Chapter 14). These successes have resulted from national control strategies based on test-and-cull aligned with livestock movement restrictions and implemented using the skin test (Radunz, 2006; More *et al.*, 2015; and see Chapter 11). Reduced performance and failure of this strategy is associated with rich *M. bovis* host communities and known wildlife maintenance hosts (Bessell *et al.*, 2012; Hardstaff *et al.*, 2014).

The dynamic of wildlife–livestock transmission varies within and between ecosystems, and is dependent on a multitude of factors including species composition, densities, contact rates, behaviours, susceptibility, pathology and excretion. Wildlife are thought to play an important role in livestock *M. bovis* outbreaks in New Zealand, where contact with infected possums (both direct and indirect) is believed to be a driving factor in a majority of *M. bovis* breakdowns in livestock (Hutchings *et al.*, 2013). In the advanced stages of infection, possums can become debilitated, unable to climb and wander about in daylight, leaving them exposed to contact with inquisitive livestock (Paterson and Morris, 1995). Inter-species transmission is thought to occur when dead or terminally ill possums are inquisitively licked or sniffed by livestock (Sauter and Morris, 1995). Consequently, lethal control of possum populations has been implemented, at a cost of US$40million per year (since 1994). This has contributed to the >95% reduction in *M. bovis*-infected cattle and managed deer herds in New Zealand (Buddle *et al.*, 2015). While it is clear that that the control strategy was a success, the contribution of possum control cannot be isolated as livestock testing and movement restrictions were also in place.

In the UK and Ireland, badgers are the wildlife species thought to play the biggest role in the epidemiology of livestock disease, with bi-directional transmission between badgers and cattle (Jenkins *et al.*, 2007b). Strain typing of isolates from badgers and cattle populations has revealed close linkages in the spatial distribution of *M. bovis* strain types in the two host species (Olea-Popelka *et al.*, 2005; Woodroffe *et al.*, 2005). This finding that spatially overlapping cattle and badger populations have similar *M. bovis* strains is consistent with inter-specific transmission, or both hosts being infected from a common source. Badgers often forage for food items (such as earthworms) on pasture used by cattle, and cattle graze badger latrines and other sites contaminated with urine, faeces or infected pus from bite wounds and scent marks

(Hutchings and Harris, 1997). Badgers will also enter farm buildings to forage on livestock feed (Garnett et al., 2002; Tolhurst et al., 2009), and proximity contact between badgers and cattle is more frequent when cattle are housed than when they are grazing (Tolhurst et al., 2009). Such behaviours provide potential for direct (via aerosols) and indirect (via environmental contamination) transmission. As with possums, M. bovis infection can alter badger behaviour, and thus transmission risk, as terminally ill badgers lose their fear of cattle and direct contact rates can increase (Gavier-Widen et al., 2001; Corner, 2006).

Badgers are a legally protected species in the UK and the risk of transmission of M. bovis from badgers to cattle remains controversial. With the national control strategy failing and M. bovis spreading and re-emerging in areas where infection in cattle had previously been eradicated, the UK undertook the Randomised Badger Culling Trial (RBCT). With a budget of £50 million, 10-year timeframe and covering 3000 km^2 (McDonald et al., 2008), the RBCT is one of the largest ever controlled veterinary epidemiology field experiments in UK history. The aim of the RBCT was to quantify the impact of culling badgers on the number of M. bovis herd breakdowns in cattle (Bourne, 2007). Somewhat counter-intuitively, the RBCT concluded that while badgers do play a role in M. bovis outbreaks in cattle, in some cases the incidence in cattle could be increased by culling of badgers (McDonald et al., 2008). In the central core of areas where badgers were proactively culled, the incidence of M. bovis in cattle decreased, whereas the incidence increased at the edge of these culled areas and increased if patchy reactive culling of badgers was applied following M. bovis breakdowns in cattle herds (Donnelly et al., 2006). The inefficiency of culling is indicative of a perturbation effect, where culling induces perturbations in the social organization of badgers, disrupting territories, enhancing movement and increasing badger-to-badger, and badger-to-cattle transmission (McDonald et al., 2008; Prentice et al., 2014). The perturbation effect is potentially amplified in disease systems with heterogeneous distributions of infection in highly structured host populations (Prentice et al., 2014). M. bovis is highly clustered in individual badger social groups (Delahay et al., 2000). Incomplete population reduction may drive relatively rapid increases in prevalence by increasing contact between dispersing infected animals and susceptible populations. Although badger–cattle transmission mechanisms remain poorly understood, the large scale and controlled nature of the RBCT experiment is the best available evidence that badgers can play a role in the epidemiology of M. bovis in livestock. Interestingly, it was the incomplete nature of the badger population reduction that enabled the results of the RBCT, as removing all the badgers would by definition remove the badger-to-cattle transmission.

In the USA, deer are believed to play a role in M. bovis outbreaks in cattle, and evidence of spillback from deer to cattle has necessitated implementation of control strategies (Palmer et al., 2004b). Deer frequently visit feeding areas in cattle farms and evidence of this has been recorded in radio collared white-tailed deer in Michigan (Berentsen et al., 2013). However, transmission between cattle and deer is thought to be indirect via shared resources, as direct contacts between the two are rare. Due to the potential of deer to act as maintenance hosts in the US, they have been a target of population reduction. In contrast to badgers, reducing deer populations in the US has been shown to reduce M. bovis incidence with no sign of a perturbation effect. As these deer exhibit a high degree of site fidelity, occupancy of overlapping home ranges and lack territorial defence behaviour, culling is unlikely to alter home ranges of adjacent deer groups and perturbation effects are not observed (Palmer et al., 2015).

Before employing disease control based on population reduction, it is important to understand the idiosyncrasies of different host populations. However, these idiosyncrasies are often unknown. Despite the investment of extensive resources in trying to understand the role of wildlife in livestock M. bovis outbreaks, livestock–wildlife transmission dynamics remain poorly understood. However, the observations that culling wildlife affects M. bovis incidence in cattle further reiterates that disease processes act at the host community and ecosystem level rather than on isolated species.

7.4 Conclusions

M. bovis has one of the widest host ranges of any known zoonotic pathogen (O'Reilly and Daborn, 1995). Compounding the complexity of multi-species transmission dynamics is the inter- and intra-species variation in pathology, excretion potential, susceptibility, and interactions between infected and susceptible individuals. With a multitude of hosts and profusion of potential transmission mechanisms, resultant patterns of transmission within ecosystems are complex and remain poorly understood. Characterization of a species' role as a maintenance or spillover host is not static – it varies with a plethora of local factors. For example, as host status is often density dependent, classifications as maintenance or spillover are likely to be indistinct as densities fluctuate with time, space and management. Consequently, the epidemiology of *M. bovis* across different host communities can be seen as highly variable, with potentially unique conditions underlying its emergence and persistence in each ecosystem. That wild boar are considered spillover hosts in North-West Italy (Dondo *et al.*, 2007) but are considered as maintenance hosts in parts of Spain (Naranjo *et al.*, 2008) reflects this variability. Similarly, deer are thought to be spillover hosts in New Zealand, yet they are considered as true maintenance hosts in Michigan. Such variations have repercussions for control and surveillance strategies, which should be tailored to fit the host community composition and structure in each region. Although it remains primarily a disease of cattle there is huge potential for wildlife to play a role in the epidemiology of *M. bovis* in livestock. Perhaps the best evidence of this is that disease control in livestock is more difficult in areas with wildlife hosts.

References

Acevedo, P., Vicente, J., Höfle, U., Cassinello, J., Ruiz-Fons, F., *et al.* (2007) Estimation of European wild boar relative abundance and aggregation: a novel method in epidemiological risk assessment. *Epidemiology and Infection* 135(3), 519–527.

Aldwell, F.E., Keen, D.L., Parlane, N.A., Skinner, M.A, de Lisle, G.W., *et al.* (2003) Oral vaccination with *Mycobacterium bovis* BCG in a lipid formulation induces resistance to pulmonary tuberculosis in brushtail possums. *Vaccine* 22, 70–76.

Berentsen, A.R., Miller, R.S., Misiewicz, R., Malmberg, J.L. and Dunbar, M.R. (2013) Characteristics of white-tailed deer visits to cattle farms: Implications for disease transmission at the wildlife-livestock interface. *European Journal of Wildlife Research* 60, 161–170.

Bessell, P.R., Orton, R., White, P.C.L., Hutchings, M.R. and Kao R.R. (2012) Risk factors for bovine tuberculosis at the national level in Great Britain. *BMC Veterinary Research* 8, 51.

Boadella, M., Vicente, J., Ruiz-Fons, F., de la Fuente, J. and Gortazar, C. (2012) Effects of culling Eurasian wild boar on the prevalence of *Mycobacterium bovis* and Aujeszky's disease virus. *Preventive Veterinary Medicine* 107(3–4), 214–221.

Bohm, M., Hutchings, M.R. and White, P.C.L. (2009) Contact networks in a wildlife–livestock host community: identifying high-risk individuals in the transmission of bovine TB among badgers and cattle. *PLOS One* 4(4), e5016.

Bourne, J. (2007) Bovine TB: The scientific evidence. *Final Report of the Independent Scientific Group on Cattle TB Presented*. Available at: www.bovinetb.info/docs/final_report.pdf (accessed 20 December 2017).

Bouvier, G., Burgisser, H. and Schneider, P.A. (1962) Observations sur les maladies du gibier et des animaux sauvages faites en 1959 et 1960. *Schweizer Archiv fur Tierheilkunde* 104, 440–450.

Buddle, B.M., de Lisle, G.W. and Corner, L.A.L. (2015) Australian brushtail possum: a highly susceptible host for *Mycobacterium bovis*. In: Makundan, H., Chambers, M., Waters, R. and Larsen, M. (eds) *Tuberculosis, Leprosy and Mycobacterial Diseases of Man and Animals: the Many Hosts of Mycobacteria*. CAB International, Wallingford, UK, pp. 325–333.

Cheeseman, C.L., Wilesmith, J.W. and Stuart, F.A. (1989) Tuberculosis: the disease and its epidemiology in the badger, a review. *Epidemiology and Infection* 103, 113–125.

Coleman, J.D. and Cooke, M.M. (2001) *Mycobacterium bovis* infection in wildlife in New Zealand. *Tuberculosis* 81, 191–202.

Coleman, J.D., Gillman, A. and Green, W.Q. (1980) Forest patterns and possum densities within podocarp/mixed hardwood forests on Mt Bryan O'Lynn, Westland. *New Zealand Journal of Ecology* 3, 69–84.

Conner, M.M., Ebinger, M.R., Blanchong, J.A. and Cross, P.C. (2008) Infectious disease in cervids of North America: Data, models, and management challenges. *Annals of the New York Academy of Sciences* 1134, 146–172.

Corner, L.A.L. (2006) The role of wild animal populations in the epidemiology of tuberculosis in domestic animals: how to assess the risk. *Veterinary Microbiology* 112(2–4), 303–312.

Corner, L.A.L., Pfeiffer, D.U., de Lisle, G.W., Morris, R.W. and Buddle B.M. (2002) Natural transmission of *Mycobacterium bovis* infection in captive brushtail possums (*Trichosurus vulpecula*). *New Zealand Veterinary Journal* 50, 154–162.

Cosgrove, M.K. Campa, H., Ramsey, D.S.L., Schmitt, S.M. and O'Brien, D.J. (2012) Modeling vaccination and targeted removal of white-tailed deer in Michigan for bovine tuberculosis control. *Wildlife Society Bulletin* 36, 676–684.

Delahay, R.J., Langton, S., Smith, G.C., Clifton-Hadley, R.S. and Cheeseman, C.L. (2000) The spatio-temporal distribution of *Mycobacterium bovis* (bovine tuberculosis) infection in a high-density badger population. *Journal of Animal Ecology* 69(3), 428–441.

Delahay, R.J., De Leeuw, A.N.S., Barlow, A.M., Clifton-Hadley, R.S. and Cheeseman, C.I. (2002) The status of *Mycobacterium bovis* infection in UK wild mammals: A review. *The Veterinary Journal* 164(2), 90–105.

Delahay, R.J., Smith, G.C., Barlow, A.M., Walker, N., Harris, A., et al. (2007) Bovine tuberculosis infection in wild mammals in the south-west region of England: a survey of prevalence and a semi-quantitative assessment of the relative risks to cattle. *The Veterinary Journal* 173, 287–301.

Delahay, R., Walker, N., Smith, G.S., Wilkinson, D., Clifton-Hadley, R.S., et al. (2013) Long-term temporal trends and estimated transmission rates for *Mycobacterium bovis* infection in an undisturbed high-density badger (*Meles meles*) population. *Epidemiology and Infection* 141, 1445–1456.

Dondo, A., Zoppi, S., Rossi, F., Chiavacci, L., Barbaro, A., et al. (2007) Mycobacteriosis in wild boar: results of 2000–2006 activity in north-western Italy. *Epidemiology et sante Animal* 51, 35–42.

Donnelly, C.A., Woodroffe, R., Cox, D.R., Bourne, J., Cheeseman, C.L., et al. (2006) Positive and negative effects of widespread badger culling on tuberculosis in cattle. *Nature* 439, 843–846.

Fitzgerald, S.D. and Kaneene, J.B. (2013) Wildlife reservoirs of bovine tuberculosis worldwide: hosts, pathology, surveillance, and control. *Veterinary Pathology* 50(3), 488–499.

Gallagher, J. and Clifton-Hadley, R.S. (2000) Tuberculosis in badgers; a review of the disease and its significance for other animals. *Research in Veterinary Science* 69, 203–217.

Gallagher, J. and Nelson, J. (1979) Cause of ill health and natural death in badgers in Gloucestershire. *The Veterinary Record* 105, 546–551.

Gallagher, J., Muirhead, R.H. and Burn, K.J. (1976) Tuberculosis in wild badgers (*Meles meles*) in Gloucerstershire: pathology. *The Veterinary Record* 98, 9–14.

Gallagher, J., Monies, R., Gavier-Widen, M. and Rule, B. (1998) Role of infected, non-diseased badgers in the pathogenesis of tuberculosis in the badger. *The Veterinary Record* 142, 710–714.

García-Jiménez, W.L., Fernandez-Llario, P., Benítez-Medina, J.M., Cerrato, R., Cuesta, J., et al. (2013) Reducing Eurasian wild boar (*Sus scrofa*) population density as a measure for bovine tuberculosis control: Effects in wild boar and a sympatric fallow deer (*Dama dama*) population in Central Spain. *Preventive Veterinary Medicine* 110, 435–446.

Garnett, B.T., Delahay, R.J. and Roper, T.J. (2002) Use of cattle farm resources by badgers (*Meles meles*) and risk of bovine tuberculosis (*Mycobacterium bovis*) transmission to cattle. *Proceedings of the Royal Society B* 269, 1487–1491.

Garnett, B.T., Delahay, R.J. and Roper, T.J. (2005) Ranging behaviour of European badgers (*Meles meles*) in relation to bovine tuberculosis (*Mycobacterium bovis*) infection. *Applied Animal Behaviour Science* 94, 331–340.

Gavier-Widen, D., Chambers, M.A., Palmer, N., Newell, D.G. and Hewinson, R.G. (2001) Pathology of natural *Mycobacterium bovis* infection in European badgers (*Meles meles*) and its relationship with bacterial excretion. *Veterinary Record* 148, 299–304.

Gortazar, C., Vicente, J., Samper, S., Garrido, J.M. and Fernandez-de-Mera, I. (2005) Molecular characterization of *Mycobacterium tuberculosis* complex isolates from wild ungulates in south-central Spain. *Veterinary Research* 36, 43–52.

Gortazar, C., Vicente, J., de la Fuente, J., Nugent, G. and Nol, P. (2015) Tuberculosis in pigs and wild boar. In: Mukundan, H., Chambers, M., Waters, R. and Larsen, M. (eds). *Tuberculosis, Leprosy and Mycobacterial Diseases of Man and Animals: The Many Hosts of Mycobacteria*. CAB International, Wallingford, UK, pp. 313–324.

Graham, J., Smith, G.C., Delahay, R.H., Bailey, T., McDonald, R.A., *et al.* (2013) Multi-state modelling reveals sex-dependent transmission, progression and severity of tuberculosis in wild badgers. *Epidemiology and Infection* 141, 1429–1436.

Griffin, J.F.T. and Buchan, G.S. (1994) Etiology, pathogenesis and diagnosis of *Mycobacterium bovis* in deer. *Veterinary Microbiology* 40, 193–205.

Griffin, J.F.T. and Mackintosh, C.G. (2000) Tuberculosis in deer: perceptions, problems and progress. *Veterinary Journal* 160, 202–219.

Hardstaff, J.L., Marion, G., Hutchings, M.R. and White, P.C.L. (2014) Evaluating the tuberculosis hazard posed to cattle from wildlife across Europe. *Research in Veterinary Science* 97, S86–S93.

Hickling, G.J. (2002) Dynamics of bovine tuberculosis in white-tailed deer in Michigan. *Wildlife Division Report No. 3363*. Michigan Department of Natural Resources Wildlife Division, Michigan.

Hlokwe, T.M., van Helden, P. and Michel, A.L. (2014) Evidence of increasing intra and inter-species transmission of *Mycobacterium bovis* in South Africa: are we losing the battle? *Preventive Veterinary Medicine* 115, 10–17.

Hunter, D.L. (1996) Tuberculosis in free-ranging, semi free-ranging and captive cervids. *Revue scientifique et technique-Office International Epizootics* 15(1), 171–181.

Hutchings, M.R. and Harris, S. (1997) Effects of farm management practices on cattle grazing behaviour and the potential for transmission of bovine tuberculosis from badgers to cattle. *The Veterinary Journal* 153(2), 149–162.

Hutchings, S.A., Hancox, N. and Livingstone, P.G. (2013) A strategic approach to eradication of bovine TB from wildlife in New Zealand. *Transboundary and Emerging Diseases* 60, 85–91.

Jackson, R. (2002) The role of wildlife in *Mycobacterium bovis* infection of livestock in New Zealand. *New Zealand Veterinary Journal* 50, 49–52.

Jackson, R., Cook, M.M., Coleman, J.D. and Morris, R.S. (1995) Naturally occurring tuberculosis caused by *Mycobacterium bovis* in brushtail possums (*Trichosurus vulpecula*). I. An epidemiological analysis of lesion distribution. *New Zealand Veterinary Journal* 43, 306–314.

Jenkins, H.E., Morrison, W.I., Cox, D.R., Donnelly, C.A., Johnstone, W.T., *et al.* (2007a) The prevalence, distribution and severity of detectable pathological lesions in badgers naturally infected with *Mycobacterium bovis*. *Epidemiology and Infection* 136, 1350–1361.

Jenkins, H.E., Woodroffe, R., Donnelly, C.A., Cox, D.R., Johnston, W.T., *et al.* (2007b) Effects of culling on spatial associations of *Mycobacterium bovis* infections in badgers and cattle. *Journal of Applied Ecology* 44, 897–908.

Johnson, L.K., Liebana, E., Nunz, A., Spencer, Y., Clifton-Hadley, R., *et al.* (2008) Histological observations of bovine tuberculosis in lung and lymph node tissues from British deer. *Veterinary Journal* 175(3), 409–412.

Keet, D.F., Michel, A.L., Bengis, R.G., Becker, P., van Dyk, D.S., *et al.* (2010) Intradermal tuberculin testing of wild African lions (*Panthera leo*) naturally exposed to infection with *Mycobacterium bovis*. *Veterinary Microbiology* 144(3–4), 384–391.

Lugton, I.W., Wilson, P.R., Morris, R.S. and Nugent, G. (1998) Epidemiology and pathogenesis of *Mycobacterium bovis* infection of red deer (*Cervus elaphus*) in New Zealand. *New Zealand Veterinary Journal* 46, 147–156.

Martín-Hernando, M.P., Höfle, U., Vicente, J., Ruiz-Fons, F., Vidal, D., *et al.* (2007) Lesions associated with *Mycobacterium tuberculosis* complex infection in the European wild boar. *Tuberculosis* 87, 360–367.

Martín-Hernando, M.P., Torres, M.J., Aznar, J., Negro, J.J., Gandía A., *et al.* (2010) Distribution of lesions in red and fallow deer naturally infected with *Mycobacterium bovis*. *Journal of Comparative Pathology* 142, 43–50.

McDonald, R.A., Delahay, R.J., Carter, S.P., Smith, G.C., Cheeseman, C.L., *et al.* (2008) Perturbing implications of wildlife ecology for disease control. *Trends in Ecology and Evolution* 23, 53–56.

McInerney, J., Small, K.J. and Caley, P. (1995) Prevalence of *Mycobacterium bovis* infection in feral pigs in the Northern Territory. *Australian Veterinary Journal* 72(1981), 448–451.

Michel, A.L., *et al.* (2006) Wildlife tuberculosis in South African conservation areas: implications and challenges. *Veterinary Microbiology* 112(2–4), 91–100.

More, S.J., Radunz, B. and Glanville, R.J. (2015). Lessons learned during the successful eradication of bovine tuberculosis from Australia. *The Veterinary Record* 177(9), 224–232.

Morris, R.S. and Pfeiffer, D.U. (1995) Directions and issues in bovine tuberculosis epidemiology and control in New Zealand. *New Zealand Veterinary Journal* 43, 256–265.

Muñoz-Mendoza, M., Marreros, N., Boadella, M., Gortazar, C., Menendez, S., *et al.* (2013) Wild boar tuberculosis in Iberian Atlantic Spain: a different picture from Mediterranean habitats. *BMC Veterinary Research* 9, 176.

Mwacalimba, K.K., Mumba, C. and Munyeme, M. (2013) Cost benefit analysis of tuberculosis control in wildlife – livestock interface areas of Southern Zambia. *Preventive Veterinary Medicine* 110, 274–279.

Naranjo, V., Gortazar, C., Vicente, J. and de la Fuente, J. (2008) Evidence of the role of European wild boar as a reservoir of *Mycobacterium tuberculosis* complex. *Veterinary Microbiology* 127, 1–9.

Neal, E. (1986) *Natural history of badgers*, Croom Helm. Facts on File, New York, USA.

Nugent, G. (2011) Maintenance, spillover and spillback transmission of bovine tuberculosis in multi-host wildlife complexes: A New Zealand case study. *Veterinary Microbiology* 151(1–2), 34–42.

Nugent, G., Whitford, J. and Young, N. (2002) Use of released pigs as sentinels for *Mycobacterium bovis*. *Journal of Wildlife Diseases* 38(4), 665–677.

Nugent, G., Buddle, B.M. and Knowles, G. (2015a) Epidemiology and control of *Mycobacterium bovis* infection in brushtail possums (*Trichosurus vulpecula*), the primary wildlife host of bovine tuberculosis in New Zealand. *New Zealand Veterinary Journal* 63(1), 28–41.

Nugent, G., Gortazar, C. and Knowles, G. (2015b) The epidemiology of *Mycobacterium bovis* in wild deer and feral pigs and their roles in the establishment and spread of bovine tuberculosis in New Zealand wildlife. *New Zealand Veterinary Journal* 63(1), 54–67.

O'Brien, D.J., Schmitt, S.M., Fierke, J.S., Hogle, S.A., Winterstein, S.R., *et al.* (2002) Epidemiology of *Mycobacterium bovis* in free-ranging white-tailed deer, Michigan, USA, 1995–2000. *Preventive Veterinary Medicine* 54, 47–63.

O'Brien, D.J., Schmirr, S.M., Fitzgerald, S.D., Berry, D.E. and Hickling, G.L. (2006) Managing the wildlife reservoir of *Mycobacterium bovis*: the Michigan, USA, experience. *Veterinary Microbiology* 112, 313–323.

O'Brien, D.J., Schmitt, S.M., Fitzgerald, S.D. and Berry, D.E. (2011) Management of bovine tuberculosis in Michigan wildlife: current status and near term prospects. *Veterinary Microbiology* 151(1–2), 179–187.

Olea-Popelka, F.J., Flynn, O., Costello, E., McGrath, G., O'Keeffe, J., *et al.* (2005) Spatial relationship between *Mycobacterium bovis* strains in cattle and badgers in four areas in Ireland. *Preventive Veterinary Medicine* 71(1), 57–70.

O'Reilly, M.L. and Daborn, C.J. (1995) The epidemiology of *Mycobacterium bovis* infections in animals and man: a review. *Tubercle and Lung Disease* 76(1), 1–46.

Palmer, M.V., Whipple, D.L. and Waters, W.R. (2001) Experimental deer-to-deer transmission of *Mycobacterium bovis*. *American Journal of Veterinary Research* 62(5), 692–696.

Palmer, M.V., Waters, W.R. and Whipple, D.L. (2004a) Shared feed as a means of deer-to-deer transmission of *Mycobacterium bovis*. *Journal of Wildlife Diseases* 40(1), 87–91.

Palmer, M.V., Waters, W.R. and Whipple, D.L. (2004b) Investigation of the transmission of *Mycobacterium bovis* from deer to cattle through indirect contact. *American Journal of Veterinary Research* 65, 1483–1489.

Palmer, M.V., *et al.* (2015) Tuberculosis in wild and captive deer. In: Mukundan, H. Chambers, M., Waters, R. and Larsen, M. (eds) *Tuberculosis, Leprosy and Mycobacterial Diseases of Man and Animals: The Many Hosts of Mycobacteria*. CAB International, Wallingford, UK, pp. 334–364.

Paterson, B.M. and Morris, R.S. (1995) Interactions between beef cattle and simulated tuberculous possums on pasture. *New Zealand Veterinary Journal* 43, 289–293.

Phillips, C.J., Foster, C.R.W., Morris, P.A. and Teverson, R. (2003) The transmission of *Mycobacterium bovis* infection to cattle. *Research in Veterinary Science* 74, 1–15.

Prentice, J.C., Marion, G., White, P.C.L., Davidson, R.S. and Hutchings, M.R. (2014) Demographic processes drive increases in wildlife disease following population reduction. *PloS One* 9(5), e86563.

Radunz, B. (2006) Surveillance and risk management during the latter stages of eradication: experiences from Australia. *Veterinary Microbiology* 112, 283–290.

Ragg, J.R., Waldrup, K.A. and Moller, H. (1995) The distribution of gross lesions of tuberculosis caused by *Mycobacterium bovis* in feral ferrets (*Mustela furo*) from Otago, New Zealand. *New Zealand Veterinary Journal* 43, 338–341.

Ramsey, D. and Cowan, P. (2003) Mortality rate and movements of brushtail possums with clinical tuberculosis (*Mycobacterium bovis*) infection. *New Zealand Veterinary Journal* 51, 179–185.

Roper, T.J., Shepherdson, D.J. and Davis, J.M. (1986) Scent marking with faces and anal secretion in the eurpoean badger(*Meles meles*): seasonal and spatial characteristics of latrine use in relation to territoriality. *Behaviour* 97(1), 94–117.

Sauter, C.M. and Morris, R.S. (1995) Behavioural studies on the potential for direct transmission of tuberculosis from feral ferrets (*Mustela furo*) and possums (*Trichosurus vulpecula*) to farmed livestock. *New Zealand Veterinary Journal* 43, 294–300.

Shury, T.K. and Bergeson, D. (2011) Lesion Distribution and Epidemiology of *Mycobacterium bovis* in Elk and White-Tailed Deer in South-Western Manitoba, Canada. *Veterinary Medicine International* 1–11.

Tolhurst, B.A., Delahay, R.J., Walker, N.J., Ward, A.I. and Roper, T.J. (2009) Behaviour of badgers (*Meles meles*) in farm buildings: opportunities for the transmission of *Mycobacterium bovis* to cattle? *Applied Animal Behaviour Science* 117, 103–113.

Tomlinson, A.J., Chambers, M.A., Wildon, G.J., McDonald, R.A. and Delahay, R.J. (2013) Sex-related heterogeneity in the life-history correlates of *Mycobacterium bovis* infection in European badgers (*Meles meles*). *Transboundary and Emerging Diseases* 60(2000), 37–45.

Vandal, O.H., Nathan, C.F. and Ehrt, S. (2009) Acid resistance in *Mycobacterium tuberculosis*. *Journal of Bacteriology* 191(15), 4714–4721.

Vicente, J., Hofle, U., Garrido, J.M., Fernandez-de-Mera, I.G., Juste, R., et al. (2006) Wild boar and red deer display high prevalences of tuberculosis-like lesions in Spain. *Veterinary Research* 37, 1–11.

Vicente, J., Hofle, U., Garrido, J.M., Fernandez-de-Mera, I.G., Acevedo, P., et al. (2007a) Risk factors associated with the prevalence of tuberculosis-like lesions in fenced wild boar and red deer in south central Spain. *Veterinary Research* 38, 451–464.

Vicente, J., Delahay, R.J., Walker, N.J. and Cheeseman, C.L. (2007b) Social organization and movement influence the incidence of bovine tuberculosis in an undisturbed high-density badger *Meles meles* population. *Journal of Animal Ecology* 76, 348–360.

Vicente, J., Barasona, J.A., Acevedo, P., Ruiz-Fons, J.F., Boadella, M., et al. (2013) Temporal trend of tuberculosis in wild ungulates from mediterranean Spain. *Transboundary and Emerging Diseases* 60, 92–103.

Weber, N., Bearhop, S., Dall, S.R.X., Delehay, R.J., McDonald, R.A., et al. (2013) Denning behaviour of the European badger (*Meles meles*) correlates with bovine tuberculosis infection status. *Behavioral Ecology and Sociobiology* 67, 471–479.

Woodroffe, R., Donnelly, C.A., Johnston, W.T., Bourne, F.J., Cheeseman, C.L., et al. (2005) Spatial association of *Mycobacterium bovis* infection in cattle and badgers *Meles meles*. *Journal of Applied Ecology* 42, 852–862.

Young, J.S., Gormley, E. and Wellington, E.M.H. (2005) Molecular detection of *Mycobacterium bovis* and *Mycobacterium bovis* BCG (Pasteur) in soil. *Applied and Enironmental Microbiology* 71(4), 1946–1952.

8 Molecular Virulence Mechanisms of *Mycobacterium bovis*

Alicia Smyth and Stephen V. Gordon*
School of Veterinary Medicine, University College Dublin, Dublin, Ireland

8.1 Introduction

Infection with *Mycobacterium bovis* is an ongoing problem both to human and animal health, costing billions annually in economic losses (Skuce *et al.*, 2011; Muller *et al.*, 2013). While eradication in some countries has met with success, infection of animals and humans with *M. bovis* is still reported globally. Understanding the virulence mechanisms that allow *M. bovis* to survive *in vivo*, cause disease and transmit to new (and diverse) hosts will be key to the ultimate eradication of *M. bovis* infection.

M. bovis is a member of the *Mycobacterium tuberculosis* complex (MTBC), the grouping of genetically related mycobacterial species that cause tuberculosis in mammals (Frothingham *et al.*, 1994; Smith *et al.*, 2006). Theobald Smith was the first to demonstrate that the causative agent of tuberculosis in cattle, and indeed other animal hosts, was not the same as the human bacillus, a finding that ultimately led to the description of the bovine-adapted species *M. bovis* (Smith, 1898; Karlson and Lessel, 1970). The hallmark member of the MTBC, *M. tuberculosis*, shares 99.95% nucleotide sequence identity with *M. bovis* (Cole *et al.*, 1998; Garnier *et al.*, 2003). *M. bovis* is the best-studied member of the MTBC that infects wild and domesticated animals, but it is certainly not the only one, with *Mycobacterium microti* found in voles (Wells, 1937, 1946), *Mycobacterium caprae* in goats and cattle (Aranaz *et al.*, 1999), *Mycobacterium orygis* in antelopes (van Ingen *et al.*, 2012), *Mycobacterium pinnipedii* in seals (Cousins *et al.*, 1993), *Mycobacterium mungi* in mongooses (Alexander *et al.*, 2010), *Mycobacterium suricattae* in meerkats (Parsons *et al.*, 2013), and the eponymous Dassie bacillus (Cousins *et al.*, 1994). A core differentiating feature of the MTBC species is their varying host preference – *M. bovis* has been found in the widest range of hosts, including humans, cattle, badgers, goats, sheep and deer (Skuce *et al.*, 2011; Muller *et al.*, 2013; Palmer, 2013; Pesciaroli *et al.*, 2014). This nomenclature for the members of the MTBC does not, however, define host range and it hinges upon whether the host in question is one to which the associated pathogen is adapted to and can successfully propagate within (a 'primary' or 'maintenance' host) or one to which the pathogen has been introduced to but is not adapted to for propagation (a 'secondary' or 'spillover' host).

When considering the virulence of the mycobacteria, there are a number of concepts that need to be considered. Firstly, one can define virulence as the degree of severity of pathology caused by a pathogen, that is, its ability to inflict damage on the host. However, the resulting pathology is not solely due to the efforts of the pathogen, but instead it is the interaction between the host and the pathogen that results in damage to the host, either due to the direct

---
* Email: stephen.gordon@ucd.ie

effects of the pathogen or the efforts of the host to control the infection. This is of importance when considering *M. bovis*, a pathogen with the ability to infect and transmit across a wide variety of hosts compared to other members of the MTBC, and suggests an intimate ability to overcome and exploit host defences to its own ends. Secondly, most virulence factors are defined as such because in their absence the pathogen is less able to negatively affect the host. However, these factors may not be involved in directly harming the host, but are essential for pathogen survival and ability to thrive, such as the ability to acquire nutrients *in vivo*. Lastly the mycobacteria have coevolved alongside their hosts over many millennia; one study suggested the emergence of the MTBC 70,000 years ago (Comas *et al.*, 2013). As the mycobacteria have adapted in order to take advantage of their animal hosts, so too have their hosts evolved under selective pressures to develop resistance to mycobacterial infection. This is most evident when examining the varying outcomes of infection with MTBC bacilli in humans, with some infections developing into disseminated disease within a few years, some showing latent infection that only progresses to full disease after many years, and some infections being eradicated by the host with no symptoms of disease evident (Lillebaek *et al.*, 2002). These outcomes reinforce the concept that the genetic and immune status of the host is significant in determining the outcome of infection and hence the underlying virulence of the mycobacteria. It is therefore important to note that although many studies have highlighted the importance of particular proteins or surface lipids in mediating disease in cultured cells or mouse models, there is likely a great deal that is unique to the interaction of mycobacteria with their respective hosts.

To summarize, we define the virulence factors as the elements required by the mycobacteria to survive and cause damage to the host, directly or indirectly. In order to quantify the virulence of an organism we can use different measures, including host mortality, bacterial burden and histopathology. When examining *M. bovis* virulence, we are interested in both the conserved factors that are shared by different mycobacterial species and the unique factors that *M. bovis* possesses that may allow it to affect such a wide range of host species. These virulence factors encompass cell wall components involved in attachment and the interaction between bacterial and host cell surfaces, secreted proteins that may guide bacterial localization and regulatory factors that influence the expression of a range of different factors. Insight into the identity of the genes underlying these factors was offered through comparative genomic analysis of *M. bovis* and other mycobacteria and it is to this topic that we shall next turn.

8.2 Genomic Analysis

A key step in defining the genetic basis of virulence and tropism in the MTBC was the elucidation of their genome sequences. Although the constituent MTBC species show a high degree of genetic similarity (>99%), there are significant differences apparent in their genomes. One of the most striking differences first identified between the genomes of *M. bovis* and *M. tuberculosis* was that *M. bovis* has a smaller genome, with large regions missing from its genome compared to *M. tuberculosis* (Garnier *et al.*, 2003). These deleted sections are known as regions of difference (RD) and they can be used to trace the evolution of the different MTBC species. It was originally thought that *M. tuberculosis* had emerged in humans following transmission of *M. bovis* into the human population with the domestication of cattle. However, the use of the RD loci as evolutionary markers revealed instead that *M. tuberculosis* more closely resembled the common progenitor of the MTBC than *M. bovis*, as the latter had suffered the greatest loss of RD loci compared to other members of the complex (Brosch *et al.*, 2002; Mostowy *et al.*, 2002). The loss of the RD loci during the evolution of *M. bovis* can be thought of as a series of deletion events, although it is not understood what role the loss of these loci had, if any, in granting some selective advantage to the bacteria in colonizing a wider range of hosts, or whether it was simply the removal of deleterious or redundant gene regions.

While multiple genome sequences of *M. bovis* and *M. tuberculosis* strains are now available, the original findings from the comparative analysis of the first strains to be sequenced,

M. tuberculosis H37Rv and *M. bovis* 2122/97, serve to set the scene. The genome sequences of both *M. bovis* and *M. tuberculosis* are collinear with no evidence of duplications or translocations, with the *M. bovis* AF2122/97 sequence 4 345 492 base pairs (bp) long and *M. tuberculosis* H37Rv strain 4 411 532 bp (Garnier et al., 2003). There are no unique genes present in *M. bovis* that are not found in *M. tuberculosis* strains; however, nine RD were deleted from *M. bovis* explaining its reduced genome size. A total of 2437 SNPs were also identified when comparing the sequencing data of *M. bovis* 2122/97 and *M. tuberculosis* H37Rv, of which 769 were non-synonymous. Although genetic coding potential has been lost from *M. bovis* as compared to *M. tuberculosis*, it is still virulent and can infect humans, although its ability to transmit between humans is limited (Magnus, 1966). It is thought that the regions lost from *M. bovis* may mostly be the removal of functionally redundant regions, although why with a reduced repertoire of genes *M. bovis* shows a wider range of host preferences is not understood. Further understanding of the regulation of genes and the responses these bacteria have to changing environments could have valuable insight into defining the ability of *M. bovis* to infect and sustain in diverse hosts. The most significant changes seem to be found in regions coding for cell wall components and secreted proteins, indicating that it is the interaction with the host that is most effected by the changes in the genome.

In addition to comparing *M. bovis* to *M. tuberculosis*, there is an excellent source for comparison with an avirulent *M. bovis* derived strain. Bacillus Calmette–Guérin (BCG) is the attenuated vaccine strain that has been used worldwide as a TB preventative control tool. Despite being the most widely used vaccine in the world, questions about its efficacy remain. Generated by repeated culture of *M. bovis* on potato slices soaked in glycerol and ox bile, this generated a new strain that was no longer able to cause disease in diverse animal hosts (Calmette, 1931). The precise molecular events that lead to the attenuation of BCG, however, remained elusive. A study of the genetic differences between virulent *M. bovis* strains and BCG using subtractive genomic hybridization identified three large deletions between *M. bovis* and BCG: RD1, RD2 and RD3 (Mahairas et al., 1996), with RD1 the only one of these deletions missing from all BCG strains and found in every virulent *M. bovis* and *M. tuberculosis* strain (Mostowy et al., 2002; Brosch et al., 2002). The role of the genes coded for by RD1–RD3 is discussed in more detail below.

8.2.1 RD1–RD3

The loss of the RD1 locus from BCG was identified as playing a key role in the loss of virulence of the vaccine strain. Complementation of BCG with RD1 restores virulence to the vaccine strain (Pym et al., 2003; Majlessi et al., 2005), although not to the full degree seen in *M. bovis* or *M. tuberculosis*. When RD1 is deleted from *M. tuberculosis* the strain is also attenuated, confirming the key role of the genes encoded by this region in virulence (Lewis et al., 2003). RD1 encodes a type VII secretion system (T7SS) that secretes a range of proteins including the potent T-cell antigens ESAT-6 and CFP-10 (Berthet et al., 1998b; Bitter et al., 2009) and hence is also known as the ESAT6 secretion system 1 (ESX-1). A site distal from RD1, the *espACD* locus is also important for the activity of the ESX-1 system, although this is still present in BCG strains.

ESAT-6 and CFP-10 are small secreted proteins (6 kDa and 10 kDa, respectively) and both belong to the ESAT-6 family of proteins, a family of secreted proteins with 23 members in the mycobacterial genome (Brodin et al., 2004). These genes occur in tandem pairs throughout the genome and although little is known about their function it is theorized that once expressed they interact to form protein complexes. Interestingly, six of the ESAT-6 protein family are missing or altered in *M. bovis* (Rv2346c, Rv2347c, Rv3619c, Rv3620c, Rv3890c and Rv3905c) (Garnier et al., 2003). The effects of these losses have not been studied, and what role they may play in mycobacterial virulence is not understood as of yet. The precise role of ESAT-6 and CFP-10 in the establishment of infection is still not completely understood, but they have a key role to play in the virulence of mycobacteria. Both proteins have been shown to have immunogenic properties and can induce T-cell responses across multiple species (Aagaard et al.,

2010; Arlehamn et al., 2012; Kassa et al., 2012). The genes for ESAT-6 and CFP-10 are co-transcribed and the proteins form a tightly binding 1:1 complex (Renshaw et al., 2002), with transport of the ESAT-6:CFP-10 heterodimer across the membrane dependent on the C-terminal region of CFP-10 (Dillon et al., 2000; Champion et al., 2006). The activity of the single proteins has also been explored and it was shown that while ESAT-6 destabilizes and lyses liposomes, CFP-10 does not appear to have this effect (Guinn et al., 2004). The ability of ESAT-6 to lyse the membrane appears key to the process whereby M. tuberculosis can escape from the phagosome into the cytosol of infected cells, as RD1 or ESAT-6 mutants of M. tuberculosis are defective in phagosome escape (van der Wel et al., 2007) and the mutants do not spread to surrounding cells (Guinn et al., 2004).

The other two deletions, RD2 and RD3, are of lesser importance to the attenuation of BCG and hence mycobacterial virulence. RD2 was lost sometime during the subculture of BCG subsequent to 1927, and while its loss does not fully attenuate the bacteria it does seem to have some contribution to virulence. RD2 contains the mpt64 gene, which codes for a known immunogenic protein. Deletion of RD2 in M. tuberculosis does not affect the growth of the bacteria, but it does decrease the bacterial burden and histopathology seen in mice (Kozak et al., 2011). Complementation of the mutant with a section of RD2 containing the mpt64 gene restored the mutant's phenotype to that of the wild type, indicating some importance for this protein in bacterial virulence (Mustafa et al., 2007). RD3 is found in M. tuberculosis H37Rv and M. bovis but is absent from BCG and 84% of clinical M. tuberculosis isolates (Mahairas et al., 1996). RD3 is a prophage so its loss from BCG may be due to phage excision, while its absence from many virulent strains would indicate it is not required for virulence.

8.3 Cell Envelope

The proteins, lipids and carbohydrates that lie at the surface of the bacterial cell are clearly crucial in host–pathogen interaction as they directly interact with host cells. Changes in the lipid profile on the cell surface therefore have significant effects on host–pathogen interactions. There are distinct differences in the lipids found on the surface of M. bovis when compared to other MTBC species, differences that could play a role in dictating host preference. Indeed, the only locus that is present in M. bovis and absent from 'modern' M. tuberculosis lineage strains is the TbD1 locus (Garnier et al., 2003). This contains the mmpS6 gene and the 5' region of mmpL6. It is thought that loss of these genes may prevent trafficking of particular lipids to the surface of the mycobacteria, but the presence of the locus in 'ancient' M. tuberculosis strains does not mark TbD1 as a strong candidate for a role in host preference.

One of the key features of the mycobacteria is their distinctive waxy cell wall, which is much thicker than that of other bacteria (Brennan, 2003). The thick waxy coat of the mycobacteria is highly impermeable and tough, acting as a shield against host defences but also harbouring an array of immune modulatory compounds. The cell wall contains covalently linked peptidoglycan, arabinogalactan and mycolic acids generating a so-called 'mycomembrane'. Interlinked with the mycolic acids are a plethora of free lipids such as phthiocerol dimycocerosate, cord factor, sulfolipid, phenolic glycolipids and phosphatidylinositol mannosides. An outer capsule of α-glucan provides the final layer. This thick protective coating makes transport of compounds into and out of the cell a complex process involving multiple import and export systems that have also been implicated in virulence due to the transport of effectors or immunomodulatory compounds. Although knocking out the genes for certain transport components may reduce the virulence of the organism it is often not clear if that component directly interacts with the host and invokes specific negative effects, or if by altering single components, larger disruptions are carried across the fundamental structure of the entire membrane, altering protein secretion and surface structures that may be directly affecting the host.

A large family of secreted and surface-exposed proteins is the Mce family, originally termed mammalian cell entry proteins as they were thought to be involved in cell invasion (Arruda et al., 1993). The genes encoding the Mce proteins are arranged into operons, numbered 1 to 4 in *M. tuberculosis*, with *M. bovis* missing the locus encoding Mce3 (Zumarraga *et al.*, 1999). While the function of Mce3 is cryptic, inactivation of the locus was shown to attenuate *M. tuberculosis* (Senaratne *et al.*, 2008), suggesting *M. bovis* may have developed compensatory mechanisms to adjust for the loss of this locus. The one clear function linked to the Mce proteins is the role of the genes of the *mce4* locus in the uptake of cholesterol and sterols; these have been suggested to be key carbon sources during persistent infection.

The pore-forming protein OmpATb has been demonstrated in both *M. tuberculosis* and *M. bovis* to be involved in virulence as its deletion results in significantly reduced multiplication of mutants in macrophages (Raynaud *et al.*, 2002b). The transcription of *ompAtb* was also increased in acidic conditions, suggesting it may play a role in surviving phagosomal maturation as the compartment acidifies. On the subject of channel proteins, an intriguing example of a dual function protein located at the cell surface is provided by the 'channel protein with necrosis-inducing toxin', CpnT, which plays roles in both nutrient uptake and induction of host cell death by *M. tuberculosis* (Danilchanka *et al.*, 2014). The CpnT protein consists of an N-terminal channel domain that is involved in the uptake of nutrients across the outer membrane, and a secreted toxic C-terminal domain that causes necrotic cell death in eukaryotic cells. The mechanism by which the C-terminal domain induces necrosis is unknown, but CpnT represents the only secreted 'toxin' described to date in the MTBC.

The 'exported repetitive protein', aka Erp or P36, is cell wall associated and secreted (Berthet *et al.*, 1998a; de Mendonca-Lima *et al.*, 2003). When it was knocked out in *M. bovis* it resulted in a mutant strain with impaired replication in macrophages and decreased lung pathology in mice that was fully restored with complementation (Bigi *et al.*, 2005). Virulence of this protein has been linked to its central domain that contains multiple repeats, so it is tempting to speculate that variation in the repeats may impact on its role in virulence. Variation in the multiple lipoproteins located at the bacterial cell surface between *M. bovis* and *M. tuberculosis* is also of note, with the genes for lipoproteins LppQ, LpqT, LpqG and LprM, all deleted or frameshifted in *M. bovis*, while the gene for lipoprotein LppA is duplicated. This variation could well be involved in altering the way the bacteria interacts with the host and its environment, facilitating different tissue tropisms or manipulation of different immune responses.

The MTBC contains many polyketide synthases (PKS), a diverse family of multifunctional enzymes that are involved in the synthesis of secondary metabolites in a wide array of bacteria (O'Hagan, 1993; Sirakova *et al.*, 2003). In mycobacteria, the PKSs are often closely associated with genes involved in fatty acid metabolism. Many PKS genes in MTBC bacilli have now been linked to pathways synthesizing lipids and glycolipid conjugates that are essential for virulence, as well as key components of the complex cell envelope (Kolattukudy *et al.*, 1997). It was shown that PKS enzymes are involved in the synthesis of lipids in the dimycocerosyl phthiocerol family (DIMs) (Trivedi *et al.*, 2005; Quadri, 2014). The role these enzymes play in virulence is not fully understood, but there are some interesting avenues to pursue in differentiating *M. bovis* from *M. tuberculosis*. For example, *M. bovis* cannot synthesize PKS6 due to a frameshift mutation in the encoding gene (Garnier *et al.*, 2003), but when the *pks6* is knocked out in *M. tuberculosis* this results in an attenuated strain in the murine model; hence, *M. bovis* may have developed compensatory systems to accommodate for the loss of PKS6, or its loss may be beneficial to the bacillus.

One of the most abundant components of the outer lipid layer are the aforementioned DIMs, primarily phthiocerol dimycocerosate (PDIM) (Azad *et al.*, 1997). These lipids on the outer surface are not covalently bound to the inner membrane, unlike the mycolic acids. Many groups have shown that knocking out the synthesis of PDIM results in an attenuated phenotype, with reduced growth or reduced bacterial burdens in infected cells and model hosts (Cox *et al.*, 1999; Camacho *et al.*, 2001). The role of PDIM was originally thought to be mainly structural, playing a part in the fluidity of the cell membrane. It was considered an indirect virulence factor as it was thought that its removal altered the ability of other proteins to affect the host, but that it did not itself have a direct influence on the ability of the bacteria to cause disease. However, later work has shown that this is not the case and that PDIM may play a significant role in the acute phase of the infection and may aid in mediating interaction between the pathogen and the host macrophage, and may in fact encourage phagocytosis of the mycobacteria (Pethe et al., 2004; Stewart et al., 2005). One significant consideration for PDIM is that it tends to be lost when the mycobacteria are repeatedly sub-cultured *in vitro* (Domenech and Reed, 2009). Once PDIM is lost, the bacterium seems to gain an advantage in growth speed, perhaps due to increased membrane permeability allowing more rapid diffusion of nutrients, meaning the PDIM-negative bacteria dominate in culture over time. This is important to consider as it has been indicated previously that attenuation of certain mutant knock-outs (Kos) may not be due to inactivation of the gene in question, but instead due to selection of mutants in PDIM-negative backgrounds. Research into the direct effects of PDIM seem to indicate that it has a role in receptor-dependent phagocytosis of mycobacteria, and that it also may influence prevention of phagosomal acidification (Astarie-Dequeker et al., 2009). There are also studies showing that it may contribute to bacterial growth and helps resist nitric oxide dependent killing, as well as playing a role in mediating the host immune response, as it was shown that in a PDIM KO there were increased levels of TNFα and IL-6 produced by murine macrophages and dendritic cells in *vitro* (Rousseau et al., 2004). The majority of these studies were performed using *M. tuberculosis*, but there are also a number of studies showing that loss of PDIM in *M. bovis* similarly effects its virulence (Hotter et al., 2005; Hotter and Collins, 2011).

M. bovis and *M. tuberculosis* both have similar levels of PDIM on their outer surface; however, certain genes that regulate synthesis and transport of PDIM are differentially regulated between the two (Golby et al., 2007). One study looking at the gene expression differences between *M. bovis* and *M. tuberculosis* when cultured *in vitro* showed that *M. bovis* had much higher expression of the *lppX-pks1* genes (Golby et al., 2007). These have been shown to be involved in the transport and synthesis of PDIM; however, there was no significant change in PDIM levels, so it was suggested that this change may reflect synthesis of PDIM-derived phenolic glycolipids (PGL). PGL compounds are not produced by H37Rv, the type strain of *M. tuberculosis* and the majority of clinical isolates, but are found in *M. bovis* and certain Beijing-lineage *M. tuberculosis* strains, with monoglycosylated mycoside B the major PGL in *M. bovis* (Brennan, 2003; Malaga et al., 2008). The loss of PGLs from many *M. tuberculosis* strains is caused by a frameshift mutation in the *pks1* gene, splitting it into two genes *pks1* and *pks15* (Constant et al., 2002). The *M. tuberculosis* strains that do have PGLs on their surface are considered hypervirulent, or more specifically hyper-lethal (Reed et al., 2004); loss of PGL from these strains decreases their virulence as evidenced by increased survival of mice infected with these variants (Reed et al., 2004).

Counter to the PGL example, sulfolipids are trehalose-containing glycolipids that are only expressed by *M. tuberculosis* and are not found in *M. bovis* (Brennan, 2003). These lipids appear to mediate pro-inflammatory responses that aid *M. tuberculosis* during infection, and that although sulfolipid KOs are not attenuated in a murine model, there was a decrease in virulence when human macrophages were used as the infection readout (Gilmore et al., 2012). Increased research into the function of sulfolipids will clarify their potential to act as species-specific virulence factors.

There are numerous cell envelope-associated proteins whose function is still unknown, or whose link to virulence is unclear, but it is highly likely that the diversity of the cell surface components will contribute to the variation in host preference, virulence and transmission of *M. bovis*.

8.4 Secretory Systems

The secretory systems of the mycobacteria are highly important as a result of the near impenetrable cell wall barrier. Specialized systems are required for protein and lipid secretion and the uptake of small molecules. *M. bovis*, in common with the other members of the complex, has the common general secretion system, also known as the Sec secretion system, consisting of a five-part membrane complex and an ATPase that recognizes the N-terminal signal sequence on unfolded proteins (Braunstein et al., 2001). This system transports proteins across the inner membrane into the periplasmic space. It has not yet been explained how the proteins then travel across the outer portion of the cell wall, and it is expected that there are additional pathways used to direct proteins across this space that are as yet unidentified. One protein known to be secreted through this pathway is MPB70, discussed below, a protein produced at significant levels by *M. bovis*. Mycobacteria also encode a second homologous SecA pathway termed SecA2 (Braunstein et al., 2001; Swanson et al., 2015). The exact role of this pathway in pathogenesis is unknown, but its removal has negative effects on *M. tuberculosis* growth *in vivo* (Braunstein et al., 2003); further work on the substrates secreted by this pathway is needed to elucidate the role of the secreted effectors in mycobacterial virulence. Mycobacteria also possess a twin arginine transporter (Tat) pathway that is also found in a number of other pathogenic bacteria where it is essential for virulence (Lee et al., 2006). The Tat pathway translocates folded proteins across the inner membrane, and its loss compromises the ability of *M. tuberculosis* to grow in vitro (Saint-Joanis et al., 2006). There is also evidence that certain substrates secreted via Tat, such as phosopholipase C enzymes, are essential for full virulence of *M. tuberculosis in vivo* (Raynaud et al., 2002a; McDonough et al., 2005).

As stated above in the description of RD1, the MTBC have a family of type VII secretion systems. Pathogenic mycobacteria including *M. bovis* possess five T7SS (Houben et al., 2014), the best characterized of which is the previously mentioned ESX-1, which is involved directly in host–pathogen interactions, and whose loss is one of the key factors of BCG attenuation (Houben et al., 2012). The other four members are not as well studied; ESX-2 and ESX-4 have no known function, while ESX-3 is involved in the balance of zinc and iron in the bacterium and in secretion of PE and PPE proteins, an important mycobacterial protein family discussed in more detail below (Serafini et al., 2009; Tufariello et al., 2016). ESX-5 has only been found in slow-growing mycobacteria, its appearance in the genetic record also seems to coincide with the differentiation between slow- and fast-growing mycobacteria (Gey Van Pittius et al., 2001). It has also been shown that ESX-5 is essential for the secretion of PPE and PE-PGRS (polymorphic GC-rich repetitive sequences) proteins, a topic we will move to next (Abdallah et al., 2009).

8.5 PE/PPE

Certain protein families are of particular interest due to their unique properties and their variation across the MTBC. While the members of the MTBC show a high degree of sequence similarity, greater than 99.9% in most cases, there are two gene families present in the MTBC that are a major source of sequence polymorphism. These are the PE and PPE gene families, PE named for the Pro-Glu residues found at residues 8 and 9 on the N terminus of the proteins and PPE for the Pro-Pro-Glu motif in the same region (Cole and Barrell, 1998; Cole, 1999). The PE family has around 100 members in *M. tuberculosis* and PPE has around 68, although the numbers vary across the MTBC, with 10% of the coding capacity of the bacteria being taken up by these gene families. These proteins appear unique to mycobacteria and are found in greater abundance in pathogenic mycobacteria. The largest family of PE proteins is the PE-PGRS protein family, with these proteins in particular seeming to have some immunologically important role (Delogu and Brennan, 2001; Sampson, 2011). The genes for PE and PPE proteins are clustered together throughout the genome, and it has been shown that some are co-transcribed and can form a stable complex. There are 40 PE/PPE gene pairs in the *M. tuberculosis* genome, and 22 of these contain PE/PPE genes exclusively, suggesting that these linked genes may have related roles (Overbeek et al., 1999; Tundup et al., 2006).

Predicted protein function based on amino acid sequence indicated that 40 of the PE/PPE genes have beta barrel-like amino acid sequences (Pajon et al., 2006). Genetic analysis of *M. bovis* and *M. tuberculosis* has shown there are blocks of sequence variation in these regions, which affects 29 different PE-PGRS and 28 PPE proteins, resulting mostly from in-frame deletions and insertions (Garnier et al., 2003). These proteins have a conserved N terminus and a highly variable C terminus, suggesting these genes as a source of variation that can be acted on by selective pressures and allowing for adaptation to changing environments or hosts (Sreevatsan et al., 1997; Cole et al., 1998).

A wide variety of functions have been associated with these proteins, with the majority associated with the cell envelope (Espitia et al., 1999; Brennan et al., 2001; Banu et al., 2002). Rv1759c (a PE-PGRS protein), binds fibronectin in M. tuberculosis, suggesting a role in tissue tropism (Espitia et al., 1999), while the orthologue in M. bovis is a pseudogene. PE-PGRS33 is a surface protein involved in the formation of mycobacterial aggregates. When it was mutated in M. bovis BCG, the resulting mutant had significantly reduced growth (Delogu et al., 2004; Cascioferro et al., 2007). PE-PGRS30 appears to have a role in arresting phagosomal maturation, as when it was knocked out in M. tuberculosis there was a marked decrease in intracellular bacterial replication, as well as decreased lung pathology in mice infected with the mutant (Iantomasi et al., 2012). Some of the PE/PPE genes are found in clusters with ESAT-6 like genes (Gey van Pittius et al., 2006). There are two PE/PPE genes located in the RD1 locus, Rv3872 gene and Rv3873, and it has been suggested that these are involved in the transport of ESAT-6 and CFP-10 out of the cell (Guinn et al., 2004). Indeed, the linkage of ESX secretion systems with PE/PPE export has been reported by a number of groups, for example, ESX-3 exporting PE5, PE15 and PE20 (Tufariello et al., 2016), while secretion of PE10 via ESX-5 is vital for capsule integrity and virulence (Ates et al., 2016). There are also numerous PE/PPE genes whose expression is upregulated at different stages during infection. During acute phases of macrophage infection with M. tuberculosis there is increased expression of several PE/PPE genes (Rv0834c, Rv3097c, Rv1361c, Rv0977, Rv1840c) (Triccas et al., 1999; Dubnau et al., 2002; Srivastava et al., 2007). There is also evidence that expression of these genes vary between M. bovis and M. tuberculosis (Golby et al., 2007). Further research is required in this area to try and clarify the role these proteins play in mycobacterial virulence, and what effect their variation may have in mediating host interactions.

8.6 Regulatory genes

Although changes in individual genes may attenuate growth or virulence in some way, more significant changes can be identified by looking at alterations in genes coding for regulatory proteins that are involved in the expression of multiple genes. Two of these that have been identified as particularly important for gene expression and phenotypic differences between M. bovis and M. tuberculosis are the PhoPR regulatory system and the RskA-SigK regulon.

8.6.1 PhoPR

PhoPR is a two-component regulatory system consisting of the PhoP response regulator and PhoR sensor kinase components (Perez et al., 2001; Lee et al., 2008). It has been demonstrated that PhoPR is an important regulator of virulence for M. tuberculosis, where it is involved in the regulation of genes for sulfolipid and di- and polyacyltrehaloses biosynthesis and secretion of ESAT-6. Three mutations in PhoPR in M. africanum L6 (a human strain) and animal-adapted species, including M. bovis, results in reduced expression of PhoP in these species (Gonzalo-Asensio et al., 2014). Introducing these mutations into M. tuberculosis results in a recombinant strain with reduced virulence in both human macrophages in vitro and in infected mice. When the mutation was corrected in M. bovis to the M. tuberculosis allele, lipid secretion was enhanced but there was no enhanced ESAT-6 secretion (Gonzalo-Asensio et al., 2014). It was instead shown that the RD8 deletion in M. bovis restored ESAT-6 secretion via a PhoPR-independent pathway, hence suggesting a selective advantage for the loss of RD8. A strain of M. bovis that was circulating between patients in a Spanish HIV ward was shown to have an IS6110 insertion upstream of the PhoPR locus, leading to increased PhoPR expression, increased virulence and improved transmission between humans, the latter being a trait that is unusual in M. bovis infections. The loss of PhoPR activity in M. bovis can therefore potentially explain why this species, despite its high degree of genetic similarity to M. tuberculosis, cannot sustain an infection in human populations. Loss of PhoPR activity altered the lipid profile of these strains and decreased their fitness for transmission between human hosts. Further study into the PhoPR genotype will identify whether mutation of this locus was beneficial for *M. bovis* infection of animal hosts, and/or what further adaptations were selected for in the aftermath to sustain *M. bovis* virulence in diverse animal hosts.

8.6.2 RskA-SigK regulon

One of the most consistent and significant differences between *M. bovis* and *M. tuberculosis* is in the levels of the secreted protein MPB70 and its membrane-bound homologue MPB83. The genes encoding these proteins share 63% sequence identity; however, MPB70 has no post-translational modifications whereas MPB83 is glycosylated and associated to the cell envelope (Wiker *et al.*, 1998). MPB70 first came to attention as the most dominant protein in the culture filtrate of *M. bovis* and some BCG strains, but produced at much lower levels in *M. tuberculosis* (Nagai *et al.*, 1981, 1986, 1991; Golby *et al.*, 2007). Later work determined that although levels of these proteins produced by *M. tuberculosis* are low under normal *in vitro* conditions, their genes are induced during intracellular growth (Schnappinger *et al.*, 2003). Further study of MPB70 identified other mycobacterial species that had similar MPB70 levels to *M. bovis* such as *M. caprae* (the goat bacillus) and *M. orygis* (the oryx bacillus).

Additional research sought to explain the molecular basis for variation in the expression of these genes. It was first identified that the genes MPB70 and MPB83 were under the control of the sigma K factor (SigK). Further work recognized that several other genes under this regulon were also expressed to a much higher degree in *M. bovis* than other MTBC species (*Mb0455c*, *Mb0456c*, *Mb0457c*, *dipZ*, *Mb2901*, and *Mb2902c*) (Golby *et al.*, 2007). Study of SigK indicated that the gene was identical across the MTBC; however, when studying the genes around SigK it was found that *Rv0444c*, encoding a potential anti-sigma factor, showed sequence variation across the complex (Said-Salim *et al.*, 2006). In *M. bovis* and *M. caprae*, two non-synonymous SNPs were found in *Rv0444c*, C320T and C551T, and as a result the amino acids encoded changed from glycine to aspartic acid and glutamic acid, respectively. Additionally, a different non-synonymous SNP was found in *M. orygis*, G698C, resulting in the stop codon being replaced by a serine. Both of these changes affected the function of the anti-sigma factor, subsequently designated RskA, meaning that negative control of SigK expression was lost in these strains and hence driving constitutive expression of the SigK regulon (Said-Salim *et al.*, 2006).

The high level of expression of the SigK regulon would result in substantial energy costs. Supporting this is the fact that 'late' strains of BCG (e.g. BCG Pasteur), derived by repeated subculture of *M. bovis*, lost high-level expression of the SigK regulon via a SNP in the start codon of SigK, and as a result show increased growth rates compared to 'early' BCG strains that retain high-level SigK expression (e.g. BCG Tokyo or Russia) (Charlet *et al.*, 2005). The fact that dysregulation of the SigK regulon occurs in some animal-adapted MTBC species, and that it has arisen in different species via independent mutations, indicates that there is a selective advantage for the overall success of some animal-adapted species to overexpress the SigK regulon.

Many of the genes of the SigK regulon are membrane associated but no particular role for them in pathogenesis or transmission has been identified. The focus has been primarily on MPB70 and MPB83, although to date no strong conclusions on their function has been made. The structure of both has been resolved and they have a novel fold similar to that of fascilin domain proteins, which in other bacteria is normally implicated in protein–protein interactions (Zinn *et al.*, 1988; Wiker *et al.*, 1998; Carr *et al.*, 2003). The studies that have been done primarily focus on the role of MPB70 and MPB83 as immunomodulatory proteins. MPB83 has been indicated to have some immunostimulatory properties as a TLR1/2 agonist and it has been indicated that it can induce TNFα and MMP-9 in human monocyte cell lines, and that blocking of TLR1/2 receptors with antibodies caused this response to be lost (Chambers *et al.*, 2010). Other experiments on murine cells also indicate that MPB83 can induce secretion of TNFα, IL-6, and IL-12p40 (Chen et al., 2012). This would suggest that MPB83 could be involved in mediation of innate immune responses.

Experiments investigating the role of MPB70 have been less clear. There is some variability in responses, but most of the work done on MPB70 has focused on its ability to induce an anamnestic immune response in patients with TB and infected animals. Roche examined T-cell responses in patients with TB and healthy individuals who had received the BCG vaccine, or were tuberculin positive and in contact with TB patients. It was found that peripheral blood mononuclear cell (PBMC) from these groups did show increases in lymphocyte proliferation following stimulation with MPB70 (Roche et al., 1994). Other groups repeated this showing T-cell responses, including proliferation and IFNγ secretion in response to MPB70, in both patients with TB and healthy individuals who had been BCG vaccinated (Mustafa et al., 1998). Similar experiments have been carried out in cattle, looking at PBMC responses to MPB70 from cattle who had been treated with M. bovis or that were BCG-Pasteur vaccinated. These indicated that PBMC from M. bovis-infected cattle showed proliferative responses, but BCG-vaccinated cattle did not, although the response seen was weaker than for other mycobacterial proteins (including ESAT-6 and MPB64) (Vordermeier et al., 1999). An experimental infection of cattle with M. bovis also showed cell proliferation in response to MPB70 in PBMC as well as increases in IFNγ secretion (Rhodes et al., 2000).

Whether the genes controlled by SigK regulon are involved in virulence, pathogenesis or transmission is unclear. While individual M. bovis mutants for SigK, MPB70, MPB83, etc. and their role in infection has not been reported, a sigK KO mutant in M. tuberculosis was not attenuated for infection of murine models (Schneider et al., 2014), but its role in the virulence of M. bovis could be very different given the evidence of a selective advantage to certain animal-adapted species in constitutive SigK activation. Worth noting in this regard is the work of Collins et al. (2005), who generated a large deletion (~10kb) at the M. bovis SigK locus and noted attenuation of the resulting mutant in guinea pigs; while multiple genes were deleted it is intriguing to speculate that some of the attenuation of this mutant may have been due to loss of SigK and hence lack of expression of genes in the SigK regulon.

8.7 Conclusions

Virulence is a complex concept, a unique configuration of factors that allow a pathogen to adapt to and inflict damage on its preferred host. Although here we have highlighted and discussed discreet factors as important in causing disease, bacterial virulence is the result of a highly organized and complex interdependent system between pathogen and host that we still only poorly understand. Host factors that can have a major role in the ability of a pathogen to cause disease include the genetic background of the host, the resident microbiome, immune status, etc. Much of the work defining pathogen virulence systems employs model organisms and in vitro cellular systems, which is a good initial step to identify the broad effects of particular proteins. However, given the varying host preferences of the MTBC, studying virulence in multiple species and with variations in the host environment could be key to understanding the true role of virulence factors.

This chapter has highlighted some of the key factors that have been discovered that contribute to the virulence of M. bovis. Almost all of these factors are shared by M. tuberculosis, and allow both bacteria to survive and cause TB in their respective hosts. However, there are also unique factors that may govern the host preferences of these species. The majority of research into mycobacterial virulence has focused on human TB and the human-adapted M. tuberculosis pathogen; however, much of this has also been relevant for our understanding of M. bovis. Future research looks certain to provide greater insight into virulence across all the constituent species of the MTBC, and hence provide the knowledge that will aid in the eradication of both human and animal TB.

Acknowledgements

A.S. is funded by the Wellcome Trust through the UCD Computational Infection Biology PhD Programme grant 102395/Z/13/Z.

References

Aagaard, C., Govaerts, M., Meikle, V., Gutierrez-Pabello, J.A., Mcnair, J., et al. (2010) Detection of bovine tuberculosis in herds with different disease prevalence and influence of paratuberculosis infection on PPDB and ESAT-6/CFP10 specificity. *Preventive Veterinary Medicine* 96, 161–169.

Abdallah, A.M., Verboom, T., Weerdenburg, E.M., Gey Van Pittius, N.C., Mahasha, P.W., et al. (2009) PPE and PE_PGRS proteins of *Mycobacterium marinum* are transported via the type VII secretion system ESX-5. *Molecular Microbiology* 73, 329–340.

Alexander, K.A., Laver, P.N., Michel, A.L., Williams, M., Van Helden, P.D., et al. (2010) Novel *Mycobacterium tuberculosis* complex pathogen, *M. mungi*. *Emerging Infectious Diseases* 16, 1296–1299.

Aranaz, A., Liebana, E., Gomez-Mampaso, E., Galan, J.C., Cousins, D., et al. (1999) *Mycobacterium tuberculosis* subsp. *caprae* subsp. nov.: a taxonomic study of a new member of the *Mycobacterium tuberculosis* complex isolated from goats in Spain. *International Journal of Systematic Bacteriology* 49(3), 1263–1273.

Arlehamn, C.S., Sidney, J., Henderson, R., Greenbaum, J.A., James, E.A., et al. (2012) Dissecting mechanisms of immunodominance to the common tuberculosis antigens ESAT-6, CFP10, Rv2031c (hspX), Rv2654c (TB7.7), and Rv1038c (EsxJ). *Journal of Immunology* 188, 5020–5031.

Arruda, S., Bomfim, G., Knights, R., Huima-Byron, T. and Riley, L.W. (1993) Cloning of an *M. tuberculosis* DNA fragment associated with entry and survival inside cells. *Science* 261, 1454–1457.

Astarie-Dequeker, C., Le Guyader, L., Malaga, W., Seaphanh, F.K., Chalut, C., et al. (2009) Phthiocerol dimycocerosates of *M. tuberculosis* participate in macrophage invasion by inducing changes in the organization of plasma membrane lipids. *PLoS Pathogens* 5, e1000289.

Ates, L.S., Van Der Woude, A.D., Bestebroer, J., Van Stempvoort, G., Musters, R.J., et al. (2016) The ESX-5 system of pathogenic mycobacteria is involved in capsule integrity and virulence through its substrate PPE10. *PLoS Pathogens* 12, e1005696.

Azad, A.K., Sirakova, T.D., Fernandes, N.D. and Kolattukudy, P.E. (1997) Gene knockout reveals a novel gene cluster for the synthesis of a class of cell wall lipids unique to pathogenic mycobacteria. *The Journal of Biological Chemistry* 272, 16741–16745.

Banu, S., Honore, N., Saint-Joanis, B., Philpott, D., Prevost, M.C., et al. (2002) Are the PE-PGRS proteins of *Mycobacterium tuberculosis* variable surface antigens? *Molecular Microbiology* 44, 9–19.

Berthet, F.X., Lagranderie, M., Gounon, P., Laurent-Winter, C., Ensergueix, D., et al. (1998a) Attenuation of virulence by disruption of the *Mycobacterium tuberculosis* erp gene. *Science* 282, 759–762.

Berthet, F.X., Rasmussen, P.B., Rosenkrands, I., Andersen, P. and Gicquel, B. (1998b) A *Mycobacterium tuberculosis* operon encoding ESAT-6 and a novel low-molecular-mass culture filtrate protein (CFP-10). *Microbiology* 144(11), 3195–3203.

Bigi, F., Gioffre, A., Klepp, L., Santangelo, M.P., Velicovsky, C.A., et al. (2005) Mutation in the P36 gene of *Mycobacterium bovis* provokes attenuation of the bacillus in a mouse model. *Tuberculosis (Edinburgh)* 85, 221–226.

Bitter, W., Houben, E.N., Bottai, D., Brodin, P., Brown, E.J., et al. (2009) Systematic genetic nomenclature for type VII secretion systems. *PLoS Pathogens* 5, e1000507.

Braunstein, M., Brown, A.M., Kurtz, S. and Jacobs Jr., W.R. (2001) Two nonredundant SecA homologues function in mycobacteria. *Journal of Bacteriology* 183, 6979–6990.

Braunstein, M., Espinosa, B.J., Chan, J., Belisle, J.T. and Jacobs Jr., W.R. (2003) SecA2 functions in the secretion of superoxide dismutase A and in the virulence of *Mycobacterium tuberculosis*. *Molecular Microbiology* 48, 453–464.

Brennan, P.J. (2003) Structure, function, and biogenesis of the cell wall of *Mycobacterium tuberculosis*. *Tuberculosis (Edinburgh)* 83, 91–97.

Brennan, M.J., Delogu, G., Chen, Y., Bardarov, S., Kriakov, J., et al. (2001) Evidence that mycobacterial PE_PGRS proteins are cell surface constituents that influence interactions with other cells. *Infection and Immunity* 69, 7326–7333.

Brodin, P., Rosenkrands, I., Andersen, P., Cole, S.T. and Brosch, R. (2004) ESAT-6 proteins: protective antigens and virulence factors? *Trends in Microbiology* 12, 500–508.

Brosch, R., Gordon, S.V., Marmiesse, M., Brodin, P., Buchrieser, C., et al. (2002) A new evolutionary scenario for the *Mycobacterium tuberculosis* complex. *Proceedings of the National Academy of Sciences of the United States of America* 99, 3684–3689.

Calmette, A. (1931) Preventive vaccination against tuberculosis with BCG. *Proceedings of the Royal Society of Medicine* 24, 1481–1490.
Camacho, L.R., Constant, P., Raynaud, C., Laneelle, M.A., Triccas, J.A., *et al*. (2001) Analysis of the phthiocerol dimycocerosate locus of *Mycobacterium tuberculosis*. Evidence that this lipid is involved in the cell wall permeability barrier. *The Journal of Biological Chemistry* 276, 19845–19854.
Carr, M.D., Bloemink, M.J., Dentten, E., Whelan, A.O., Gordon, S.V., *et al*. (2003) Solution structure of the *Mycobacterium tuberculosis* complex protein MPB70: from tuberculosis pathogenesis to inherited human corneal disease. *The Journal of Biological Chemistry* 278, 43736–43743.
Cascioferro, A., Delogu, G., Colone, M., Sali, M., Stringaro, A., *et al*. (2007) PE is a functional domain responsible for protein translocation and localization on mycobacterial cell wall. *Molecular Microbiology* 66, 1536–1547.
Chambers, M.A., Whelan, A.O., Spallek, R., Singh, M., Coddeville, B., *et al*. (2010) Non-acylated *Mycobacterium bovis* glycoprotein MPB83 binds to TLR1/2 and stimulates production of matrix metalloproteinase 9. *Biochemical and Biophysical Research Communications* 400, 403–408.
Champion, P.A., Stanley, S.A., Champion, M.M., Brown, E.J. and Cox, J.S. (2006) C-terminal signal sequence promotes virulence factor secretion in *Mycobacterium tuberculosis*. *Science* 313, 1632–1636.
Charlet, D., Mostowy, S., Alexander, D., Sit, L., Wiker, H.G., *et al*. (2005) Reduced expression of antigenic proteins MPB70 and MPB83 in *Mycobacterium bovis* BCG strains due to a start codon mutation in sigK. *Molecular Microbiology* 56, 1302–1313.
Chen, S.T., Li, J.Y., Zhang, Y., Gao, X. and Cai, H. (2012) Recombinant MPT83 derived from *Mycobacterium tuberculosis* induces cytokine production and upregulates the function of mouse macrophages through TLR2. *Journal of Immunology* 188, 668–677.
Cole, S.T. (1999) Learning from the genome sequence of *Mycobacterium tuberculosis* H37Rv. *FEBS Letters* 452, 7–10.
Cole, S.T. and Barrell, B.G. (1998) Analysis of the genome of *Mycobacterium tuberculosis* H37Rv. *Novartis Foundation Symposium* 217, 160–172; discussion 172–177.
Cole, S.T., Brosch, R., Parkhill, J., Garnier, T., Churcher, C., *et al*. (1998) Deciphering the biology of *Mycobacterium tuberculosis* from the complete genome sequence. *Nature* 393, 537–544.
Collins, D.M., Skou, B., White, S., Bassett, S., Collins, L., *et al*. (2005) Generation of attenuated *Mycobacterium bovis* strains by signature-tagged mutagenesis for discovery of novel vaccine candidates. *Infection and Immunity* 73, 2379–2386.
Comas, I., Coscolla, M., Luo, T., Borrell, S., Holt, K.E., *et al*. (2013) Out-of-Africa migration and neolithic coexpansion of *Mycobacterium tuberculosis* with modern humans. *Nature Genetics* 45, 1176–1182.
Constant, P., Perez, E., Malaga, W., Laneelle, M.A., Saurel, O., *et al*. (2002) Role of the pks15/1 gene in the biosynthesis of phenolglycolipids in the *Mycobacterium tuberculosis* complex. Evidence that all strains synthesize glycosylated p-hydroxybenzoic methyl esters and that strains devoid of phenolglycolipids harbor a frameshift mutation in the pks15/1 gene. *The Journal of Biological Chemistry* 277, 38148–38158.
Cousins, D.V., Williams, S.N., Reuter, R., Forshaw, D., Chadwick, B., *et al*. (1993) Tuberculosis in wild seals and characterisation of the seal bacillus. *Australian Veterinary Journal* 70, 92–97.
Cousins, D.V., Peet, R.L., Gaynor, W.T., Williams, S.N. and Gow, B.L. (1994) Tuberculosis in imported hyrax (*Procavia capensis*) caused by an unusual variant belonging to the *Mycobacterium tuberculosis* complex. *Veterinary Microbiology* 42, 135–145.
Cox, J.S., Chen, B., Mcneil, M. and Jacobs Jr., W.R. (1999) Complex lipid determines tissue-specific replication of *Mycobacterium tuberculosis* in mice. *Nature* 402, 79–83.
Danilchanka, O., Sun, J., Pavlenok, M., Maueroder, C., Speer, A., *et al*. (2014) An outer membrane channel protein of *Mycobacterium tuberculosis* with exotoxin activity. *Proceedings of the National Academy of Sciences of the United States of America* 111, 6750–6755.
De Mendonca-Lima, L., Bordat, Y., Pivert, E., Recchi, C., Neyrolles, O., *et al*. (2003) The allele encoding the mycobacterial erp protein affects lung disease in mice. *Cellular Microbiology* 5, 65–73.
Delogu, G. and Brennan, M.J. (2001) Comparative immune response to PE and PE_PGRS antigens of *Mycobacterium tuberculosis*. *Infection and Immunity* 69, 5606–5611.
Delogu, G., Pusceddu, C., Bua, A., Fadda, G., Brennan, M.J., *et al*. (2004) Rv1818c-encoded PE_PGRS protein of *Mycobacterium tuberculosis* is surface exposed and influences bacterial cell structure. *Molecular Microbiology* 52, 725–733.

Dillon, D.C., Alderson, M.R., Day, C.H., Bement, T., Campos-Neto, A., *et al.* (2000) Molecular and immunological characterization of *Mycobacterium tuberculosis* CFP-10, an immunodiagnostic antigen missing in *Mycobacterium bovis* BCG. *Journal of Clinical Microbiology* 38, 3285–3290.

Domenech, P. and Reed, M.B. (2009) Rapid and spontaneous loss of phthiocerol dimycocerosate (PDIM) from *Mycobacterium tuberculosis* grown in vitro: implications for virulence studies. *Microbiology* 155, 3532–3543.

Dubnau, E., Fontan, P., Manganelli, R., Soares-Appel, S. and Smith, I. (2002) *Mycobacterium tuberculosis* genes induced during infection of human macrophages. *Infection and Immunity* 70, 2787–2795.

Espitia, C., Laclette, J.P., Mondragon-Palomino, M., Amador, A., Campuzano, J., *et al.* (1999) The PE-PGRS glycine-rich proteins of *Mycobacterium tuberculosis*: a new family of fibronectin-binding proteins? *Microbiology* 145(12), 3487–3495.

Frothingham, R., Hills, H.G. and Wilson, K.H. (1994) Extensive DNA sequence conservation throughout the *Mycobacterium tuberculosis* complex. *Journal of Clinical Microbiology* 32, 1639–1643.

Garnier, T., Eiglmeier, K., Camus, J.C., Medina, N., Mansoor, H., *et al.* (2003) The complete genome sequence of *Mycobacterium bovis*. *Proceedings of the National Academy of Sciences of the United States of America* 100, 7877–7882.

Gey Van Pittius, N.C., Gamieldien, J., Hide, W., Brown, G.D., Siezen, R.J., *et al.* (2001) The ESAT-6 gene cluster of *Mycobacterium tuberculosis* and other high G+C Gram-positive bacteria. *Genome Biology* 2, RESEARCH0044.

Gey Van Pittius, N.C., Sampson, S.L., Lee, H., Kim, Y., Van Helden, P.D., *et al.* (2006) Evolution and expansion of the *Mycobacterium tuberculosis* PE and PPE multigene families and their association with the duplication of the ESAT-6 (esx) gene cluster regions. *BMC Evolutionary Biology* 6, 95.

Gilmore, S.A., Schelle, M.W., Holsclaw, C.M., Leigh, C.D., Jain, M., *et al.* (2012) Sulfolipid-1 biosynthesis restricts *Mycobacterium tuberculosis* growth in human macrophages. *ACS Chemical Biology* 7, 863–870.

Golby, P., Hatch, K.A., Bacon, J., Cooney, R., Riley, P., *et al.* (2007) Comparative transcriptomics reveals key gene expression differences between the human and bovine pathogens of the *Mycobacterium tuberculosis* complex. *Microbiology* 153, 3323–3336.

Gonzalo-Asensio, J., Malaga, W., Pawlik, A., Astarie-Dequeker, C., Passemar, C., *et al.* (2014) Evolutionary history of tuberculosis shaped by conserved mutations in the PhoPR virulence regulator. *Proceedings of the National Academy of Sciences of the United States of America* 111, 11491–11496.

Guinn, K.M., Hickey, M.J., Mathur, S.K., Zakel, K.L., Grotzke, J.E., *et al.* (2004) Individual RD1-region genes are required for export of ESAT-6/CFP-10 and for virulence of *Mycobacterium tuberculosis*. *Molecular Microbiology* 51, 359–370.

Hotter, G.S. and Collins, D.M. (2011) *Mycobacterium bovis* lipids: virulence and vaccines. *Molecular Microbiology* 151, 91–98.

Hotter, G.S., Wards, B.J., Mouat, P., Besra, G.S., Gomes, J., *et al.* (2005) Transposon mutagenesis of Mb0100 at the ppe1-nrp locus in *Mycobacterium bovis* disrupts phthiocerol dimycocerosate (PDIM) and glycosylphenol-PDIM biosynthesis, producing an avirulent strain with vaccine properties at least equal to those of *M. bovis* BCG. *Journal of Bacteriology* 187, 2267–2277.

Houben, D., Demangel, C., Van Ingen, J., Perez, J., Baldeon, L., *et al.* (2012) ESX-1-mediated translocation to the cytosol controls virulence of mycobacteria. *Cellular Microbiology* 14, 1287–1298.

Houben, E.N., Korotkov, K.V. and Bitter, W. (2014) Take five – Type VII secretion systems of Mycobacteria. *Biochimica et Biophysica Acta* 1843, 1707–1716.

Iantomasi, R., Sali, M., Cascioferro, A., Palucci, I., Zumbo, A., *et al.* (2012) PE_PGRS30 is required for the full virulence of *Mycobacterium tuberculosis*. *Cellular Microbiology* 14, 356–367.

Karlson, A.G. and Lessel, E.F. (1970) *Mycobacterium bovis* nom. nov. *International Journal of Systematic and Evolutionary Microbiology* 20, 273–282.

Kassa, D., Ran, L., Geberemeskel, W., Tebeje, M., Alemu, A., *et al.* (2012) Analysis of immune responses against a wide range of *Mycobacterium tuberculosis* antigens in patients with active pulmonary tuberculosis. *Clinical and Vaccine Immunology* 19, 1907–1915.

Kolattukudy, P.E., Fernandes, N.D., Azad, A.K., Fitzmaurice, A.M. and Sirakova, T.D. (1997) Biochemistry and molecular genetics of cell-wall lipid biosynthesis in mycobacteria. *Molecular Microbiology* 24, 263–270.

Kozak, R.A., Alexander, D.C., Liao, R., Sherman, D.R. and Behr, M.A. (2011) Region of difference 2 contributes to virulence of *Mycobacterium tuberculosis*. *Infection and Immunity* 79, 59–66.

Lee, P.A., Tullman-Ercek, D. and Georgiou, G. (2006) The bacterial twin-arginine translocation pathway. *Annual Review of Microbiology* 60, 373–395.

Lee, J.S., Krause, R., Schreiber, J., Mollenkopf, H.J., Kowall, J., et al. (2008) Mutation in the transcriptional regulator PhoP contributes to avirulence of *Mycobacterium tuberculosis* H37Ra strain. *Cell Host Microbe* 3, 97–103.

Lewis, K.N., Liao, R., Guinn, K.M., Hickey, M.J., Smith, S., et al. (2003) Deletion of RD1 from *Mycobacterium tuberculosis* mimics bacille Calmette-Guérin attenuation. *The Journal of Infectious Diseases* 187, 117–123.

Lillebaek, T., Dirksen, A., Baess, I., Strunge, B., Thomsen, V.O., et al. (2002) Molecular evidence of endogenous reactivation of *Mycobacterium tuberculosis* after 33 years of latent infection. *The Journal of Infectious Diseases* 185, 401–404.

Magnus, K. (1966) Epidemiological basis of tuberculosis eradication. 3. Risk of pulmonary tuberculosis after human and bovine infection. *Bulletin of the World Health Organization* 35, 483–508.

Mahairas, G.G., Sabo, P.J., Hickey, M.J., Singh, D.C. and Stover, C.K. (1996) Molecular analysis of genetic differences between *Mycobacterium bovis* BCG and virulent *M. bovis*. *Journal of Bacteriology* 178, 1274–1282.

Majlessi, L., Brodin, P., Brosch, R., Rojas, M.J., Khun, H., et al. (2005) Influence of ESAT-6 secretion system 1 (RD1) of *Mycobacterium tuberculosis* on the interaction between mycobacteria and the host immune system. *Journal of Immunology* 174, 3570–3579.

Malaga, W., Constant, P., Euphrasie, D., Cataldi, A., Daffe, M., et al. (2008) Deciphering the genetic bases of the structural diversity of phenolic glycolipids in strains of the *Mycobacterium tuberculosis* complex. *The Journal of Biological Chemistry* 283, 15177–15184.

Mcdonough, J.A., Hacker, K.E., Flores, A.R., Pavelka Jr., M.S. and Braunstein, M. (2005) The twin-arginine translocation pathway of *Mycobacterium smegmatis* is functional and required for the export of mycobacterial beta-lactamases. *Journal of Bacteriology* 187, 7667–7679.

Mostowy, S., Cousins, D., Brinkman, J., Aranaz, A. and Behr, M.A. (2002) Genomic deletions suggest a phylogeny for the *Mycobacterium tuberculosis* complex. *The Journal of Infectious Diseases* 186, 74–80.

Muller, B., Durr, S., Alonso, S., Hattendorf, J., Laisse, C.J., et al. (2013) Zoonotic *Mycobacterium bovis*-induced tuberculosis in humans. *Emerging Infectious Diseases* 19, 899–908.

Mustafa, A.S., Amoudy, H.A., Wiker, H.G., Abal, A.T., Ravn, P., et al. (1998) Comparison of antigen-specific T-cell responses of tuberculosis patients using complex or single antigens of *Mycobacterium tuberculosis*. *Scandinavian Journal of Immunology* 48, 535–543.

Mustafa, T., Wiker, H.G., Morkve, O. and Sviland, L. (2007) Reduced apoptosis and increased inflammatory cytokines in granulomas caused by tuberculous compared to non-tuberculous mycobacteria: role of MPT64 antigen in apoptosis and immune response. *Clinical and Experimental Immunology* 150, 105–113.

Nagai, S., Matsumoto, J. and Nagasuga, T. (1981) Specific skin-reactive protein from culture filtrate of *Mycobacterium bovis* BCG. *Infection and Immunity* 31, 1152–1160.

Nagai, S., Miura, K., Tokunaga, T. and Harboe, M. (1986) MPB70, a unique antigenic protein isolated from the culture filtrate of BCG substrain Tokyo. *Developments in Biological Standardization* 58(B), 511–516.

Nagai, S., Wiker, H.G., Harboe, M. and Kinomoto, M. (1991) Isolation and partial characterization of major protein antigens in the culture fluid of *Mycobacterium tuberculosis*. *Infection and Immunity* 59, 372–382.

O'hagan, D. (1993) Biosynthesis of fatty acid and polyketide metabolites. *Natural Product Reports* 10, 593–624.

Overbeek, R., Fonstein, M., D'souza, M., Pusch, G.D. and Maltsev, N. (1999) The use of gene clusters to infer functional coupling. *Proceedings of the National Academy of Sciences of the United States of America* 96, 2896–2901.

Pajon, R., Yero, D., Lage, A., Llanes, A. and Borroto, C.J. (2006) Computational identification of beta-barrel outer-membrane proteins in *Mycobacterium tuberculosis* predicted proteomes as putative vaccine candidates. *Tuberculosis (Edinburgh)* 86, 290–302.

Palmer, M.V. (2013) *Mycobacterium bovis*: characteristics of wildlife reservoir hosts. *Transboundary and Emerging Diseases* 60(1), 1–13.

Parsons, S.D., Drewe, J.A., Gey Van Pittius, N.C., Warren, R.M. and Van Helden, P.D. (2013) Novel cause of tuberculosis in meerkats, South Africa. *Emerging Infectious Diseases* 19, 2004–2007.

Perez, E., Samper, S., Bordas, Y., Guilhot, C., Gicquel, B., *et al.* (2001) An essential role for phoP in *Mycobacterium tuberculosis* virulence. *Molecular Microbiology* 41, 179–187.

Pesciaroli, M., Alvarez, J., Boniotti, M.B., Cagiola, M., Di Marco, V., *et al.* (2014) Tuberculosis in domestic animal species. *Research in Veterinary Science* 97(Suppl), S78–S85.

Pethe, K., Swenson, D.L., Alonso, S., Anderson, J., Wang, C., *et al.* (2004) Isolation of *Mycobacterium tuberculosis* mutants defective in the arrest of phagosome maturation. *Proceedings of the National Academy of Sciences of the United States of America* 101, 13642–13647.

Pym, A.S., Brodin, P., Majlessi, L., Brosch, R., Demangel, C., *et al.* (2003) Recombinant BCG exporting ESAT-6 confers enhanced protection against tuberculosis. *Nature Medicine* 9, 533–539.

Quadri, L.E. (2014) Biosynthesis of mycobacterial lipids by polyketide synthases and beyond. *Critical Reviews in Biochemistry and Molecular Biology* 49, 179–211.

Raynaud, C., Guilhot, C., Rauzier, J., Bordat, Y., Pelicic, V., *et al.* (2002a) Phospholipases C are involved in the virulence of *Mycobacterium tuberculosis*. *Molecular Microbiology* 45, 203–217.

Raynaud, C., Papavinasasundaram, K.G., Speight, R.A., Springer, B., Sander, P., *et al.* (2002b) The functions of OmpATb, a pore-forming protein of *Mycobacterium tuberculosis*. *Molecular Microbiology* 46, 191–201.

Reed, M.B., Domenech, P., Manca, C., Su, H., Barczak, A.K., *et al.* (2004) A glycolipid of hypervirulent tuberculosis strains that inhibits the innate immune response. *Nature* 431, 84–87.

Renshaw, P.S., Panagiotidou, P., Whelan, A., Gordon, S.V., Hewinson, R.G., *et al.* (2002) Conclusive evidence that the major T-cell antigens of the *Mycobacterium tuberculosis* complex ESAT-6 and CFP-10 form a tight, 1:1 complex and characterization of the structural properties of ESAT-6, CFP-10, and the ESAT-6*CFP-10 complex. Implications for pathogenesis and virulence. *The Journal of Biological Chemistry* 277, 21598–21603.

Rhodes, S.G., Gavier-Widen, D., Buddle, B.M., Whelan, A.O., Singh, M., *et al.* (2000) Antigen specificity in experimental bovine tuberculosis. *Infection and Immunity* 68, 2573–2578.

Roche, P.W., Triccas, J.A., Avery, D.T., Fifis, T., Billman-Jacobe, H., *et al.* (1994) Differential T cell responses to mycobacteria-secreted proteins distinguish vaccination with bacille Calmette-Guérin from infection with *Mycobacterium tuberculosis*. *The Journal of Infectious Diseases* 170, 1326–1330.

Rousseau, C., Winter, N., Pivert, E., Bordat, Y., Neyrolles, O., *et al.* (2004) Production of phthiocerol dimycocerosates protects *Mycobacterium tuberculosis* from the cidal activity of reactive nitrogen intermediates produced by macrophages and modulates the early immune response to infection. *Cellular Microbiology* 6, 277–287.

Said-Salim, B., Mostowy, S., Kristof, A.S. and Behr, M.A. (2006) Mutations in *Mycobacterium tuberculosis* Rv0444c, the gene encoding anti-SigK, explain high level expression of MPB70 and MPB83 in *Mycobacterium bovis*. *Molecular Microbiology* 62, 1251–1263.

Saint-Joanis, B., Demangel, C., Jackson, M., Brodin, P., Marsollier, L., *et al.* (2006) Inactivation of Rv2525c, a substrate of the twin arginine translocation (Tat) system of *Mycobacterium tuberculosis*, increases beta-lactam susceptibility and virulence. *Journal of Bacteriology* 188, 6669–6679.

Sampson, S.L. (2011) Mycobacterial PE/PPE proteins at the host-pathogen interface. *Clinical and Developmental Immunology* 2011, 497203.

Schnappinger, D., Ehrt, S., Voskuil, M.I., Liu, Y., Mangan, J.A. *et al.*, (2003) Transcriptional Adaptation of *Mycobacterium tuberculosis* within macrophages: insights into the phagosomal environment. *The Journal of Experimental Medicine* 198, 693–704.

Schneider, J.S., Sklar, J.G. and Glickman, M.S. (2014) The rip1 protease of *Mycobacterium tuberculosis* controls the SigD regulon. *Journal of Bacteriology* 196, 2638–2645.

Senaratne, R.H., Sidders, B., Sequeira, P., Saunders, G., Dunphy, K., *et al.* (2008) *Mycobacterium tuberculosis* strains disrupted in mce3 and mce4 operons are attenuated in mice. *Journal of Medical Microbiology* 57, 164–170.

Serafini, A., Boldrin, F., Palu, G. and Manganelli, R. (2009) Characterization of a *Mycobacterium tuberculosis* ESX-3 conditional mutant: essentiality and rescue by iron and zinc. *Journal of Bacteriology* 191, 6340–6344.

Sirakova, T.D., Dubey, V.S., Cynamon, M.H. and Kolattukudy, P.E. (2003) Attenuation of *Mycobacterium tuberculosis* by disruption of a mas-like gene or a chalcone synthase-like gene, which causes deficiency in dimycocerosyl phthiocerol synthesis. *Journal of Bacteriology* 185, 2999–3008.

Skuce R.A. and McDowell, S. (2011) Bovine tuberculosis (TB): a review of cattle-to-cattle transmission, risk factors and susceptibility. Agri-food and Biosciences Institute, Belfast, Northern Ireland, UK. Available at: https://www.daera-ni.gov.uk/sites/default/files/publications/dard/afbi-literature-review-tb-review-cattle-to-cattle-transmission.pdf (accessed 21 February 2018).

Smith, T. (1898) A comparative study of bovine tubercle bacilli and of human bacilli from sputum. *The Journal of Experimental Medicine* 3, 451–511.

Smith, N.H., Kremer, K., Inwald, J., Dale, J., Driscoll, J.R., *et al.* (2006) Ecotypes of the *Mycobacterium tuberculosis* complex. *Journal of Theoretical Biology* 239, 220–225.

Sreevatsan, S., Pan, X., Stockbauer, K.E., Connell, N.D., Kreiswirth, B.N., *et al.* (1997) Restricted structural gene polymorphism in the *Mycobacterium tuberculosis* complex indicates evolutionarily recent global dissemination. *Proceedings of the National Academy of Sciences of the United States of America* 94, 9869–9874.

Srivastava, V., Rouanet, C., Srivastava, R., Ramalingam, B., Locht, C., *et al.* (2007) Macrophage-specific *Mycobacterium tuberculosis* genes: identification by green fluorescent protein and kanamycin resistance selection. *Microbiology* 153, 659–666.

Stewart, G.R., Patel, J., Robertson, B.D., Rae, A. and Young, D.B. (2005) Mycobacterial mutants with defective control of phagosomal acidification. *PLoS Pathogens* 1, 269–278.

Swanson, S., Ioerger, T.R., Rigel, N.W., Miller, B.K., Braunstein, M., *et al.* (2015) Structural similarities and differences between two functionally distinct seca proteins, *Mycobacterium tuberculosis* SecA1 and SecA2. *Journal of Bacteriology* 198, 720–730.

Triccas, J.A., Berthet, F.X., Pelicic, V. and Gicquel, B. (1999) Use of fluorescence induction and sucrose counterselection to identify *Mycobacterium tuberculosis* genes expressed within host cells. *Microbiology* 145(10), 2923–2930.

Trivedi, O.A., Arora, P., Vats, A., Ansari, M.Z., Tickoo, R., *et al.* (2005) Dissecting the mechanism and assembly of a complex virulence mycobacterial lipid. *Molecular Cell* 17, 631–643.

Tufariello, J.M., Chapman, J.R., Kerantzas, C.A., Wong, K.W., Vilcheze, C., *et al.* (2016) Separable roles for *Mycobacterium tuberculosis* ESX-3 effectors in iron acquisition and virulence. *Proceedings of the National Academy of Sciences of the United States of America* 113, E348–E357.

Tundup, S., Akhter, Y., Thiagarajan, D. and Hasnain, S.E. (2006) Clusters of PE and PPE genes of *Mycobacterium tuberculosis* are organized in operons: evidence that PE Rv2431c is co-transcribed with PPE Rv2430c and their gene products interact with each other. *FEBS Letters* 580, 1285–1293.

Van Der Wel, N., Hava, D., Houben, D., Fluitsma, D., Van Zon, M., *et al.* (2007) *M. tuberculosis* and *M. leprae* translocate from the phagolysosome to the cytosol in myeloid cells. *Cell* 129, 1287–1298.

Van Ingen, J., Rahim, Z., Mulder, A., Boeree, M.J., Simeone, R., *et al.* (2012) Characterization of *Mycobacterium orygis* as *M. tuberculosis* complex subspecies. *Emerging Infectious Diseases* 18, 653–655.

Vordermeier, H.M., Cockle, P.C., Whelan, A., Rhodes, S., Palmer, N., *et al.* (1999) Development of diagnostic reagents to differentiate between *Mycobacterium bovis* BCG vaccination and *M. bovis* infection in cattle. *Clinical and Diagnostic Laboratory Immunology* 6, 675–682.

Wells, A.Q. (1937) Tuberculosis in wild voles. *The Lancet* 229, 1221.

Wells, A.Q. (1946) The murine type of tubercle bacilli (the vole acid-fast bacillus). *MRC Special Report Series.* Medical Research Council, London, UK.

Wiker, H.G., Lyashchenko, K.P., Aksoy, A.M., Lightbody, K.A., Pollock, J.M., *et al.* (1998) Immunochemical characterization of the MPB70/80 and MPB83 proteins of *Mycobacterium bovis*. *Infection and Immunity* 66, 1445–1452.

Zinn, K., Mcallister, L. and Goodman, C.S. (1988) Sequence analysis and neuronal expression of fasciclin I in grasshopper and Drosophila. *Cell* 53, 577–587.

Zumarraga, M., Bigi, F., Alito, A., Romano, M.I. and Cataldi, A. (1999) A 12.7 kb fragment of the *Mycobacterium tuberculosis* genome is not present in *Mycobacterium bovis*. *Microbiology* 145(4), 893–897.

9 The Pathology and Pathogenesis of *Mycobacterium bovis* Infection

Francisco J. Salguero*

Department of Pathology and Infectious Diseases, School of Veterinary Medicine, University of Surrey, Guildford, UK

9.1 Introduction

Mycobacterium bovis is able to infect a wide variety of domestic and wild animals, including humans (O'Reilly and Daborn, 1995). *M. bovis* is a member of the *Mycobacterium tuberculosis* complex (MTBC), which also includes *M. tuberculosis*, *M. bovis*, *M. africanum*, *M. microti*, *M. caprae*, *M. canetti*, *M. pinnipedii* and *M. mungi* (Rodriguez-Campos *et al.*, 2014).

Bovine tuberculosis is the infectious disease of cattle caused by *M. bovis* or *M. caprae* (Domingo *et al.*, 2014). The disease follows a chronic course with the formation of a granulomatous, caseous and necrotizing inflammatory process affecting mainly the respiratory tract (lungs and draining lymph nodes) or other locations, including the gastrointestinal tract and secondary lymphoid organs.

Once the bacteria enter the host, the infection can remain subclinical for long periods of time. The lesions will start to form, and can develop into a localized or generalized form of the disease affecting multiple organs. The route of infection will determine the location and spectrum of the lesions observed in bovine tuberculosis (Domingo *et al.*, 2014). The most common route of infection is via inhalation of droplet nuclei or other aerosol material, causing lesions in the upper and lower respiratory tract, including the lungs, and the associated lymphoid tissues (Neill *et al.*, 1994, 2001). Depending on the infection dose, *M. bovis* may also induce typical lesions in the upper respiratory tract mucosa and the retropharyngeal lymph nodes (Cassidy *et al.*, 1999). Interestingly, animals experimentally infected intratracheally with *M. bovis* in addition to those that are infected naturally can also show lesions in a variety of lymph nodes in the head and neck area (Dean *et al.*, 2014, 2015; Ameni *et al.*, 2017; Salguero *et al.*, 2017).

The tonsils are an interesting site of infection by *M. bovis*, with a significant number of animals naturally and experimentally infected with *M. bovis* showing either lesions or viable bacteria isolated by culture in this organ (Cassidy *et al.*, 1999; Liébana *et al.*, 2008).

If the pathogen enters the organism via ingestion of contaminated pasture, water or feed, a gastrointestinal form of the disease will be established with frequent lesions in the mesenteric and hepatic lymph nodes (Menzies and Neill, 2000). Other routes of infection (e.g. genital, intramammary or transplacental) can be also observed but with very low frequency due to the epidemiological situation of most countries that have active control or eradication programmes (Domingo *et al.*, 2014).

Bovine tuberculosis continues to be a very important disease for cattle farming and as a public health concern because of its zoonotic

---

* Email: f.salguerobodes@surrey.ac.uk

potential. Even though the disease has been known for centuries, its pathogenesis is still not fully understood and the mechanisms of diagnosis and control in different scenarios are under constant revision. This chapter reviews the pathology of *M. bovis* infection in cattle and other animal species and the main aspects of the pathogenesis of the immune response in the host after infection.

9.2 Macroscopic Pathology of *M. bovis* Infection

The typical gross pathological lesion of bovine tuberculosis is known as a tubercle, which is a circumscribed yellowish granulomatous inflammatory nodule of variable size that is more or less encapsulated by connective tissue and often contains a central core of necrotic tissue with varying degrees of mineralization (Aranday-Cortés *et al.*, 2013; Domingo *et al.*, 2014). The localization of the granulomatous nodules depends largely on the route of infection. Adult cattle typically show respiratory lesions, circumscribed to the lung parenchyma (Fig. 9.1) and regional lymph nodes within the thoracic cavity. The association of lung and mediastinal lymph nodes in the pathogenesis of tuberculosis has been described many years ago (Ghon, 1912) as illustrated by the identification of the primary complex, or Ghon complex, defined as the presence of both primary pulmonary lesion and caseous lymph node lesion.

The primary lesion is often localized within the dorsal area of one of the lung lobes. This lesion generally progresses towards an encapsulated and mineralized lesion. However, if the infected animal is immunocompromised, or the immune response is ineffective, the primary infection may generalize during the initial stages, in a process known as 'early generalization'. Generalization via haematogenous or lymphatic dissemination can also occur after re-infection or in the post-primary phase, therefore called 'late generalization' (Domingo *et al.*, 2014).

The primary lesion can progress and generalize, inducing a 'miliary' form with abundant nodules of small size throughout the lung and pleura (primary generalization). The lesion can grow, showing different forms depending on the development and involvement of adjacent tissues, including: (i) an 'acinar' form showing numerous small yellowish nodules affecting primary pulmonary lobules; (ii) a 'cavernous' form when the bronchial lumen is dilated due to the accumulation of caseum coming from the lesion or when the caseum breaks out into a bronchus; and (iii) an 'ulcerative' form in the trachea and bronchi when bacilli infect small erosions within the airway epithelium.

Typical tubercles can also be observed in extra-thoracic lymph nodes in the head and neck area (parotid, medial and lateral retropharyngeal and submandibular) (Aranday-Cortés *et al.*, 2013; Dean *et al.*, 2014, 2015; Ameni *et al.*, 2017; Salguero *et al.*, 2017). In calves, bovine tuberculosis is usually transmitted by ingestion and lesions involve the mesenteric

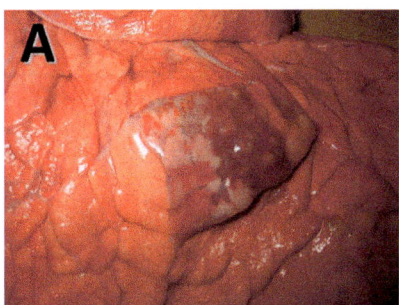 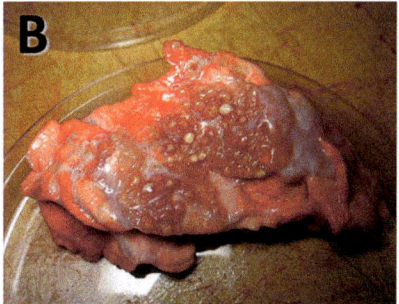

Fig. 9.1. Gross pathology of *Mycobacterium bovis* infection in cattle. (a) Multiple sub-pleural lesions can be observed in the dorsal part of the right middle lung lobe. (b) After sectioning, multiple coalescing granulomatous lesions observable with caseous necrosis in the centre and inflammatory reaction surrounding the areas of necrosis.

lymph nodes with possible spread to other organs (Terefe, 2014).

Detection of tuberculosis by slaughter surveillance requires that the infected animal have visible lesions at inspected sites. A detailed post-mortem examination in the abattoir or post-mortem room is crucial to identify tuberculosis-like lesions in a variety of organs, including the liver, spleen, kidney, mammary gland, etc. Several studies have reported that the detection of tuberculosis infection in the abattoir increases with enhanced meat inspection procedures, such as multiple slicing of organs and tissues (Corner, 1994; Whipple et al., 1996). Macroscopic detection of granulomatous lesions can produce a tentative diagnosis of bovine tuberculosis. Histopathological examination of the lesions may increase the confidence of the diagnosis, but the bacteriological isolation of M. bovis is the final answer to a definitive diagnosis (Corner, 1994). The inspection and culture of lymph nodes are crucial for the diagnosis of bovine tuberculosis and there is a recent hypothesis proposing tuberculosis to be a lymphatic disease with a pulmonary portal (Behr and Waters, 2013).

9.3 The Hallmark Microscopic Lesion of Bovine Tuberculosis: The Granuloma

The microscopic lesion observed in tuberculosis, regardless of the tissue and the host, is the granuloma. The granuloma is a distinctive morphological lesion typical of a chronic inflammatory reaction with abundant epithelial-like (epithelioid) macrophages (Palmer et al., 2015). Lymphocytes, plasma cells, neutrophils and Langhans-type multi-nucleated giant cells (MNGCs), formed through the fusion of multiple macrophages, are also observed within the granuloma. These cell types are often observed surrounding a caseous necrotic core.

Following mycobacterial infection, monocytes, lymphocytes, neutrophils and tissue-resident macrophages are recruited, mediated by cytokines and chemokines (Mattila et al., 2013) in an attempt to control the infection, forming cellular aggregates (Aranday-Cortés et al., 2013). Granulomas in cattle show different stages of formation, suggesting dissemination from primary foci as described in human tuberculosis (van Rhijn et al., 2008).

The granuloma structure has been described as a physical barrier to mycobacterial growth and spread (Aranday-Cortés et al., 2013). Experimental infection in cattle has allowed the qualitative classification of granulomas during the course of bovine tuberculosis infection (Wangoo et al., 2005; Johnson et al., 2006; Palmer et al., 2007; Aranday-Cortés et al., 2013). Microscopically, the granulomas are classified into four different stages of development (Wangoo et al., 2005) (Fig. 9.2). Early lesions, categorized as stage I ('initial') small granulomas are formed by an accumulation of neutrophils, epithelioid macrophages, a small number of lymphocytes and a few Langhans-type multi-nucleated giant cells. Necrosis is absent in stage I granulomas. The lesion will progress to stage II ('solid') granulomas with a similar structure to stage I, but with a central infiltrate of neutrophils and lymphocytes together with a thin capsule surrounding the lesion. The lesion will start to form a central area of caseous necrosis and progress to stage III ('necrotic') granuloma where the central caseous necrosis is surrounded by multiple epithelioid cells, multi-nucleated giant cells and lymphocytes. Stage III granulomas exhibit a complete fibrous capsule with a central area of necrosis and occasionally minimal mineralization. The necrotic core is surrounded by epithelioid macrophages and MNGCs, and a peripheral zone of macrophages, clustered lymphocytes and isolated neutrophils (Aranday-Cortés et al., 2013). Finally, stage IV ('mineralized') granulomas are completely surrounded by a relatively thick capsule of fibrous tissue and display obvious central areas of necrosis with extensive mineralization. Necrotic cores are surrounded by macrophages and MNGCs and a peripheral zone of macrophages and dense clusters of lymphocytes just inside the fibrotic capsule. Stage IV granulomas may be multi-centric with several granulomas coalescing to form one very large granuloma displaying multiple necrotic cores. Large stage IV granulomas are often surrounded by a small amount of 'satellite' stage I and stage II granulomas (Aranday-Cortés et al., 2013).

The presence of acid-fast bacilli (AFB) in tissue sections with the Ziehl-Neelsen stain show a

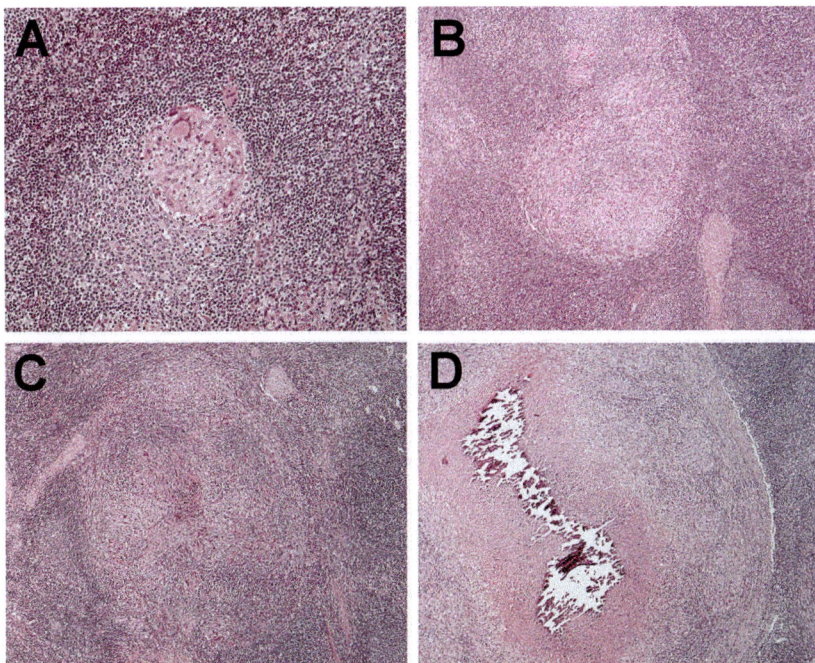

Fig. 9.2. (a) Stage I granuloma showing clustered epithelioid macrophages with some Langhans-type multi-nucleated giant cells (MNGCs). (H&E, 200×) (b) Stage II granuloma with abundant epithelioid macrophages, visible MNGCs and an incomplete fibrous capsule. (H&E, 100×) (c) Stage III granuloma showing a complete fibrous capsule and central necrosis. (H&E, 40×) (d) Stage IV granuloma with a complete fibrous encapsulation, extensive central necrosis and mineralization. (H&E, 40×)

small amount of AFB in stage I and II granulomas, mostly within the cytoplasm of macrophages, epithelioid cells and MNGCs (Fig. 9.3), and a higher number of bacteria within the necrotic cores of stage III and IV granulomas.

The four types of granulomas have been found in the lung and lymph nodes from natural and experimentally infected cattle, showing no remarkable differences in different tissues when studying conventional H&E-stained slides. The presence and quantification of granulomas of different stages have been used as an important tool to evaluate strain pathogenicity and vaccine efficacy in cattle (Johnson *et al.*, 2006; Dean *et al.*, 2014, 2015; Salguero *et al.*, 2017).

Several studies have been carried out to study in depth the cell composition of granulomas in bovines infected by *M. bovis*. Different techniques (e.g. immunohistochemistry [IHC] or *in situ* hybridization [ISH]) have been used to characterize and quantify the presence of macrophages, lymphocytes and their

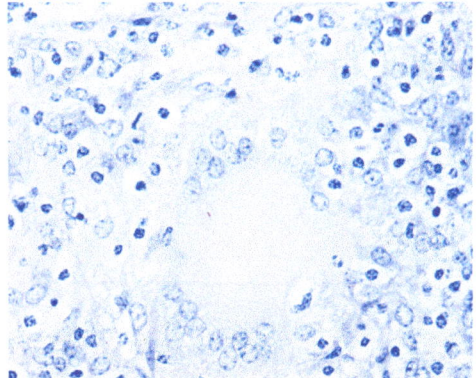

Fig. 9.3. Acid-fast bacilli within the cytoplasm of a MNGC. (Ziehl-Neelsen, 600×)

subpopulations within tissue sections (Liébana *et al.*, 2008; Aranday-Cortés *et al.*, 2013; Palmer *et al.*, 2015, 2016; Salguero *et al.*, 2017).

Immunohistochemical detection of CD68 has been used to characterize and locate macrophages, epithelial cells and MNGCs within the granulomas at different stages of development. In general, the number of CD68+ cells is quite high in stage I granulomas and decreases throughout the development of the lesion. In stage I and II, a high percentage of the cells within the granulomas are CD68+, whereas in stages III and IV the CD68+ cells display a rim of macrophages surrounding the necrotic centres and a few cells in the outer layers of the granuloma (Aranday-Cortés et al., 2013) (Fig. 9.4).

CD3+ T lymphocytes appear to be scattered within the stage I and II granulomas, while being distributed in the outer layers of the stage III and IV granulomas (Fig. 9.5), but not immediately adjacent to the necrotic cores. The immunohistochemical detection of CD4+ and CD8+ T lymphocytes using formalin-fixed paraffin-embedded (FFPE) tissues has been very difficult to standardize. However, it has been possible to study these two cell populations using zinc salt fixatives (Hicks et al., 2006; Aranday-Cortés et al., 2013). Experimental studies have shown that both CD4+ and CD8+ are present within the granulomas in a similar way to CD3+ cells, scattered within stage I and II granulomas and within the outer layers of the granuloma in stage III and IV (Aranday-Cortés et al., 2013) (also see Chapter 10).

The role of B lymphocytes in the immune response of bovine tuberculosis and the distribution of these cells within the tuberculous granuloma has been historically unappreciated. However, it has been shown that B cells can modulate the host response to *M. tuberculosis* in murine models in a variety of ways (Maglione and Chan, 2009). We have found interspersed B cells within the stage I and II granulomas in bovine tuberculosis, but also abundant numbers of B cells in stage III and IV granulomas, often producing satellite nests of B cells around the outside of the fibrous capsule (Aranday-Cortés et al., 2013) (Fig. 9.6). These structures resemble active follicles found in secondary lymphoid organs, with B cells at many different stages of maturation present, and it has been proposed that these clusters of cells might coordinate the host local immune responses to control the growth of mycobacteria in the lung (Ulrichs et al., 2004) (see Chapter 10).

9.4 Local Immunity Against *M. bovis*

The initial immunologic events following pathogenic mycobacteria infection include cytokine- and chemokine-mediated recruitment of monocytes, neutrophils and macrophages (Lawn and Zumla, 2011). Macrophages must interact with activated T cells to organize the granuloma and act as a functional unit to control the infection (Mattila et al., 2013).

The pathogenesis of bovine tuberculosis can be compared with human tuberculosis, and

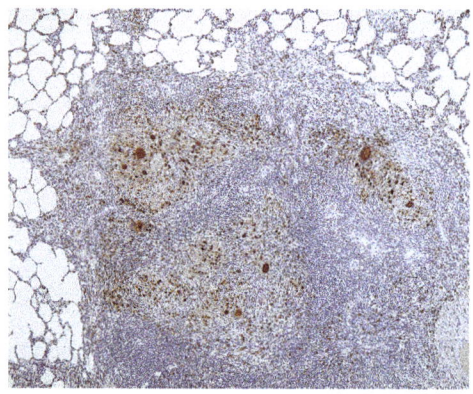

Fig. 9.4. CD68+ staining in stage I and II granulomas in the lung of a cow experimentally infected with *M. bovis*. Heavy positive staining can be observed within the cytoplasm of macrophages and multi-nucleated giant cells. (IHC, 100×)

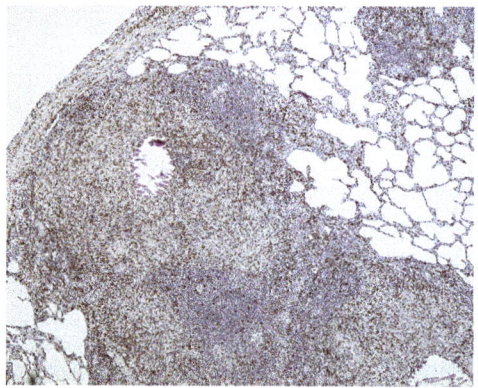

Fig. 9.5. CD3+ staining in stage IV granulomas in the lung of an infected cow with *M. bovis*. Abundant positive T cells can be observed mostly in the outer layers of the granulomas. (IHC, 100×)

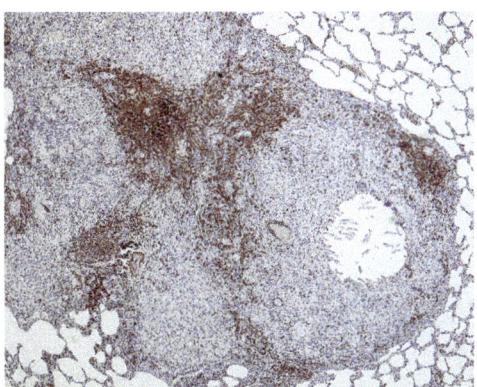

Fig. 9.6. CD79a⁺ staining in stage I, II and IV granulomas in the lung of a cow experimentally infected with *M. bovis*. Scattered CD79a⁺ cells can be observed within the rim of inflammatory cells surrounding the necrotic core of the stage IV granuloma and interspersed within the stage I and II granulomas. The formation of a nest of B cells can be observed in the lesion with a high number of CD79a⁺ cells. (IHC, 100×)

both diseases have improved our understanding of the mechanisms involved in mammalian infection with pathogenic mycobacteria (Waters *et al.*, 2014; Waters and Palmer, 2015). Following inhalation, the bacilli are deposited within the terminal respiratory bronchioles and alveolar lumina, where they are phagocytized by resident alveolar macrophages (Palmer *et al.*, 2016). Infected macrophages will start producing cytokines, chemokines and enzymes (Aranday-Cortés *et al.*, 2013; Palmer *et al.*, 2015, 2016; Salguero *et al.*, 2017) (see Chapter 10). Macrophages produce both pro- and anti-inflammatory cytokines, inducing the activation of innate immune response with the involvement of neutrophils, monocytes, macrophages and dendritic cells (Etna *et al.*, 2014). After the innate immune response, the adaptive response is initiated as dendritic cells containing bacilli may migrate from the primary site of infection within the lung to local lymph nodes, activating naïve T lymphocytes through cytokine production and antigen presentation (Palmer *et al.*, 2016) (see Chapter 10). After activation and expansion, T lymphocytes migrate to the lesion in the lung, giving shape to the granuloma together with epithelioid macrophages and MNGCs (Etna *et al.*, 2014).

The granuloma is a very dynamic structure where cells can migrate from and to the lesion. Studies using zebra fish (*Danio rerio*) as a model of tuberculosis have shown that mycobacteria can leave and enter granulomas using infected macrophages as vehicles, and this process can contribute to the dissemination of bacilli to other tissues and organs (Bold and Ernst, 2009; Volkman *et al.*, 2010). Granulomas develop individually and the disease is controlled at the level of the granuloma (Lin *et al.*, 2014).

Modern techniques have been used recently to study the local immune response in-depth within tuberculous granulomas. Among them, a combination of laser-capture micro-dissection (LCMD) and quantitative polymerase chain reaction (qPCR), has proven to be very useful to quantify the expression of cytokine and chemokine mRNA within individual lesions (Aranday-Cortés *et al.*, 2013). Classic IHC and a novel chromogenic ISH technique (RNAScope) linked to digital image analysis has also been used recently to quantify the expression of cytokine/chemokine mRNA and protein by different cell population within the lesions (Aranday-Cortés *et al.*, 2013; Palmer *et al.*, 2015, 2016; Salguero *et al.*, 2017).

The early stages of the granuloma (stages I and II) express large amounts of IL-17A (Aranday-Cortés *et al.*, 2013), a cytokine that has been proposed as a possible biomarker for bovine tuberculosis and playing a very important role in the maturation of the granuloma (Blanco *et al.*, 2011; Waters *et al.*, 2015). This upregulation in early stage granulomas is also observed for CXCL9 and CXCL10. These high levels of CXCL9 and CXCL10 are related to the recruitment of more inflammatory cells at the initial stages of the disease to assist in the destruction and control of the pathogen in the site of infection (Aranday-Cortés *et al.*, 2013). The level of these chemokines decrease in the late granuloma stages when the response has been overwhelmed and the recruitment of cells is less important than the production of a physical barrier, through walling the bacteria within a fibrous capsule, to control the pathogen (Algood *et al.*, 2003; Widdison *et al.*, 2009).

There is a consistent high level of expression of IFN-γ in all stages of granuloma formation (Fig. 9.7), as the host mounts a typical Th1 response against *M. bovis* (Pollock *et al.*, 2001;

Thacker *et al.*, 2007; Aranday-Cortés *et al.*, 2013). Interestingly, certain levels of TNF-α expression are observed in all stages of the granuloma (Fig. 9.8). TNF-α is mainly produced by macrophages, MNGCs and dendritic cells, contributing to the development of the Th1 immune response as well as having an important role in maintaining the structure of the granuloma (Algood *et al.*, 2003; Welsh *et al.*, 2005; Boddu-Jasmine *et al.*, 2008; Blanco *et al.*, 2011; Aranday-Cortés *et al.*, 2013). The activation of macrophages in the early stages of the granuloma is also related to a high expression of iNOS by epithelioid cells and MNGCs in stage I and II granulomas and within the epithelioid cells forming a rim adjacent to the necrotic cores in advanced stage III and IV granulomas (Fig. 9.9) (Aranday-Cortés *et al.*, 2013). TGF-β is also expressed in all stages of granuloma formation (Aranday-Cortés *et al.*, 2013), although the expression is upregulated in late stage granulomas when the disease is really advanced (Wangoo *et al.*, 2005), coinciding with the presence of thick fibrotic capsules surrounding the granulomas. This cytokine has been described as a potent stimulator of collagen production by fibroblasts.

9.5 Laboratory Animal Models of Bovine Tuberculosis

Due to significant ethical and practical considerations, laboratory animal models of disease have been used extensively to study *M. tuberculosis* infection. These animal models have also been used frequently for vaccination trials and novel anti-tuberculosis drug discovery. Similar models have been used to study *M. bovis* infection, although the pathology and pathogenesis of the disease can present different features than those observed in the natural hosts. *M. bovis* can infect a wide variety of laboratory animals, including

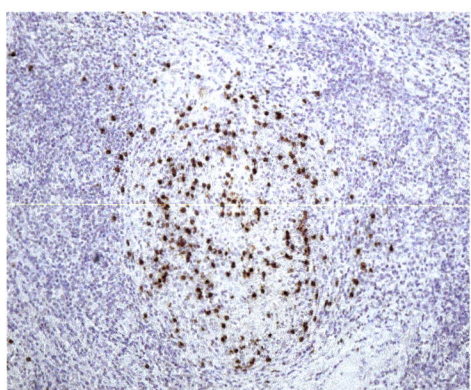

Fig. 9.7. Staining of INF-γ in a stage II granuloma from the mediastinal lymph node of a cow experimentally infected with *M. bovis*. Abundant IFN-γ positive cells can be observed within the granuloma. (IHC, 400×)

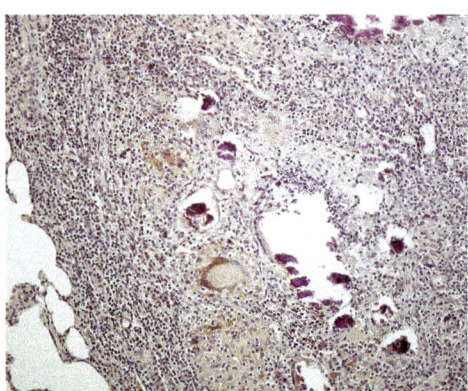

Fig. 9.8. Staining of TNF-α in a stage IV granuloma from the lung of a cow experimentally infected with *M. bovis*. The expression of TNF-α can be observed within the cytoplasm of few epithelioid macrophages and a multi-nucleated giant cell. (IHC, 400×)

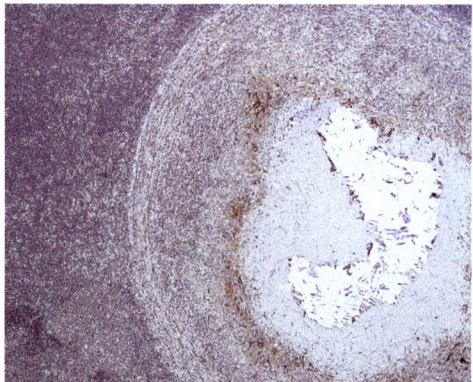

Fig. 9.9. Staining of TGF-β in a stage IV granuloma from the mediastinal lymph node of a cow experimentally infected with *M. bovis*. Abundant epithelioid macrophages are expressing TGF-β within a rim of inflammatory cells adjacent to the necrotic core. (IHC, 40×)

mice, rabbits, guinea pigs and non-human primates.

Rabbits are relatively more susceptible to progressive disease when infected with *M. bovis* compared to *M. tuberculosis* (Converse *et al.*, 1996). This species can develop cavitations at later stages of the disease, an important aspect of human disease.

The mouse is not a natural host of *M. tuberculosis* or *M. bovis*, but it has proven to be a useful tool to investigate the interaction between the pathogen and the immune system of mammals because of the wide array of immunological reagents available for this species (Aranday-Cortés *et al.*, 2012; Orme and Basaraba, 2014). The choice of the specific mouse strain amongst the many available is critical to a successful outcome. The inhalation model induces a mononuclear inflammatory cell infiltration in the lungs following infection in C57BL/6 mouse. The mononuclear cells accumulate in the alveolar spaces and lymphocytes migrate from blood vessels in response to the chemokine and cytokine signals. The granulomas are typically solid with abundant foamy macrophages laden with numerous AFBs as seen with the Ziehl-Neelsen stain (Fig. 9.10). The lesions develop and usually coalesce into larger granulomas occupying vast areas of the lung parenchyma, without forming fibrotic capsules surrounding the granulomas. MNGCs are not present and the necrotic areas are usually small and circumscribed to few cells. Mineralization of the lesions does not occur. The structure of the lesion in the mouse is often described as 'unorganized', although there is some degree of organization taking place with the large sheets of epithelioid macrophages and aggregates of T cells around the periphery of the granuloma (Orme and Basaraba, 2014).

The guinea pig has been used historically to model and diagnose both human and animal tuberculosis. The pathology of tuberculosis in this species has been described in detail and multiple similarities with the human disease have been described, including the development of caseation and necrosis, hallmarks of progressive tuberculosis (Turner *et al.*, 2003; Basaraba, 2008; Orme and Basaraba, 2014). Lesions develop from small aggregates of mononuclear inflammatory cell infiltrates to larger granulomas with a necrotic core surrounded by large numbers of foamy macrophages and lymphocytes (Fig. 9.11). Adjacent to the core, intact macrophages and possibly fibroblasts initiate the calcification, resulting in the mineralization of the lesions. The lesions grow rapidly and can coalesce resulting in often fatal lung consolidation (Orme and Basaraba, 2014).

Non-human primates are the model species that are thought to most closely mimic the naturally occurring human disease (Orme and Basaraba, 2014). Several features of *M. tuberculosis* infection in rhesus macaques (*Macaca mulatta*) and cynomolgus macaques (*Macaca fascicularis*) can also be described as similar to those induced by *M. bovis* in cattle (Peña and Ho, 2015).

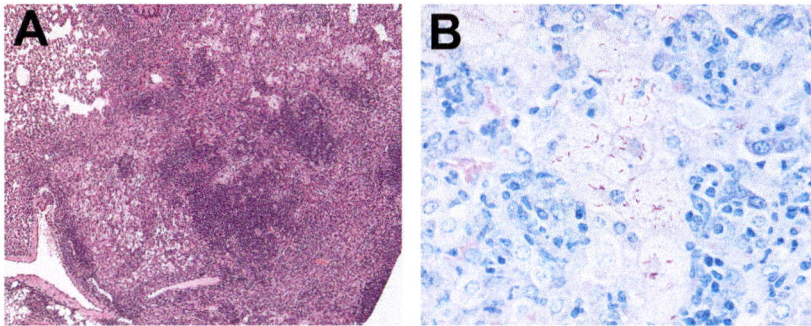

Fig. 9.10. (a) Granulomatous disorganized and diffuse lesion, poorly demarcated within the lung of a mouse experimentally infected with *M. bovis*. (H&E, 100×). (b) Abundant AFBs within the cytoplasm of 'foamy' macrophages at the periphery of the granulomatous lesion. (Ziehl-Neelsen, 600×)

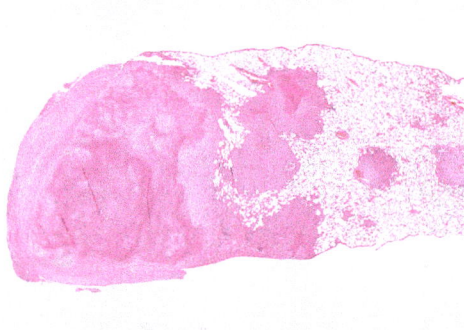

Fig. 9.11. Multifocal granulomas within the lung of a guinea pig infected with *M. tuberculosis*. The granulomas are in different stages of development showing solid lesions with no necrosis (small) and extensive necrosis and fibrotic capsule (large). (H&E, 20×)

9.6 Comparative Pathology of *M. bovis* Infection in Other Domestic and Wildlife Species

The range of hosts susceptible to *M. bovis* is very broad and includes humans, domestic and wild ruminants, swine and carnivores (Palmer *et al.*, 2015).

9.6.1 Domestic animals

Small ruminants

M. bovis infection in sheep and goats is closely related to tuberculosis in cattle in terms of immunological responses and pathological characteristics (Marianelli *et al.*, 2010; Bezos *et al.*, 2011; Domingo *et al.*, 2014). Tuberculosis in small ruminants is primarily a chronic infection causing exudative granulomatous caseous inflammatory lesions in the lungs and associated lymph nodes, although lesions can also occur in the upper respiratory tract (Domingo *et al.*, 2014). Generalized forms affecting other organs such as the spleen, liver and kidneys are infrequent (Daniel *et al.*, 2009). Goats can develop liquefactive necrosis with the formation of cavernous lesions, similarly to human tuberculosis, making this animal a good experimental model of the human disease (Marianelli *et al.*, 2010; Gonzalez-Juarrero *et al.*, 2013).

Companion animals (dogs, cats and horses)

There are few data on the prevalence of tuberculosis in dogs and cats worldwide. Depending on the route of infection, the lesions will be localized in the respiratory, gastrointestinal or integumentary system (Gunn-Moore *et al.*, 2010). Historically, cats were usually infected by drinking contaminated milk, while dogs were infected by aerosol from infected owners (Jennings, 1949). Dogs typically start with lesions in the lungs, but they disseminate quickly. The most common form of tuberculosis in cats is the cutaneous form, with respiratory and gastrointestinal forms less frequently observed (Gunn-Moore *et al.*, 2010, 2011; Rufenacht *et al.*, 2011). This cutaneous form probably arises from infected bite wounds, local spread, haematogenous dissemination to the skin or even contaminated surgical wounds (Jennings, 1949; Gunn-Moore *et al.*, 2010; Roberts *et al.*, 2014; Murray *et al.*, 2015). The lesions are typically firm, raised dermal nodules with ulceration with draining sinus tracts and subcutaneous tissue inflammation (Gunn-Moore *et al.*, 2011; Rufenacht *et al.*, 2011) (Fig. 9.12). The skin lesions are often associated with localized or generalized granulomatous lymphadenitis. The infection can disseminate to the lung from the skin site inducing a typical haematogenous interstitial pneumonia. Pleurisy and pericardial effusion are also common in animals with respiratory infection (Snider, 1971). Histologically, the lesions are typical multifocal to coalescing granulomas composed of multiple macrophages and epithelioid cells. MNGCs are very uncommon and neutrophils are often observed in large numbers, mostly due to secondary infections in the skin lesions. In general, the lesions are less prone to encapsulate and mineralization is very rare. The number of AFBs is quite low with some exceptions (Fig. 9.12).

The digestive route of infection is the most common in the horse, with lesions frequently found in head and neck lymph nodes, the gastrointestinal tract and the mesenteric lymph nodes. The lesions are often disseminated with miliary inflammation in the liver, spleen and lungs. The lesions in the horse are typically proliferative and less caseous than in cattle. Mineralization is very rare and the lesions can be mistaken for neoplastic masses (Domingo *et al.*, 2014).

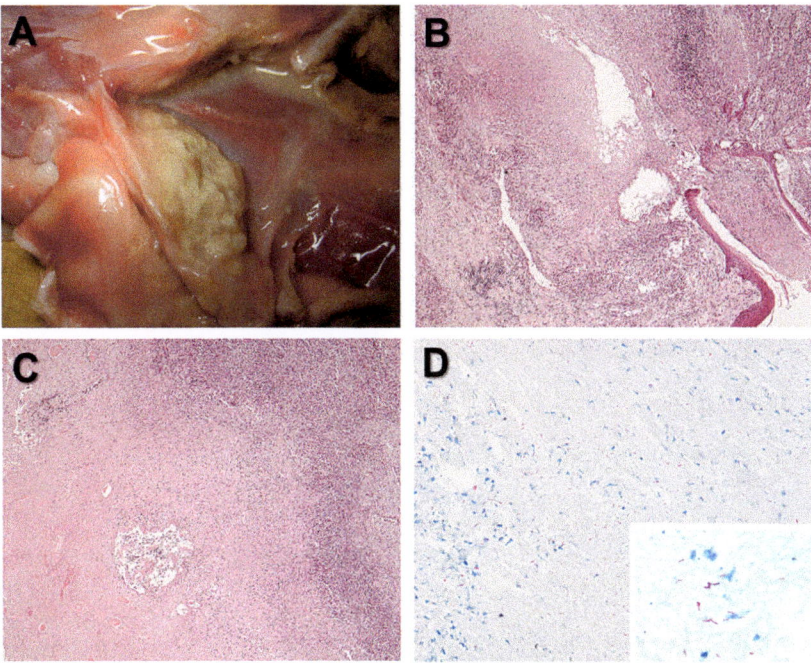

Fig. 9.12. (a) Pyogranulomatous severe panniculitis from a cat naturally infected with *M. bovis*. (b) Skin lesion from a cat infected with *M. bovis*, showing extensive dermatitis and inflammatory cell infiltration in the subcutis, with disruption of the normal epithelium, close to a fistula. (H&E, 40×) (c) Granulomatous inflammation within extensive necrotic core within the axillar lymph node. (HE, 40×) (d) Abundant acid-fast bacilli within the necrotic centre of the lymph node. (Ziehl-Neelsen, 400×; inset, 1000×)

South American camelids

The bacteria from the MTBC can induce extensive pathology in llamas and alpacas. The respiratory system and associated lymph nodes are the most frequently affected organs. The lung lesions can be very extensive, affecting more than 50% of the lung surface (Crawshaw *et al.*, 2013). The lesions are very caseous with soft, yellowish creamy material at section. Lesions often coalesce to form larger granulomas showing cavitations (Garcia-Bocanegra *et al.*, 2010). Pleurisy is also frequently observed. The lymph nodes are much enlarged, containing the same white or yellowish creamy caseous material. Histologically, the lesions show large areas of necrosis with multiple AFBs within, surrounded by a rim of inflammatory cells including macrophages, neutrophils, lymphocytes and plasma cells (Fig. 9.13). Other organs, including the liver, skin, gastrointestinal tract and mammary gland, can show multifocal lesions (Richey *et al.*, 2011). The extensive lesions in infected camelids in the UK, associated with the high within-herd prevalence of *M. bovis*-infected animals in some outbreaks, suggests that these species can be amplifier hosts and can spread the disease amongst themselves and possibly to other species, including cattle and man (Twomey *et al.*, 2009). Immunohistochemical characterization of the lesions has proven to be very difficult due to the lack of specific reagents and the phylogenetic distance of these species to others more extensively studied, such as cattle. This same problem exists for wildlife species described in this chapter.

9.6.2 Wild animals

Several examples occur where a variety of wild animal species represent major reservoirs of infection for domestic livestock (Fitzgerald and Kaneene, 2012). These include cervids in North America and the Mediterranean basin,

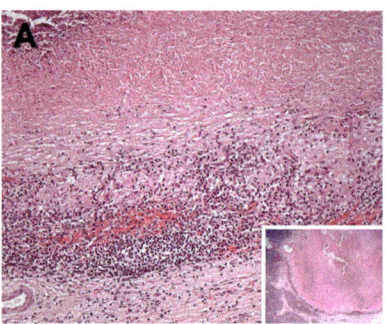 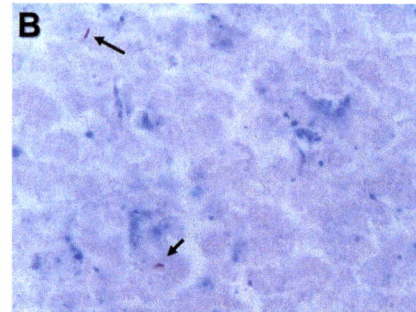

Fig. 9.13. (a) Detail of the outer layer of a granuloma from the mesenteric lymph node of an alpaca infected with *M. bovis*. The necrotic area (upper part of Fig) is surrounded by abundant inflammatory infiltrate, mostly composed of lymphocytes, a few macrophages and no multi-nucleated giant cells. (inset) Extensive necrotic core of the lesion. (H&E, 200×; inset 20×) (b) Few acid-fast bacilli (arrows) are observed within the necrotic centre of the lymph node. (Ziehl-Neelsen, 600×)

mustelids in the British Isles, swine in southern Europe, marsupials in New Zealand and bovids in Africa (see Chapter 6). The pathology and pathogenesis of *M. bovis* infection in these species have been studied with some limitations due to the lack of reagents and reduced number of experimental studies.

Eurasian badgers

The Eurasian badger (*Meles meles*) is an important wildlife reservoir of bovine tuberculosis in the UK and the Republic of Ireland (Chambers *et al.*, 2017), and their role in the maintenance and spread of the disease is a matter of considerable scientific, political and public interest (Brooks-Pollock *et al.*, 2014). Badgers infected with *M. bovis* have been also found in other countries in continental Europe (Sobrino *et al.*, 2008). The pathology associated with tuberculosis in badgers is centred on the respiratory system, with more than 50% of the lesions restricted to the lungs and 35% of the badgers showing lymph node involvements (Gallagher and Clifton-Hadley, 2000). The pulmonary lesions are variable, typically caseous granulomas showing different sizes from large nodules and lobar pneumonia to disseminated miliary lesions. The lesions in the lymph nodes are typical of a granulomatous lymphadenitis, with yellowish areas with enlarged and oedematous granulomas. Very rarely, the lesions will develop mineralization. Lesions can also be found in the kidneys resulting in elongated radial lesions, liver or spleen, as pale sawdust-like and disseminated (Fitzgerald and Kaneene, 2012). Badgers appear to have a containment phase of the disease, similarly to latency in humans, which can last for years (Gallagher and Clifton-Hadley, 2000). In contrast, many badgers show no visible (gross) lesions (NVL) with positive bacterial culture from either the lung or lymph nodes, making the diagnosis and epidemiology of the disease more complicated. Histologically, the granulomas are solid, composed mainly of epithelioid macrophages with fewer lymphocytes, no apparent MNGCs (Fig. 9.14) and with limited areas of necrosis (Corner *et al.*, 2011). Badgers can also be infected with non-tuberculous mycobacteria, nematodes or fungal adiaspiromycosis, inducing granulomatous lesions in the lung.

Cervids

White-tail deer are a cervid species heavily involved in the epidemiology of *M. bovis* infection in the US. The typical gross pathology in this species consists of multiple caseous granulomas with purulent centres in affected lungs or lymph nodes. The caseous centre is normally very soft and can resemble abscesses (Fitzgerald and Kaneene, 2012). The typical lymph node affected is the medial retropharyngeal frequently with other tissues involved. The thoracic lesions normally consist of multiple pulmonary granulomas disseminated throughout the lung parenchyma and often extending to the parietal and visceral pleura (Fitzgerald and Kaneene, 2012).

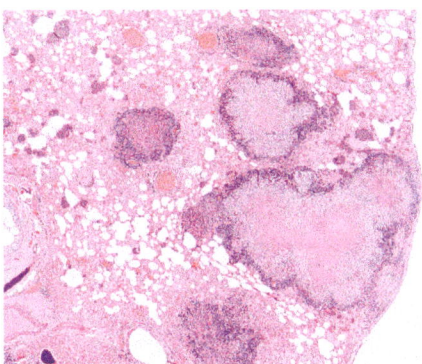
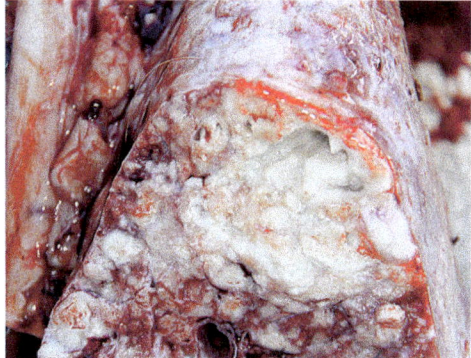

Fig. 9.14. Multifocal granulomas at different stage of development in a badger infected with *M. bovis*. Some of the lesions are small and solid, while other show a central area of necrosis surrounded by a rim of epithelioid cells, no multinucleated giant cells and lymphocytes at the outer layers of the lesion. No evident capsule can be identified. (H&E, 40×)

Fig. 9.15. Large coalescent caseous granulomas in the lung of a fallow deer infected with *M. bovis*. Yellowish creamy material can be observed within the lesion. Courtesy of 'Red de Recursos Faunisticos' group, University of Extremadura, Spain.

Microscopically, the pulmonary and lymphoid granulomas are typical caseous lesions with an outer layer of lymphocytes, histiocytes and MNGCs surrounding a necrotic core that may contain large areas of mineralization (Fitzgerald and Kaneene, 2012).

The role of wild cervids as reservoirs of tuberculosis in some regions of Spain has also been described (Gortazar *et al*., 2003; Aranaz *et al*., 2004; Hermoso de Mendoza *et al*., 2006). In fallow deer, we have observed a high prevalence of tuberculosis with animals showing parynchematous caseous lung lesions varying from 1–10 cm in diameter, often coalescing (Fig. 9.15). Generalized disease is frequent with large and encapsulated granulomas similar to abscesses in lymph nodes of variable size, sometimes up to 20 cm, and containing creamy yellowish caseous material (García-Jiménez *et al*., 2012). The number of AFBs within the lesions is far greater than those observed in cattle with tuberculosis (Martin-Hernando *et al*., 2010; García-Jiménez *et al*., 2012). Red and fallow deer show the largest number of poorly encapsulated granulomas often containing many hundreds of bacilli (De Lisle *et al*., 2002; Johnson *et al*., 2008; Martin-Hernando *et al*., 2010; García-Jiménez *et al*., 2012). The presence of these poorly encapsulated granulomas has been pointed out as a potential source of environmental contamination from deer species in the British Isles and onward transmission to other animal species (Johnson *et al*., 2008).

The characteristic cellular composition of early stage granulomas is associated with an initial immune response from the host. The majority of cells in these granulomas are macrophages and T lymphocytes. Interestingly, stage I and II granulomas express high levels of IFN-γ (García-Jiménez *et al*., 2012) associated with an early Th1 response by the host and positively correlated with an increase in pathogenicity in *M. bovis* infection in cattle (Villarreal-Ramos *et al*., 2003). The presence of abundant B cells in the outer layers of late-stage granulomas, forming nests similar to those observed in cattle, might contribute to the coordination of host immune responses with the CD3+ T cells (Ulrichs *et al*., 2004).

Wild boar

Several wild ungulate species contribute to *M. bovis* infection maintenance in a multi-host system in the Mediterranean habitat of southern Europe, but wild boar is the single most important reservoir in these regions (Hermoso de Mendoza *et al*., 2006; García-Jiménez *et al*., 2013a). The typical macroscopic lesion pattern in wild boar with tuberculosis are characterized by localized and delimited granulomas in the head lymph nodes (Fig. 9.16) and rare generalizations (Bollo *et al*., 2000; Zanella *et al*., 2008).

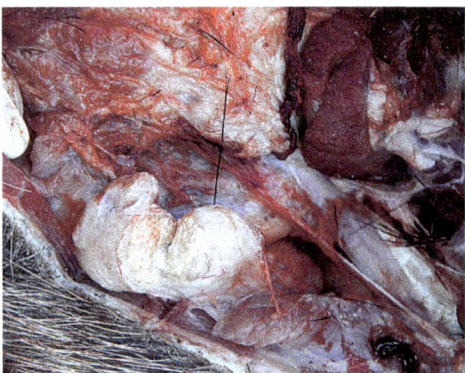

Fig. 9.16. Solid well-encapsulated lesion in the mandibular lymph node from a wild boar infected with *M. bovis*. The lesion is also heavily mineralized and 'gritty' on sectioning. Courtesy of 'Red de Recursos Faunisticos' group, University of Extremadura, Spain.

Similar patterns have been observed in domestic pigs with *M. bovis* infection. These patterns may change in non-natural or artificial managements (Martin-Hernando *et al.*, 2010) or after infections with other mycobacteria as *M. caprae* (García-Jiménez *et al.*, 2013b). The histopathological features of the granulomas in swine are similar to those observed in cattle and the differentiation of granulomas by development stage has also been used in this species (García-Jiménez *et al.*, 2013a, 2013b). Occasionally, wild boar show small lesions heavily mineralized with a very thick rim of fibrous capsule and with poor cell component in lymph nodes, normally associated to high health status in the group.

Using IHC techniques to determine the presence of different cell populations and cytokine expression within granulomas, it has been shown that wild boar show large numbers of macrophages in early stage granulomas and T-cell distribution similar to lesions in cattle.

There is a high expression of iNOS in stage I, II and III granulomas and to a lesser extent in a rim surrounding the necrotic cores in stage IV granulomas, as an attempt from the animal to control the mycobacterial infection and spread (García-Jiménez *et al.*, 2013a). These features are different from what is observed in fallow deer granulomas (García-Jiménez *et al.*, 2012).

Typical responses in wild boar include very active phagocytosis and bacterial lysis sustained by macrophages and iNOS in initial stages (García-Jiménez *et al.*, 2013a). The involvement of B cells is not significant as observed in cattle, and the typical nests of B cells have not been found (García-Jiménez *et al.*, 2013a).

African buffalo and lechwe

African buffalo (*Syncerus caffer*) and lechwe antelope (*Kobus leche*) have both been found to be important wildlife reservoirs of bovine tuberculosis in South Africa and Zambia, respectively (Fitzgerald and Kaneene, 2012). Macroscopic lesions in buffalo are mostly restricted to retropharyngeal, bronchial and mediastinal lymph nodes, and interestingly few animals show gross visible lesions in the lung (Laisse *et al.*, 2011). Gross lesions are typically single or multiple granulomas with a caseous core and mineralization. Microscopically, the lymph nodes show a variety of inflammatory cells including epithelioid macrophages, lymphocytes and MNGCs, with a variable degree of necrosis, fibrous encapsulation and mineralization (Laisse *et al.*, 2011). The number of AFBs within the lesions is very low, and the lesions in general are similar to those observed in cattle or North American cervids (Laisse *et al.*, 2011).

In the lechwe antelopes, the typical site of infection is the lung, followed by thoracic lymph nodes (Gallagher and Macadam, 1972). The lung lesions are typical of central necrosis and light mineralization with the presence of abundant AFBs. The lymph nodes show concentric areas of mineralization (Gallagher and Macadam, 1972).

Brushtail possum

The possum serves as the principal reservoir of tuberculosis in New Zealand (Fitzgerald and Kaneene, 2012). Possums are highly susceptible to *M. bovis* infection and the disease is fatal within months (Ryan *et al.*, 2006). The disseminated form of tuberculosis in this species results in axillary and inguinal lymph nodes, which can fistulize, draining infective AFBs through the skin posing an important implication in the epidemiology of the disease (Cooke *et al.*, 1995).

9.7 Concluding Remarks

There are many studies on the pathology of *M. bovis* infection in a variety of animals in the literature. Some aspects of the disease are well understood, but others are not. *M. bovis* can induce a disease indistinguishable from *M. tuberculosis* infection in man and the study of *M. bovis* infection in animals has been invaluable to understand the pathogenesis of human tuberculosis and vice versa. The hallmark lesion induced by pathogenic mycobacteria in the host is the granuloma, a dynamic structure with a continuous movement of cells into and out of the structure, orchestrated by the host as well as by the pathogen (Ramakrishnan, 2012). Differential cell composition, bacterial burden and cytokine expression patterns at the protein and mRNA levels may result from the independent nature of the granuloma microenvironment (Orme and Basaraba, 2014). With new molecular techniques available linked to 'classic' pathology, thorough studies can now be performed to maximize the outputs and compare the changes occurring in different granulomas within different organs and structures from one single animal. New pathology data coming from domestic animals and wildlife reservoirs will be very valuable to produce new control strategies of tuberculosis disease induced by *M. bovis* in different epidemiological scenarios.

Acknowledgements

The author would like to acknowledge UE FP7 grant 228394 NADIR, Defra (SE3227), as well as many colleagues at the TB research group from Animal and Plant Health Agency, the Department of Pathology and Infectious Diseases from the University of Surrey, and the 'Red de Recursos Faunisticos' group from University of Extremadura, Spain and Ingulados S.L. for their valuable collaboration.

References

Algood, H.M.S., Chan, J. and Flynn, J.A.L. (2003) Chemokines and tuberculosis. *Cytokine and Growth Factor Review* 14, 467–477.

Ameni, G., Tafess, K., Zewde, A., Eguale, T., Tilahun, M., *et al.* (2017) Vaccination of calves with *Mycobacterium bovis* bacillus Calmette-Guerin reduces the frequency and severity of lesions of bovine tuberculosis under a natural transmission setting in Ethiopia. *Transboundary and Emerging Diseases*, in press. DOI: 10.1111/tbed.12618.

Aranaz, A., De Juan, L., Montero, N., Sánchez, C., Galka, M., *et al.* (2004) Bovine tuberculosis (*Mycobacterium bovis*) in wildlife in Spain. *Journal of Clinical Microbiology* 42, 2602–2608.

Aranday-Cortés, E., Hogarth, P.J., Kaveh, D.A., Whelan, A.O., Villarreal-Ramos, B., *et al.* (2012) Transcriptional profiling of disease-induced host responses in bovine tuberculosis and the identification of potential diagnostic biomarkers. *PLoS ONE* 7, e30626.

Aranday-Cortés, E., Bull, N.C., Villarreal-Ramos, B., Gough, J., Hicks, D. *et al.* (2013) Upregulation of IL-17A, CXCL9 and CXCL10 in early-stage granulomas induced by *Mycobacterium bovis* in cattle. *Transboundary and Emerging Diseases* 60, 525–537.

Basaraba, R.J. (2008) Experimental tuberculosis: the role of comparative pathology in the discovery of improved tuberculosis treatment strategies. *Tuberculosis (Edinb.)* 88, S35–S47.

Behr, M.A. and Waters, W.R. (2013) Is tuberculosis a lymphatic disease with a pulmonary portal? *Lancet Infectious Diseases* 13, 70253–70256.

Bezos, J., Alvarez, J., de Juan, L., Romero, B., Rodríguez, S., *et al.* (2011) Assessment of in vivo and in vitro tuberculosis diagnostic tests in *Mycobacterium caprae* naturally infected caprine flocks. *Preventive Veterinary Medicine* 100(3–4), 187–192.

Blanco, F.C., Bianco, M.V., Meikle, V., Garbaccio, S., Vagnoni, L., *et al.* (2011) Increased IL-17 expression is associated with pathology in a bovine model of tuberculosis. *Tuberculosis (Edinb.)* 91, 57–63.

Boddu-Jasmine, H.C., Witchell, J., Vordermeier, M., Wangoo, A. and Goyal, M. (2008) Cytokine mRNA expression in cattle infected with different dosages of *Mycobacterium bovis*. *Tuberculosis (Edinb.)* 88, 610–615.

Bold, T.D. and Ernst, J.D. (2009) Who benefits from granulomas, mycobacteria or host? *Cell* 136, 17–19.

Bollo, E., Ferroglio, E., Dini, V., Mignone, W., Biolatti, B. and Rossi, L. (2000) Detection of *Mycobacterium tuberculosis* complex in lymph nodes of wild boar (*Sus scrofa*) by a target-amplified test system. *Journal of Veterinary Medicine Series B* 47, 337–342.

Brooks-Pollock, E., Roberts, G.O. and Keeling, M.J. (2014) A dynamic model of bovine tuberculosis spread and control in Great Britain. *Nature* 511, 228–231.

Cassidy, J.P., Bryson, D.G. and Neill, S.D. (1999) Tonsillar lesions in cattle naturally infected with *Mycobacterium bovis*. *The Veterinary Record* 144, 139–142.

Chambers, M.A., Adwell, F., Williams, G.A., Palmer, S., Gowtage, S., *et al.* (2017) The effect of oral vaccination with *Mycobacterium bovis* BCG on the development of tuberculosis in captive European badgers (*Meles meles*). *Frontiers in Cellular and Infection Microbiology* 7(6), eCollection 2017.

Converse, P.J., Dannenberg, A.M. Jr., Estep, J.E., Sugisaki, K., Abe, Y., *et al.* (1996) Cavitary tuberculosis produced in rabbits by aerosolised virulent tubercle bacilli. *Infection and Immunity* 64, 4776–4787.

Cooke, M.M., Jackson, R., Coleman, J.D. and Alley, J.R. (1995) Naturally occurring tuberculosis caused by *Mycobacterium bovis* in brushtail possums (*Trichosurus vulpecula*): pathology. *New Zealand Veterinary Journal* 43, 315–321.

Corner, L.A. (1994) Post mortem diagnosis of *M. bovis* infection in cattle. *Veterinary Microbiology* 40, 53–63.

Corner, L.A.L., Murphy, D. and Gormley, E. (2011) *Mycobacterium bovis* infection in the Eurasian badger (*Meles meles*): the disease, pathogenesis, epidemiology and control. *Journal of Comparative Pathology* 144, 1–24.

Crawshaw, T.R., de la Rua-Domenech, R. and Brown, E. (2013) Recognising the gross pathology of tuberculosis in South American camelids, deer, goats, pigs and sheep. *In Practice* 35, 490–502.

Daniel, R., Evans, H., Rolfe, S., de la Rua-Domenech, R., Crawshaw, T., *et al.* (2009) Outbreak of tuberculosis caused by *Mycobacterium bovis* in golden Guernsey goats in Great Britain. *The Veterinary Record* 165, 335–342.

Dean, G., Whelan A., Clifford, D., Salguero, F.J., Xing, Z., *et al.* (2014) Comparison of the immunogenicity and protection against bovine tuberculosis following immunization by BCG-priming and boosting with adenovirus or protein based vaccines. *Vaccine* 32, 1304–1310.

Dean, G.S., Clifford, D., Whelan, A.O., Tchilian, E.Z., Beverely, P.C., *et al.* (2015) Protection induced by simultaneous subcutaneous and endobronchial vaccination with BCG/BCG and BCG/Adenovirus expressing Ag85A against *Mycobacterium bovis* in cattle. *PLoS One* 10(11), e0142270.

De Lisle, G.W., Bengis, R.G., Schmitt, S.M. and O'Brien, D.J. (2002) Tuberculosis in free-ranging wildlife: detection, diagnosis and management. *OIE Revue Scientifique et Technique* 21, 317–334.

Domingo, M., Vidal, E. and Marco, A. (2014) Pathology of bovine tuberculosis. *Research in Veterinary Science* 97, S20–S29.

Etna, M.P., Giacomini, E., Severa, M. and Coccia, E.M. (2014) Pro- and anti-inflammatory cytokines in TB: A two-edged sword in TB pathogenesis. *Seminars in Immunology* 26, 543–551.

Fitzgerald, S.D. and Kaneene, J.B. (2012) Wildlife reservoirs of bovine tuberculosis worldwide: hosts, pathology, surveillance and control. *Veterinary Pathology* 50, 488–499.

Gallagher, J. and Clifton-Hadley, R.S. (2000) Tuberculosis in badgers: a review of the disease and its significance for other animals. *Research in Veterinary Science* 69, 203–217.

Gallagher, J. and Macadam, I. (1972) Pulmonary tuberculosis in free-living lechwe antelope in Zambia. *Tropical Animal Health and Production* 4, 204–213.

Garcia-Bocanegra, I., Barranco, I., Rodriguez-Gomez, I.M., Perez, B., Gomez-Laguna, J., *et al.* (2010) Tuberculosis in alpacas (*Lama pacos*) caused by *Mycobacterium bovis*. *Journal of Clinical Microbiology* 48, 1960–1964.

García-Jiménez, W.L., Fernández-Llario, P., Gómez, L., Benítez-Medina, J.M., García-Sánchez, A., *et al.* (2012) Histological and immunohistochemical characterisation of *Mycobacterium bovis* induced granulomas in naturally infected Fallow deer (*Dama dama*). *Veterinary Immunology and Immunopathology* 149, 66–75.

García-Jimenez, W.L., Salguero, F.J., Fernandez-Llario, P., Martinez, R., Risco, D., *et al.* (2013a) Immunopathology of granulomas produced by *Mycobacterium bovis* in naturally infected wild boar. *Veterinary Immunology and Immunopathology* 156, 54–63.

García-Jiménez, W.L., Benítez-Medina, J.M., Fernández-Llario, P., Abecia, J.A., García-Sánchez, A., *et al.* (2013b) Comparative pathology of the natural infections by *Mycobacterium bovis* and by *Mycobacterium caprae* in wild boar (*Sus scrofa*). *Transboundary and Emerging Diseases* 60, 102–109.

Ghon, A. (1912) *Der primare Lungenherd bei der Tuberkulose der Kinder*. Urbach & Schwarzenberg, Berlin, Germany.

Gonzalez-Juarrero, M., Bosco-Lauth, A., Podell, B., Soffler, C., Brooks, E., *et al.* (2013) Experimental aerosol *Mycobacterium bovis* model of infection in goats. *Tuebrculosis (Edinb)* 93, 558–564.

Gortazar, C., Vicente, J. and Gavier-Widén, D. (2003) Pathology of bovine tuberculosis in the European wild boar (*Sus scrofa*). *Veterinary Record* 152, 779–780.

Gunn-Moore, D.A., Dean, R. and Shaw, S. (2010) Mycobacterial infections in cats. *In Practice* 32, 444–452.

Gunn-Moore, D.A., McFarland, S., Brewer, J., Crawshaw, T., Clifton-Hadley, R.S., *et al.* (2011) Mycobacterial disease in cats in Great Britain, 1 bacterial species, geographical distribution and clinical presentation of 339 cases. *Journal of Feline Medicine and Surgery* 13, 934–944.

Hermoso de Mendoza, J., Parra, A., Tato, A., Alonso, J.M., Rey, J.M., *et al.* (2006) Bovine tuberculosis in wild boar (*Sus scrofa*), red deer (*Cervus elaphus*) and cattle (*Bos taurus*) in a Mediterranean ecosystem (1992–2004). *Preventive Veterinary Medicine* 74, 239–247.

Hicks, D.J., Johnson, L., Mitchell, S.M., Gough, J., Cooley, W.A., *et al.* (2006) Evaluation of zinc salt based fixatives for preserving antigenic determinants for immunohistochemical demonstration of murine immune system cell markers. *Biotechnology and Histochemistry* 81, 23–30.

Jennings, A.R. (1949) The distribution of tuberculous lesions in the dog and the cat, with reference to the pathogenesis. *Veterinary Record* 27, 380–384.

Johnson, L., Gough, J., Spencer, Y., Hewinson, G., Vordermeier, M. and Wangoo, A. (2006) Immunohistochemical markers augment evaluation of vaccine efficacy and disease severity in bacillus Calmette-Guerin (BCG) vaccinated cattle challenged with *Mycobacterium bovis*. *Veterinary Immunology and Immunopathology* 111, 219–229.

Johnson, L.K., Liebana, E., Nunez, A., Spencer, Y., Clifton-Hadley, R., *et al.* (2008) Histological observations of the bovine tuberculosis in lung and lymph node tissues from British deer. *Veterinary Journal* 175, 409–412.

Laisse, C.J.M., Gavier-Widen, D., Ramis, G., Bila, C.G., Machado, A., *et al.* (2011) Characterization of tuberculosis lesions in naturally infected African buffalo (*Syncerus caffer*). *Journal of Veterinary Diagnostic Investigation* 23, 1022–1027.

Lawn, S.D. and Zumla, A.I. (2011) Tuberculosis. *Lancet* 378, 57–72.

Liébana, E., Johnson, L., Gough, J., Durr, P., Jahans, K., *et al.* (2008) Pathology of naturally occurring bovine tuberculosis in England and Wales. *The Veterinary Journal* 176, 354–360.

Lin, P.L., Ford, C.B., Coleman, M.T., Myers, A.J., Gawande, R., *et al.* (2014) Sterilization of granulomas is common in active and latent tuberculosis despite within-host variability in bacterial killing. *Nature Medicine* 20, 75–79.

Maglione, P.J. and Chan, J. (2009) How B cells shape the immune response against *Mycobacterium tuberculosis*. *European Journal of Immunology* 39, 676–686.

Marianelli, C., Cifani, N., Capucchio, M.T., Fiasconaro, M., Russo, M., La Mancusa, F., *et al.* (2010) A case of generalized bovine tuberculosis in a sheep. *Journal of Veterinary Diagnostic Investigation* 22, 445–448.

Martin-Hernando, M.P., Torres, M.J., Aznar, J., Negro, J.J., Gandia, A. and Gortazar, C. (2010) Distribution of lesions in red and fallow deer naturally infected with *Mycobacterium bovis*. *Journal of Comparative Pathology* 142, 43–50.

Mattila, J.T., Ojo, O.O., Kepka-Lenhart, D., Marino, S., Kim, J.H., *et al*. (2013) Microenvironments in tuberculous granulomas are delineated by distinct populations of macrophage subsets and expression of nitric oxide synthase and arginase isoforms. *Journal of Immunology* 191, 773–784.

Menzies, F.D. and Neill, S.D. (2000) Cattle-to-cattle transmission of bovine tuberculosis. *The Veterinary Journal* 160, 92–106.

Murray, A., Dineen, A., Kelly, P., McGoey, K., Madigan, G., *et al.* (2015) Nosocomial spread of *Mycobacterium bovis* in domestic cats. *Journal of Feline Medicine and Surgery* 17(2), 173–80.

Neill, S.D., Pollock, J.M., Bryson, D.B. and Hanna, J. (1994) Pathogenesis of *Mycobacterium bovis* infection in cattle. *Veterinary Microbiology* 40, 41–52.

Neill, S.D., Bryson, D.G. and Pollock, J.M. (2001) Pathogenesis of tuberculosis in cattle. *Tuberculosis* 81, 79–86.

O'Reilly, L.M. and Daborn, C.J. (1995) The epidemiology of *Mycobacterium bovis* infections in animals and man. A review. *Tubercle and Lung Disease,* 1–46.

Orme, I.M. and Basaraba, R.J. (2014) The formation of the granuloma in tuberculosis infection. *Seminars in Immunology* 26, 601–609.

Palmer, M.V., Waters, W.R. and Thacker, T.C. (2007) Lesion development and immunohistochemical changes in granulomas from cattle experimentally infected with *Mycobacterium bovis*. *Veterinary Pathology* 44, 863–874.

Palmer, M.V., Thacker, T.C. and Waters, W.R. (2015) Analysis of cytokine expression using a novel chromogenic in-situ hybridisation method in pulmonary granulomas of cattle infected experimentally by aerosolized *Mycobaterium bovis*. *Journal of Comparative Pathology* 153, 150–159.

Palmer, M.V., Thacker, T.C. and Waters, W.R. (2016) Differential cytokine expression in granulomas from lungs and lymph nodes of cattle experimentally infected with aerosolized *Mycobacterium bovis*. *PLoS One* 11(11), e0167471.

Peña, J.C. and Ho, W.Z. (2015) Monkey models of tuberculosis: lessons learned. *Infection and Immunity* 83, 852–862.

Pollock, J.M., McNair, J., Welsh, M.D., Girvin, R.M., Kennedy, H.E., et al. (2001) Immune responses in bovine tuberculosis. *Tuberculosis (Edinb.)* 81, 103–107.

Ramakrishnan, L. (2012) Revisiting the role of the granuloma in tuberculosis. *Nature Reviews in Immunology* 12(5), 352–366

Richey, M.J., Foster, A.P., Crawshaw, T.R. and Shok, A. (2011) *Mycobacterium bovis* mastitis in an alpaca and its implications. *Veterinary Record* 169, 214.

Roberts, T., O'Connor, C., Nuñez-Garcia, J., de la Rua-Domenech, R. and Smith, N.H. (2014) Unusual cluster of *Mycobacterium bovis* infection in cats. *Veterinary Record* 174(13), 326.

Rodriguez-Campos, S., Smith, N.H., Boniotti, M.B. and Aranaz, A. (2014) Overview and phylogeny of *Mycobacterium tuberculosis* complex organisms: implications for diagnostics and legislation of bovine tuberculosis. *Research in Veterinary Science* 97, S5–S19.

Rufenacht, S., Bogil-Stuber, K., Bodmer, T., Bornand Jaunin, V., Gonin Jmaa, D.C. and Gunn-Moore, D.A. (2011) Feline *Mycobacterium microti* infection: a case report and literature review. *Journal of Feline Medicine and Surgery* 13, 195–204.

Ryan, T.J., Livingstone, P.G., Ramsey, D.S.L., de Lisle, G.W., Nugent, G., et al. (2006) Advances in understanding disease epidemiology and implications for control and eradication of tuberculosis in livestock: the experience from New Zealand. *Veterinary Microbiology* 112, 211–219.

Salguero, F.J., Gibson, S., García-Jiménez, W., Gough, J., Strickland, T.S., et al. (2017) Differential cell composition and cytokine expression within lymph node granulomas from BCG-vaccinated and non-vaccinated cattle experimentally infected with *Mycobacterium bovis*. *Transboundary and Emerging Diseases*, 64(6), 1734–1749.

Snider, W.R. (1971) Tuberculosis in canine and feline populations: review of the literature. *American Review of Respiratory Diseases* 104, 877–887.

Sobrino, R., Martin-Hernando, M.P., Vicnete, J., Aurtenetxe, O., Garrido, J.M. and Gortazar, C. (2008) Bovine tuberculosis in a badger (*Meles meles*) in Spain. *Veterinary Record* 163, 159–160.

Terefe, D. (2014) Gross pathological lesions of bovine tuberculosis and efficiency of meat inspection procedure to detect infected cattle in Adama municipal abattoir. *Journal of Veterinary Medicine and Animal Health* 6, 48–53.

Thacker, T.C., Palmer, M.V. and Waters, W.R. (2007) Associations between cytokine gene expression and pathology in *Mycobacterium bovis* infected cattle. *Veterinary Immunology and Immunopathology* 119, 204–213.

Turner, O.C., Basraba, R.J. and Orme, I.M. (2003) Immunopathogenesis of pulmonary granulomas in the guinea pig after infection with *Mycobacterium tuberculosis*. *Infection and Immunity* 71, 864–871.

Twomey, D.F., Crawshaw, T.R., Foster, A.P., Higgins, R.J., Smith, N.H., et al. (2009) Suspected transmission of *Mycobacterium bovis* between alpacas. *Veterinary Record* 165, 121–122.

Ulrichs, T., Kosmiadi, G.A., Trusov, V., Jörg, S., Pradl, L., et al. (2004) Human tuberculous granulomas induce peripheral lymphoid follicle-like structures to orchestrate local host defence in the lung. *Journal of Pathology* 204, 217–228.

Van Rhijn, I., Godfroid, J., Michel, A. and Rutten, V. (2008) Bovine tuberculosis as a model for human tuberculosis. Advantages over small animal models. *Microbes and Infection* 10, 711–715.

Villarreal-Ramos, B., McAulay, M., Chance, V., Martin, M., Morgan, J. and Howard, C.J. (2003) Investigation of the role of CD8+ T cells in bovine tuberculosis in vivo. *Infection and Immunity* 71, 4297–4303.

Volkman, H.E., Pozos, T.C., Zheng, J., Davis, J., Rawls, J.F. and Ramakrishnan, L. (2010) Tuberculous granuloma induction via interaction of a bacterial secreted protein with host epithelium. *Science* 327, 466.

Wangoo, A., Johnson, L., Gough, J., Ackbar, R., Inglut, S., *et al.* (2005) Advanced granulomatous lesions in *Mycobacterium bovis*-infected cattle are associated with increased expression of type I procollagen, γδ (WC1+) T cells and CD 68+ cells. *Journal of Comparative Pathology* 133, 223–234.

Waters, W.R. and Palmer, M.V. (2015) *Mycobacterium bovis* infection of cattle and white-tailed deer: Translational research of relevance to human tuberculosis. *ILAR Journal* 56, 26–43.

Waters, W.R., Maggioli, M.F., McGill, J.L., Lyashchenko, K.P. and Palmer, M.V. (2014) Relevance of bovine tuberculosis research to the understanding of human disease: historical perspectives, approaches, and immunologic mechanisms. *Veterinary Immunology and Immunopathology* 159, 113–132.

Waters, W.R., Maggioli, M.F., Palmer, M.V., Thacker, T.C., McGill, J.L., *et al.* (2015) Interleukin 17A as a biomarker for bovine tuberculosis. *Clinical and Vaccine Immunology* 23, 168–180.

Welsh, M.D., Cunningham, R.T., Corbett, D.M., Girvin, R.M., McNair, J., *et al.* (2005) Influence of pathological progression on the balance between cellular and humoral immune responses in bovine tuberculosis. *Immunology* 114, 101–111.

Whipple, L.D., Boline, A.C. and Miller, M.J. (1996) Distribution of lesion in cattle infected with *Mycobacterium bovis*. *Journal of Veterinary Diagnostic Investigation* 8, 351–354.

Widdison, S., Watson, M. and Coffey, T.J. (2009) Correlation between lymph node pathology and chemokine expression during bovine tuberculosis. *Tuberculosis (Edinb.)* 89, 417–422.

Zanella, G., Duvauchelle, A., Hars, J., Moutou, F., Boschiroli, M.L. and Durand, B. (2008) Patterns of lesions of bovine tuberculosis in wild red deer and wild boar. *Veterinary Record* 163, 43–47.

10 Innate Immune Response in Bovine Tuberculosis

Jacobo Carrisoza-Urbina,[1] Xiangmei Zhou[2] and José A. Gutiérrez-Pabello[1],*

[1]*Departamento de Microbiología e Inmunología, Facultad de Medicina Veterinaria y Zootecnia, Universidad Nacional Autónoma de México, México;* [2]*Veterinary Pathology Department, College of Veterinary Medicine, China Agricultural University, P. R. China*

10.1 Introduction

The innate immune system is the first line of defense against pathogens, of which some of its functions include participation in activation and direction of adaptive immunity, as well as maintaining the integrity and tissue repair (Kumar *et al.*, 2011). The innate system is integrated by macrophages, dendritic cells (DCs), neutrophils and natural killer (NK) cells. These cells use pathogen-recognition receptors (PRRs) for their activity, which are responsible for identifying the presence of conserved structures between microorganisms known as pathogen-associated molecular patterns (PAMPs); similarly, they recognize molecules from damaged cells known as damage-associated molecular patterns (DAMs). During a mycobacterial infection, the innate immune system is able to recognize bacilli through PRRs; this allows the activation of intracellular signalling cascades, the production of pro-inflammatory cytokines, such as tumor necrosis factor-alpha (TNF-α), type 1 interferons (IFNs), interleukin (IL) 1β, IL-18 and IL-12. At the same time, chemokines and antimicrobial proteins are also produced, and antigen presentation is initiated. This inflammatory microenvironment allows the concentration of cells of the innate response at the site of infection, which later allow the activation of the adaptive immune system that is essential for restraining the infection. However, virulent mycobacteria can evade the immune system by replicating inside macrophages, allowing disease pathology to develop (Plüddemann *et al.*, 2011; Yuk and Jo, 2014).

The induced immune response in infection by *Mycobacterium bovis* is a complex process, and its study in cattle has mainly focused on the adaptive immune response (MacHugh *et al.*, 2009), therefore comprehension of the innate immune system in bovine tuberculosis is limited. Nevertheless, studies in humans and mice have shown the importance of the innate immune system in the outcome of mycobacterial infections, helping to control the bacterial load and organizing and directing the magnitude of the adaptive immune response (Magee *et al.*, 2012). In this chapter we will analyze the components of the innate immune response involved in *M. bovis* infection, such as: PRRs; cells of the innate immune system; inflammasomes; and autophagy and apoptosis processes. Furthermore, we will describe the importance of innate

---

* Email: jagp@unam.mx

immunity in natural resistance to bovine tuberculosis.

10.2 Pathogen-Recognition Receptors

Cells of the innate immune system have different types of PRRs: (i) Toll-like receptors (TLRs); (ii) complement receptor 3 (CR3); (iii) the nucleotide-binding oligomerization domain (NOD); (iv) retinoic acid-inducible gene 1-like receptor (RIG-1); (v) mannose-binding receptor; and (vi) dendritic cell-specific intercellular adhesion molecule-3-grabbing non-integrin (DC-SIGN). These receptors are mainly expressed on the cell surface, the endosomal compartments or in the macrophage and dendritic cell cytoplasm. Although there are different receptors for *M. bovis* recognition, TLRs are the most studied receptors participating in the innate response to tuberculosis. TLRs permit macrophage activation and production of pro-inflammatory mediators and oxygen- and nitrogen-reactive intermediates that act to restrict bacterial growth. Among the receptors that compose the TLR family, TLR1, TLR2, TLR4, TLR8 and TLR9 have been associated with the recognition of *Mycobacterium tuberculosis* (Mortaz *et al.*, 2015). However, the TLR type and the activated inflammatory response are dependent on the host species, as well as the species and *Mycobacterium* strain present during the infection. For example, TLR4 activation was described in human neutrophils infected with different mycobacterial species. Under these latter experimental conditions, *M. tuberculosis* H37Rv induced increased expression of CD32, CD64, CXCR3 and TLR4, as well as TNF-α secretion and a decrease of early apoptosis in infected cells, whereas *M. bovis* bacillus Calmette–Guérin (BCG) infection only showed increased CD32 expression and *M. indicus pranii* could not activate an immune response in neutrophils (Ma *et al.*, 2016). On the other hand, *M. indicus pranii* infection in macrophages induced a higher activation of TLR2 compared to *M. bovis* BCG, suggesting that atypical mycobacteria may have increased levels of TLR2 ligands compared to *M. bovis* BCG (Kumar *et al*, 2014). In a bovine model, *M. bovis* and *M. tuberculosis* induced a significant increase in the expression of TLR2 and RIG-1 type receptors in alveolar macrophages. Comparatively, *M. bovis* was able to maintain the expression of TLR2 for a longer time period than *M tuberculosis* (Magee *et al.*, 2014). Similarly, there is evidence of TLR activation in a MyD88-dependent and -independent fashion in cattle and sheep bronchial epithelial cells infected with *M. bovis* and *M. tuberculosis* (Ma *et al.*, 2016). It is evident that each *Mycobacterium* species induces specific changes depending on the infected host. Furthermore, while *M. bovis* is capable of causing tuberculosis in different animal species including humans, *M. tuberculosis* mainly infects humans and it does not cause or induce a transient infection in cattle. These data suggest key differences in the innate response among bacterial species, possibly related to the host species-specific TLRs and to genetic differences between the mycobacterial species and strains (Widdison *et al.*, 2008; Ma *et al.*, 2016).

10.3 Cells of the Innate Immune Response in Bovine Tuberculosis

10.3.1 Macrophages

Macrophages are specialized phagocytic cells involved in the homeostasis, development and repair of damaged tissue, and are considered the first line of defense against mycobacteria. During a classical *M. bovis* infection, alveolar macrophages and DCs phagocytize the bacilli, initiating the immune response in order to control bacterial dissemination (Hussain Bhat and Mukhopadhyay, 2015).

Different studies have demonstrated that bovine monocyte-derived macrophages phagocytize virulent and avirulent *M. bovis* strains. Bacteria phagocytized by resting macrophages range from 1.25 to 2.64 per macrophage, suggesting that phagocytosis was very similar regardless of bacterial virulence (Gutiérrez-Pabello and Adams, 2003). Infection of bovine macrophages with BCG or virulent *M. bovis* revealed a functional difference in controlling growth of both strains among cattle. Virulent *M. bovis* grew to higher colony-forming unit numbers in macrophages from 24 different donors compared to BCG. Levels of nitric oxide

(NO) released in response to *M. bovis* were significantly increased compared to levels released by uninfected cells. Macrophage activation by the classical pathway induced large NO release; however, lipopolysaccharide (LPS) pretreatment followed by *M. bovis* infection showed a higher NO production. Under these conditions *M. bovis* replication was significantly decreased. Neutralizing NO production with n^G-monomethyl-L-arginine monoacetate (MMLA) in *M. bovis* and LPS treatments confirmed that macrophage microbicidal activity against *M. bovis* was NO dependent. These results demonstrated that NO generation is a key process in anti-mycobacterial activity in bovine macrophages (Esquivel-Solís et al., 2013).

Macrophages induced to acquire an alternative activation status by incubation with IL-4 decreased basal production of NO induced by LPS alone or in combination with INF-γ. Short-term incubation (4 hours) with IL-4 showed an increase in the number of bacilli phagocytized, independently of the strain virulence. The virulent strain played an important role in phagocytosis inducing a higher number of bacilli phagocytized in comparison with BCG; however, this number was affected in those treatments where IL-4 incubation was maintained for 24 hours, reducing the phagocytosis levels with no differences between bacterial strains. This effect was more evident when a virulent *M. bovis* strain was used. The number of intracellular survival bacilli phagocytized showed a higher intracellular proliferation in cells incubated for 4 hours with IL-4; however, when the stimulation was maintained for 24 hours, macrophages further reduced their microbicidal ability. LPS alone or in combination with *M. bovis* infection increased pro-inflammatory cytokine gene expression of bovine macrophages, whereas IL-4 treatment reversed the effect of classical activation by decreasing mRNA levels of the inflammatory mediators. Collectively this body of evidence indicates that macrophage alternative activation induced functional changes that resulted in modification of the rate of phagocytosis, decreased NO production and iNOS mRNA levels, and as a consequence increased pathogen intracellular survival suggesting that alternatively activated macrophages are in general more permissive to *M. bovis* growth (Castillo-Velázquez et al., 2011).

10.3.2 Dendritic cells

DCs are specialized cells in antigen presentation, capable of activating different cells of the immune system such as NK, T γδ cells and naive T cells that are important for the initiation and maintenance of the immune response (Fabrik et al., 2013; Pearce and Everts, 2015). DCs, just like macrophages, express PRRs that serve for bacterial recognition. Hence, once DCs phagocytize bacilli, antigens are processed and uploaded into the major histocompatibility complex (MHC) molecules for presentation in the lymph nodes (Hope et al., 2004).

Mycobacterial interaction with DCs may exert a dual role in innate immune response modulation. For instance, the *M. bovis* mannosylated lipoarabinomannan (ManLAM) is recognized by the DC-SIGN receptor (Hope et al., 2004; Fabrik et al., 2013; Stamm et al., 2015), which induces the expression of the potent immunosuppressant IL-10, affecting the antigen presentation process by inhibiting the migration and maturation of DCs (Hope et al., 2004; Fabrik et al., 2013). In this way, the onset of the immune response is delayed and is insufficient to eradicate mycobacteria. On the other hand, the interplay between DCs and mycobacteria increases the expression of DC surface molecules such as MHC-II, CD80, CD86 and CD40, that leads to T cells activation in an attempt to eliminate the bacterial invader (Hope et al., 2004; Pearce and Everts, 2015).

Indeed, mycobacteria have the ability to modulate the cytokine profile of DCs. Dendritic cell infection with *M. tuberculosis* or *M. bovis* BCG has been associated with a higher expression of IL-12, TNF-α, IL-1 and IL-6 (Hope et al., 2004), which are essential in the control of tuberculosis. IL-12 participates in the acquired immune response through increasing IFN-γ and TNF-α secretion by T cells; this, in turn, increases the microbicidal activity of macrophages and NK cells in order to destroy the bacilli (Hope et al., 2004; Denis and Buddle, 2008).

It has also been demonstrated that DCs have a higher capacity to phagocytize *M. bovis*; however, once internalized in these cells, *M. bovis* also shows enhanced replication since the DCs release between five and ten times lower amounts of NO, IL-1β and TNF-α compared to macrophages. Survival and replication of mycobacteria within DCs could result in the transport of bacteria to the lymph nodes and therefore, bacterial dissemination (Denis and Buddle, 2008).

10.3.3 Natural killer cells

NK cells are large granular lymphocytes with diverse functions that include cytotoxicity and cytokine production, and that interact with DCs and other myeloid cells to remove damaged and infected cells (Bastos et al., 2008; Boysen and Storset, 2009). NK cells respond to target cells through the activation and inhibition of receptors. In addition, NK directly recognize PAMPs, TLRs and PRRs.

Bovine active NK cells have high expression levels of CD2 (Boysen and Storset, 2009; Siddiqui et al., 2012). Activated NK cells use granule exocytosis and release of cytotoxic proteins (perforins and granulysins) to reduce mycobacteria viability, inducing target cell death (Siddiqui et al., 2012). It has been demonstrated that bovine NK cells can reduce M. bovis replication in bovine macrophages through direct contact with the infected cell and IL-12 stimulation (Denis et al., 2007; Bastos et al., 2008; Boysen and Storset, 2009). The ability to control M. bovis growth was associated with an increase in IL-12 and nitric oxide release in M. bovis-infected macrophages, which in turn cooperated to amplify a Th1 response, NK cell activation and macrophage apoptosis. An increase in granulysin, IFN-γ and perforin was associated with the cytotoxic activity of activated bovine NK cells against M bovis BCG-infected alveolar and monocyte-derived macrophages (Endsley et al., 2006). On the other hand, neonatal BCG vaccination induced a significant increase in NK cells of peripheral blood and within lymph nodes (Siddiqui et al., 2012).

10.3.4 Neutrophils

Neutrophils are professional phagocytes that play an essential role in the innate immune response. Recent findings have identified that these cells also participate in the activation and regulation of adaptive immune responses at different levels, including regulation of B and T lymphocytes, and even control the homeostasis of NK cells. Neutrophils also produce large amounts of cytokines and neutrophil extracellular traps (NETs). All these activities support a key role for neutrophils in the protection against intracellular pathogens, such as viruses and mycobacteria (Mantovani et al., 2011; Mocsai, 2013).

During infection with mycobacteria, neutrophils are recruited within a few hours at the site of infection, where they phagocytize the bacilli (Lowe et al., 2012). Once they encounter M. bovis antigens, neutrophils are able to release cytokines and chemokines that attract inflammatory cells, including T lymphocytes (Shu et al., 2014). Bovine neutrophils infected with M. bovis show an increase in CD32, CD64 and TLR4 expression, as well as increased TNF-α and IL-10 secretion. Secretion products of infected neutrophils promoted macrophage activation through the classical pathway, producing pro-inflammatory cytokines and chemokines (Wang et al., 2013). Another effect on human neutrophils infected with M. tuberculosis was the formation of NETs. These structures are part of the innate immune response, being phagocytized by macrophages, promoting their activation and the production of cytokines and interleukins, such as IL-6, TNF-α, IL-1β and IL-10, confirming the importance of neutrophils and their close interaction with macrophages during mycobacteria infections (Braian et al., 2013).

Neutrophils are able to phagocytize bacteria by direct recognition and opsonization, promoting rapid phagosome fusion with lysosomes and killing bacteria through oxidation reactions by producing reactive oxygen and nitrogen species. However, it is controversial whether neutrophils can eliminate phagocytized mycobacteria, especially virulent strains, because it has been reported that neutrophils are the main cells found in the bronchoalveolar washings and sputum of patients with active tuberculosis, which have an increased load of bacilli. Virulent strains of M. tuberculosis can live in neutrophils despite the microbicidal components of these cells, and it has been shown that they can escape neutrophil-induced death by necrosis (netosis) (Corleis et al., 2012). M. bovis is capable of surviving and escaping from bovine neutrophils, in addition to inducing autophagy in an undetermined way (Wang et al., 2013).

The success or failure of mycobacterial removal *in vivo* by neutrophils depends on the resistance or susceptibility of each individual, and the ability of mycobacteria to survive within these cells. Therefore, it has been proposed that neutrophils are able to control infection during early stages; however, depending on the circumstances, neutrophils can act as 'trojan horses', where their inability to eliminate the infecting mycobacteria may promote the spread of bacilli to distal sites of the infection focus (Corleis *et al.*, 2012; Lowe *et al.*, 2012).

10.3.5 γδ T cells

γδ T lymphocytes constitute between 50–60% of the T cells in the bloodstream of young ruminants, and decrease down to 12% in adult animals. Two subgroups of these cells have been identified based on the expression of the WC1 antigen (workshop cluster antigen-1): WC1.1 and WC1.2, where the first subgroup is characterized by IFN-γ secretion and the second subgroup is more sensitive to mitogen stimulation (Price *et al.*, 2010). These cells have characteristics of both innate and adaptive immune systems, so they are considered as transient T cells of the immune response. Their participation in the innate immune response has been demonstrated by their ability to recognize PAMs and DAMs in the absence of antigen presenting cells (Vantourout and Hayday, 2013).

In vitro studies have demonstrated the participation of γδ T cells in the immune response to bovine tuberculosis. Bovine γδ T cells respond to a sonicated extract of *M. bovis* by increasing the expression of CD25 and the secretion levels of IFN-γ. An *in vivo* study in calves where these cells were depleted by a monoclonal anti-WC1 prior to infection with *M. bovis*, caused a decrease in the IFN-γ concentration, an increase in the IL-4 production and a lack of G_2 type-specific immunoglobulin antibodies, suggesting that γδ T cells are involved in the early differentiation of a Th1 type response (Kennedy *et al.*, 2002; Price and Hope, 2009). It has also been identified that there is a direct interaction at the infection site between γδ T cells and DCs, which increases IFN-γ production due to the presence of IL-2 and IL-15 (Alvarez *et al.*, 2009). In the early stages of bovine granuloma formation, a correlation of the amount of γδ T cells with the degree of organization was seen (Plattner *et al.*, 2009).

Calves vaccinated with *M. bovis* BCG rapidly increased the proportion of WC1+ γδ T cells, and also showed increased levels of INF-γ in peripheral blood. Subsequently, it was shown that this latter IFN-γ production was related to the number of WC1+ γδ T cells, and not to the CD8+ CD4+ lymphocyte population (Guzman *et al.*, 2012).

Despite recent progress in the study of bovine WC1+ γδ T cells, their function and importance in the immune response remains unknown. However, bovines offer an alternative as a model for studying these cells and vaccine design against tuberculosis.

10.4 Cell Death Mechanisms Involved in the Innate Immune Response to Bovine Tuberculosis

10.4.1 Autophagy

Macroautophagy or autophagy is an evolutionarily conserved process in eukaryotes, where damaged and surplus cytosolic components are removed in order to provide nutrients during starvation periods. The participation of this phenomenon in tuberculosis pathogenesis was identified by physiological induction or rapamycin treatment of macrophages infected with *M. bovis* BCG or *M. tuberculosis*, which led to maturation of mycobacterial phagosomes into phagolysosomes, hence reducing intracellular bacterial viability. IFN-γ treatment of *Mycobacterium*-infected macrophages further enhanced autophagy induction (Gutierrez *et al.*, 2004).

Subsequent studies have confirmed the importance of autophagy in controlling the growth of *M. tuberculosis* and *M. bovis* in macrophages. Furthermore, this process has been observed in bovine neutrophils infected with *M. bovis*, where a higher percentage of cells showing autophagy was identified compared to macrophages from infected cattle. These results suggest that autophagy is one of the central innate mechanisms available to cells for controlling mycobacteria.

Current studies have attempted to identify how mycobacteria induce autophagy. It has been demonstrated that autophagy is differentially induced by mycobacterial species; *M. smegmatis* induced a higher autophagy response than *M. bovis* BCG. In addition, it is postulated that mycobacterial lipid components are responsible for autophagy induction (Zullo and Lee, 2012). Cytosolic detection of bacterial products plays a crucial role in initiating the innate immune response, including autophagy activation. The *M. bovis*-induced AIM2 inflammasome activation decreases autophagy in immortalized and primary murine macrophages. This relies on the inflammasome sensor AIM2 which conjugates with cytosolic DNA to inhibit the STING-dependent pathway involved in selective autophagy. The DNA sensor of IFN-γ inducible protein 204 (IFI204) plays an important role for autophagy marker LC3 expression during *M. bovis* infection (Liu et al., 2016, 2017). Hence, a growing body of evidence points to autophagy as an innate immunity mechanism that plays an important role in the control of mycobacterial, including *M. bovis*, infections.

10.4.2 Apoptosis

Apoptosis is a type of regulated cell death that also has been reported to participate in the innate immune response controlling the growth of intracellular pathogens, including mycobacteria. This type of cell death is characterized by not generating an inflammatory response. Morphologically, apoptotic cells exhibit cellular and nuclear shrinkage, chromatin condensation, DNA fragmentation and the formation of apoptotic bodies. Two pathways are known by which apoptosis is activated during physiological or pathological conditions that are dependent or independent of caspase activation; the extrinsic pathway, which is initiated by ligand binding, such as via TNF-α or FasL binding to its respective receptor located on the cell surface, and the intrinsic pathway activated by intracellular death signals where the mitochondria plays a fundamental role (Parandhaman and Narayanan, 2014).

The participation of apoptosis in tuberculosis has been shown in several studies where it has been demonstrated that mycobacterial species modulate apoptosis. Virulent strains of *M. tuberculosis* and *M. bovis* were able to inhibit apoptosis in a mouse model (Hinchey et al., 2007; Rodrigues et al., 2009). In fact, the expression of several genes encoding for pro-apoptotic proteins (e.g. CASP8, CASP7, IDB, CYCS) and inhibitory for apoptosis (e.g. BCL2A1, CFLAR, BCL2, BCL2L1, BIRC2, BIRC3, XIAP, MCL1 and PRKX) was increased at 2, 6, 24 and 48 hours after infecting bovine alveolar macrophages with *M. bovis*, demonstrating the regulation of genes involved in apoptosis during the early stages of infection with *M. bovis* (Nalpas et al., 2015). Moreover, microarray analysis of *M. bovis*-infected macrophages identified an increased number of downregulated genes compared to uninfected controls, suggesting that *M. bovis* infection is associated with host gene repression (Widdison et al., 2011; Magee et al., 2012; Nalpas et al., 2015). Macrophages from healthy and infected animals can both be fully activated by *M. bovis* infection, yet there are differences between these macrophages: changes (fold-changes) in global transcriptome induced by *in vitro* challenge of *M. bovis* were higher in healthy cows than in tuberculosis-positive cows, suggesting that healthy macrophages responded marginally better to *in vitro* infection (Lin et al., 2015).

Results from different studies using an *in vitro* model of macrophage infection have demonstrated that virulent and avirulent strains of *M. bovis* are capable of inducing macrophage apoptosis (Gutiérrez-Pabello et al., 2002; Vega-Manriquez et al., 2007; Castillo-Velázquez et al., 2011; Esquivel-Solís et al., 2013). Macrophage apoptosis was time and multiplicity of infection (MOI) dependent. Rates of apoptosis, measured via chromatin condensation and DNA fragmentation, progressed rapidly after infection and increased significantly post-infection. Also, the number of bacteria per macrophage had a direct effect on the apoptotic counts. Macrophages infected with an MOI of 25:1 developed chromatin condensation and DNA fragmentation at 4 and 8 hours, respectively, whereas changes in chromatin condensation induced by MOIs of 10:1 and 1:1 required a longer time and resulted in fewer apoptotic cells. In addition, it was not only infected cells that underwent apoptosis but also uninfected bystander cells, suggesting a possible role of macrophage-secreted mediators in the induction of apoptosis (Gutiérrez-Pabello et al., 2002).

It has been postulated that host resistance and the virulence of the strain influenced the degree of macrophage apoptosis. Macrophages from resistant donors underwent apoptosis as a consequence of *M. bovis* infection at higher levels than from susceptible donors. At the same time, virulent strains showed a tendency to induce a higher percentage of apoptosis than BCG. Although experimental results indicate a possible role of host resistance and bacterial virulence in macrophage apoptosis, further investigation is required to validate these observations (Esquivel-Solís et al., 2013).

Induction of bovine macrophage apoptosis has been described using whole *M. bovis* cells; however, experimental data also indicates that *M. bovis* cell-free protein extract and individual proteins can also induce macrophage apoptosis. Furthermore, bovine macrophage apoptosis can occur in the absence of caspase activation with participation of the mitochondrial apoptosis inducing factor (AIF). These results strongly suggest that *M. bovis* infection drives the release of AIF into the cytosol and its translocation to the nucleus, where it participates in chromatin condensation and DNA fragmentation in a caspase-independent pathway (Vega-Manriquez et al., 2007). Recent studies suggested that *M. bovis* infection results in loss of Ca^{2+} from the ER and an increase in the intracellular redox state which results in accumulation of unfolded or misfolded proteins in the ER resulting in ER stress. *M. bovis* effectively induced apoptosis in murine macrophages via ER stress. The STING-TBK1-IRF3 pathway mediates cross-talk between ER stress and apoptosis during *M. bovis* infection which can control intracellular bacteria effectively (Cui et al., 2016). Taken together, these observations illustrate the importance of macrophage apoptosis in the pathogenesis of bovine tuberculosis and the role of apoptosis as a bovine innate immune mechanism.

10.5 Inflammasome

The innate immune system has the ability to combat microbial infections and at the same time handle pathological inflammation. The inflammasome is a multiprotein complex that plays a central role in this process, regulating the production and action of pro-inflammatory cytokines such as IL-1β, IL-18, IL-33, and a type of cell death (pyroptosis) in response to pathogens and internal warning signs.

The inflammasome allows the release of active IL-1β and has been considered to be part of resistance to tuberculosis since interleukin deficient mice infected with *M. tuberculosis* exhibit acute mortality and increased pulmonary bacterial load (Mayer-Barber et al., 2010). In macrophages and dendritic cells, one pathway to IL-1β production is due to inflammasome activation; another route is through serine proteinases such as proteinase-3, elastase and G-cathepsin from neutrophils and macrophages involved in pro-IL-1β cleavage (Netea et al., 2010).

Because IL-1β is synthesized as a pro-IL-1β biological precursor, it needs to be activated by cleavage of caspase 1, allowing its maturation and exit into the extracellular space. This process is regulated by the multiprotein complexes referred as inflammasomes, which are: (i) IPAF (protease activator factor); (ii) NLRP1 (oligomerization domain by nucleotide binding containing protein 1); and (iii) NLRP3 and AIM2 (absent receiver in melanoma 2). It is known that virulent strains of *M. tuberculosis* activate the NLRP3 through the recognition of ESAT-6 protein (Mishra et al., 2010). Also, virulent *M. bovis* activates NLRP7 in THP-1 macrophages, and induces pyroptosis, TNF-α and CCL3 expression, whereas the non-virulent *M. bovis* BCG strain is unable to activate the inflammasome (Zhou et al., 2016). Moreover, it also has been shown that *M. bovis* can activate the AIM2 inflammasome, which recognizes double-stranded DNA (Yang et al., 2013).

In a mouse model of *M. tuberculosis* infection it was demonstrated that the IL-1 regulation was induced through INF-γ produced by T lymphocytes, and that this process was mediated by NO, which inhibited the NLRP3 inflammasome assembly through thiol nitrosylation; this in turn inhibited persistent neutrophil recruitment, preventing tissue damage (Mishra et al., 2012).

During chronic infections like tuberculosis, inflammasomes are a double-edged sword. On the one hand, they help innate immunity to increase pro-inflammatory signals with the purpose to identify and eliminate pathogens, but on the other hand they promote development of immunopathology. A fine balance is required in order to favour host survival. The AIM2 cytosolic DNA sensor may conjugate competitively with cytosolic *M. bovis* DNA to restrict *M. bovis*-induced STING-TBK1-dependent autophagy activation and IFN-β secretion (Liu et al., 2016).

10.6 Role of Interferon-β in Infection of *M. bovis*

Until now, several cytokines have been shown to participate in the innate host response against *M. tuberculosis*, where they can either function to enhance host resistance or may play a role in aggravating the infection (O' Garra et al., 2013). The critical role of inflammatory cytokines such as IL-1β has been established in the control of *M. tuberculosis* activity by augmenting the antimicrobial function of macrophages (Fremond et al., 2007). On the other hand, an important cytokine IFN-β has been reported to have pro-bacterial activity and is associated with the development of tuberculosis in many studies on animal models and humans (Manca et al., 2005; Stanley et al., 2006; Berry et al., 2010; Trinchieri, 2010). Recent studies showed that this pro-bacterial activity of IFN-β is correlated with its anti-inflammatory characteristics as it antagonizes the production and function of IL-1β and IL-18 through increased IL-10 production and also inhibits the NLRP3 inflammasome. Furthermore, IFN-β also fails to initiate an appropriate Th1 response with reduced expression of MHC-II and IFN-γ receptors (IFNGR).

IL-1 is an important and extensively studied cytokine. It plays a pivotal role in the induction of the inflammatory and immune response against virulent mycobacterial strains, but it is suppressed by type I IFN (Mayer-Barber et al., 2011; Novikov et al., 2011). IFN-β–induced inhibition of IL-1 production has been reported by Guarda et al. (2011) and Ma et al. (2014) through two distinct pathways. IFN-β signalling, via the STAT1 transcription factor, repressed the activity of nucleotide-binding domain and leucine-rich repeat containing proteins 1 and 3 (NLRP1 and NLRP3) inflammasomes, hence suppressing the caspase-1-dependent IL-1β maturation. In addition, IFN-β induced IL-10 in a STAT1-dependent manner, and then IL-10, via autocrine action, led to reduced production of pro-IL-1α and pro-IL-1β through STAT3 signalling. Mayer-Barber et al. (2011) reported that IFN-β inhibited IL-1 production by both subsets, whereas CD4+ T-cell–derived IFN-γ suppressed IL-1 expression selectively in inflammatory monocytes. The data provided cellular evidence for the anti-inflammatory effects of IFN-β as well as pro-bacterial functions during mycobacterial infection. In another report by the same group (Mayer-Barber et al., 2014), it was revealed that IL-1β prostaglandin E2 (PGE2) is another important pathway by which IFN-β antagonizes IL-1 production during mycobacterial infection. The absence of IFN-β signalling resulted in increased PGE2 and IL-1β and decreased IL-1Ra. *M. tuberculosis*-infected wild-type bone marrow-derived macrophages produced significantly less PGE2 when exogenous IFN-β was present. Novikov et al. (2011) demonstrated that IFN-β selectively limits the production of IL-1β. This regulation occurs at the level of IL-1β mRNA expression, rather than caspase-1 activation or autocrine IL-1 amplification, and this regulation is only evident in the virulent mycobacterial strains as avirulent strains fail to trigger the same response. Reciprocal control of type 1 IFNs by IL-1β PGE2-mediated pathway has also been reported, and PGE2 treatment led to reduced production of type 1 IFNs and increased protection against *M. tuberculosis* infection (Xu et al., 1998; Mayer-Barber et al., 2014). Briken et al. (2013) reviewed the role of IFN-β after its induction by mycobacterial infection, showing it could suppress NLRP3-inflammasome activation while increasing the action of AIM2 (absent in melanoma)-inflammasome. In contrast, a recent study reported the AIM2 cytosolic DNA sensor may conjugate competitively with cytosolic *M. bovis* DNA to restrict *M. bovis*-induced STING-TBK1-dependent IFN-β secretion (Liu et al., 2016). IFN-β release increases in macrophages exposed to *M. bovis* and this requires the activation of the DNA sensor of IFN-γ inducible protein 204 (IFI204). Knockdown of the IFI204 in immortalized and primary murine macrophages blocked IFN-β production (Liu et al., 2017). The balance between IL-1 and IFN-β is important in defining the outcome of bovine tuberculosis and their role in the therapy of tuberculosis requires further research.

10.7 Natural Resistance to *M. bovis*

Tuberculosis does not always develop in individuals who are exposed to pathogenic mycobacteria. Some individuals may not exhibit evidence of infection and this may be due to the multifactorial risk of tuberculous mycobacteria, where host factors, pathogens and the environment are involved. Among the factors involved in the host, it is known that genetics and innate and acquired immunity have an essential role in this natural resistance to tuberculosis.

Natural disease resistance to bacterial intracellular pathogens was identified in cattle using a *Brucella abortus in vivo* challenge of non-vaccinated pregnant cows. Results from this experiment segregated cattle into two groups, one that was resistant (R) to infection and a susceptible (S) group that developed active infection and aborted. The frequency of natural resistance to brucellosis was shown to be 18% in cross-bred cattle. Selective breeding of naturally resistant cows increased this frequency to 53.6% in the F1 progeny (Adams and Templeton, 1998). A macrophage bactericidal assay was established to test if superior bactericidal activity of macrophages from brucellosis resistance cattle was also operational against *M. bovis* BCG, *Salmonella* Dublin and *Salmonella* Typhimurium, and would hence have use as *in vitro* correlate of the resistance phenotype. A value of 65% bacterial survival for *M. bovis* BCG correlated highly with actual numbers of animals designated as resistant, and therefore was considered a phenotypic marker of the resistant trait (Qureshi et al., 1996).

Macrophages from R and S cattle also differed significantly ($p<0.01$) in controlling virulent *M. bovis* intracellular growth. A virulent *M. bovis* strain survived better in both R and S macrophages than BCG; however, macrophages from R cattle were superior to those from S cattle in controlling *in vitro* intracellular replication (Gutiérrez-Pabello and Adams, 2003).

Experimental evidence identified that *M. bovis*-infected macrophages from R cattle produced more nitric oxide and were slightly more prone to undergo apoptosis than S cells. The blockade of nitric oxide production enhanced the replication of *M. bovis* in both R and S cells but had no effect on apoptosis induction. As a result, NO was identified as a major determinant of macrophage resistance to *M. bovis* infection in cattle (Esquivel-Solís et al., 2013). Alternative activation modified the macrophage response against *M. bovis*. Macrophage IL-4 treatment increased the number of bacilli phagocytized in both R and S macrophages; however, intracellular survival was augmented mainly in S macrophages. Alternative activation decreased gene expression of pro-inflammatory cytokines, NO production and DNA fragmentation mainly in R macrophages, in this way minimizing the functional differences that existed between R and S macrophages (Castillo-Velázquez et al., 2011).

A macrophage pro-inflammatory gene expression profile was a common feature after *M. bovis* infection regardless of bacterial virulence; however, superior expression of pro-inflammatory genes in S macrophages was induced by the attenuated strain, whereas in R macrophages increased pro-inflammatory gene expression was driven by the virulent *M. bovis* strain. A macrophage pro-inflammatory profile is intended to control *M. bovis* intracellular growth. However, the host resistant phenotype plays a determinant role in it, since R macrophages had better intracellular bacterial control than S cells.

Genetic polymorphisms associated with innate immunity are also involved in resistance and susceptibility to tuberculosis. For example, gene polymorphisms in genes encoding TLRs, vitamin D receptors, as well as immunity effector molecules like TNFα, have been associated with a higher susceptibility to tuberculosis infection (Azad et al., 2012). In the case of Holstein cattle from China, it has been documented that a TLR1 gene polymorphism has been associated with a higher susceptibility to active tuberculosis (Sun et al., 2012). Similarly, it has been found that the genetic variability in *Bos indicus* cattle confers a more resistant phenotype on them compared to *Bos taurus* cattle (Ameni et al., 2007). Bermingham et al. (2014) showed that while variation in the resistance and susceptibility to tuberculosis in Holstein Friesian cattle is polygenic, they could identify two major regions that were associated with resistance to disease coding for the phosphatase tyrosine receptor and IIIB myosin (Bermingham *et al.*, 2014).

Vitamin D is another factor involved in the response to tuberculosis. Among the factors that have been found associated with a variation in susceptibility to the disease are lower levels of 25-hydroxyvitamin D in serum, and genetic polymorphisms in the vitamin D receptors and vitamin D-binding proteins, especially when they are combined with low serum levels of calciferol, the precursor of the active form of vitamin D. Vitamin D treatment improves the *in vitro* bactericidal capacity of macrophages, increasing phagosome fusion with lysosomes, autophagy, antimicrobial peptide production (e.g. cathelicidins) and oxidative capacity (Cassidy and Martineau, 2014). In bovine monocytes infected with *M. bovis*, active vitamin D increased the production of the nitric oxide synthase enzyme, NOS and the RANTES chemokine (regulated upon the activation of normal T-cell, expressed and secreted) (Nelson *et al.*, 2010).

Selective breeding of naturally resistant cattle may have a profound effect improving herd health status. A reduction in antibiotic usage and a better response to vaccines are some of the arguments to support this statement. Exploiting natural disease resistance to inform selective breeding programmes is one of the tools that the cattle industry may use to improve livestock production efficiency.

10.8 Conclusions

The presence of pathogenic bacteria, like *M. bovis*, in host tissues triggers alarm signals that brings the innate immune response into play. Physical, chemical, molecular and cellular barriers are turned on to identify and stop invaders. In this scenario, bacteria and innate immune components interplay to drive induction of a pro-inflammatory response that sets up a survival competition among host and pathogen. Under these conditions non-opsonic receptors, inflammatory cytokines and chemokines allow the influx of different types of cells, phagocytosis and the production of antimicrobial molecules that provide protection against mycobacteria, inhibiting bacilli growth (Liu *et al.*, 2013; Hilda *et al.*, 2014). However, it is important to consider that in the end, bacterial virulence and the host natural disease resistance determines the net profit or loss in this biological transaction. In this chapter we attempted to provide an overview of the innate immune response of cattle to *M. bovis* infection; however, this is a complex process that still requires much further investigation.

References

Adams, L.G. and Templeton, J.W. (1998) Genetic resistance to bacterial diseases of animals. *Revue Scientifique et Technique (International Office of Epizootics)* 17(1), 200–219.

Alvarez, A.J., Endsley, J.J., Werling, D. and Estes, M.D. (2009) WC1 γδ T cells indirectly regulate chemokine production during *Mycobacterium bovis* Infection in SCID-bo mice. *Transboundary and Emerging Diseases* 56(6–7), 275–284.

Ameni, G., Aseffa, A., Engers, H., Young, D., Gordon, S., *et al.* (2007) High prevalence and increased severity of pathology of bovine tuberculosis in Holsteins compared to Zebu breeds under field cattle husbandry in central Ethiopia. *Clinical and Vaccine Immunology* 14(10), 1356–1361.

Azad, A.K., Sadee, W. and Schlesinger, L.S. (2012) Innate immune gene polymorphisms in tuberculosis. *Infection and Immunity* 80(10), 3343–3359.

Bastos, R.G., Johnson, W.C., Mwangi, W., Brown, W.C. and Goff, W.L. (2008) Bovine NK cells acquire cytotoxic activity and produce IFN-γ after stimulation by *Mycobacterium bovis* BCG- or *Babesia bovis*-exposed splenic dendritic cells. *Veterinary Immunology and Immunopathology* 124(3–4), 302–312.

Bermingham, M.L., Bishop, S.C., Woolliams, J.A., Pong-Wong, R., Allen, A.R., *et al.* (2014) Genome-wide association study identifies novel loci associated with resistance to bovine tuberculosis. *Heredity* 112(5), 543–551.

Berry, M.P., Graham, C.M., McNab, F.W., Xu, Z., Bloch, S.A., *et al.* (2010) An interferon-inducible neutrophil driven blood transcriptional signature in human tuberculosis. *Nature* 466, 973–977.

Boysen, P. and Storset, A.K. (2009) Bovine natural killer cells. *Veterinary Immunology and Immunopathology*, 130(3–4), 163–177.

Braian, C., Hogea, V. and Stendahl, O. (2013) *Mycobacterium tuberculosis* induced neutrophil extracellular traps activate human macrophages. *Journal of Innate Immunity* 5(6), 591–602.

Briken, V., Sarah, E.A., Shah, S. (2013) *Mycobacterium tuberculosis* and the host cell inflammasome: a complex relationship. *Frontiers in Cellular and Infection Microbiology* 62, 1–6.

Cassidy, J.P. and Martineau, A.R. (2014) Innate resistance to tuberculosis in man, cattle and laboratory animal models: nipping disease in the bud? *Journal of Comparative Pathology* 151(4), 291–308.

Castillo-Velázquez, U., Aranday-Cortés, E. and Gutiérrez-Pabello, J.A. (2011) Alternative activation modifies macrophage resistance to *Mycobacterium bovis*. *Veterinary Microbiology* 151(1), 51–59.

Corleis, B., Korbel, D., Wilson, R., Bylund, J., Chee, R. and Schaible, U.E. (2012) Escape of *Mycobacterium tuberculosis* from oxidative killing by neutrophils. *Cellular Microbiology* 14(7), 1109–1121.

Cui, Y., Zhao, D., Sreevatsan, S., Liu, C., Yang, W., *et al.* (2016) *Mycobacterium bovis* induces endoplasmic reticulum stress mediated–apoptosis by activating IRF3 in a murine macrophage cell line. *Frontiers in Cellular and Infection Microbiology* 6, 182.

Denis, M. and Buddle, B.M. (2008) Bovine dendritic cells are more permissive for *Mycobacterium bovis* replication than macrophages, but release more IL-12 and induce better immune T-cell proliferation. *Immunology Cell Biology* 86(2), 185–191.

Denis, M., Keen, D.L., Parlane, N.A., Storset, A.K. and Buddle, B.M. (2007) Bovine natural killer cells restrict the replication of *Mycobacterium bovis* in bovine macrophages and enhance IL-12 release by infected macrophages. *Tuberculosis* 87(1), 53–62.

Endsley, J.J., Endsley, M.A. and Estes, D.M. (2006) Bovine natural killer cells acquire cytotoxic/effector activity following activation with IL-12/15 and reduce *Mycobacterium bovis* BCG in infected macrophages. *Journal of Leukocyte Biology* 79, 71–79.

Esquivel-Solís, H., Vallecillo, A.J., Benítez-Guzmán, A., Adams, L.G., López-Vidal, Y., *et al.* (2013) Nitric oxide not apoptosis mediates differential killing of *Mycobacterium bovis* in bovine macrophages. *PLoS ONE* 8(5), e63464.

Fabrik, I., Härtlova, A., Rehulka, P. and Stulik, J. (2013) Serving the new masters – dendritic cells as hosts for stealth intracellular bacteria. *Cellular Microbiology* 15(9), 1473–1483.

Fremond, C.M., Togbe, D., Doz, E., Rose, S., Vasseur, V., *et al.* (2007) IL-1 receptor-mediated signal is an essential component of MyD88-dependent innate response to *Mycobacterium tuberculosis* infection. *Journal of Immunology* 179, 1178–1189.

Guarda, G., Braun, M., Staehli, F., Tardivel, A., Mattmann, C., *et al.* (2011) Type I interferon inhibits interleukin-1 production and inflammasome activation. *Immunity* 34, 213–223.

Gutierrez, M.G., Master, S.S., Singh, S.B., Taylor, G.A., Colombo, M.I. and Deretic, V. (2004) Autophagy is a defense mechanism inhibiting BCG and *Mycobacterium tuberculosis* survival in infected macrophages. *Cell* 119(6), 753–766.

Gutiérrez-Pabello, J.A., McMurray, D.N. and Adams, L.G. (2002) Upregulation of thymosin beta-10 by *Mycobacterium bovis* infection of bovine macrophages is associated with apoptosis. *Infection and Immunity* 70(4), 2121–2127.

Guzman, E., Price, S., Poulsom, H. and Hope, J. (2012) Bovine γδ T cells: Cells with multiple functions and important roles in immunity. *Veterinary Immunology and Immunopathology* 148(1), 161–167.

Hilda, J.N., Narasimhan, M. and Das, S.D. (2014) Neutrophils from pulmonary tuberculosis patients show augmented levels of chemokines MIP-1α, IL-8 and MCP-1 which further increase upon in vitro infection with mycobacterial strains. *Human Immunology* 75(8), 914–922.

Hinchey, J., Lee, S., Jeon, B.Y., Basaraba, R.J., Venkataswamy, M.M., *et al.* (2007) Enhanced priming of adaptive immunity by a proapoptotic mutant of *Mycobacterium tuberculosis*. *Journal of Clinical Investigation* 117(8), 2279–2288.

Hope, J.C., Thom, M.L., McCormick, P.A. and Howard, C.J. (2004) Interaction of antigen presenting cells with mycobacteria. *Veterinary Immunology and Immunopathology* 100(3–4), 187–195.

Hussain Bhat, K. and Mukhopadhyay, S. (2015) Macrophage takeover and the host-bacilli interplay during tuberculosis. *Future Microbiology* 10(5), 853–872.

Kennedy, H.E., Welsh, M.D., Bryson, D.G., Cassidy, J.P., Forster, F.I., *et al.* (2002) Modulation of immune responses to *Mycobacterium bovis* in cattle depleted of WC1+gammadelta T cells. *Infection and Immunity* 70(3), 1488–1500.

Kumar, H., Kawai, T. and Akira, S. (2011) Pathogen recognition by the innate immune system. *International Reviews of Immunology* 30(1), 16–34.

Kumar, P., Tyagi, R., Das, G. and Bhaskar, S. (2014) *Mycobacterium indicus pranii* and *Mycobacterium bovis* BCG lead to differential macrophage activation in Toll-like receptor-dependent manner. *Immunology* 143(2), 258–268.

Lin, J.J., Zhao, D., Wang, J., Wang, Y., Li, H., *et al*. (2015) Transcriptome changes upon in vitro challenge with Mycobacterium bovis in monocyte-derived macrophages from bovine tuberculosis-infected and healthy cows. *Veterinary Immunology and Immunopathology* 163, 146–156.

Liu, H., Liu, Z., Chen, J., Chen, L., He, X., *et al*. (2013) Induction of CCL8/MCP-2 by mycobacteria through the activation of TLR2/PI3K/Akt signaling pathway. *PLoS One* 8(2), e56815.

Liu, C., Yue, R., Yang, Y., Cui, Y., Yang, L., *et al*. (2016) AIM2 inhibits autophagy and IFN-β production during *M. bovis* infection. *Oncotarget* 7(30), 46972–46987.

Liu, C., Xin, S., Yang, L., Zhao, D. and Zhou, X. (2017) The central role of ifi204 in ifn-beta release and autophagy activation during *Mycobacterium bovis* infection. *Frontiers in Cellular and Infection Microbiology* 7, 169.

Lowe, D.M., Redford, P.S., Wilkinson, R.J., O'Garra, A. and Martineau, A.R. (2012) Neutrophils in tuberculosis: friend or foe? *Trends in Immunology* 33(1), 14–25.

Ma, Y., Han, F., Liang, J., Yang, J., Shi, J., *et al*. (2016) A species-specific activation of Toll-like receptor signaling in bovine and sheep bronchial epithelial cells triggered by mycobacterial infections. *Molecular Immunology* 71, 23–33.

Ma, J., Yang, B., Yu, S., Zhang, Y., Zhang, X., *et al*. (2014) Tuberculosis antigen-induced expression of IFN-α in tuberculosis patients inhibits production of IL-1β. *FASEB Journal* 28, 3238–3248.

MacHugh, D.E., Gormley, E., Park, S.D.E., Browne, J.A., Taraktsoglou, M., *et al*. (2009) Gene expression profiling of the host response to *Mycobacterium bovis* infection in cattle. *Transboundary and Emerging Diseases* 56(6–7), 204–214.

Magee, D.A., Taraktsoglou, M., Killick, K.E., Nalpas, N.C., Browne, J.A., *et al*. (2012) Global gene expression and systems biology analysis of bovine monocyte-derived macrophages in response to in vitro challenge with *Mycobacterium bovis*. *PLoS One* 7(2), e32034.

Magee, D.A., Conlon, K.M., Nalpas, N.C., Browne, J.A., Pirson, C., *et al*. (2014) Innate cytokine profiling of bovine alveolar macrophages reveals commonalities and divergence in the response to *Mycobacterium bovis* and *Mycobacterium tuberculosis* infection. *Tuberculosis* 94(4), 441–450.

Manca, C., Tsenova, L., Freeman, S., Barczak, A.K., Tovey, M., *et al*. (2005) Hypervirulent *M. tuberculosis* W/Beijing strains upregulate type I IFNs and increase expression of negative regulators of the Jak-Stat pathway. *Journal of Interferon and Cytokine Research* 25, 694–701.

Mantovani, A., Cassatella, M.A., Costantini, C. and Jaillon, S. (2011) Neutrophils in the activation and regulation of innate and adaptive immunity. *Nature Reviews Immunology* 11(8), 519–531.

Mayer-Barber, K.D., Barber, D.L., Shenderov, K., White, S.D., Wilson, M.S., *et al*. (2010) Caspase-1 independent IL-1beta production is critical for host resistance to *Mycobacterium tuberculosis* and does not require TLR signaling in vivo. *Journal of Immunology* 184(7), 3326–3330.

Mayer-Barber, K.D., Andrade, B.B., Barber, D.L., Hieny, S., Feng, C.G., *et al*. (2011) Innate and adaptive interferons suppress IL-1a and IL-1b production by distinct pulmonary myeloid subsets during *Mycobacterium tuberculosis* infection. *Immunity* 35, 1023–1034.

Mayer-Barber, K.D., Andrade, B.B., Oland, S.D., Amaral, E.P., Barber, D.L., *et al*. (2014) Host-directed therapy of tuberculosis based on interleukin-1 and type I interferon crosstalk. *Nature* 511(7507), 99–103.

Mishra, B.B., Moura-Alves, P., Sonawane, A., Hacohen, N., Griffiths, G., *et al*. (2010) *Mycobacterium tuberculosis* protein ESAT-6 is a potent activator of the NLRP3/ASC inflammasome. *Cellular Microbiology* 12(8), 1046–1063.

Mishra, B.B., Rathinam, V.A.K., Martens, G.W., Martinot, A.J., Kornfeld, H., *et al*. (2012) Nitric oxide controls the immunopathology of tuberculosis by inhibiting NLRP3 inflammasome–dependent processing of IL-1β. *Nature Immunology* 14(1), 52–60.

Mocsai, A. (2013) Diverse novel functions of neutrophils in immunity, inflammation, and beyond. *Journal of Experimental Medicine* 210(7), 1283–1299.

Mortaz, E., Adcock, I.M., Tabarsi, P., Masjedi, M.R., Mansouri, D., *et al*. (2015) Interaction of pattern recognition receptors with *Mycobacterium tuberculosis*. *Journal of Clinical Immunology* 35(1), 1–10.

Nalpas, N.C., Magee, D.A., Conlon, K.M., Browne, J.A., Healy, C., *et al*. (2015) RNA sequencing provides exquisite insight into the manipulation of the alveolar macrophage by tubercle bacilli. *Scientific Reports* 5, 13629.

Nelson, C.D., Reinhardt, T.A., Thacker, T.C., Beitz, D.C. and Lippolis, J.D. (2010) Modulation of the bovine innate immune response by production of 1alpha,25-dihydroxyvitamin D(3) in bovine monocytes. *Journal of Dairy Science* 93(3), 1041–1049.

Netea, M.G., Simon, A., van de Veerdonk, F., Kullberg, B.-J., Van der Meer, J.W.M. and Joosten, L.A.B. (2010) IL-1β Processing in host defense: beyond the inflammasomes. *PLoS Pathogens* 6(2), e1000661.

Novikov, A., Cardone, M., Thompson, R., Shenderov, K., Kirschman, K.D., et al. (2011) *Mycobacterium tuberculosis* triggers host type I IFN signaling to regulate IL-1β production in human macrophages. *Journal of Immunology* 187, 2540–2547.

O' Garra, A., Redford, P.S., McNab, F.W., Bloom, C.I., Wilkinson, R.J. and Berry, M.P. (2013) The immune response in tuberculosis. *Annual Review of Immunology* 31, 475–527.

Pabello, J.A.G. and Adams, L.G. (2003) Sobrevivencia de *Mycobacterium bovis* en macrófagosde bovinos naturalmente resistentes y susceptiblesa patógenos intracelulares. *Veterinaria México* 34(3), 277–281.

Parandhaman, D.K. and Narayanan, S. (2014) Cell death paradigms in the pathogenesis of *Mycobacterium tuberculosis* infection. *Frontiers in Cellular and Infection Microbiology* 4, 31.

Pearce, E.J. and Everts, B. (2015) Dendritic cell metabolism. *Nature Reviews Immunology* 15(1), 18–29.

Plattner, B.L., Doyle, R.T. and Hostetter, J.M. (2009) Gamma-delta T cell subsets are differentially associated with granuloma development and organization in a bovine model of mycobacterial disease. *International Journal of Experimental Pathology* 90(6), 587–597.

Plüddemann, A., Mukhopadhyay, S. and Gordon, S. (2011) Innate immunity to intracellular pathogens: macrophage receptors and responses to microbial entry. *Immunological Reviews* 240(1), 11–24.

Price, S.J. and Hope, J.C. (2009) Enhanced secretion of interferon-γ by bovine γδ T cells induced by coculture with *Mycobacterium bovis*-infected dendritic cells: evidence for reciprocal activating signals. *Immunology* 126(2), 201–208.

Price, S., Davies, M., Villarreal-Ramos, B. and Hope, J. (2010) Differential distribution of WC1+ gammadelta TCR+ T lymphocyte subsets within lymphoid tissues of the head and respiratory tract and effects of intranasal *M. bovis* BCG vaccination. *Veterinary Immunology and Immunopathology* 136, 133–137.

Qureshi, T., Templeton, J.W. and Adams, L.G. (1996) Intracellular survival of *Brucella abortus*, *Mycobacterium bovis* BCG, *Salmonella dublin*, and *Salmonella typhimurium* in macrophages from cattle genetically resistant to *Brucella abortus*. *Veterinary Immunology and Immunopathology* 50(1–2), 55–65.

Rodrigues, M.F., Barsante, M.M., Alves, C.C.S., Souza, M.A., Ferreira, A.P., et al. (2009) Apoptosis of macrophages during pulmonary *Mycobacterium bovis* infection: correlation with intracellular bacillary load and cytokine levels. *Immunology* 128(1 Suppl), e691–9.

Shu, D., Heiser, A., Wedlock, D.N., Luo, D., de Lisle, G.W. and Buddle, B.M. (2014) Comparison of gene expression of immune mediators in lung and pulmonary lymph node granulomas from cattle experimentally infected with *Mycobacterium bovis*. *Veterinary Immunology and Immunopathology* 160(1–2), 81–89.

Siddiqui, N., Price, S. and Hope, J. (2012) BCG vaccination of neonatal calves: Potential roles for innate immune cells in the induction of protective immunity. *Comparative Immunology, Microbiology and Infectious Diseases* 35(3), 219–226.

Stanley, S.A., Johndrow, J.E., Manzanillo, P., Cox, J.S. (2006) The type I IFN response to infection with *Mycobacterium tuberculosis* requires ESX-1-mediated secretion and contributes to pathogenesis. *Journal of Immunology* 178, 3143–3152.

Stamm, C.E., Collins, A.C. and Shiloh, M.U. (2015) Sensing of *Mycobacterium tuberculosis* and consequences to both host and bacillus. *Immunology Review* 264, 204–219.

Sun, L., Song, Y., Riaz, H., Yang, H., Hua, G., Guo, A. and Yang, L. (2012) Polymorphisms in Toll-like receptor 1 and 9 genes and their association with tuberculosis susceptibility in Chinese Holstein cattle. *Veterinary Immunology and Immunopathology* 147(3), 195–201.

Trinchieri, G. (2010) Type I interferon: friend or foe? *Journal of Experimental Medicine* 207(10), 2053–2063.

Vantourout, P. and Hayday, A. (2013) Six-of-the-best: unique contributions of γδ T cells to immunology. *Nature Reviews Immunology* 13(2), 88–100.

Vega-Manriquez, X., López-Vidal, Y., Moran, J., Adams, L. and Gutiérrez-Pabello, J.A. (2007) Apoptosis-inducing factor participation in bovine macrophage *Mycobacterium bovis* induced caspase-independent cell death. *Infection and Immunity* 75(3), 1223–1228.

Wang, J., Zhou, X., Pan, B., Yang, L., Yin, X., et al. (2013) Investigation of the effect of *Mycobacterium bovis* infection on bovine neutrophils functions. *Tuberculosis* 93(6), 675–687.

Widdison, S., Watson, M., Piercy, J., Howard, C. and Coffey, T.J. (2008) Granulocyte chemotactic properties of *M. tuberculosis* versus *M. bovis*-infected bovine alveolar macrophages. *Molecular Immunology* 45(3), 740–749.

Widdison, S., Watson, M. and Coffey, T. J. (2011) Early response of bovine alveolar macrophages to infection with live and heat-killed *Mycobacterium bovis*. *Developmental & Comparative Immunology* 35(5), 580–591.

Xu, H., Moraitis, M., Reedstrom, R.J. and Matthews, K.S. (1998) Protein chemistry and structure: kinetic and thermodynamic studies of purine repressor binding to corepressor and operator DNA. *Journal of Biological Chemistry* 273, 8958–8964.

Zhou, Y., Shah, S.Z., Yang, L., Zhang, Z., Zhou, X. and Zhao, D. (2016) Virulent *Mycobacterium bovis* Beijing strain activates the NLRP7 inflammasome in THP-1 macrophages. *PLoS One* 11(4), e0152853.

Yang, Y., Zhou, X., Kouadir, M., Shi, F., Ding, T., *et al.* (2013) The AIM2 Inflammasome is involved in macrophage activation during infection with virulent *Mycobacterium bovis* strain. *Journal of Infectious Diseases* 208(11), 1849–1858.

Yuk, J.-M. and Jo, E.-K. (2014) Host immune responses to mycobacterial antigens and their implications for the development of a vaccine to control tuberculosis. *Clinical and Experimental Vaccine Research* 3(2), 155–167.

Zullo, A.J. and Lee, S. (2012) Mycobacterial induction of autophagy varies by species and occurs independently of mammalian target of rapamycin inhibition. *Journal of Biological Chemistry* 287(16), 12668–12678.

11 Adaptive Immunity

Jayne Hope[1,]* and Dirk Werling[2]
[1]The Roslin Institute, University of Edinburgh, Edinburgh, UK;
[2]The Royal Veterinary College, Hatfield, UK

Immunity to mycobacterial infections is an interplay between innate and adaptive immune responses; both cellular and humoral mechanisms are involved. While it is clear that the response to mycobacterial infection is driven and shaped by the initial innate immune response, defining the mechanisms of adaptive immunity underpins on-going efforts to develop effective tuberculosis (TB) vaccines for humans and cattle. Importantly, definition of correlates of protective immunity that can be measured readily will facilitate the development and screening of vaccine candidates and assessment of their success. However, it must also be stressed that in the case of mycobacterial infection, these correlates of protective immunity must be defined carefully. They not only include an 'absence of clinical symptoms', a definition used for many other veterinary vaccines, but must be defined as 'protection to infection', given the socioeconomic importance of infection with *Mycobacterium bovis*. In addition, since measurement of the adaptive immune response through tuberculin skin testing or assessment of antigen-specific IFN-γ release forms the basis of currently used diagnostic tests (Waters *et al* 2011; Pai *et al*., 2014), increased knowledge of the immune response associated with infection or induced by vaccination is required for improved surveillance.

11.1 Cell-Mediated Immune Responses

Studies in cattle have demonstrated that the cell-mediated adaptive immune response of adult cattle is similar to that observed in humans (Goddeeris, 1998), although the presence of distinct disease-associated Th1-Th2 bias is less clear in the bovine immune response. There is also a significant similarity in the primary mechanisms of anti-mycobacterial immunity between humans and cattle (Pollock *et al*., 2001; Ottenhoff *et al*., 2005), including those responses induced by bacillus Calmette–Guérin (BCG) vaccination (Semple *et al*., 2011; Siddiqui *et al*., 2012). These include roles for CD4[+], CD8[+] and γδ TCR[+] T cells, function and sources of IFN-γ, roles for IL-17 and IL-22, and antigen-specific memory T lymphocytes. In addition, there is growing evidence for involvement of non-conventional lymphocytes including mucosal-associated invariant T (MAIT) cells and lipid-responsive CD1-restricted T cells. While our understanding of the immune mechanisms induced by infection of cattle is less advanced compared to that in humans (or from murine studies), it is evident that similar responses are observed across the two species, implying that bovine models may provide insights relevant to human medicine and vice versa (reviewed by Waters *et al*., 2011).

---

* Email: Jayne.hope@roslin.ed.ac.uk

11.1.1 CD4⁺ T cells

Most individuals exposed to *M. tuberculosis* or *M. bovis* develop antigen-specific T-cell responses; this immune response is dominated by CD4⁺ T cells, although CD8⁺ T cells and populations of non-conventional T cells (see section 11.2) are also implicated. These T-cell responses are evident in the periphery within 2 to 3 weeks and may be maintained for long duration. While CD4⁺ T-cell responses are known to be central to immunity to mycobacterial infections, they are also considered to contribute to the pathological damage observed within infected tissues.

The diversity of both myeloid cell populations and T-lymphocyte subsets indicates that there is a level of complexity in immune control. Nevertheless, a significant body of evidence suggests that Th1 CD4⁺ T cells, through their interactions with mycobacteria-infected antigen-presenting cells, are key to immune control of infection.

Evidence for the central role of CD4⁺ T cells was provided by studies of mice and non-human primates depleted of CD4⁺ T cells – such animals were highly susceptible to *Mycobacterium tuberculosis* infection and even succumb to BCG-induced disease. Alongside this, the increased susceptibility and associated morbidity and mortality of HIV-positive individuals following exposure to *M. tuberculosis* suggests that CD4⁺ T cells are essential for immune control. A number of studies across species indicate that the major protective role of CD4⁺ T cells in anti-mycobacterial immunity is in containment rather than clearance, and that the cytokine IFN-γ is of importance. Early studies in IFN-γ-depleted mice (Cooper *et al.*, 1993; Flynn *et al.*, 1993), complemented by evidence from humans with defects in the IFN-γ/IL-12 axis (van de Vosse *et al.*, 2004), demonstrated that IFN-γ is essential for the containment of infection. In cattle, a key feature of *Mycobacterium bovis* infection is an early and persistent production of IFN-γ (Pollock *et al.*, 2001) consistently detectable 2 to 3 weeks after experimental infection. As with *M. tuberculosis* infection of humans, CD4, CD8 and γδ T cells (as well as natural killer [NK] cells) contribute to the IFN-γ response to *M. bovis* infection in cattle (Pollock *et al.*, 2001; Endsley *et al.*, 2009). However, Th1 CD4⁺ T cells are the predominant cellular source of IFN-γ across species (Walravens *et al.*, 2002; Ottenhoff *et al.*, 2005). Recently, Green *et al.* (2013) demonstrated that CD4⁺-derived IFN-γ is essential for host survival from *M. tuberculosis* infection. Thus, CD4 T cells and an intact Th1 response are essential for control of mycobacterial infections in both species, but they are not sufficient for clearance.

The expression of IFN-γ by CD4⁺ T cells has also been demonstrated as central to the success of current vaccination regimes. Indeed, the most effective tuberculosis vaccines elicit specific IFN-γ responses, and vaccines which do not induce IFN-γ generally fail to induce protective immunity against TB in both murine models and in experimental challenge of cattle (reviewed by Hope and Vordermeier, 2005). However, IFN-γ is not the only mechanism underpinning CD4⁺-dependent immune responses, since not all vaccines that induce IFN-γ are protective against tuberculosis, and vaccine-induced IFN-γ levels do not necessarily correlate with the level of protection induced (Mittrucker *et al.*, 2007; Abebe, 2012; Waters *et al.*, 2012).

However, IFN-γ may also contribute to the pathological consequences of infection. Indeed, expression of IFN-γ has also been shown to correlate positively with disease, fever and weight loss in humans (Tsao *et al.*, 2002), and an increased frequency of antigen-specific CD4⁺ IFN-γ⁺ cells correlated with increased pathology scores and bacterial burden following *M. bovis* infection of calves (Sopp *et al.*, 2006). This highlights the complex nature of the immune response to infection, the balance between protective immunity and pathology and the multiparametric nature of the immune response. In addition to the secretion of IFN-γ, other cytokines and functional capacities of CD4⁺ T cells likely contribute to their effector mechanisms in immune control. Here, polyfunctional T cells, and other Th-cell-derived cytokines (in addition to IFN-γ) may play an important role.

11.1.1 Polyfunctional T cells

The expression of additional cytokines by so-called 'polyfunctional T cells' may be important in the immune response to mycobacterial infections. Polyfunctional T cells, by definition, simultaneously produce two or more cytokines in response to antigen, and higher frequencies of these cells have been associated with control of chronic infections such as HIV, hepatitis C, leishmaniasis and malaria in humans (Wilkinson and Wilkinson, 2010), as well as PCV2 in pigs (Koinig et al., 2015). A number of studies of M. tuberculosis infection in humans indicate a protective role for polyfunctional T cells but these cells may also be associated with disease progression (Sutherland et al., 2009; Wilkinson et al., 2010; Geluk et al., 2012). It is clear that the pattern of co-expression of multiple cytokines by these polyfunctional T cells is important for their potential protective effect. In humans with active TB, T cells predominantly express IFN-γ with TNF-α or TNF-α alone, whereas in humans with latent TB, where it is assumed infection is controlled, or in successfully treated patients, higher frequencies of polyfunctional T cells expressing IFN-γ, TNF-α and IL-2 can be observed (Geluk et al., 2012). Similarly, bovine polyfunctional CD4$^+$ T cells which expressed IFN-γ, IL-2 and TNF-α were shown to have an effector phenotype (CD44^{hi} CD62L^{lo} CD45RO$^+$) and were associated with pathology rather than protection (Whelan et al., 2011). In line with the observation that more diverse cytokine profiles reflect progression towards disease rather than immunological control, Rhodes et al. (2014) demonstrated that cattle producing both antigen-specific IFN-γ *and* IL-2 were more likely to present with visible pathology at post mortem than those that expressed IFN-γ alone.

11.1.2 Tissue responses to infection

The balance between protective immunity and pathology is likely driven by the ability of mycobacteria to manipulate the CD4$^+$ T-cell response either directly or indirectly via antigen-presenting cells. In tissues this may be evidenced by slow, weak stimulation of antigen-specific T cells enabling early growth and persistence of mycobacteria within immune privileged sites (granulomas). The delayed tissue response to M. tuberculosis infection is well documented in mice; the first antigen-specific T cells arrive in lung-draining lymph nodes (mediastinal) after ~10 days (Reiley et al., 2008) and then in the lungs several weeks following exposure (Reiley et al., 2008). This delay contributes to the inability of the host to clear the organism. While the specific mechanisms are not yet well understood, this delay likely reflects the time taken for infected dendritic cells (DC) and recruited macrophages (MO) to reach the lungs.

Both M. tuberculosis and M. bovis have been shown to alter the functional capacity of DC and MO, which likely alters their capacity to recruit and activate T cells (Hope et al., 2004; Piercy et al., 2007; Wolf et al., 2007). Using TCR transgenic mice, the initial recognition of mycobacterial antigens was shown to occur in draining lymph nodes rather than in the lung (Chackerian et al., 2002a; Reiley et al., 2008; Wolf et al., 2008). In addition, it has been hypothesized that poor stimulation/activation of T cells occurs in the inflamed lung environment potentially through limited availability of antigen (Bold et al., 2011; Egen et al., 2011). This leads to poor cytokine secretion and lack of engagement with infected MO (Robinson et al., 2015). Whether this occurs in cattle infected with M. bovis has not been determined. However, given that the kinetics of T-cell responses to infection are similar in cattle and humans (Waters et al., 2011), and reflected by those observed in mice, it seems likely that M. bovis also affects the timing and development of antigen-specific CD4$^+$ T-cell responses in the bovine respiratory tract tissues. However, in contrast to the murine environment, the bovine airway mucosal system is already developed and contains significant numbers of DC at the time of birth (Hope and Werling, unpublished data). This is an important consideration for vaccine design and the definition of immune correlates of protection. The response of circulating T cells is relatively easily measured in both humans and cattle but may not reflect events occurring at local infection sites where inflammation and low antigen availability may be of importance. Therefore, consideration of adjuvants, routes of immunization as well as antigen/epitope availability is of crucial importance to protect the lung from infection.

Related to this is recent evidence that antigens other than the immunodominant antigens of M. tuberculosis and M. bovis (e.g. ESAT-6 and CFP-10) may be recognized by specific CD4$^+$ T cells. It has been estimated that only ~5 to 20% of murine lung T cells recognized ESAT-6 and/or CFP-10 (Brandt et al., 1996; Winslow et al., 2003; Wolf et al., 2008). Indeed, unbiased genome-wide analysis revealed that CD4⁺ T cells in latently infected humans recognize a much wider range of antigens (Tang et al., 2011; Lindestam Arlehamn et al., 2013; Commandeur et al., 2013), many of which were cryptic epitopes. The majority of these were recognized by CXCR3⁺CCR6⁺ IFN-γ⁻ expressing Th1 cells (Lindestam Arlehamn et al., 2013). Further understanding the nature of the T-cell response and its regulation by *M. tuberculosis* and *M. bovis* is needed for the design of vaccines and regimes that protect the lung effectively.

11.1.3 Regulation of CD4⁺ T-cell responses

Tissue-specific CD4⁺ T-cell responses are likely limited by other cell populations or immunoregulatory cytokines such as IL-10 and TGF-β. These pathways are important to limit immunopathology, but they may also contribute to the persistence of bacilli in bovine lymph nodes (Widdison et al., 2006). Regulatory T cells (Tregs) proliferate rapidly in *M. tuberculosis*-infected lymph nodes (Shafiani et al., 2010) and limit priming and activation of activated effectors in the lung. Depletion of Tregs from mice increased Th1 priming and reduced bacterial burden (Scott-Browne et al., 2007). Tregs induced by infection may also overcome the protective effects of BCG vaccination and reduce recruitment of CD4⁺ and CD8⁺ T cells to the lungs of mice (Ordway et al., 2011). While FoxP3⁺ Tregs have not yet been described in bovine TB, they were described to expand in calves infected with *M. avium* subsp. *paratuberculosis* and hypothesized to limit secretion of IFN-γ by Th1 CD4⁺ T cells (Bull et al., 2014).

11.1.4 Effector memory T-cell and central memory T-cell subsets

Immune protection against a range of diseases relies upon the induction and maintenance of memory cells capable of responding rapidly and efficiently upon subsequent infection. This immunological memory may be induced following natural infection or vaccines. Upon the first encounter with antigen the number of specific T lymphocytes increases over tenfold (Hou et al., 1994; Murali-Krishna et al., 1998; Whitmire et al., 1998; Pollock et al., 2001). This is associated with differentiation into effector cells which express important molecules for pathogen control including TNF-α, IFN-γ, perforin and granulysin. Following this, the majority of T cells undergo apoptosis and only a few memory cells will develop (Wilkinson et al., 2009; Totté et al., 2010). In humans, memory T-cell subsets have been defined based on cell surface antigen expression. Central memory T cells (Tcm) have the phenotype CD62L⁺CCR7⁺, preferentially localize to lymphoid tissues and secrete principally IL-2. By contrast, effector memory T cells (Tem) are CD62L⁻CCR7⁻ and secrete only low levels of IL-2 upon stimulation (Sallusto et al., 1999; Champagne et al., 2001; Woodland and Kohlmeier, 2009; Sallusto et al., 2010). In cattle, populations of Tm have been similarly identified by expression of CD45RO, CD62L and CCR7 (Blunt et al., 2015; Maggioli et al., 2015a), contrasting with some of the earlier observations that CD62L is not a memory marker in cattle (Howard et al., 1992), potentially indicating that induced expression of CD62L is indicative of antigen exposure.

The secretion of IFN-γ by effector T cells and Tem in response to stimulation with mycobacterial antigens is the read-out of interferon-gamma release assays, and this correlates with infection with mycobacteria in both humans and cattle. In addition, in a number of studies the frequency of Tcm (measured by 'cultured ELISPOT', which detects antigen-specific IFN-γ release in long-term cultures of T cells; Maggioli et al., 2015b) correlates with vaccine-induced immunity measured as a reduction in bacterial burden and tissue pathology (Vordermeier et al., 2006, 2009; Hope et al., 2011). Studies with samples from human patients have demonstrated that the responding cells within these long-term cultures (up to 14 days) are mainly Tcm and that this response, in contrast to effector responses, correlates with protection from infectious challenge (Todryk et al., 2009). In cattle, Tcm (CD45RO⁺CCR7⁺CD62L^{hi}) are the primary cell type responding in long-term cultured IFN-γ ELISPOT responses to *M. bovis* infection (Blunt et al., 2015; Maggioli et al., 2015a). The functional relevance of Tcm in driving natural or vaccine-induced protection remains to be determined for both humans (reviewed by Henao-Tamayo *et al.*, 2014) and cattle. However, the correlation between measurements of antigen-specific Tcm with vaccine-induced protection may assist the prioritization of vaccine candidates for efficacy testing within calves.

11.1.5 Key cytokines secreted by CD4+ T cells: IL-17 and IL-22

Key roles for a number of effector molecules have been identified in both humans and animals (Henao-Tamayo *et al.*, 2014). Notably, IL-17 and IL-22 have been described as important across a large number of studies. As mentioned for IFN-γ, roles for IL-17A have been described in both immune protection and pathology/disease progression (Torrado and Cooper, 2010; Cooper, 2010). The kinetics, cellular source and relative production of other cytokines likely affect the outcome of IL-17 expression. In both mice and humans, significant IL-17 responses are elicited by *M. tuberculosis* (Khader and Cooper, 2008; Jurado *et al.*, 2012). Early expression of IL-17 was shown to be required for rapid accumulation of protective memory cells (Khader *et al.*, 2008), and was associated with early recruitment of neutrophils and granuloma formation (Umemura *et al.*, 2007; Okamoto Yoshida *et al.*, 2010). Effective Th1 responses to BCG vaccination in mice require IL-17 (Khader *et al.*, 2007) and secondary/memory responses to infection of mice with *M. tuberculosis* appear also to depend on IL-17 (Freches *et al.*, 2013). In cattle, increased levels of vaccine-induced IL-17 observed prior to infectious challenge were associated with protective immunity (Vordermeier *et al.*, 2009). However, a correlation between IL-17 expression (Aranday-Cortes *et al.*, 2013) and the development of macroscopic TB lesions (Blanco *et al.*, 2011) as well as with mycobacterial burden (Waters *et al.*, 2016) have also been reported post-infection. Thus, in the bovine model, IL-17 has been suggested as both a biomarker for infection as well as a correlate or predictor of vaccine-induced protection in cattle (Aranday-Cortes *et al.*, 2012). In mice, γδ and other non-CD4+ T cells are the primary producers of IL-17, whereas in humans both γδ T cells and CD4+ Th17 cells produce IL-17 during *M. tuberculosis* infection.

Roles for IL-22 in immune protection have also been indicated, although these are less well-described in the literature. *In vitro*, IL-22 expressing human NK cells were able to inhibit intracellular growth of *M. tuberculosis* (Dhiman *et al.*, 2009, 2012) within macrophages and are associated with BCG-induced immune responses (Dhiman *et al.*, 2012). As with IL-17, expression of IL-22 in BCG-vaccinated cattle correlated with vaccine-induced protection (Bhuju *et al.*, 2012) and could act as a predictor of vaccine success. In contrast, assessment of IL-22 post-infection revealed utility as a biomarker of infection (Aranday-Cortes *et al.*, 2012). Recently, the cellular sources of IL-22 and IL-17 have been elucidated in cattle studies (Steinbach *et al.*, 2016). In *M. bovis*-infected animals, antigen-specific IL-22 and IL-17A responses were observed in both CD4+ T-cell and γδ T-cell populations. Low frequencies of IL-17+IL-22+ double positive cells were observed within the γδ T-cell population. Salguero *et al.* (2016) also recently demonstrated IL-17A and IL-22 expression within tuberculous lesions in cattle, particularly in early lesions, suggesting roles for these cytokines in directing the tissue response to infection.

11.2 Non-Conventional T Cells

11.2.1 γδ T cells

T lymphocytes expressing the γδ T-cell receptor (γδ T cells) are significantly more abundant in a number of livestock species including ruminants, pigs and poultry (reviewed by Guzman *et al.*, 2012; McGill *et al.*, 2014a; Baldwin and Telfer, 2015). In particular, neonatal calves have very high numbers of γδ T cells (up to 60% of the circulating peripheral blood mononuclear cells), which decrease with age (Hein and Mackay, 1991; Jutila *et al.*, 2008). In contrast, the frequency of γδ T cells within the peripheral lymphocyte pool in humans and mice is as low as ~5–10% (Kabelitz, 2011). It is now well recognized that γδ T cells function at the innate–adaptive interface and have functions in both arms of the immune response. In cattle, T regulatory functions are also ascribed to γδ T cells that have been shown able to suppress both CD4 and CD8⁺ T-cell responses (Hoek et al., 2009; Guzman et al., 2014). Subpopulations of cells expressing the γδ TCR are found in cattle: a small subset express CD8 and CD2 whereas the majority are defined by expression of the Workshop Cluster 1 (WC1) molecule (Mackay et al., 1989; Clevers et al., 1990; Morrison and Davis, 1991), a transmembrane glycoprotein and member of the scavenger receptor cysteine rich (SCRC) superfamily, which includes CD163, CD5, CD6 and DMBT1 (Sarrias et al., 2004). The WC1 molecules, encoded in cattle by 13 genes, act as co-receptors and as pattern recognition receptors (Chen et al., 2012). Within the WC1⁺ T cells are subpopulations expressing combinations of the 13 WC1-gene-encoded molecules. Broadly, these have been defined as WC1.1 and WC1.2 which have been shown to respond differentially to pathogenic stimulation: the WC1.1 molecules are responsive to leptospires and mycobacteria and produce IFN-γ, whereas WC1.2 respond to anaplasmas and produce IL-10 and TGF-β (Lahmers et al., 2004; Rogers et al., 2005).

In the context of *M. bovis* infection, it is the WC1⁺ subpopulation of γδ T cells that has been shown to respond, although recent studies indicate that WC1⁻ γδ T cells are also responsive (McGill et al., 2014a). γδ T cells undergo dynamic changes in distribution after *M. bovis* infection, with a marked decrease in the circulating pool shortly after infection (Pollock et al., 1996). Following the initial decrease in circulating WC1⁺ T cells following infection with *M. bovis*, their frequency increased with a concomitant increase in CD25 expression (Pollock et al., 1996). These data suggest that γδ T cells are actively responding to *M. bovis* infection and equipped to move rapidly to sites of active immune responses. WC1⁺ γδ T cells are among the first cells to accumulate at the site of DTH responses following PPD injection of *M. bovis*-infected cattle (Doherty et al., 1996). There is a body of evidence demonstrating that γδ T cells traffic to sites of mycobacterial infection *in vivo* and accumulate within tuberculous lesions of cattle (Cassidy et al., 1998; Palmer et al., 2007; Salguero et al., 2016). These cells are also associated with vaccine-induced responses in cattle. Soon after BCG vaccination there are dynamic changes in circulating bovine γδ T cells and γδ T cells infiltrate rapidly the respiratory tract-associated lymph nodes, lungs and the head-associated lymphoid tissues (Price et al., 2010). These cells were shown to be predominantly of the WC1.1⁺ phenotype associated with high-level IFN-γ secretion (Price et al., 2010). In studies of mice infected with BCG, a similar infiltration of γδ T cells into the respiratory tract-associated tissues was observed (Dieli et al., 2003). It has been hypothesized that the efficacy of BCG vaccination in neonatal calves is, at least in part, due to the IFN-γ secreted by WC1+ γδ T cells which are increased not only in frequency, but also functional activity in young cattle (Price et al., 2006). In human neonates vaccinated with BCG, enhanced IFN-γ secretion by γδ T cells is associated with early life-immunity (Mazzola et al., 2007).

In vitro, γδ T cells from *M. bovis*-infected cattle were shown to proliferate and produce IFN-γ in response to stimulation with a range of *M. bovis* antigens, including both protein and non-protein antigens such as lipoarabinomannan and isopentenyl pyrophosphate (Rhodes et al., 2001; Smyth et al., 2001; Welsh et al., 2002; Maue et al., 2005). Subsets of bovine γδ T cells can also respond to *M. bovis*-infected antigen-presenting cells (APCs) (Price and Hope, 2009). This interaction between APC and WC1⁺ γδ T cells is reciprocal in nature, with both γδ and APC function/phenotype alterations evident (Price and Hope, 2009). It has been hypothesized that this licences the APC for improved Th1 stimulation. Similar studies in humans and mice also reveal cross-talk between γδ and APCs (Kabelitz, 2011). The hypothesis that early γδ responses influence the downstream immune response is supported by evidence from WC1⁺ T-cell depleted calves which, upon infection with *M. bovis*, show reduced secretion of antigen-specific IFN-γ and alterations in immunoglobulin subclasses indicative of a skew towards a Th2 response (Kennedy et al., 2002). However, the depleted cattle showed no alteration in the extent of TB lesions.

γδ T-cell deficient mice are able to temporarily control BCG (Ladel et al., 1995) and low-dose *M. tuberculosis* infection (D'Souza et al., 1997) but exhibit a more severe inflammatory response as compared to control mice, suggesting a regulatory role for γδ T cells in granuloma formation and maintenance. In line with this, depletion of WC1⁺ γδ T cells from SCID-bo mice prior to *M. bovis* infection significantly altered the architecture of the developing granuloma (Smith *et al.*, 1999).

Additional functions of γδ T cells in the immune response to mycobacteria include IL-17 production (Lockhart *et al.*, 2006; Umemura *et al.*, 2007; McGill *et al.*, 2014b), direct cytotoxicity (Stenger *et al.*, 1998; Skinner *et al.*, 2003) and Treg activity (Guzman *et al.*, 2014). Each of these has been demonstrated in both murine and bovine systems. However, further studies are required to define fully these functions with *M. bovis* infection in cattle.

11.2.2 MAIT cells

Mucosal invariant T cells (MAIT cells) are an innate-like subset of T cells with functional roles at the innate–adaptive interface. In humans, these are defined by the expression of the semi-invariant TCRα chain TRAV1-2 (Porcelli *et al.*, 1993; Tilloy *et al.*, 1999). These cells are restricted by the non-polymorphic major histocompatibility complex class I-like molecule MR1 and express high levels of CD26 (Sharma *et al.*, 2015). MAIT cells can respond to infected cells through the secretion of IFN-γ and TNF-α and display cytotoxic capacity. Studies in MR-1-deficient mice provided evidence for an early role of MAIT cells in anti-mycobacterial immunity (Chua *et al.*, 2012). In parallel it was demonstrated that MAIT cells contributed to the enhanced killing of *M. tuberculosis* by murine macrophages. In humans, a role for MAIT cells is supported by the observation that patients with active pulmonary TB have fewer MAIT cells in the peripheral blood: this may reflect specific trafficking of these cells to sites of infection (Gold *et al.*, 2010; Le Bourhis *et al.*, 2010). Interestingly, the number of MAIT cells in the blood is restored in individuals undergoing treatment for tuberculosis (Sharma *et al.*, 2015) providing further evidence for a role for MAIT cells in control of mycobacterial infections.

Goldfinch *et al.* (2010) demonstrated that there was a high level of homology between the murine, human, bovine, and ovine MR1 and MAIT TCRα chain sequences, suggesting evolutionary conservation of the MR1/MAIT system between these species. No current data exists regarding the role of MAIT cells in *M. bovis* infection, but this should be the subject of further study.

11.2.3 Lipid-restricted T cells

A significant body of evidence suggests a role for non-conventional lipid-specific T cells in the response of humans to infection with *M. tuberculosis*. Lipids are presented to T cells by members of the CD1 family (Van Rhijn and Moody, 2015). In humans, CD1 genes are divided into group 1 (CD1a, b and c) and group 2 (CD1d), with group 1 CD1 genes thought to present lipids to T cells that exhibit adaptive-like characteristics. By contrast, the majority of CD1d-restricted cells have features of innate–effector cells and are thought primarily to serve an immuno-regulatory role, bridging the innate and adaptive immune systems (Behar and Porcelli, 2007; Van Rhijn *et al.*, 2013).

A diverse array of mycobacterial lipids has been identified as ligands for *M. tuberculosis*-specific group 1 CD1-restricted T cells in humans. Relatively high frequencies of CD1-restricted T cells are observed following *M. tuberculosis* infection or BCG vaccination (Kawashima *et al.*, 2003; Ulrichs *et al.*, 2003). In addition, CD1-restricted T cells have the capacity to migrate to the site of infection in the lung (Montamat-Sicotte *et al.*, 2011), have mycobacteriocidal activity and the capacity to produce key cytokines such as IFN-γ (Stenger *et al.*, 1998; Gilleron *et al.*, 2004). Taken together, these data suggest that CD1-restricted lipid-reactive T cells are an important aspect of the response to *M. tuberculosis* infection. Alongside this is evidence that CD1d-restricted iNKT cells respond to *M. tuberculosis*-infected cells and that incorporation of iNKT-activating glycolipids as adjuvants can improve the immunogenicity and vaccine efficacy of BCG (Chackerian *et al.*, 2002b; Gansert *et al.*, 2003; Venkataswamy *et al.*, 2009).

In cattle, one CD1a, five CD1b, no CD1c and two CD1d orthologues have been described (Van Rhijn *et al.*, 2006), indicating that both group 1 and 2 like lipid-specific T cells may be present. (Van Rhijn *et al.*, 2009) demonstrated that *M. bovis*-specific, lipid-reactive T cells were present following *in vitro* recall stimulation. More recently, Pirson *et al.* (2015) showed that phosphoatidylinositol mannoside-specific T cells were present in a proportion of *M. bovis*-infected cattle. These were predominantly of the phenotype NKp46$^+$CD3$^+$. This population of non-conventional T cells has been described to have features of both the innate- and adaptive immune response and shown be present in other infectious diseases of cattle (Connelley *et al.*, 2014). Further study of the roles of lipid-specific T cells in the immune response of cattle to *M. bovis* and BCG vaccination is required to determine whether the presence or functional activity of these cells correlates with natural or vaccine-induced protective immunity and whether they could be useful targets for new vaccine strategies for enhanced immunity.

11.3 CD8$^+$ T Lymphocytes

While it is generally accepted that CD4$^+$ T cells are essential for immunity to TB, it is also clear that infection of humans and animals is associated with induction of CD8$^+$ T cells. These cells are recruited to the sites of infection and likely play roles through cytolysis and cytokine secretion (Einarsdottir *et al.*, 2009; Behar, 2013). In cattle, antigen-specific CD8$^+$ T cells were demonstrated to induce the release of viable *M. bovis* from infected bovine macrophages, indicating CTL activity (Liebana *et al.*, 2000). Activated CD8$^+$ T cells are also shown to be present in early-stage bovine tuberculous granulomas, indicating a potential role for these cells in the initial containment of the bacilli (Liebana *et al.*, 2007). Bovine T cells also express a homologue of human granulysin, a potent antimicrobial protein stored in association with perforin in cytotoxic granules (Endsley *et al.*, 2004). Induced expression of the bovine granulysin gene in CD8$^+$ T cells (as well as in CD4$^+$ and γδ T cells) resulted in anti-mycobacterial activity (Endsley *et al.*, 2004, 2007). Evidence for a role of CD8$^+$ in the immune response of cattle to *M. bovis* infection was also presented in studies where these cells were depleted early following infection. Calves depleted of CD8$^+$ T cells had significantly lower antigen-specific IFN-γ expression, suggesting a key role for these cells in cytokine responses to infection. By contrast, there were no significant differences in the extent of TB lesions in lower respiratory tract tissues between depleted and non-depleted calves (Villarreal-Ramos *et al.*, 2003). Thus, CD8$^+$ T cells are involved in the bovine immune response to *M. bovis* infection; however, further studies are required to determine their exact roles in protection and pathogenesis. Antigen-specific CD8$^+$ T cells were also induced in BCG-vaccinated cattle and may play a role in vaccine-induced protective immunity (Charleston *et al.*, 2001; Howard *et al.*, 2002).

11.4 Humoral Immunity

Studies of the adaptive immune response to mycobacteria have focussed largely on T cells given the intracellular nature of the pathogens. However, it is becoming clear that previously under-studied cell populations may play important roles in immunity. The role for B cells has largely been considered to be supportive, rather than required (reviewed by Maglione and Chan, 2009), although recent evidence suggests that B cells may be more important than first thought. A large number of studies have assessed the humoral response to infection in the context of measuring antibodies for diagnostic purposes, particularly in humans to differentiate latent from active TB (Scriba *et al.*, 2016). For the most part, these studies show that the antibody response to infection with *M. tuberculosis* is highly variable with a high degree of overlap between healthy and infected individuals (Fletcher *et al.*, 2016). In cattle, serological diagnostic tests have suffered from relatively poor sensitivity. However, recent advances in antigen discovery and the development of novel detection systems have led to serological assays that show promise in delivering highly sensitive tests (Buddle *et al.*, 2009; Whelan *et al.*, 2010; see also Chapter 13). Vaccination of infants with BCG can induce modest levels of antibodies. In a cohort of infants vaccinated with BCG at birth, higher levels of Ag85A-specific antibodies were associated with a reduced risk of developing TB disease (Fletcher *et al.*, 2016).

Potential mechanisms by which B cells may function in immune responses to mycobacterial infection include antigen presentation and cytokine secretion. In addition, indirect effects of antibodies such as the regulation of APC function via Fc receptors, regulatory actions of immune complexes and antibody-dependent cytotoxicity likely contribute to the induction of immune responses (Achkar et al., 2015). Currently little is known regarding the role for B cells in *M. bovis* infection in cattle, although these cells have been demonstrated to be present within TB granulomas (Aranday-Cortes et al., 2013; Salguero et al., 2016). Likewise, B-cell aggregates are consistently detected in association with tuberculous lesions in mice, non-human primates and humans infected with *M. tuberculosis*. These tertiary structures contain naive, memory and plasma B cells as well as intermixed $CD4^+$ and $CD8^+$ T cells, follicular dendritic cells and *M. tuberculosis*-infected APCs (Ulrichs et al., 2004). In mice, formation of B-cell follicles within infected lung tissues is dependent upon IL-23 and CXCL13, and CXCL13 production is dependent upon IL-17A and IL-22 in this response (Khader et al., 2011). The presence of ectopic germinal centres indicates that the *M. tuberculosis* complex – and the ensuing inflammation – induces active B-cell clusters that modulate the host response. Thus, these follicles provide at least a partial framework for coordinated immune control of mycobacterial growth in the affected tissues (Ulrichs et al., 2004).

In cattle, early granulomas (stages I and II) displayed scattered B cells, whereas more advanced granulomas (stages III and IV) showed clusters of $CD79a^+$ cells located peripherally and outside of the fibrous capsule (Salguero et al., 2016). In BCG-vaccinated, *M. bovis*-infected cattle, although few stage II and IV granulomas were observed, the numbers of B cells were significantly increased compared to non-vaccinated *M. bovis* cattle. Further studies in cattle are required to elucidate the roles for B cells and to determine whether they could or should be targets for vaccine-driven intervention strategies.

11.5 Co-Infection Alters the Adaptive Immune Response

Co-infection of individuals with mycobacteria and other pathogenic organisms affects the nature of the adaptive immune response. The best cited example of this is co-infection of humans with *M. tuberculosis* and HIV, where the progressive loss of CD4+ T cells as HIV infection develops into AIDS has significant negative consequences on the growth of *M. tuberculosis*. Early co-infection studies suggested that co-infection of cattle with bovine viral diarrhoea virus (BVDV) and mycobacteria impacts on the results of the interferon-gamma release assay, due to the effect of BVDV on type I interferon production, specifically in the case on non-cytopathic BVDV.

Concurrent infection with parasitic worms or with other environmental mycobacteria has been reported to significantly alter the capacity to respond to BCG vaccination or to control *M. tuberculosis* infection in humans and in murine studies (Stanford et al., 1981; Flaherty et al., 2006; Babu and Nutman, 2016). Under experimental conditions it has been demonstrated that co-infection of cattle with *M. avium* complex organisms (including *M. avium* subsp. *paratuberculosis*) and *M. bovis* leads to altered antigen specificity of the T-cell response (Howard et al., 2002; Thom et al., 2008), leading to a masking of diagnostic accuracy (Barry et al., 2011). There is a significant body of evidence suggesting that co-infection with liver fluke (*Fasciola hepatica*) has a major impact on the outcome of infection with *M. bovis* and the accuracy of diagnostic tests for bovine TB. In the UK, areas with high bovine TB prevalence are generally associated with high endemic prevalence of helminthic infections (Salimi-Bejestani et al., 2005). It has been reported that co-infection with *F. hepatica* significantly altered the diagnosis of *M. bovis* by both the tuberculin skin test and the IFN-γ blood test (Flynn et al., 2007, 2009). In a large-scale epidemiological study, Claridge et al. (2012) estimated that co-infection would lead to significant under-estimation of bovine TB in the UK dairy herd. The reduced sensitivity of the diagnostic tests was shown to be associated with alterations in the ratio of IL-4 and IFN-γ, and therefore hypothesized to be due to altered Th bias or immunosuppression induced by *F. hepatica* infection. A downregulation of the Th1 immune response due to *Fasciola* co-infection has also been shown to be associated with an increase in bacterial loads in mice infected with *Salmonella enterica* serovar Dublin or *Bordetella pertussis* (Aitken et al., 1978; Brady et al., 1999).

More recently, it has been demonstrated that although there was a significant reduction in the expression of antigen-specific IFN-γ in cattle co-infected with *F. hepatica* and *M. bovis*, the co-infected animals had a lower burden of *M. bovis* compared to cattle infected only with *M. bovis* (Garza-Cuartero *et al.*, 2016). This appeared to be associated with a downregulation of pro-inflammatory cytokines and the activation of alternatively-activated macrophages. This may suggest that helminth infection limits the pro-inflammatory environment, favouring a slower development of mycobacteria, with reduced bacterial loads, but which presents a higher barrier for immune-based diagnostic assays.

11.6 Adaptive Immune Responses in Other Mammalian Models of Mycobacterial Disease

In addition to mice, other small mammals, such as cotton rats, rats and rabbits, as well as larger mammals such as guinea pigs, goats, pigs and badgers, are used as models to assess vaccine efficacy for mycobacteria and to examine aspects of the adaptive immune response with a view to identification of correlates of immune protection. While these models have value and, broadly, immune responses appear to be mediated by similar mechanisms, each has limitations. These include access to species-specific reagents in addition to differences in host cell immune populations and different tissue responses. For example, in the mini-pig model, studies are not only impacted on by the presence of a CD4/CD8-double positive T-cell population in peripheral blood, but also by the fact that it is not possible to reproduce an exudative lesion, and thus typical TB pathology, even after locally inoculating up to 1×10^3 bacilli (Gil *et al.*, 2010). In guinea pigs, the main characteristic of infection is an extreme reaction against the bacilli, which has a very important parallelism with the exudative lesions of humans although curiously, this exudative response is very much dominated by eosinophils. However, after BCG vaccination, an early B-cell influx (Ordway *et al.*, 2008), accompanied by CD4 and CD8 T-cell activation, was observed. In this model secondary lesions occur as a consequence of blood dissemination and a notable feature is the major destruction of pulmonary lymph nodes. Investigations in the CD8/CD8 response, and their kinetics in response to infection have been performed (reviewed in (Orme and Ordway, 2016).

Overall, in order to accurately measure the induction and maintenance of natural or vaccine-induced immunity in cattle against *M. bovis* infection it would appear that these models are inaccurate and that *in vivo* studies in the natural host are preferable. Importantly, cattle can act as a good model for human disease (despite differences in the virulence of *M. tuberculosis* and *M. bovis* in cattle) (Waters *et al.*, 2011).

11.7 Summary

Detailed knowledge of the adaptive immune response to mycobacterial infection is required to inform the development of improved vaccines and diagnostic tests. Key to this is the capability to understand which parameters can potentially be used as correlates of immune protection but also those which reflect infection and disease progression. Accurate assessment requires the use of appropriate animal models of disease and immunological reagents and can be informed further by mathematical models. The knowledge reflected in this chapter and across the related chapters in this book suggest that we are in a strong position to harness and integrate a wide range of information to aid future disease control not only for bovine TB but across species to human disease.

References

Abebe, F. (2012) Is interferon-gamma the right marker for bacille Calmette-Guérin-induced immune protection? the missing link in our understanding of tuberculosis immunology. *Clinical and Experimental Immunology* 169(3), 213–219.

Achkar, J.M., Chan, J. and Casadevall, A. (2015) B cells and antibodies in the defense against *Mycobacterium tuberculosis* infection. *Immunological Reviews* 264(1), 167–181.

Aitken, M.M., Jones, P.W., Hall, G.A., Hughes, D.L. and Collis, K.A. (1978) Effects of experimental *Salmonella* Dublin infection in cattle given *Fasciola hepatica* thirteen weeks previously. *Journal of Comparative Pathology* 88(1), 75–84.

Aranday-Cortes, E., Hogarth, P.J., Kaveh, D.A., Whelan, A., Villarreal-Ramos, B., et al. (2012) Transcriptional profiling of disease-induced host responses in bovine tuberculosis and the identification of potential diagnostic biomarkers. *PLoS One* 7(2), e30626.

Aranday-Cortes, E., Bull, N.C., Villarreal-Ramos, B., Gough, J., Hicks, D., et al. (2013) Upregulation of IL-17A, CXCL9 and CXCL10 in early-stage granulomas induced by *Mycobacterium bovis* in cattle. *Transboundary and Emerging Diseases* 60(6), 525–537.

Babu, S. and Nutman, T.B. (2016) Helminth-tuberculosis co-infection: an immunologic perspective. *Trends in Immunology* 37(9), 597–607.

Baldwin, C.L. and Telfer, J.C. (2015) The bovine model for elucidating the role of $\gamma\delta$ T cells in controlling infectious diseases of importance to cattle and humans. *Molecular Immunology* 66(1), 35–47.

Barry, C., Corbett, D., Bakker, D., Andersen, P., McNair, J. and Strain, S. (2011) The effect of *Mycobacterium avium* complex infections on routine *Mycobacterium bovis* diagnostic tests. *Veterinary Medicine International* 2011, 1–7.

Behar, S.M. (2013) *Antigen-Specific CD8+ T Cells and Protective Immunity to Tuberculosis*. Springer, New York, USA, pp. 141–163.

Behar, S.M. and Porcelli, S.A. (2007) CD1-restricted T cells in host defense to infectious diseases. *Current Topics in Microbiology and Immunology* 314, 215–250.

Bhuju, S., Aranday-Cortes, E., Villarreal-Ramos, B., Xing, Z., Singh, M. and Vordermeier, H.M. (2012) Global gene transcriptome analysis in vaccinated cattle revealed a dominant role of IL-22 for protection against bovine tuberculosis. *PLoS Pathogens* 8(12), e1003077.

Blanco, F.C., Bianco, M.V., Meikle, V., Garbaccio, S., Vagnoni, L., et al. (2011) Increased IL-17 expression is associated with pathology in a bovine model of tuberculosis. *Tuberculosis* 91(1), 57–63.

Blunt, L., Hogarth, P.J., Kaveh, D.A., Webb, P., Villarreal-Ramos, B. and Vordermeier, H.M. (2015) Phenotypic characterization of bovine memory cells responding to mycobacteria in IFNγ enzyme linked immunospot assays. *Vaccine* 33(51), 7276–7282.

Bold, T.D., Banaei, N., Wolf, A.J. and Ernst, J.D. (2011) Suboptimal activation of antigen-specific CD4+ effector cells enables persistence of *M. tuberculosis* in vivo. *PLoS Pathogens* 7(5), e1002063.

Brady, M.T., O'Neill, S.M., Dalton, J.P. and Mills, K.H. (1999) *Fasciola hepatica* suppresses a protective Th1 response against *Bordetella pertussis*. *Infection and Immunity* 67(10), 5372–5378.

Brandt, L., Oettinger, T., Holm, A., Andersen, A.B. and Andersen, P. (1996) Key epitopes on the ESAT-6 antigen recognized in mice during the recall of protective immunity to *Mycobacterium tuberculosis*. *Journal of Immunoassay* 157(8), 3527–3533.

Buddle, B., Livingstone, P. and de Lisle, G. (2009) Advances in ante-mortem diagnosis of tuberculosis in cattle. *New Zealand Veterinary Journal* 57(4), 173–180.

Bull, T.J., Vrettou, C., Linedale, R., McGuinnes, C., Strain, S., et al. (2014) Immunity, safety and protection of an adenovirus 5 prime – modified vaccinia virus Ankara boost subunit vaccine against *Mycobacterium avium* subspecies *paratuberculosis* infection in calves. *Veterinary Research* 45(1), 112.

Cassidy, J.P., Bryson, D.G., Pollock, J.M., Evans, R.T., Forster, F. and Neill, S.D. (1998) Early lesion formation in cattle experimentally infected with *Mycobacterium bovis*. *Journal of Comparative Pathology* 119(1), 27–44.

Chackerian, A.A., Alt, J.M., Perera, T.V., Dascher, C.C. and Behar, S.M. (2002a) Dissemination of *Mycobacterium tuberculosis* is influenced by host factors and precedes the initiation of T-cell immunity. *Infection and Immunity* 70(8), 4501–4509.

Chackerian, A., Alt, J., Perera, V. and Behar, S.M. (2002b) Activation of NKT cells protects mice from tuberculosis. *Infection and Immunity* 70(11), 6302–6309.

Champagne, P., Ogg, G.S., King, A.S., Knabenhans, C., Ellefsen, K., et al. (2001) Skewed maturation of memory HIV-specific CD8 T lymphocytes. *Nature* 410(6824), 106–111.

Charleston, B., Hope, J.C., Carr, B.V. and Howard, C.J. (2001) Masking of two in vitro immunological assays for *Mycobacterium bovis* (BCG) in calves acutely infected with non-cytopathic bovine viral diarrhoea virus. *Veterinary Record* 149(16), 481–484.

Chen, C., Herzig, C.T., Alexander, L.J., Keele, J., McDaneld, T., *et al.* (2012) Gene number determination and genetic polymorphism of the gamma delta T cell co-receptor WC1 genes. *BMC Genetics* 13(1), 86.

Chua, W.-J., Truscott, S.M., Eickhoff, C.S., Blazevic, A., Hoft, D.F. and Hansen, T.H. (2012) Polyclonal mucosa-associated invariant T cells have unique innate functions in bacterial infection. *Infection and Immunity* 80(9), 3256–3267.

Claridge, J., Diggle, P., McCann, C.M., Mulcahy, G., Flynn, R., *et al.* (2012) *Fasciola hepatica* is associated with the failure to detect bovine tuberculosis in dairy cattle. *Nature Communications* 3, 853.

Clevers, H., Machugh, N.D., Bensaid, A., Dunlap, S., Baldwin, C., *et al.* (1990) Identification of a bovine surface antigen uniquely expressed on CD4−CD8− T cell receptor γ/δ+ T lymphocytes. *European Journal of Immunogenetics* 20(4), 809–817.

Commandeur, S., van Meijgaarden, K.E., Prins, C., Pichugin, A., Dijkman, K., *et al.* (2013) An unbiased genome-wide *Mycobacterium tuberculosis* gene expression approach to discover antigens targeted by human T cells expressed during pulmonary infection. *Journal of Immunology* 190(4), 1659–1671.

Connelley, T.K., Longhi, C., Burrells, A., Degnan, K., Hope, J., *et al.* (2014) NKp46$^+$CD3$^+$ cells: A novel nonconventional T cell subset in cattle exhibiting both NK cell and T Cell features. *Journal of Immunology* 192(8), 3868–3880.

Cooper, A.M. (2010) Editorial: be careful what you ask for: is the presence of IL-17 indicative of immunity? *Journal of Leukocyte Biology* 88(2), 221–223.

Cooper, A.M., Dalton, D.K., Stewart, T.A., Griffin, J.P., Russell, D.G. and Orme, I.M. (1993) Disseminated tuberculosis in interferon gamma gene-disrupted mice. *The Journal of Experimental Medicine* 178(6), 2243–2247.

Dhiman, R., Indramohan, M., Barnes, P.F., Nayak, R., Paidipally, P., *et al.* (2009) IL-22 produced by human NK cells inhibits growth of *Mycobacterium tuberculosis* by enhancing phagolysosomal fusion. *Journal of Immunology* 183(10), 6639–6645.

Dhiman, R., Periasamy, S., Barnes, P.F., Jaiswal, A., Paidipally, P., *et al.* (2012) NK1.1+ cells and IL-22 regulate vaccine-induced protective immunity against challenge with *Mycobacterium tuberculosis*. *Journal of Immunology* 189(2), 897–905.

Dieli, F., Ivanyi, J., Marsh, P., Williams, A., Naylor, I., *et al.* (2003) Characterization of lung γδ T cells following intranasal infection with *Mycobacterium bovis* Bacillus Calmette-Guérin. *Journal of Immunology* 170(1), 463–469.

Doherty, M.L., Bassett, H.F., Quinn, P.J., Davis, W.C., Kelly, A.P. and Monaghan, M.L. (1996) A sequential study of the bovine tuberculin reaction. *Immunology* 87(1), 9–14.

D'Souza, C.D., Cooper, A.M., Frank, A.A., Mazzaccaro, R.J., Bloom, B.R. and Orme, I.M. (1997) An anti-inflammatory role for gamma delta T lymphocytes in acquired immunity to *Mycobacterium tuberculosis*. *Journal of Immunology* 158(3), 1217–1221.

Egen, J.G., Rothfuchs, A.G., Feng, C.G., Horwitz, M.A., Sher, A. and Germain, R.N. (2011) Intravital imaging reveals limited antigen presentation and T cell effector function in mycobacterial granulomas. *Immunity* 34(5), 807–819.

Einarsdottir, T., Lockhart, E. and Flynn, J.L. (2009) Cytotoxicity and secretion of gamma interferon are carried out by distinct CD8 T cells during *Mycobacterium tuberculosis* infection. *Infection and Immunity* 77(10), 4621–4630.

Endsley, J.J., Furrer, J.L., Endsley, M.A., McIntosh, M.A., Maue, A.C., *et al.* (2004) Characterization of bovine homologues of granulysin and NK-lysin. *Journal of Immunology* 173(4), 2607–2614.

Endsley, J.J., Hogg, A., Shell, L.J., McAulay, M., Coffey, T.J., *et al.* (2007) *Mycobacterium bovis* BCG vaccination induces memory CD4+ T cells characterized by effector biomarker expression and antimycobacterial activity. *Vaccine* 25(50), 8384–8394.

Endsley, J.J., Waters, W.R., Palmer, M.V., Nonnecke, B.J., Thacker, T.C. *et al.* (2009) The calf model of immunity for development of a vaccine against tuberculosis. *Veterinary Immunology and Immunopathology* 128(1–3), 199–204.

Flaherty, D.K., Vesosky, B., Beamer, G.L., Stromberg, P. and Turner, J. (2006) Exposure to *Mycobacterium avium* can modulate established immunity against *Mycobacterium tuberculosis* infection generated by *Mycobacterium bovis* BCG vaccination. *Journal of Leukocyte Biology* 80(6), 1262–1271.

Fletcher, H.A., Snowden, M.A., Landry, B., Rida, W., Satti, I., *et al.* (2016) T-cell activation is an immune correlate of risk in BCG vaccinated infants. *Nature Communications* 7(May), 11290.

Flynn, J.L., Chan, J., Triebold, K.J., Dalton, D.K., Stewart, T.A. and Bloom, B.R. (1993) An essential role for interferon gamma in resistance to *Mycobacterium tuberculosis* infection. *The Journal of Experimental Medicine* 178(6), 2249–2254.

Flynn, R.J., Mannion, C., Golden, O., Hacariz, O. and Mulcahy, G. (2007) Experimental *Fasciola hepatica* infection alters responses to tests used for diagnosis of bovine tuberculosis. *Infection and Immunity* 75(3), 1373–1381.

Flynn, R.J., Mulcahy, G., Welsh, M., Cassidy, J.P., Corbett, D., et al. (2009) Co-Infection of cattle with *Fasciola hepatica* and *Mycobacterium bovis* – immunological consequences. *Transboundary and Emerging Diseases* 56(6–7), 269–274.

Freches, D., Korf, H., Denis, O., Havaux, X., Huygen, K. and Romano, M. (2013) Mice genetically inactivated in interleukin-17A receptor are defective in long-term control of *Mycobacterium tuberculosis* infection. *Immunology* 140(2), 220–231.

Gansert, J.L., Kießler, V., Engele, M., Wittke, F., Röllinghoff, M., et al. (2003) Human NKT cells express granulysin and exhibit antimycobacterial activity. *Journal of Immunology* 170(6), 3154–3161.

Garza-Cuartero, L., O'Sullivan, J., Blanco, A., McNair, J., Welsh, M., et al. (2016) *Fasciola hepatica* infection reduces *Mycobacterium bovis* burden and mycobacterial uptake and suppresses the pro-inflammatory response. *Parasite Immunology* 38(7), 387–402.

Geluk, A., van den Eeden, S.J.F., van Meijgaarden, K.E., Dijkman, K., Franken, K.L.M.C. and Ottenhoff, T.H.M. (2012) A multistage-polyepitope vaccine protects against *Mycobacterium tuberculosis* infection in HLA-DR3 transgenic mice. *Vaccine* 30(52), 7513–7521.

Gil, O., Díaz, I., Vilaplana, C., Tapia, G., Díaz, J., et al. (2010) Granuloma encapsulation is a key factor for containing tuberculosis infection in minipigs. *PLoS One* 5(4), e10030.

Gilleron, M., Stenger, S., Mazorra, Z., Wittke, F., Mariotti, S., et al. (2004) Diacylated sulfoglycolipids are novel mycobacterial antigens stimulating CD1-restricted T cells during infection with *Mycobacterium tuberculosis*. *The Journal of Experimental Medicine* 199(5), 649–659.

Goddeeris, B. (1998) Immunology of cattle. In: Pastoret, P.-P., Griebel, P., Bazin, H. and Govaerts, A. (eds) *Handbook of Vertebrate Immunology*. Academic Press, San Diego, USA, pp. 439–484.

Gold, M.C., Cerri, S., Smyk-Pearson, S., Cansler, M., Vogt, T., et al. (2010) Human mucosal associated invariant T cells detect bacterially infected cells. *PLoS Biology* 8(6), e1000407.

Goldfinch, N., Reinink, P., Connelley, T., Koets, A., Morrison, I. and Van Rhijn, I. (2010) Conservation of mucosal associated invariant T (MAIT) cells and the MR1 restriction element in ruminants, and abundance of MAIT cells in spleen. *Veterinary Research* 41(5), 62.

Green, A.M., Difazio, R. and Flynn, J.L. (2013) IFN-γ from CD4 T cells is essential for host survival and enhances CD8 T cell function during *Mycobacterium tuberculosis* infection. *Journal of Immunology* 190(1), 270–277.

Guzman, E., Price, S., Poulsom, H. and Hope, J. (2012) Bovine γδ T cells: cells with multiple functions and important roles in immunity. *Veterinary Immunology and Immunopathology* 148, 161–167.

Guzman, E., Hope, J., Taylor, G., Smith, A.L., Cubillos-Zapata, C. and Charleston, B. (2014) Bovine γδ T cells are a major regulatory T cell subset. *Journal of Immunology* 193(1), 208–222.

Hein, W.R. and Mackay, C.R. (1991) Prominence of gamma delta T cells in the ruminant immune system. *Immunol Today* 12(1), 30–34.

Henao-Tamayo, M., Ordway, D.J. and Orme, I.M. (2014) Memory T cell subsets in tuberculosis: what should we be targeting? *Tuberculosis* 94(5), 455–461.

Hoek, A., Rutten, V.P.M.G., Kool, J., Arkesteijn, G., Bouwstra, R., et al. (2009) Subpopulations of bovine WC1(+) gammadelta T cells rather than CD4(+)CD25(high) Foxp3(+) T cells act as immune regulatory cells ex vivo. *Veterinary Research* 40(1), 6.

Hope, J.C. and Vordermeier H.M. (2005) Vaccines for bovine tuberculosis: current views and future prospects. *Expert Review of Vaccines* 4(6), 891–903.

Hope, J.C., Thom, M.L., McCormick, P.A. and Howard, C.J. (2004) Interaction of antigen presenting cells with mycobacteria. *Veterinary Immunology and Immunopathology* 100(3–4), 187–195.

Hope, J.C., Thom, M.L., McAulay, M., Mead, E., Vordermeier, H.M., et al. (2011) Identification of surrogates and correlates of protection in protective immunity against *Mycobacterium bovis* infection induced in neonatal calves by vaccination with *M. bovis* BCG pasteur and *M. bovis* BCG Danish. *Clinical and Vaccine Immunology* 18(3), 373–379.

Hou, S., Hyland, L., Ryan, K.W., Portner, A. and Doherty, P.C. (1994) Virus-specific CD8+ T-cell memory determined by clonal burst size. *Nature* 369(6482), 652–654.

Howard, C.J., Sopp, P. and Parsons, K.R. (1992) L-selectin expression differentiates T cells isolated from different lymphoid tissues in cattle but does not correlate with memory. *Immunology* 77(2), 228–234.

Howard, C.J., Kwong, L.S., Villarreal-Ramos, B., Sopp, P. and Hope, J.C. (2002) Exposure to *Mycobacterium avium* primes the immune system of calves for vaccination with *Mycobacterium bovis* BCG. *Clinical and Experimental Immunology* 130(2), 190–195.

Jurado, J.O., Pasquinelli, V., Alvarez, I.B., Pena, D., Rovetta, A., *et al.* (2012) IL-17 and IFN-γ expression in lymphocytes from patients with active tuberculosis correlates with the severity of the disease. *Journal of Leukocyte Biology* 91(6), 991–1002.

Jutila, M.A., Holderness, J., Graff, J.C., Hedges, J., Abrahamsen, M., *et al.* (2008) Antigen-independent priming: a transitional response of bovine γδ T-cells to infection. *Animal Health Research Reviews* 9(1), 47–57.

Kabelitz, D. (2011) γδ T-cells: cross-talk between innate and adaptive immunity. *Cellular and Molecular Life Sciences* 68(14), 2331–2333.

Kawashima, T., Norose, Y., Watanabe, Y., Enomoto, Y., Narazaki, H., *et al.* (2003) Cutting edge: major CD8 T cell response to live Bacillus Calmette-Guérin is mediated by CD1 molecules. *Journal of Immunology* 170(11), 5345–5348.

Kennedy, H.E., Welsh, M.D., Bryson, D.G., Cassidy, J., Forster, F., *et al.* (2002) Modulation of immune responses to *Mycobacterium bovis* in cattle depleted of WC1(+) gamma delta T cells. *Infection and Immunity* 70(3), 1488–1500.

Khader, S.A. and Cooper, A.M. (2008) IL-23 and IL-17 in tuberculosis. *Cytokine* 41(2), 79–83.

Khader, S.A., Bell, G.K., Pearl, J.E., Fountain, J.J., Rangel-Moreno, J., *et al.* (2007) IL-23 and IL-17 in the establishment of protective pulmonary CD4+ T cell responses after vaccination and during *Mycobacterium tuberculosis* challenge. *Natural Immunity* 8(4), 369–377.

Khader, S.A., Guglani, L., Rangel-Moreno, J., Gopal, R., Junecko, B.A., *et al.* (2011) IL-23 is required for long-term control of *Mycobacterium tuberculosis* and B cell follicle formation in the infected lung. *Journal of Immunology* 187(10), 5402–5407.

Koinig, H.C., Talker, S.C., Stadler, M., Ladinig, A., Graage, R., *et al.* (2015) PCV2 vaccination induces IFN-γ/TNF-α co-producing T cells with a potential role in protection. *Veterinary Research* 46(1), 20.

Ladel, C.H., Hess, J., Daugelat, S., Mombaerts, P., Tonegawa, S. and Kaufmann, S.H.E. (1995) Contribution of α/β and γ/δ T lymphocytes to immunity against *Mycobacterium bovis* Bacillus Calmette Guérin: studies with T cell receptor-deficient mutant mice. *European Journal of Immunogenetics* 25(3), 838–846.

Lahmers, K.K., Norimine, J., Abrahamsen, M.S., Palmer, G.H. and Brown, W.C. (2004) The CD4+ T cell immunodominant anaplasma marginale major surface protein 2 stimulates T cell clones that express unique T cell receptors. *Journal of Leukocyte Biology* 77(2), 199–208.

Le Bourhis, L., Martin, E., Péguillet, I., Guihot, A., Froux, N., *et al.* (2010) Antimicrobial activity of mucosal-associated invariant T cells. *Natural Immunity* 11(8), 701–708.

Liebana, E., Aranaz, A., Aldwell, F.E., McNair, J., Neill, S., *et al.* (2000) Cellular interactions in bovine tuberculosis: release of active mycobacteria from infected macrophages by antigen-stimulated T cells. *Immunology* 99(1), 23–29.

Liebana, E., Marsh, S., Gough, J., Nunez, A., Vordermeier, H.M., *et al.* (2007) Distribution and activation of T-lymphocyte subsets in tuberculous bovine lymph-node granulomas. *Veterinary Pathology* 44(3), 366–372.

Lindestam Arlehamn, C.S., Gerasimova, A., Mele, F., Henderson, R., Swann, J., *et al.* (2013) Memory T cells in latent *Mycobacterium tuberculosis* infection are directed against three antigenic islands and largely contained in a CXCR3+CCR6+ Th1 subset. *PLoS Pathogen* 9(1), e1003130.

Lockhart, E., Green, A.M. and Flynn, J.L. (2006) IL-17 production is dominated by γδ T cells rather than CD4 T cells during *Mycobacterium tuberculosis* infection. *Journal of Immunology* 177(7), 4662–4669.

Mackay, C.R. and Beya, M.-F. (1989) Matzinger P. γ/δ T cells express a unique surface molecule appearing late during thymic development. *European Journal of Immunogenetics* 19(8), 1477–1483.

Maggioli, M.F., Palmer, M.V., Thacker, T.C., Vordermeier, H.M. and Waters, W.R. (2015a) Characterization of effector and memory T cell subsets in the immune response to bovine tuberculosis in cattle. *PLoS One* 10(4), 1–20.

Maggioli, M.F., Palmer, M.V., Vordermeier, H.M., Whelan, A.O., Fosse, J.M., *et al.* (2015b) Application of long-term cultured interferon-gamma; enzyme-linked immunospot assay for assessing effector and memory T cell responses in cattle. *Journal of Visualized Experiments* 101, e52833.

Maglione, P.J. and Chan, J. (2009) How B cells shape the immune response against *Mycobacterium tuberculosis*. *European Journal of Immunogenetics* 39(3), 676–686.

Maue, A.C., Waters, W.R., Davis, W.C., Palmer, M.V., Minion, F.C. and Estes, D.M. (2005) Analysis of immune responses directed toward a recombinant early secretory antigenic target six-kilodalton protein-culture filtrate protein 10 fusion protein in *Mycobacterium bovis*-infected cattle. *Infection and Immunity* 73(10), 6659–6667.

Mazzola, T.N., Da Silva, M.T.N., Moreno, Y.M.F., Lima, S.C.B.S., Carniel, E.F., *et al.* (2007) Robust γδ+ T cell expansion in infants immunized at birth with BCG vaccine. *Vaccine* 25(34), 6313–6320.

McGill, J.L., Sacco, R.E., Baldwin, C.L., Telfer, J.C., Palmer, M.V. and Waters, W.R. (2014a) The role of gamma delta T cells in immunity to *Mycobacterium bovis* infection in cattle. *Veterinary Immunology and Immunopathology* 159(3–4), 133–143.

McGill, J.L., Sacco, R.E., Baldwin, C.L., Telfer, J.C., Palmer, M.V. and Waters, W.R. (2014b) Specific recognition of mycobacterial protein and peptide antigens by T cell subsets following infection with virulent *Mycobacterium bovis*. *Journal of Immunology* 192(6), 2756–2769.

Mittrucker, H.W., Steinhoff, U., Kohler, A., Krause, M., Lazar, D., *et al.* (2007) Poor correlation between BCG vaccination-induced T cell responses and protection against tuberculosis. *Proceedings of the National Academy of Sciences* 104(30), 12434–12439.

Montamat-Sicotte, D.J., Millington, K.A., Willcox, C.R., Hingley-Wilson, S., Hackforth, S., *et al.* (2011) A mycolic acid-specific CD1-restricted T cell population contributes to acute and memory immune responses in human tuberculosis infection. *The Journal of Clinical Investigation* 121(6), 2493–2503.

Morrison, W.I. and Davis, W.C. (1991) Individual antigens of cattle. differentiation antigens expressed predominantly on CD4- CD8- T lymphocytes (WC1, WC2). *Veterinary Immunology and Immunopathology* 27(1–3), 71–76.

Murali-Krishna, K., Altman, J.D., Suresh, M., Sourdive, D.J., Zajac, A.J., *et al.* (1998) Counting antigen-specific CD8 T cells: a reevaluation of bystander activation during viral infection. *Immunity* 8(2), 177–187.

Okamoto Yoshida, Y., Umemura, M., Yahagi, A., O'Brien, R.L., Ikuta, K., *et al.* (2010) Essential role of IL-17A in the formation of a mycobacterial infection-induced granuloma in the lung. *Journal of Immunology* 184(8), 4414–4422.

Ordway, D., Henao-Tamayo, M., Shanley, C., Smith, E., Palanisamy, G., *et al.* (2008) Influence of *Mycobacterium bovis* BCG vaccination on cellular immune response of guinea pigs challenged with *Mycobacterium tuberculosis*. *Clinical and Vaccine Immunology* 15(8), 1248–1258.

Ordway, D.J., Shang S., Henao-Tamayo, M., Obregon-Henao, A., Nold, L., *et al.* (2011) *Mycobacterium bovis* BCG-mediated protection against W-Beijing strains of *Mycobacterium tuberculosis* is diminished concomitant with the emergence of regulatory T Cells. *Clinical and Vaccine Immunology* 18(9), 1527–1535.

Orme, I.M. and Ordway, D.J. (2016) Mouse and guinea pig models of tuberculosis. *Microbiology Spectrum* 4(4), chapter 7.

Ottenhoff, T.H.M., Verreck, F.A.W., Hoeve, M.A. and van de Vosse, E. (2005) Control of human host immunity to mycobacteria. *Tuberculosis (Edinb)* 85(1–2), 53–64.

Pai, M., Denkinger, C.M., Kik, S.V., Rangaka, M.X., Zwerling, A., *et al.* (2014) Gamma interferon release assays for detection of *Mycobacterium tuberculosis* infection. *Clinical Microbiology Reviews* 27(1), 3–20.

Palmer, M.V., Waters, W.R. and Thacker, T.C. (2007) Lesion development and immunohistochemical changes in granulomas from cattle experimentally infected with *Mycobacterium bovis*. *Veterinary Pathology* 44(6), 863–874.

Piercy, J., Werling, D. and Coffey, T.J. (2007) Differential responses of bovine macrophages to infection with bovine-specific and non-bovine specific mycobacteria. *Tuberculosis* 87(5), 415–420.

Pirson, C., Engel, R., Jones, G.J., Holder, T., Holst, O. and Vordermeier, H.M. (2015) Highly purified mycobacterial phosphatidylinositol mannosides drive cell-mediated responses and activate NKT cells in cattle. *Clinical and Vaccine Immunology* 22(2), 178–184.

Pollock, J.M., Pollock, D.A., Campbell, D.G., Girvin, R.L., Crockard, A.D., *et al.* (1996) Dynamic changes in circulating and antigen-responsive T-cell subpopulations post-*Mycobacterium bovis* infection in cattle. *Immunology* 87(2), 236–241.

Pollock, J.M., McNair, J., Welsh, M.D., Girvin, R.L., Kennedy, H.E., *et al.* (2001) Immune responses in bovine tuberculosis. *Tuberculosis* 81(1–2), 103–107.

Porcelli, S., Yockey, C.E., Brenner, M.B. and Balk, S.P. (1993) Analysis of T cell antigen receptor (TCR) expression by human peripheral blood CD4-8- alpha/beta T cells demonstrates preferential use of several V beta genes and an invariant TCR alpha chain. *The Journal of Experimental Medicine* 178(1), 1–16.

Price, S.J. and Hope, J.C. (2009) Enhanced secretion of interferon-γ by bovine γδ T cells induced by coculture with *Mycobacterium bovis*-infected dendritic cells: evidence for reciprocal activating signals. *Immunology* 126(2), 201–208.

Price, S.J., Sopp, P., Howard, C.J. and Hope, J.C. (2006) Workshop cluster 1+ γδ T-cell receptor+ T cells from calves express high levels of interferon-γ in response to stimulation with interleukin-12 and -18. *Immunology* 120(1), 57–65.

Price, S., Davies, M., Villarreal-Ramos, B. and Hope, J. (2010) Differential distribution of WC1 + γδ TCR + T lymphocyte subsets within lymphoid tissues of the head and respiratory tract and effects of intranasal *M. bovis* BCG vaccination. *Veterinary Immunology and Immunopathology* 136(1–2), 133–137.

Reiley, W.W., Calayag, M.D., Wittmer, S.T., Huntington, J.L., Pearl, J.E. *et al.* (2008) ESAT-6-specific CD4 T cell responses to aerosol *Mycobacterium tuberculosis* infection are initiated in the mediastinal lymph nodes. *Proceedings of the National Academy of Sciences* 105(31), 10961–10966.

Rhodes, S.G., Hewinson, R.G. and Vordermeier, H.M. (2001) Antigen recognition and immunomodulation by γδ T cells in bovine tuberculosis. *Journal of Immunology* 166(9), 5604–5610.

Rhodes, S.G., McKinna, L.C., Steinbach, S., Dean, G.S., Villarreal-Ramos, B., *et al.* (2014) Use of antigen-specific interleukin-2 to differentiate between cattle vaccinated with *Mycobacterium bovis* BCG and cattle infected with *M. bovis*. *Clinical and Vaccine Immunology* 21(1), 39–45.

Robinson, R.T., Orme, I.M. and Cooper, A.M. (2015) The onset of adaptive immunity in the mouse model of tuberculosis and the factors that compromise its expression. *Immunological Reviews* 264(1), 46–59.

Rogers, A.N., Vanburen, D.G., Hedblom, E.E., Tilahun, M.E., Telfer, J.C. and Baldwin, C.L. (2005) Gammadelta T cell function varies with the expressed WC1 coreceptor. *Journal of Immunology* 174(6), 3386–3393.

Salguero, F.J., Gibson, S., Garcia-Jimenez, W., Gough, J., Strickland, T.S., *et al.* (2016) Differential cell composition and cytokine expression within lymph node granulomas from BCG-vaccinated and non-vaccinated cattle experimentally infected with *Mycobacterium bovis*. *Transboundary and Emerging Diseases* 64(6), 1734–1749.

Salimi-Bejestani, M.R., Daniel, R.G., Felstead, S.M., Cripps, P.J., Mahmoody, H. and Williams, D.J.L. (2005) Prevalence of *Fasciola hepatica* in dairy herds in England and Wales measured with an ELISA applied to bulk-tank milk. *Veterinary Record* 156(23), 729–731.

Sallusto, F., Lenig, D., Förster, R., Lipp, M. and Lanzavecchia, A. (1999) Two subsets of memory T lymphocytes with distinct homing potentials and effector functions. *Nature* 401(6754), 708–712.

Sallusto, F., Lanzavecchia, A., Araki, K. and Ahmed, R. (2010) From vaccines to memory and back. *Immunity* 33(4), 451–463.

Sarrias, M.R., Gronlund, J., Padilla, O., Madsen, J., Holmskov, U. and Lozano, F. (2004) The scavenger receptor cysteine-rich (SRCR) domain: an ancient and highly conserved protein module of the innate immune system. *Critical Reviews in Immunology* 24(1), 1–38.

Scott-Browne, J.P., Shafiani, S., Tucker-Heard, G., Ishida-Tsubota, K., Fontenot, J.D., *et al.* (2007) Expansion and function of Foxp3-expressing T regulatory cells during tuberculosis. *The Journal of Experimental Medicine* 204(9), 2159–2169.

Scriba, T.J., Coussens, A.K. and Fletcher, H.A. (2016) Human immunology of tuberculosis. *Microbiology Spectrum* 4(5). DOI: 10.1128/microbiolspec.TBTB2-0016-2016.

Semple, P.L., Watkins, M., Davids, V., Krensky, A.M., Hanekom, W.A., *et al.* (2011) Induction of granulysin and perforin cytolytic mediator expression in 10-Week-Old infants vaccinated with BCG at birth. *Clinical and Developmental Immunology* 2011, 438463.

Shafiani, S., Tucker-Heard, G., Kariyone, A., Takatsu, K. and Urdahl, K.B. (2010) Pathogen-specific regulatory T cells delay the arrival of effector T cells in the lung during early tuberculosis. *The Journal of Experimental Medicine* 207(7), 1409–1420.

Sharma, P.K., Wong, E.B., Napier, R.J., Bishai, W.R., Ndung'u, T., *et al.* (2015) High expression of CD26 accurately identifies human bacteria-reactive MR1-restricted MAIT cells. *Immunology* 145(3), 443–453.

Siddiqui, N., Price, S. and Hope, J. (2012) BCG vaccination of neonatal calves: potential roles for innate immune cells in the induction of protective immunity. *Comparative Immunology, Microbiology and Infectious Diseases* 35(3), 219–216.

Skinner, M.A., Parlane, N., McCarthy, A. and Buddle, B.M. (2003) Cytotoxic T-cell responses to *Mycobacterium bovis* during experimental infection of cattle with bovine tuberculosis. *Immunology* 110(2), 234–241.

Smith, R.A., Kreeger, J.M., Alvarez, A.J., Goin, J.C., Davis, W.C., et al. (1999) Role of CD8+ and WC-1+ gamma/delta T cells in resistance to *Mycobacterium bovis* infection in the SCID-bo mouse. *Journal of Leukocyte Biology* 65(1), 28–34.

Smyth, A.J., Welsh, M.D., Girvin, R.M. and Pollock, J.M. (2001) In vitro responsiveness of gammadelta T cells from *Mycobacterium bovis*-infected cattle to mycobacterial antigens: predominant involvement of WC1(+) cells. *Infection and Immunity* 69(1), 89–96.

Sopp, P., Howard, C.J. and Hope, J.C. (2006) Flow cytometric detection of gamma interferon can effectively discriminate *Mycobacterium bovis* BCG-vaccinated cattle from *M. bovis*-infected cattle. *Clinical and Vaccine Immunology* 13(12), 1343–1348.

Stanford, J.L., Shield, M.J. and Rook, G.A. (1981) How environmental mycobacteria may predetermine the protective efficacy of BCG. *Tubercle* 62(1), 55–62.

Steinbach, S., Vordermeier, H.M. and Jones, G.J. (2016) CD4+ and $\gamma\delta$ T cells are the main producers of IL-22 and IL-17A in lymphocytes from *Mycobacterium bovis*-infected cattle. *Science Reporter* 6(May), 29990.

Stenger, S., Hanson, D.A., Teitelbaum, R., Dewan, P., Niazi, K.R., et al. (1998) An antimicrobial activity of cytolytic T cells mediated by granulysin. *Science* 282(5386), 121–125.

Sutherland, J.S., Adetifa, I.M., Hill, P.C., Adegbola, R.A. and Ota, M.O.C. (2009) Pattern and diversity of cytokine production differentiates between *Mycobacterium tuberculosis* infection and disease. *European Journal of Immunogenetics* 39(3), 723–729.

Tang, S.T., van Meijgaarden, K.E., Caccamo, N., Guggino, G., Klein, M.R., et al. (2011) Genome-Based in silico identification of new *Mycobacterium tuberculosis* antigens activating polyfunctional CD8+ T Cells in human tuberculosis. *Journal of Immunology* 186(2), 1068–1080.

Thom, M., Howard, C., Villarreal-Ramos, B., Mead, E., Vordermeier, M. and Hope, J. (2008) Consequence of prior exposure to environmental mycobacteria on BCG vaccination and diagnosis of tuberculosis infection. *Tuberculosis* 88(4), 324–334.

Tilloy, F., Treiner, E., Park, S.H., Garcia, G., Lemonnier, F., et al. (1999) An invariant T cell receptor alpha chain defines a novel TAP-independent major histocompatibility complex class Ib-restricted alpha/beta T cell subpopulation in mammals. *The Journal of Experimental Medicine* 189(12), 1907–1921.

Todryk, S.M., Pathan, A.A., Keating, S., Porter, D.W., Berthoud, T., et al. (2009) The relationship between human effector and memory T cells measured by ex vivo and cultured ELISPOT following recent and distal priming. *Immunology* 128(1), 83–91.

Torrado, E. and Cooper, A.M. (2010) IL-17 and Th17 cells in tuberculosis. *Cytokine and Growth Factor Reviews* 21(6), 455–462.

Totté, P., Duperray, C. and Dedieu, L. (2010) CD62L defines a subset of pathogen-specific bovine CD4 with central memory cell characteristics. *Developmental and Comparative Immunology* 34(2), 177–182.

Tsao, T.C.Y., Huang, C.C., Chiou, W.K., Yang, P.Y., Hsieh, M.J. and Tsao, K.C. (2002) Levels of interferon-gamma and interleukin-2 receptor-alpha for bronchoalveolar lavage fluid and serum were correlated with clinical grade and treatment of pulmonary tuberculosis. *The International Journal of Tuberculosis and Lung Disease* 6(8), 720–727.

Ulrichs, T., Moody, D.B., Grant, E., Kaufmann, S.H.E. and Porcelli, S.A. (2003) T-cell responses to CD1-presented lipid antigens in humans with *Mycobacterium tuberculosis* infection. *Infection and Immunity* 71(6), 3076–3087.

Ulrichs, T., Kosmiadi, G.A., Trusov, V., Jorg, S., Pradl, L., et al. (2004) Human tuberculous granulomas induce peripheral lymphoid follicle-like structures to orchestrate local host defence in the lung. *The Journal of Pathology* 204(2), 217–228.

Umemura, M., Yahagi, A., Hamada, S., Begum, M.D., Watanabe, H., et al. (2007) IL-17-mediated regulation of innate and acquired immune response against pulmonary *Mycobacterium bovis* bacille Calmette-Guérin infection. *Journal of Immunology* 178(6), 3786–3796.

Van Rhijn, I. and Moody, D.B. (2015) CD1 and mycobacterial lipids activate human T cells. *Immunology Reviews* 264(1), 138–153.

Van Rhijn, I., Koets, A.P., Im, J.S., Piebes, D., Reddington, F., et al. (2006) The bovine CD1 family contains group 1 CD1 proteins, but no functional CD1d. *Journal of Immunology* 176(8), 4888–4893.

Van Rhijn, I., Nguyen, T.K.A., Michel, A., Cooper, D., Govaerts, M., *et al.* (2009) Low cross-reactivity of T-cell responses against lipids from *Mycobacterium bovis* and *M. avium paratuberculosis* during natural infection. *European Journal of Immunogenetics* 39(11), 3031–3041.

Van Rhijn, I., Ly, D. and Moody, D.B. (2013) *CD1a, CD1b, and CD1c in Immunity against Mycobacteria*. Springer, New York, pp. 181–197.

van de Vosse, E., Hoeve, M.A. and Ottenhoff, T.H. (2004) Human genetics of intracellular infectious diseases: molecular and cellular immunity against mycobacteria and salmonellae. *The Lancet Infectious Diseases* 4(12), 739–749.

Venkataswamy, M.M., Baena, A., Goldberg, M.F., Bricard, G., Im, J.S., *et al.* (2009) Incorporation of NKT cell-activating glycolipids enhances immunogenicity and vaccine efficacy of *Mycobacterium bovis* Bacillus Calmette-Guerin. *Journal of Immunology* 183(3), 1644–1656.

Villarreal-Ramos, B., McAulay, M., Chance, V., Martin, M., Morgan, J. and Howard, C.J. (2003) Investigation of the role of CD8+ T cells in bovine tuberculosis in vivo. *Infection and Immunity* 71(8), 4297–4303. DOI: 10.1128/IAI.71.8.4297-4303.2003.

Vordermeier, H.M., Huygen, K., Singh, M., Hewinson, R.G. and Xing, Z. (2006) Immune responses induced in cattle by vaccination with a recombinant adenovirus expressing mycobacterial antigen 85A and *Mycobacterium bovis* BCG. *Infection and Immunity* 74(2), 1416–1418.

Vordermeier, H.M., Villarreal-Ramos, B., Cockle, P.J., McAulay, M., Rhodes, S.G., *et al.* (2009) Viral booster vaccines improve *Mycobacterium bovis* BCG-Induced protection against bovine tuberculosis. *Infection and Immunity* 77(8), 3364–3373.

Walravens, K., Wellemans, V., Weynants, V., Boelaert, F., DeBergeyck, V., *et al.* (2002) Analysis of the antigen-specific IFN-gamma producing T-cell subsets in cattle experimentally infected with *Mycobacterium bovis*. *Veterinary Immunology and Immunopathology* 84(1–2), 29–41.

Waters, W.R.R., Palmer, M.V.M.V., Thacker, T.C., Davis, W.C., Sreevatsan, S., *et al.* (2011) Tuberculosis immunity: opportunities from studies with cattle. *Clinical and Developmental Immunology* 2011, 768542.

Waters, W.R., Palmer, M.V., Buddle, B.M. and Vordermeier, H.M. (2012) Bovine tuberculosis vaccine research: historical perspectives and recent advances. *Vaccine* 30(16), 2611–2622.

Waters, W.R., Maggioli, M.F., Palmer, M.V., Thacker, T.C., McGill, J.L., *et al.* (2016) Interleukin-17A as a biomarker for bovine tuberculosis. In: Pasetti, M.F. (ed.) *Clinical and Vaccine Immunology* 23(2), 168–180.

Welsh, M.D., Kennedy, H.E., Smyth, A.J., Girvin, R.M., Andersen, P. and Pollock, J.M. (2002) Responses of bovine WC1(+) gammadelta T cells to protein and nonprotein antigens of *Mycobacterium bovis*. *Infection and Immunity* 70(11), 6114–6120.

Whelan, C., Whelan, A.O., Shuralev, E., *et al.* (2010) Performance of the enferplex TB assay with cattle in great Britain and assessment of its suitability as a test to distinguish infected and vaccinated animals. *Clinical and Vaccine Immunology* 17(5), 813–817.

Whelan, A.O., Villarreal-Ramos, B., Vordermeier, H.M., Hogarth, P.J., Ashford, D.A., *et al.* (2011) Development of an antibody to bovine IL-2 reveals multifunctional CD4 TEM cells in cattle naturally Infected with bovine tuberculosis. *PLoS One* 6(12), e29194.

Whitmire, J.K., Asano, M.S., Murali-Krishna, K., Suresh, M. and Ahmed, R. (1998) Long-term CD4 Th1 and Th2 memory following acute lymphocytic choriomeningitis virus infection. *Journal of Virology* 72(10), 8281–8288.

Widdison, S., Schreuder, L.J., Villarreal-Ramos, B., Howard, C.J., Watson, M. and Coffey, T.J. (2006) Cytokine expression profiles of bovine lymph nodes: effects of *Mycobacterium bovis* infection and bacille calmette-guerin vaccination. *Clinical and Experimental Immunology* 144(2), 281–289.

Wilkinson, K.A. and Wilkinson, R.J. (2010) Polyfunctional T cells in human tuberculosis. *European Journal of Immunogenetics* 40(8), 2139–2142.

Wilkinson, K.A., Seldon, R., Meintjes, G., Rangaka, M.X., Hanekom, W.A., *et al.* (2009) Dissection of regenerating T-Cell responses against tuberculosis in HIV-infected adults sensitized by *Mycobacterium tuberculosis*. *American Journal of Respiratory and Critical Care Medicine* 180(7), 674–683.

Winslow, G.M., Roberts, A.D., Blackman, M.A. and Woodland, D.L. (2003) Persistence and turnover of antigen-specific CD4 T cells during chronic tuberculosis infection in the mouse. *Journal of Immunoassay* 170(4), 2046–2052.

Wolf, A.J., Linas, B., Trevejo-Nuñez, G.J., Kincaid, E., Tamura, T., *et al.* (2007) *Mycobacterium tuberculosis* infects dendritic cells with high frequency and impairs their function in vivo. *Journal of Immunology* 179(4), 2509–2519.

Wolf, A.J., Desvignes, L., Linas, B., Banaiee, N., Tamura T., *et al.* (2008) Initiation of the adaptive immune response to *Mycobacterium tuberculosis* depends on antigen production in the local lymph node, not the lungs. *The Journal of Experimental Medicine* 205(1), 105–115.

Woodland, D.L. and Kohlmeier, J.E. (2009) Migration, maintenance and recall of memory T cells in peripheral tissues. *Nature Reviews Immunology* 9(3), 153–161.

12 Immunological Diagnosis

Ray Waters[1],* and Martin Vordermeier[2]

[1]*National Animal Disease Center, Agricultural Research Service, United States Department of Agriculture, Ames, Iowa, USA;* [2]*Tuberculosis Research Group, Animal and Plant Health Agency, Addlestone, UK*

12.1 Introduction

Bovine tuberculosis (TB) is generally considered a slowly progressive disease of extended duration (lasting years), and most cattle do not exhibit readily apparent clinical signs of infection until late in the course of disease (Waters, 2015). Currently, agent-based strategies for the detection of tuberculous cattle, such as detection of bacilli within bodily excretions, are generally unreliable for use as ante-mortem tests, possibly due to the paucibacillary nature of the disease resulting in a transient and low level of bacterial shedding (Good and Duignan, 2011). Thus, traditional clinical and microbiological techniques are rarely used for the ante-mortem diagnosis of bovine TB. Fortunately, *Mycobacterium bovis* is highly immunogenic in cattle, eliciting robust cell-mediated immune (CMI) responses early in the course of disease, thereby providing a useful surrogate of infection for a disease in which ante-mortem detection of the organism is difficult.

An immunological basis for the diagnosis of TB was first realized shortly after Koch's discovery of tuberculin in 1890. With his studies, Koch noted that injection of tuberculin into *Mycobacterium tuberculosis*-infected humans often resulted in systemic reactions including hyperthermia. Using this information, veterinarians discovered that subcutaneous injection of tuberculin also evoked a transient rise in body temperature in tuberculous cattle and this reaction could be of use as an immune-based diagnostic assay. The cumbersome subcutaneous test was eventually replaced by a more sensitive and practical intradermal tuberculin test. Along with slaughter inspection followed by epidemiologic trace-back studies to determine herds of origin for tuberculous carcasses, application of the intradermal tuberculin test for removal of test positive cattle has led to the complete eradication of bovine TB in Australia and near eradication of TB in Canada, most states within the USA, New Zealand, and several European Union countries (Cousins and Roberts, 2001; Good and Duignan *et al.*, 2011; Farnham *et al.*, 2012; Rivière *et al.*, 2014; More *et al.*, 2015). Despite these advances, eradication and control efforts are seriously hindered by the emergence of wildlife reservoirs of *M. bovis* in multiple countries, large-scale dairy calf and replacement heifer rearing operations resulting in congregation and widespread dispersal of single source-infected animals, and increasing trade of cattle (as a result of globalization of economies) from regions with moderate bovine TB prevalence to regions with very low prevalence (e.g. ~1 million cattle shipped annually from Mexico to the US). Thus, modern approaches requiring novel and improved ante-mortem tests and testing algorithms will be required to offset the emerging challenges in the control and eradication of bovine TB.

---

* Email: wwaters@iastate.edu

12.2 Immunopathogenesis as Related to Development of Diagnostic Tests

Bovine peripheral blood CD4, CD8 and γδ T cells from *M. bovis*-infected cattle proliferate and display an overt activated phenotype (i.e. increased CD25, CD26, CD44, CD45RO and CD69 expression) upon stimulation with mycobacterial antigens (Rhodes *et al.*, 2000; Waters *et al.*, 2003; Maue *et al.*, 2005; El-Naggar *et al.*, 2015). Antigen-specific activation is also accompanied by a robust and diverse cytokine response ranging from pro-inflammatory (e.g. IFN-γ, IL-17, and IL-1) to immunosuppressive, regulatory and tissue remodeling responses (e.g. IL-10 and TGF-β) (Rhodes *et al.*, 2000; Vordermeier *et al.*, 2002; Jones *et al.*, 2010a; Aranday-Cortes *et al.*, 2012; McGill *et al.*, 2014; Shu *et al.*, 2014; Palmer *et al.*, 2015; Waters *et al.*, 2015a). To add to the complexity, polyfunctional T cells expressing various combinations of IFN-γ, IL-2 and TNF-α are also elicited by *M. bovis* infection/ bacillus Calmette–Guérin (BCG) vaccination (Whelan *et al.*, 2011; Dean *et al.*, 2015; Maggioli *et al.*, 2015a); yet, the nature of protective versus detrimental polyfunctional T-cell responses to infection and vaccination remains unclear. With that said, initial studies indicate that increasing responses by CD4$^+$ cells co-producing IFN-γ$^+$ and TNFα$^+$ (particularly the CD45RO$^+$, CCR7$^+$, CD62L^{hi} subset) are associated with the degree of pathology (disease severity), possibly correlating with antigen load (Maggioli and Waters, unpublished observations). Studies with *M. tuberculosis* infection in HIV-infected humans suggest that CD4 T cells secreting IL-2 alone or with other cytokines correlate with beneficial responses (Day *et al.*, 2008; Wilkinson and Wilkinson, 2010), whereas a high proportion of IFN-γ$^+$TNFα$^+$ cells is detected in patients with active but not latent disease (Chiacchio *et al.*, 2014; Salgame *et al.*, 2015). Thus, the complexity and diversity of the immune response to TB provides many opportunities for the discovery and development of diagnostically useful biomarkers of infection.

An essential component of the response to *M. tuberculosis* infection in mice and humans is the production of IFN-γ by T helper 1 (Th1) CD4 T cells (Cooper and Torrado, 2012). Immune deficiencies affecting CD4 T cells and IL-12/IFN-γ/STAT1 signaling pathways result in more severe disease in TB-infected individuals (Cooper *et al.*, 2007; Diedrich and Flynn, 2011). As such, it is not surprising that IFN-γ and delayed-type hypersensitivity (DTH) responses are useful correlates of infection for bovine TB (reviewed by Schiller *et al.*, 2010 for cattle and Walzl *et al.*, 2011 for humans). For diagnostic purposes in cattle, IFN-γ responses are generally measured in whole blood cultures for convenience and after overnight (i.e. 16–24 hour) stimulation with antigen (i.e. IFN-γ release assay, IGRA). Measure of IFN-γ by peripheral blood mononuclear cells (PBMCs) in long-term cultures (i.e. ~14 days) is also useful as a measure of vaccine-elicited protection (Whelan *et al.*, 2008b). For instance, BCG alone or in combination with viral-vectored subunit vaccines elicit long-term cultured IFN-γ responses that correlate with reduced colonization and severity of tuberculous lesions upon subsequent challenge with virulent *M. bovis* (Vordermeier *et al.*, 2009; Waters *et al.*, 2009). Recent studies have demonstrated that the responding cells within these long-term cultures are primarily CD4$^+$ central memory T cells (Blunt *et al.*, 2015; Maggioli *et al.*, 2015b). Thus, contingent on the type of assay performed, a measure of IFN-γ responses is valuable both as a surrogate of infection and protection. Additional host biomarkers beyond IFN-γ have also emerged as potential candidates for use in blood-based TB tests for humans (reviewed by Walzl *et al.*, 2011; Salgame *et al.*, 2015) and cattle (e.g. IL-1β, IL-2, TNF-α, nitric oxide, IP-10, IL-17 and IL-22) (Waters *et al.*, 2003, 2012; Vordermeier *et al.*, 2009; Jones *et al.*, 2010a; Blanco *et al.*, 2011, 2013; Bhuju *et al.*, 2012; Rhodes *et al.*, 2014; Goosen *et al.*, 2015).

12.3 Current Ante-mortem Testing Schemes

A major impediment for the control of bovine TB is the relatively poor accuracy of current ante-mortem tests compounded by difficulties in the ability to reliably detect tuberculous lesions and the agent (primarily *M. bovis*) in all infected animals due, in part, to the focal nature of the disease. For instance, the accuracy of tuberculin skin test (TST) ranges from

52–100% (sensitivity) and 55–99% (specificity) contingent on the type of TST applied, interpretation criteria, study population, prevalence and other factors (de la Rua-Domenech et al., 2006; Schiller et al., 2010; Bezos et al., 2014). Particularly in countries with a low prevalence of bovine TB, traditional slaughter inspection has a low sensitivity for detection of tuberculous cattle (e.g. <20% in Australia in the 1980s [Corner et al., 1990], 31.4% in Catalonia, Spain [Garcia-Saenz et al., 2015] and 28.5% in Texas, USA [Chioino, 2003; APHIS, 2009]). Even with enhanced inspection, visual detection of tuberculous lesions at post mortem is seldom greater than 60% (Corner et al., 1990; Buddle et al., 2015). For these reasons, the determination of bovine TB test accuracy is difficult, especially in countries with a low prevalence of disease in which TB-affected herds are scarce.

Specific applications for ante-mortem bovine TB testing currently include routine surveillance to identify TB-affected herds, movement tests, epidemiologic trace-back testing resulting from detection of a tuberculous carcass at slaughter, and in TB-affected herds to delineate animals going to a slaughter plant (test negative) versus being condemned for rendering (test positive). While a few new tests have emerged (Bezos et al., 2014), TST and IGRAs remain as the principal tests used in bovine TB control programmes. The intradermal TST may be applied as a single injection of M. bovis purified protein derivative (PPD) in the caudal fold or at the base of the tail (i.e. caudal fold test, CFT) or in the mid-cervical region (i.e. single intradermal test, SIT). A major confounding variable for use of M. bovis PPD alone for skin test is that test specificity is often jeopardized by prior exposure to ubiquitous non-tuberculous Mycobacteria species. Thus, a comparative test may be applied in which Mycobacterium avium-derived PPD and M. bovis-derived PPD are delivered at adjacent sites on the neck (designated as either comparative cervical test [CCT] or single intradermal comparative cervical test [SICCT]). The CFT is currently used as a primary test for cattle in the southern hemisphere and North America, whereas the SICCT is used as the primary test in the UK and Ireland. The SIT is used in many countries in continental Europe. To improve specificity, CCT and/or IGRAs may be used as secondary tests (i.e. as a follow-up to CFT or SIT), thereby reducing the number of animals falsely identified as TB-infected by the primary test. In known-infected herds, IGRAs may also be used in parallel with a skin test for prioritization of animal removal and for decision making on which animals may be sent to slaughter as likely non-infected, thereby salvaging value for the farmer and reducing indemnity costs for regulatory agencies. While approved by the OIE for use as a primary test, IGRAs are currently not routinely used as a primary test (Bezos et al., 2014). Further details on TST and IGRAs and their specific applications in bovine TB control programmes are provided in recent reviews of the subject (de la Rua-Domenech et al., 2006; Schiller et al., 2010; Bezos et al., 2014; Buddle et al., 2015).

Tuberculins, including PPDs, are a poorly defined and complex mix of proteins, lipids and carbohydrates of inherently poor specificity as many of the compounds within PPDs are antigenically cross-reactive amongst the various mycobacterial species. Given the complex nature of PPDs, standardization and potency evaluation of various lots for use in TST and IGRAs is difficult (Bakker et al., 2005; Good et al., 2011). PPD potency is routinely evaluated in guinea pigs by comparison to an international standard using a multiple comparative skin test; however, these results may not correlate to a similar potency in cattle (Dobbelaer et al., 1983; Good et al., 2011). Tuberculin activity may also be evaluated with blood samples from M. bovis-infected or sensitized cattle by comparison of activity in serial dilutions of PPDs using IGRAs to determine the relative potency 30 (RP30) defined as 'the protein concentration (µg/ml) or as activity (iu/ml) of a given PPD needed to obtain 30 per cent of the response (RP30) of the peak value of a reference PPD (OD_{max})' (Schiller et al., 2010). Potencies of PPDs may also be evaluated in DTH assays (in vivo) in cattle, although this approach is cumbersome due to the requirement of costly experimental infection studies or access to naturally infected cattle. While a combination of guinea pig and cattle testing for PPD potency in comparison to international standards is optimal (OIE, 2009), PPD potency testing in cattle is rarely conducted due to costs and logistical demands (Bezos et al., 2014).

12.4 Application of Specific Antigens for use in TST and IGRAs for Diagnostic Purposes and as a DIVA Strategy

Extensive studies have been carried out over the past 20 years to discover and develop specific antigens for use in TSTs and IGRAs, as well as a means to differentiate infected from vaccinated animals (DIVA) (reviewed by Schiller *et al.*, 2010; Vordermeier *et al.*, 2011; Bezos *et al.*, 2014). Specific antigens may be used in place of PPDs or in addition to PPDs (i.e. side-by-side tests), particularly with IGRAs (Andersen *et al.*, 2000). While numerous antigens have been evaluated, ESAT-6 and CFP10 are currently considered the most immunodominant antigens both for CMI-based tests and as DIVA reagents with BCG-based vaccines (Anderson *et al.*, 2000; Pollock *et al.*, 2001; Vordermeier *et al.*, 2001). Pollock and Andersen were the first to demonstrate the diagnostic potential of recombinant ESAT-6 in IGRAs in cattle (Pollock and Andersen, 1997a) and improved accuracy using recombinant ESAT-6 and CFP10 in combination (van Pinxteren *et al.*, 2000). The same group then showed the potential, with limitations, for use of ESAT-6 protein as a skin-test reagent in cattle (Pollock *et al.*, 2003). Later, it was demonstrated that ESAT-6 along with MPB64 and MPB83 elicits IFN-γ responses in *M. bovis*-infected but not BCG-vaccinated cattle (Vordermeier *et al.*, 1999, 2000), and, importantly, peptides of ESAT-6 and CFP10 can be used as antigens in IGRAs (Vordermeier *et al.*, 2001). Further, addition of peptides from other *M. bovis* antigens (e.g. Rv3873, Rv3879c, Rv0288, and Rv3019c [Cockle *et al.*, 2006] or Rv3615c [Sidders *et al.*, 2008; Casal *et al.*, 2012]) improved the sensitivity of ESAT-6/CFP10-based IGRAs. One caveat to using an ESAT-6/CFP10 approach, however, is the potential, albeit uncommon, for cross-reactivity of ESAT-6 and CFP10 peptides with *Mycobacterium kansasii* homologues, thereby confounding interpretation of the test in animals infected with or sensitized to *M. kansasii* (Vordermeier *et al.*, 2007). With that said, infection/sensitization with *M. kansasii* may confound interpretation of PPD-based tests as well (Waters *et al.*, 2006a).

The elucidation of the genome of a number of mycobacterial species including *M. tuberculosis*, *M. bovis*, BCG and *M. avium* subsp. *paratuberculosis* over the last two decades has allowed a more rational approach to mine for antigens recognized by bovine T cells (see section 12.5 for more details on approaches). However, the approaches taken were not unbiased, as a number of hypotheses were tested. For example, antigen prioritization strategies involved listing potential antigens due to their expression levels, whether they were predicted to be secreted or were likely to be induced by hypoxia. These approaches have been recently reviewed in a detailed manuscript (Vordermeier *et al.*, 2016). The leading candidates coming out of these antigen-mining activities at present for antigens for diagnostic and DIVA applications are ESAT-6/CFP10/Rv3615c +/− Rv3020c for use in both TST and IGRAs (Sidders *et al.*, 2008; Whelan *et al.*, 2010a; Vordermeier *et al.*, 2011; Jones *et al.*, 2012). Antigen preparations may include recombinant proteins or overlapping peptides. A potential concern with this approach is the relatively high cost of antigen production, particularly for use as a skin-test reagent requiring ~30 mg/dose; however, applying economy of scale will reduce costs considerably to a degree comparable to that of tuberculin. Chen *et al.* (2014) and Parlane *et al.* (2015) have recently developed a low cost and high production method to produce polyester beads displaying ESAT-6/CFP10/Rv3615c +/− Rv3020c proteins on the surface in a spherical design that theoretically enhances antigen uptake and presentation by antigen presenting cells. These antigens could be used in TST, IGRA or other CMI-based tests. The high output method of production for these beads displaying antigen is of particular benefit for regulatory release of large batches of product. Initial trials using ESAT-6/CFP10/Rv3615c +/− Rv3020c as recombinant proteins, peptide cocktails or as displayed on polyester beads are encouraging and further studies are underway in several countries (e.g. New Zealand, UK and USA) to better determine the accuracy and practicality of this approach in the field with both IGRA and TST assays.

12.5 Antigen-Mining Strategies for Discovery of Additional Specific Antigens of Diagnostic Use

12.5.1 Mapping diagnostic antigens

One of the main tasks of TB diagnostic test development is the identification (mining) of strong and specific antigens recognized by T cells from tuberculous animals (infected mainly, but not exclusively, with *M. bovis*) but not from individuals sensitized by environmental mycobacterial species, *M. avium* subsp. *paratuberculosis* or BCG (if vaccination is being considered). A number of empirical approaches have been applied that led to the discovery of the antigens introduced in section 12.4 (e.g. ESAT-6, CFP-10, Rv3615c, Rv3020c and others) and we will discuss these approaches in this section.

12.5.2 Hypothesis-driven approaches to antigen mining

The elucidation of the genomes for relevant mycobacterial species (including *M. bovis* [Garnier et al., 2003], *M. tuberculosis* [Cole et al., 1998], *M. bovis* BCG [Brosch et al., 2007], *M. avium* subsp. *avium* and *M. avium* subsp. *paratuberculosis* [Li et al., 2005]) and the advent of microarray technology has revolutionized antigen-mining strategies. The following paragraphs summarize the most widely applied of these approaches.

Comparative genomic analysis

Comparative genomic analysis has been used to identify *M. bovis* genes that are deleted from the genome of BCG (either as individual gene deletions or present in deleted gene regions, the so-called RD regions), or that contain mutations resulting in either truncations or modified amino acid sequences after frame-shifting. (Pollock and Andersen 1997a, 1997b; Ravn et al., 1999; van Pinxteren et al., 2000; Vordermeier et al., 2001). Thus, antigens such as ESAT-6 and CFP-10 have the capacity to differentiate *M. bovis*-infected cattle from BCG-vaccinated cattle (Buddle et al., 1999; Vordermeier et al., 1999, 2001). The DIVA potential of other gene products encoded in the RD1 region and other regions (RD2 and RD14) deleted from the BCG genome (Garnier et al., 2003; Brosch et al., 2007) has also been assessed (Cockle et al., 2002, 2006) but none of the antigens identified in these studies complemented ESAT-6 and CFP-10 in increasing overall test sensitivity in cattle. Thus, alternative approaches to comparative genomic analysis were needed to identify potential DIVA antigens to complement ESAT-6/CFP-10 and increase overall test sensitivity.

Comparative transcriptome analysis

This approach has been used to explore the link between gene-expression levels and antigenicity. *M. tuberculosis* and *M. bovis* gene products that were consistently expressed at high levels under a variety of culture conditions (known as the abundant invariome) (Sidders et al., 2007) were tested in cattle. These studies identified one antigen, Rv3615c, which was recognized by a significant proportion of infected animals but not in BCG vaccinates (Sidders et al., 2008). Furthermore, Rv3615c responses were detected in a proportion of cattle not detected by ESAT-6/CFP-10 (i.e. Rv3615c complemented ESAT-6/CFP-10 to increase overall test sensitivity; Sidders et al., 2008).

Bacterial cell biology

In TB research, it has long been held that secretion of antigenic proteins by mycobacteria induces strong cellular immune responses in the host. To identify potential DIVA reagents, 119 *M. bovis* proteins predicted to be secreted were screened in infected cattle and BCG vaccinates (Jones et al., 2010b, 2010c). These studies confirmed the immune dominance of members of the ESAT-6 protein family (Jones et al., 2010b). The ESAT-6 family member Rv3020c, associated with the esx-3 secretion site, showed DIVA potential in cattle (Jones et al., 2010c). However, subsequent evaluation of these proteins in a larger cohort of infected animals failed to demonstrate complementation of the ESAT-6/

CFP-10 and Rv3615c reagents (Jones and Vordermeier, unpublished data).

12.5.3 Non-biased genome-wide approaches

We have over the past 15 years assessed the immunogenicity of 626 *M. bovis*/*M. tuberculosis*-derived proteins, either in the form of recombinant proteins or, more frequently, as overlapping sets of synthetic peptides. The high-throughput readout system to generate these data was the blood-based IGRA introduced in previous sections of this review. This analysis allowed us to define antigenicity in infected cattle based on the frequency a particular antigen was recognized (responder frequency). As shown in Fig. 12.1, a response hierarchy could be established in this manner ranging from no recognition (responder frequency = 0%) to frequencies of around 90% (Fig. 12.1). When the results were stratified according to protein functionality or membership of particular protein families, we could confirm the dominance of ESAT-6-family members, predicted secreted proteins and members of the PE/PPE families (Vordermeier and Jones, unpublished data). However, the studies, while contributing to populate our response hierarchy (Fig. 12.1), as well as earlier and more empirical approaches, were not unbiased as they depended on an underlying assumption on what rendered a protein immunogenic, such as being secreted, highly expressed or being a PE or PPE protein. Therefore, it is to date not possible to conclude fully that particular functionalities of proteins can be related to their immunogenicity. Thus, unbiased, proteome-wide immunogenicity mapping to define the T-cell antigenome of *M. bovis* in cattle would be highly beneficial to provide a platform to rationally explore the specificity of immunogenic proteins.

An unbiased approach taken towards this goal was to prepare proteins based on a Gateway library from *M. tuberculosis* and to screen these proteins with blood from infected or uninfected cattle using IGRA (Jones et al., 2013). In this approach, however, protein quality (e.g. purity) had to be de-prioritized in favour of quantity. While this study lead to the identification of potential new subunit vaccine candidates (Jones et al., 2013), it also highlighted several limitations of this approach, namely, that due to low purity, the cut-off for classifying a positive response had to be increased to mitigate against false-positive responses, which in turn most likely resulted in potential antigens being missed out due to the decreased sensitivity of the readout system. This system was also not able to produce a library of proteins that covered the whole proteome within a reasonable period and protein amounts required for T-cell screening.

Recently, an alternative approach was applied to human TB, namely the combination of robust computational methods to predict proteome-wide peptides binding to human HLA molecules combined with high throughput peptide synthesis and ELISPOT-based T-cell assays. The study by the group of Sette (Lindestam Arlehamn et al., 2013) established an immunological footprint of *M. tuberculosis* CD4 T-cell recognition, thereby demonstrating that $CXCR3^+$/$CCR6^+$ memory T cells are highly focused in their recognition towards three immunodominant antigenic islands mapping to ESAT-6 family members associated esx secretion systems (Lindestam Arlehamn et al., 2013). To implement a similar strategy for cattle depends on the availability of similarly robust bovine MHC class

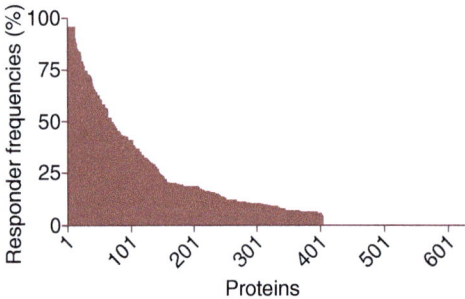

Fig. 12.1. Hierarchy of T-cell responses to 626 *M. bovis*/*M. tuberculosis* proteins. Results are shown as responder frequencies (proportion of tested animals responding to a given protein). Responses were established using whole blood cultures from *M. bovis*-infected cattle to measure antigen-specific IFN-γ responses.

II (BoLA) binding prediction algorithms, which are not available to date to cover MHC diversity in cattle compared to the human or murine systems. We have used, with moderate success, a method to predict human HLA binding proteins (ProPred) (Vordermeier et al., 2003), or a BoLA DRB3 structure-based prediction method (Hepitom) (Jones et al., 2011) to predict bovine promiscuously recognized peptides (i.e. peptides recognized in the context of multiple BoLA class II alleles). However, the accuracy of either method, particularly in respect to the specificity of detecting promiscuously recognized peptides was not optimal, requiring impractically large peptide sets to cover the whole proteome (Jones et al., 2011). Nevertheless, better prediction methods are under development and it is highly likely that such genome-wide mapping studies can soon be undertaken to define the *M. bovis* T-cell antigenome in cattle.

12.5.4. Predicting specificity

While predicting antigenicity or immunogenicity is a challenge, so is the prediction of antigens that are specific for *M. bovis*. The absence of a particular protein within a genome (e.g. antigens encoded on gene regions deleted from the BCG genome compared to *M. bovis*) does not guarantee specificity as the areas of cross-reactivity can be harboured within short stretches (<10–20 amino acid residues long) within an antigen that can be shared with other, otherwise undeleted antigens (Cockle et al., 2002). The actual amino acid differences between a peptide being 'specific' or 'cross-reactive' can be minute and unpredictable, as was shown for peptides from highly homologous PE or PPE proteins (Vordermeier et al., 2012). However, not surprisingly, the fewer identical or homologous amino acids located within an epitopic region of a peptide, the higher the chance of it being specific (Vordermeier et al., 2012). This highlights not only the possibility of selecting individual specific peptides out of otherwise cross-reactive proteins (Jones et al., 2010), but also the need for continued 'wet' experimental immunological investigation of cross-reactivity and specificity.

12.6 Biomarkers: Promising Candidates and Alternative Approaches

12.6 Emerging biomarkers for CMI-based assays beyond IFN-γ

Numerous biomarkers beyond IFN-γ are being evaluated for use in the immunodiagnosis of *M. tuberculosis* infection of humans (reviewed by Chegou et al., 2014). As mentioned in the immunopathogenesis section (section 12.3), several cytokines and chemokines have been identified as biomarkers of *M. bovis* infection as well as surrogates of protection in response to vaccination in cattle. Of these, Th-17-associated cytokines are attractive as multiple studies have implicated cytokines from this T-cell subset in both protective responses elicited by vaccination and/or responses associated with lesion severity after *M. bovis* infection in cattle (Vordermeier et al., 2009; Blanco et al., 2011, 2013; Aranday-Cortes et al., 2012; Bhuju et al., 2012; Rizzi et al., 2012; Shu et al., 2014; Waters et al., 2015a). Indeed, using RNA-seq followed by RT-qPCR, we have recently demonstrated that Th17-related cytokine genes (i.e. IL-17A, IL-17F, IL-22, IL-19, and IL-27) follow similar kinetics and levels as compared to IFN-γ in the response to BCG vaccination and subsequent infection with virulent *M. bovis* (Waters et al., 2015a). Using ELISA to measure protein, the IL-17A and IFN-γ responses were highly correlated and exhibited similar diagnostic capacity. Also, reduced IL-17A responses by BCG vaccinates (i.e. exhibiting significant protection upon necropsy) at 2.5 weeks after *M. bovis* challenge correlated with reduced disease burden. Thus, measure of Th17-associated cytokines may also be useful both as a biomarker of infection and as a surrogate of protection in the immune response to bovine TB.

Other biomarkers for measure of CMI responses (e.g. IL-2, IP-10, IL-1β, TNF-α, and nitric oxide) have also been evaluated for diagnostic applications in cattle, although only in proof of principle studies (Waters et al., 2003, 2012; Jones et al., 2010a; Rhodes et al., 2014). Rhodes et al. (2014) demonstrated that IL-2 responses to ESAT-6/CFP10 or PPD are detectable in whole blood assays after infection with virulent *M. bovis* but not after vaccination with

BCG, thereby affording an ability to differentiate infected from non-infected or BCG-vaccinated animals (Rhodes et al., 2014). In a systematic meta-analysis on the diagnosis of latent M. tuberculosis infection of humans, it was determined that use of IL-2 release assays provides some benefit, particularly when combined with IGRAs (Mamishi et al., 2014). Soluble IL-2 receptor-alpha is also released in PBMC culture supernatants after mycobacterial antigen stimulation in M. bovis-infected cattle, and may have potential as a biomarker of infection (Nualláin et al., 1997).

There is also considerable interest in use of IP-10 (IFN-γ-induced protein 10 or CXCL10) as a diagnostic biomarker of M. tuberculosis infection in humans as measured in sera, urine, or antigen-stimulated cultures (Chegou et al., 2014; Tonby et al., 2015). Similarly, IP-10 has shown promise as a biomarker of M. bovis infection in cattle (Waters et al., 2012) and African buffaloes (Syncerus caffer) (Goosen et al., 2015). One potential concern with use of IP-10 as a specific marker of infection is that this chemokine is often produced in large quantities as a result of inflammation or due to various infections resulting in high levels of IP-10 in sera; thus, while IP-10 has shown promise for diagnostic purposes and to monitor antimicrobial therapy with M. tuberculosis infection in humans (Tonby et al., 2015), it may also be falsely elevated in response to other infections or inflammatory conditions (Waters et al., 2012; Clifford et al., 2015), thereby confounding interpretation of agent-specific assays using IP-10 as a readout. Antibodies for detection of numerous bovine cytokines and chemokines are increasingly being developed and becoming readily available through multiple commercial companies. Thus, further studies will be warranted to evaluate the clinical and diagnostic potential of emerging immune markers as related to bovine TB.

Multi-parameter readouts of CMI responses have also shown diagnostic potential with both bovine and human TB (Jones et al., 2010a; Tebruegge et al., 2015). Using a multi-parameter approach, Tebruegge et al. (2015) demonstrated that combinations of TNF-α/IL-1Rα and TNF-α/IL-10 correctly classified latent versus active TB in 95.5% and 100% of cases in children, respectively. While numerous cytokines were evaluated and there was considerable overlap between treatment groups for the majority of cytokines, the use of IP-10, TNF-α and IL-2 achieved a high level of accuracy in the distinction between TB-infected versus non-infected humans in this study (Tebruegge et al., 2015). With bovine TB, Jones et al. (2010a) demonstrated that the combined use of IL-1β, TNF-α, and IFN-γ in response to ESAT-6/CFP10 increased the sensitivity of the assay by 11% as compared to use of IFN-γ alone; however, there was a concomitant decrease in specificity by 14% (Jones et al., 2010a). Thus, balancing gains in sensitivity must be balanced by the potential for loss in specificity when using multi-parameter approaches. Interestingly, in the Jones et al. (2010a) study, applying only IFN-γ and IL-1β in parallel increased the sensitivity of the assay by 5% without a loss in specificity. Multi-parameter approaches may be particularly useful for 'test-and-removal' applications in which identification of all infected animals is a priority over specificity of the assay, as use of multiple parameters may increase the odds over detecting a response to a single parameter. However, the overall costs of multiple parameter test applications will have to be balanced against their benefit in control programmes. A potential pitfall of the multi-parameter approach is that variables such as co-infection with other pathogens (e.g.; parasites [Flynn et al., 2009]), age of the animal (i.e. non-specific production of cytokine by NK cells in young animals [Olsen et al., 2005]), and stage of the disease may be amplified by use of multiple versus single readout tests.

12.6.2 Whole blood assays and 'in-tube' strategies

Whole blood assays for the detection of IFN-γ responses to TB have been used in cattle for over 25 years (i.e. Bovigam [Rothel et al., 1990]) and humans for almost 20 years (i.e. Quantiferon [Streeton et al., 1998]). A limitation of the initial Quantiferon assay for humans was the requirement for shipment of blood samples to a laboratory for transfer of the blood to vessels (i.e. tubes, microtiter plates, etc.) for antigen stimulation. Thus, there was a requirement for easily accessible satellite laboratories to process the sample in a timely manner. The 'in-tube' approach for immediate antigen stimulation partially resolved this limitation with the third generation of the Quantiferon assay (Mahomed et al., 2006). Similar approaches, while in development, are not currently available for use with samples from cattle. Particularly in large countries with diverse environmental conditions and shipping networks, improved methods to assure sample viability are critical for the continued use of CMI-based tests requiring live and fully functional leukocytes. The variability in sample conditions associated with shipment in many countries (e.g. hot or cold conditions within aeroplane cargo holds, physical turbulence of the container, and time to antigen stimulation) adversely impacts the reliability of the Bovigam assay. An 'in-tube' approach including use of portable field-ready incubators could remedy this pitfall. For instance, the stimulation phase could be initiated in the field and samples sent to satellite laboratories for plasma harvest after the necessary incubation time. Then, stimulated plasma samples could be either sent to regional laboratories or simply analysed at the satellite laboratory for IFN-γ or other biomarkers within the samples. Once the logistical and technical hurdles are overcome, an 'in-tube' approach for immediate antigen stimulation may prove particularly useful for assays that are less robust than IGRAs and/or assays that utilize multi-parameter readouts.

While whole blood assays have greatly improved the convenience and technical compatibility of CMI-based tests for diagnostic laboratories, detection of biomarkers within the sample continues to require laboratory-based assays such as ELISA or ELISPOT. Thus, development of point-of-care assays for use in the field could prove useful for animal/patient-side applications and for remote locales. Indeed, user-friendly lateral flow assays for the detection of IP-10 and CCL4 in antigen-stimulated whole blood samples from humans, including ambient shipping/storage of reagents and lightweight stand-alone readers, are in development for use in remote and resource-limited settings (Corstjens et al., 2016). In addition, biomarker detection from dried blood spots on filter paper is another technology applicable for field use (reviewed by Chegou et al., 2014), as demonstrated by Skogstrand et al. (2012) in proof of concept studies using a Luminex-based assay.

Once host biomarker signatures of TB infection are validated, similar approaches could be used for humans and cattle.

12.6.3 Alternative approaches including flow cytometry and gene-expression profiling

Novel methods for detecting CMI responses are also being explored for diagnostic purposes. For instance, flow cytometric-based tests are in development for the diagnosis of TB in humans (reviewed by Rovina et al., 2013). Specifically, flow cytometry approaches may be used to determine cytokine production, phenotype/activation marker status of responding cells, polyfunctionality and immunosuppressive markers – all of which are useful for clinical and diagnostic applications. With cattle, El-Naggar et al. (2015) recently demonstrated the utility of a flow cytometric-based assay to detect M. bovis PPD- and ESAT-6/CFP10-specific intracellular IFN-γ responses by naturally infected cattle. For this assay, whole blood stimulation also included use of monoclonal antibodies specific for bovine CD28 and CD49d as co-stimulatory molecules to improve the capacity of lymphocytes to respond to specific antigen. Use of co-stimulatory molecules and measurement of intracellular IFN-γ reduced the stimulation phase of the assay from 18 hours to 6 hours. Downsides to this approach are the requirement for flow cytometry instrumentation and expertise, as well as the necessity of immediate delivery of samples to a laboratory for cell viability assurance. Use of an 'in-tube' approach in which both antigens and co-stimulatory molecules are contained in the blood collection vessel may improve the convenience of the assay; however, samples would still need to be delivered within 2 hours to the laboratory for initiation of the intracellular cytokine staining protocol. Clinical use of flow cytometry is rapidly increasing in hospitals for use in infectious, neoplastic, hematologic and immune deficiency disorders; thus, improvements in this approach are on the horizon.

Another tactic for measure of CMI responses for diagnostic applications is to evaluate expression (i.e. mRNA typically using RT-qPCR) of cytokines and chemokines in response to antigen stimulation. Kasprowicz et al. (2011) demonstrated the diagnostic potential of this approach by evaluating monokine-induced by IFN-γ (MIG) and IP-10 responses to ESAT-6/CFP10 by leukocytes in whole blood samples from humans in response to HIV, cytomegalovirus, and TB infection. In regard to TB diagnosis, the mRNA response correlated with the *ex vivo* ELISPOT protein response and, importantly, the assay could be performed with small volumes of whole blood. With cattle, global gene-expression studies have defined numerous candidate biomarkers, particularly in the context of protective versus non-protective responses to BCG vaccination (Bhuju et al., 2012). Of these, genes encoding IL-22, IFN-γ, the zinc metallothionein MT-3, IL-13 and CCL3 were strongly up-regulated in response to PPD in vaccinated and protected versus vaccinated and non-protected calves. Functional analysis of the RNA-seq data indicated that the most significantly modulated network of expression was the cytokine-to-cytokine receptor interaction pathway. These studies, as well as other unpublished results in our laboratories, provide numerous candidate markers for further validation by follow-up RT-qPCR and, if available, protein assays (e.g. Th17-associated genes [Waters et al., 2015a]).

Evaluation of gene expression in non-stimulated blood cells may also be used to identify candidate biomarkers to discriminate active versus latent TB and risk for recurrent disease (Jacobsen et al., 2007; Maertzdorf et al., 2011; Mihret et al., 2014). With this approach, TB can also be distinguished from other pulmonary diseases such as sarcoidosis, pneumonias and lung cancers using transcriptional signatures of blood leukocytes from humans (Bloom et al., 2013). Most recently, Jenum et al. (2016) identified a host biomarker signature consisting of *BPI, CD3E, CD14, FPR1, IL4, TGFBR2, TIMP2* and *TNFRSF1B* that differentiated children with active TB from asymptomatic siblings. Signatures associated with a tendency towards active disease consisted of *FCGR1A, FPR1, MMP9, RAB24, TNFRSF1A* and *TIMP2*, whereas *BLR1, CD8A, IL7R* and *TGFBR2* were associated with a decreased likelihood of TB-associated disease in this population, thereby providing useful information for the clinical management of TB in children. This approach is particularly appealing as it does not require an antigen-stimulation phase. Thus, immune markers are measured directly from blood leukocytes. Using global gene expression, Zak et al. (2016) recently identified a gene signature predictive of development of active TB. The signature predicted disease development with a sensitivity/specificity of 66.1%/80.6%, respectively. In addition to mRNA, micro RNAs (miRNA) expressed in the blood of infected patients have been explored for the development of improved diagnostic tests and to distinguish active versus latent TB as well as to distinguish HIV co-infection from other pulmonary diseases (Miotto et al., 2013). Using a bovine microRNA microarray, Golby et al. (2014) demonstrated that miR-155 is a potentially useful biomarker of *M. bovis* infection as well as a prognostic marker (in regard to protective BCG vaccination) to identify animals with advanced pathology.

While biomarker discovery studies have traditionally utilized transcriptomics, other approaches such as evaluation of the proteome and epigenome are also being developed to define markers associated with clinical stages of TB in humans (Esterhuyse et al., 2015). In a large study evaluating serum protein markers in HIV$^+$ and HIV$^-$ patients with TB (active versus latent) and other respiratory diseases, Achkar et al. (2015) established that soluble CD14 and SEPP1 were present in TB serum panels from both HIV$^+$ and HIV$^-$ patients. Several other promising candidate biomarkers of TB infection discovered in this study included: GP1BA (pulmonary inflammation); SELL and LUM (leukocyte homing); TNXB, COMP, PEPD and QSOX1 (morphogenesis and extracellular matrix remodeling); and APOC1 (lipid transport and regulation). With cattle, Seth et al. (2009) and Lamont et al. (2014) have identified multiple host proteins in sera associated with *M. bovis* infection of cattle; of which, vitamin D binding protein had the greatest diagnostic potential. Using metabolomics profiling, Lau et al. (2015) identified four metabolites increased in plasma from human TB patients as compared to plasma from community-acquired pneumonia patients and non-affected controls. Thus, emerging technologies will likely prove useful for the discovery of biomarkers of diagnostic relevance for bovine TB.

12.7 Antibody-Based Assays

Antibody-based assays are appealing due to ease and convenience of sample collection, storage and analysis. Until recently, the poor sensitivity of antibody-based tests has prevented widespread development and use of these assays for the diagnosis of TB in cattle (Pollock *et al.*, 2001). Several serologic tests designed to detect antibodies to sero-dominant *M. bovis* antigens (e.g. MPB83, MPB70, ESAT-6 and CFP10) have recently emerged for field validation studies in cattle (Lyashchenko *et al.*, 2000; Whelan *et al.*, 2008a, 2010b; Green *et al.*, 2009; Waters *et al.*, 2011). Indeed, a commercial ELISA to MPB83/MPB70 (*M. bovis* Ab Test, IDEXX Laboratories, Westbrook, Maine; Waters *et al.*, 2011) is approved for use in cattle for bovine TB control programs by the Office International des Epizooties and US Department of Agriculture; however, applications of this test are currently limited to ancillary applications such as confirmation of infection and potentially to detect *M. bovis*-infected cattle anergic to TST. A commercial immunochromatographic test (Dual-Path Platform VetTB Assay, Chembio Diagnostic Systems, Medford, New York; Lyashchenko *et al.*, 2013) is also approved for use in deer and elephants in several countries and may be applied for TB diagnosis in multiple other zoo and alternative livestock species. With serologic tests for bovine TB, injection of PPDs for skin tests significantly boosts antibody responses to specific antigens in *M. bovis*-infected cattle, including animals without detectable antibody responses prior to skin test(s) (Lightbody *et al.*, 1998, 2000; Waters *et al.*, 2006b, 2011; Casal *et al.*, 2014). PPD-boosted antibody responses are targeted to specific antigens (e.g. MPB83 and MPB70) and accompanied by an increase in avidity of antibodies to MPB83/70 (Waters *et al.*, 2015b). Thus, it is generally recommended that serologic tests for bovine TB in cattle be applied after skin test. Recently, Casal *et al.* (2014) demonstrated that use of serology applied after skin test in combination with TST increases the number of tuberculosis-positive animals detected within TB-affected cattle herds as compared to that of skin test alone. Currently, the best promise for developing an improved antibody-based test is the discovery of antigens that are recognized early after infection and preferably without the requirement for injection of PPD for skin test to achieve detectable levels.

It should also be noted that proteome-wide definition of the *M. bovis* B-cell antigenome in cattle still awaits elucidation to a similar degree as the use of protein arrays has been undertaken for *M. tuberculosis* in humans or non-human primates (Kunnath-Velayudhan *et al.*, 2010, 2012). Furthermore, the apparent sero-dominance of antigens such as MPB70 and MPB83 may be due to a bias introduced into antigen screening by using sera from skin-test positive reactors, whose antibody responses are boosted by an application of a prior tuberculin test (as alluded to in the previous paragraph). As MPB83 is the main intact protein that can be demonstrated in bovine PPD by SDS-PAGE and immune-blotting (Whelan and Vordermeier, unpublished data), it is perhaps not surprising that this protein, together with responses to its homologue MPB70, are dominant in bovine TB. Recent data using sera from skin-test negative cattle with confirmed TB (but IGRA-positive) suggest that this is the case. While MPB83 responses were still very frequent, they were less so compared to sera from skin-test positive cattle. By contrast, recognition of less dominant antigens observed in skin-test positive cattle became more frequent using sera from skin-test negative TB cattle (Waters *et al.*, 2017). Thus, we hypothesize that proteome-wide antigen mining for sero-dominant antigens using sera from skin-test negative TB animals could yield additional relevant targets for sero-diagnosis that could increase the sensitivity of serology to detect tuberculous cattle.

12.8 Host Markers in Sera, Urine, Saliva and Other Bodily Fluids

Historically, much of the work on evaluation of pre-formed biomarkers in serum has been limited to evaluation of traditional markers of inflammation such as C-reactive protein, mannose-binding lectin, alpha-1-acid glycoprotein, serum adenosine deaminase, complement components, fibronectin, erythrocyte sedimentation rate, prolidase activity, various cytokines and other commonly measured hematologic parameters (reviewed by Walzl et al., 2011; Thakur et al., 2012; Wallis et al., 2013). Phalane et al. (2013) evaluated a panel of 33 host immunological markers in saliva and sera from TB patients in Cape Town, South Africa. As compared to non-infected subjects, fractalkine, IL-17, IL-6, IL-9, MIP-1β, CRP, VEGF and IL-5 levels in saliva and IL-6, IL-2, SAP and SAA levels in serum were significantly higher in TB patients. Of note, there were large differences between markers in saliva versus sera.

12.9 Conclusions

Over the past 20 years, numerous advances have been made in the discovery and development of antigens and immune biomarkers for potential use in the diagnosis of bovine TB. With that said, only a handful of these antigens (e.g. ESAT-6, CFP10, Rv3615c, MPB83 and MPB70) and none of the biomarkers have been utilized even for limited use in commercial diagnostic tests. Thus, a critical need for the next decade will be to take the next step in immune assay development by critically evaluating novel immune biomarkers/antigens in practical platforms with a wide range of samples from naturally infected cattle for direct comparison to existing official tests (in particular, traditional TST and IGRAs). This next step will likely require collaborations and investment from funding agencies, biologics companies, livestock stakeholders, policymakers, and federal/regional veterinary field staff.

References

Achkar, J.M., Cortes, L., Croteau, P., Yanofsky, C., Mentinova, M., et al. (2015) Host protein biomarkers identify active tuberculosis in HIV uninfected and co-infected individuals. *EBioMedicine* 2(9), 1160–1168.

Andersen, P., Munk, M.E., Pollock, J.M. and Doherty, T.M. (2000) Specific immune-based diagnosis of tuberculosis. *Lancet* 356(9235), 1099–1104.

APHIS (2009) Analysis of Bovine Tuberculosis Surveillance in Accredited Free States. Available at: https://www.aphis.usda.gov/vs/nahss/cattle/tb_2009_evaluation_of_tb_in_accredited_free_states_jan_09.pdf (accessed 1 February 2016).

Aranday-Cortes, E., Hogarth, P.J., Kaveh, D.A., Whelan, A.O., Villarreal-Ramos, B., et al. (2012) Transcriptional profiling of disease-induced host responses in bovine tuberculosis and the identification of potential diagnostic biomarkers. *PLoS One* 7(2), e30626.

Bakker, D., Eger, A., McNair, J., Riepema, K., Willemsen, P.T., et al. (2005) Comparison of commercially available PPDs: practical considerations for diagnosis and control of bovine tuberculosis. *Proceedings of the 4th International Conference on Mycobacterium bovis.* Dublin, August 22 to 26, 2005.

Bezos, J., Casal, C., Romero, B., Schroeder, B., Hardegger, R., et al. (2014) Current ante-mortem techniques for diagnosis of bovine tuberculosis. *Research in Veterinary Science* 97(Suppl), S44–52.

Bhuju, S., Aranday-Cortes, E., Villarreal-Ramos, B., Xing, Z., Singh, M., et al. (2012) Global gene Transcriptome analysis in vaccinated cattle revealed a dominant role of IL-22 for protection against bovine tuberculosis. *PLoS Pathogens* 8(12), e1003077.

Blanco, F.C., Bianco, M.V., Meikle, V., Garbaccio, S., Vagnoni, L., et al. (2011) Increased IL-17 expression is associated with pathology in a bovine model of tuberculosis. *Tuberculosis (Edinburgh)* 91(1), 57–63.

Blanco, F.C., Bianco, M.V., Garbaccio, S., Meikle, V., Gravisaco, M.J., et al. (2013) *Mycobacterium bovis* mce2 double deletion mutant protects cattle against challenge with virulent *M. bovis. Tuberculosis (Edinburgh)* 93(3), 363–372.

Bloom, C.I., Graham, C.M., Berry, M.P., Rozakeas, F., Redford, P.S., et al. (2013) Transcriptional blood signatures distinguish pulmonary tuberculosis, pulmonary sarcoidosis, pneumonias and lung cancers. *PLoS One* 8(8), e70630.

Blunt, L., Hogarth, P.J., Kaveh, D.A., Webb, P., Villarreal-Ramos, B., et al. (2015) Phenotypic characterization of bovine memory cells responding to mycobacteria in IFNγ enzyme linked immunospot assays. *Vaccine* 33(51), 7276–7282.

Brosch, R., Gordon, S.V., Garnier, T., Eiglmeier, K., Frigui, W., *et al.* (2007) Genome plasticity of BCG and impact on vaccine efficacy. *Proceedings of the National Academy of Sciences* USA 104(13), 5596–5601.

Buddle, B.M., Parlane, N.A., Keen, D.L., Aldwell, F.E., Pollock, J.M., *et al.* (1999) Differentiation between *Mycobacterium bovis* BCG-vaccinated and *M. bovis*-infected cattle by using recombinant mycobacterial antigens. *Clinical and Diagnostic Laboratory Immunology* 6(1), 1–5.

Buddle, B.M., de Lisle, G.W., Waters, W.R. and Vordermeier, H.M. (2015) *Diagnosis of Mycobacterium bovis infection in cattle.* In: Mukundan, H., Chambers, M.A., Waters, W.R. and Larsen, M.H. (eds) *Tuberculosis, Leprosy, and Mycobacterial Diseases of Man and Animals: The Many Hosts of Mycobacteria.* CAB International, Wallingford, UK, pp. 168–184.

Casal, C., Bezos, J., Díez-Guerrier, A., Álvarez, J., Romero, B., *et al.* (2012) Evaluation of two cocktails containing ESAT-6, CFP-10 and Rv-3615c in the intradermal test and the interferon-γ assay for diagnosis of bovine tuberculosis. *Preventive Veterinary Medicine* 105, 149–154.

Casal, C., Díez-Guerrier, A., Álvarez, J., Rodriguez-Campos, S., Mateos, A., *et al.* (2014) Strategic use of serology for the diagnosis of bovine tuberculosis after intradermal skin testing. *Veterinary Microbiology* 170, 342–351.

Chegou, N.N., Heyckendorf, J., Walzl, G., Lange, C. and Ruhwald, M. (2014) Beyond the IFN-γ horizon: biomarkers for immunodiagnosis of infection with *Mycobacterium tuberculosis*. *European Respiratory Journal* 43(5), 1472–1486.

Chen, S., Parlane, N.A., Lee, J., Wedlock, D.N., Buddle, B.M., *et al.* (2014) New skin test for detection of bovine tuberculosis based on antigen-displaying polymer inclusions produced by recombinant *Escherichia coli*. *Applied and Environmental Microbiology* 80, 2526–2535.

Chiacchio, T., Petruccioli, E., Vanini, V., Cuzzi, G., Pinnetti, C., *et al.* (2014) Polyfunctional T-cells and effector memory phenotype are associated with active TB in HIV-infected patients. *Journal of Infection* 69(6), 533–545.

Chioino, C. (2003) *Evaluation of U.S. System for Control and Eradication of Tuberculosis in Cattle.* USDA APHIS VS Policy and Planning Division, Riverdale, Maryland.

Clifford, V., Tebruegge, M., Zufferey, C., Germano, S., Denholm, J., *et al.* (2015) Serum IP-10 in the diagnosis of latent and active tuberculosis. *Journal of Infection* 71(6), 696–698.

Cockle, P.J., Gordon, S.V., Lalvani, A., Buddle, B.M., Hewinson, R.G., *et al.* (2002) Identification of novel *Mycobacterium tuberculosis* antigens with potential as diagnostic reagents or subunit vaccine candidates by comparative genomics. *Infection and Immunity* 70(12), 6996–7003.

Cockle, P.J., Gordon, S.V., Hewinson, R.G. and Vordermeier, H.M. (2006) Field evaluation of a novel differential diagnostic reagent for detection of *Mycobacterium bovis* in cattle. *Clinical and Vaccine Immunology* (10), 1119–1124.

Cole, S.T., Brosch, R., Parkhill, J., Garnier, T., Churcher, C., *et al.* (1998) Deciphering the biology of *Mycobacterium tuberculosis* from the complete genome sequence. *Nature* 393(6685), 537–544.

Cooper, A.M. and Torrado, E. (2012) Protection versus pathology in tuberculosis: recent insights. *Current Opinions in Immunology* 24(4), 431–437.

Cooper, A.M., Solache, A. and Khader, S.A. (2007) Interleukin-12 and tuberculosis: an old story revisited. *Current Opinions in Immunology* 19(4), 441–447.

Corner, L.A., Melville, L., McCubbin, K., Small, K.J., McCormick, B.S., *et al.* (1990) Efficiency of inspection procedures for the detection of tuberculous lesions in cattle. *Australian Veterinary Journal* 67(11), 389–392.

Corstjens, P.L., Tjon Kon Fat, E.M., de Dood, C.J., van der Ploeg-van Schip, J.J., Franken, K.L., *et al.* (2016) Multi-center evaluation of a user-friendly lateral flow assay to determine IP-10 and CCL4 levels in blood of TB and non-TB cases in Africa. *Clinical Biochemistry* 49(1), 22–31.

Cousins, D.V. and Roberts J.L. (2001) Australia's campaign to eradicate bovine tuberculosis: the battle for freedom and beyond. *Tuberculosis (Edinburgh)* 81(1–2), 5–15.

Day, C.L., Mkhwanazi, N., Reddy, S., Mncube, Z., van der Stok, M., *et al.* (2008) Detection of polyfunctional *Mycobacterium tuberculosis*-specific T cells and association with viral load in HIV-1-infected persons. *Journal of Infectious Diseases* 197(7), 990–999.

Dean, G.S., Clifford, D., Whelan, A.O., Tchilian, E.Z., Beverley, P.C., *et al.* (2015) Protection induced by simultaneous subcutaneous and Endobronchial vaccination with BCG/BCG and BCG/Adenovirus expressing Antigen 85A against *Mycobacterium bovis* in Cattle. *PLoS One* 10(11), e0142270.

de la Rua-Domenech, R., Goodchild, A.T., Vordermeier, H.M., Hewinson, R.G., Christiansen, K.H., *et al.* (2006) Ante mortem diagnosis of tuberculosis in cattle: a review of the tuberculin tests, gamma-interferon assay and other ancillary diagnostic techniques. *Research in Veterinary Science* 81(2), 190–210.

Diedrich, C.R. and Flynn, J.L. (2011) HIV-1/*Mycobacterium tuberculosis* coinfection immunology: how does HIV-1 exacerbate tuberculosis? *Infection and Immunity* 79(4), 1407–1417.

Dobbelaer, R., O'Reilly, L.M., Génicot, A. and Haagsma, J. (1983) The potency of bovine PPD tuberculins in guinea pigs and in tuberculous cattle. *Journal of Biological Standardization* 11(3), 213–220.

El-Naggar, M.M., Abdellrazeq, G.S., Sester, M., Khaliel, S.A., Singh, M., *et al.* (2015) Development of an improved ESAT-6 and CFP-10 peptide-based cytokine flow cytometric assay for bovine tuberculosis. *Comparative Immunology, Microbiology and Infectious Diseases* 42, 1–7.

Esterhuyse, M.M., Weiner, J. 3rd, Caron, E., Loxton, A.G., Iannaccone, M., *et al.* (2015) Epigenetics and proteomics join Transcriptomics in the quest for tuberculosis biomarkers. *MBio* 6(5), e01187–15.

Farnham, M.W., Norby, B., Goldsmith, T.J. and Wells, S.J. (2012) Meta-analysis of field studies on bovine tuberculosis skin tests in United States cattle herds. *Preventive Veterinary Medicine* 103(2–3), 234–242.

Flynn, R.J., Mulcahy, G., Welsh, M., Cassidy, J.P., Corbett, D., *et al.* (2009) Co-Infection of cattle with *Fasciola hepatica* and *Mycobacterium bovis*- immunological consequences. *Transboundary and Emerging Diseases* 56(6–7), 269–274.

Garcia-Saenz, A., Napp, S., Lopez, S., Casal, J. and Allepuz, A. (2015) Estimation of the individual slaughterhouse surveillance sensitivity for bovine tuberculosis in Catalonia (North-Eastern Spain). *Preventive Veterinary Medicine* 121(3–4), 332–337.

Garnier, T., Eiglmeier, K., Camus, J.C., Medina, N., Mansoor, H., *et al.* (2003) The complete genome sequence of *Mycobacterium bovis*. *Proceedings of the National Academy of Sciences* USA 100(13), 7877–7882.

Golby, P., Villarreal-Ramos, B., Dean, G., Jones, G.J. and Vordermeier, M. (2014) MicroRNA expression profiling of PPD-B stimulated PBMC from *M. bovis*-challenged unvaccinated and BCG vaccinated cattle. *Vaccine* 32(44), 5839–5844.

Good, M. and Duignan, A. (2011) Perspectives on the history of bovine TB and the role of Tuberculin in bovine TB eradication. *Veterinary Medicine International* 2011, 410470.

Good, M., Clegg, T.A., Murphy, F. and More, S.J. (2011) The comparative performance of the single intradermal comparative tuberculin test in Irish cattle, using tuberculin PPD combinations from different manufacturers. *Veterinary Microbiology* 151(1–2), 77–84.

Goosen, W.J., Cooper, D., Miller, M.A., van Helden, P.D. and Parsons, S.D. (2015) IP-10 Is a sensitive biomarker of antigen recognition in whole-blood stimulation assays used for the diagnosis of *Mycobacterium bovis* infection in African Buffaloes (*Syncerus caffer*). *Clinical and Vaccine Immunology* 22(8), 974–978.

Green, L.R., Jones, C.C., Sherwood, A.L., Garkavi, I.V., Cangelosi, G.A., *et al.* (2009) Single-antigen serological testing for bovine tuberculosis. *Clinical and Vaccine Immunology* 16, 1309–1313.

Jacobsen, M., Repsilber, D., Gutschmidt, A., Neher, A., Feldmann, K., *et al.* (2007) Candidate biomarkers for discrimination between infection and disease caused by *Mycobacterium tuberculosis*. *Journal of Molecular Medicine (Berlin)* 85, 613–621.

Jenum, S., Dhanasekaran, S., Lodha, R., Mukherjee, A., Kumar Saini, D., *et al.* (2016) Approaching a diagnostic point-of-care test for pediatric tuberculosis through evaluation of immune biomarkers across the clinical disease spectrum. *Scientific Reports* 6, 18520.

Jones, G.J., Pirson, C., Hewinson, R.G. and Vordermeier, H.M. (2010a) Simultaneous measurement of antigen-stimulated interleukin-1 beta and gamma interferon production enhances test sensitivity for the detection of *Mycobacterium bovis* infection in cattle. *Clinical and Vaccine Immunology* 17(12), 1946–1951.

Jones, G.J., Gordon, S.V., Hewinson, R.G. and Vordermeier, H.M. (2010b) Screening of predicted secreted antigens from *Mycobacterium bovis* reveals the immunodominance of the ESAT-6 protein family. *Infection and Immunity* 78(3), 1326–1332.

Jones, G.J., Hewinson, R.G. and Vordermeier, H.M. (2010c) Screening of predicted secreted antigens from *Mycobacterium bovis* identifies potential novel differential diagnostic reagents. *Clinical and Vaccine Immunology* 17(9), 1344–1348.

Jones, G.J., Bagaini, F., Hewinson, R.G. and Vordermeier, H.M. (2011) The use of binding-prediction models to identify *M. bovis*-specific antigenic peptides for screening assays in bovine tuberculosis. *Veterinary Immunology and Immunopathology* 141(3–4), 239–245.

Jones, G.J., Whelan, A., Clifford, D., Coad, M. and Vordermeier, H.M. (2012) Improved skin test for differential diagnosis of bovine tuberculosis by the addition of Rv3020c-derived peptides. *Clinical and Vaccine Immunology* 19(4), 620–622.

Jones, G.J., Khatri, B.L., Garcia-Pelayo, M.C., Kaveh, D.A., Bachy, V.S., et al. (2013) Development of an unbiased antigen-mining approach to identify novel vaccine antigens and diagnostic reagents for bovine tuberculosis. *Clinical and Vaccine Immunology* 20(11), 1675–1682.

Kasprowicz, V.O., Mitchell, J.E., Chetty, S., Govender, P., Huang, K.H., et al. (2011) A molecular assay for sensitive detection of pathogen-specific T-cells. *PLoS One* 6(8), e20606.

Kunnath-Velayudhan, S., Salamon, H., Wang, H.Y., Davidow, A.L., Molina, D.M., et al. (2010) Dynamic antibody responses to the *Mycobacterium tuberculosis* proteome. *Proceedings of the National Academy of Sciences* USA 107(33), 14703–14708.

Kunnath-Velayudhan, S., Davidow, A.L., Wang, H.Y., Molina, D.M., Huynh, V.T., et al. (2012) Proteome-scale antibody responses and outcome of *Mycobacterium tuberculosis* infection in nonhuman primates and in tuberculosis patients. *Journal of Infectious Diseases* 206(5), 697–705.

Lamont, E.A., Janagama, H.K., Ribeiro-Lima, J., Vulchanova, L., Seth, M., et al. (2014) Circulating *Mycobacterium bovis* peptides and host response proteins as biomarkers for unambiguous detection of subclinical infection. *Journal of Clinical Microbiology* 52(2), 536–543.

Lau, S.K., Lee, K.C., Curreem, S.O., Chow, W.N., To, K.K., et al. (2015) Metabolomic profiling of plasma from patients with tuberculosis by use of untargeted mass spectrometry reveals novel biomarkers for diagnosis. *Journal of Clinical Microbiology* 53(12), 3750–3759.

Li, L., Bannantine, J.P., Zhang, Q., Amonsin, A., May, B.J., et al. (2005) The complete genome sequence of *Mycobacterium avium* subspecies *paratuberculosis*. *Proceedings of the National Academy of Sciences* USA 102(35), 12344–12349.

Lightbody, K.A., Skuce, R.A., Neill, S.D. and Pollock, J.M. (1998) Mycobacterial antigen-specific antibody responses in bovine tuberculosis: an ELISA with potential to confirm disease status. *Veterinary Record* 142, 295–300.

Lightbody, K.A., McNair, J., Neill, S.D. and Pollock, J.M. (2000) IgG isotype antibody responses to epitopes of the *Mycobacterium bovis* protein MPB70 in immunised and in tuberculin skin test-reactor cattle. *Veterinary Microbiology* 75, 177–188.

Lindestam Arlehamn, C.S., Gerasimova, A., Mele, F., Henderson, R., Swann, J., et al. (2013) Memory T cells in latent *Mycobacterium tuberculosis* infection are directed against three antigenic islands and largely contained in a CXCR3+CCR6+ Th1 subset. *PLoS Pathogens* 9(1), e1003130.

Lyashchenko, K.P., Singh, M., Colangeli, R. and Gennaro, M.L. (2000) A multi-antigen print immunoassay for the development of serological diagnosis of infectious diseases. *Journal of Immunological Methods* 242, 91–100.

Lyashchenko, K.P., Greenwald, R., Esfandiari, J., O'Brien, D.J., Schmitt, S.M., et al. (2013) Rapid detection of serum antibody by dual-path platform VetTB assay in white-tailed deer infected with *Mycobacterium bovis*. *Clinical and Vaccine Immunology* 20, 907–911.

Maertzdorf, J., Repsilber, D., Parida, S.K., Stanley, K., Roberts, T., et al. (2011) Human gene expression profiles of susceptibility and resistance in tuberculosis. *Genes and Immunity* 12, 15–22.

Maggioli, M., Palmer, M., Whelan, A., Vordermeier, H.M. and Waters, W.R. (2015a) Polyfunctional cytokine responses by central memory CD4+ T cells in response to bovine tuberculosis. *Host Response to Tuberculosis and Granulomas in Infectious and Non-Infectious Disease, Proceedings of Keystone Symposia*, Santa Fe, January 22–27, 2015.

Maggioli, M.F., Palmer, M.V., Thacker, T.C., Vordermeier, H.M. and Waters, W.R. (2015b) Characterization of effector and memory T cell subsets in the immune response to bovine tuberculosis in cattle. *PLoS One* 10(4), e0122571.

Mahomed, H., Hughes, E.J., Hawkridge, T., Minnies, D., Simon, E., et al. (2006) Comparison of mantoux skin test with three generations of a whole blood IFN-gamma assay for tuberculosis infection. *International Journal of Tuberculosis and Lung Disease* 10(3), 310–316.

Mamishi, S., Pourakbari, B., Teymuri, M., Rubbo, P.A., Tuaillon, E., et al. (2014) Diagnostic accuracy of IL-2 for the diagnosis of latent tuberculosis: a systematic review and meta-analysis. *European Journal of Clinical Microbiology and Infectious Diseases* 33(12), 2111–2119.

Maue, A.C., Waters, W.R., Davis, W.C., Palmer, M.V., Minion, F.C., et al. (2005) Analysis of immune responses directed toward a recombinant early secretory antigenic target six-kilodalton protein-culture filtrate protein 10 fusion protein in *Mycobacterium bovis*-infected cattle. *Infection and Immunity* 73(10), 6659–6667.

McGill, J.L., Sacco, R.E., Baldwin, C.L., Telfer, J.C., Palmer, M.V. and Waters, W.R. (2014) Specific recognition of mycobacterial protein and peptide antigens by γδ T cell subsets following infection with virulent *Mycobacterium bovis*. *Journal of Immunology* 192(6), 2756–2769.

Mihret, A., Loxton, A.G., Bekele, Y., Kaufmann, S.H., Kidd, M., *et al.* (2014) Combination of gene expression patterns in whole blood discriminate between tuberculosis infection states. *BMC Infectious Diseases* 14, 257.

Miotto, P., Mwangoka, G., Valente, I.C., Norbis, L., Sotgiu, G., *et al.* (2013) miRNA signatures in sera of patients with active pulmonary tuberculosis. *PLoS One* 8(11), e80149.

More, S.J., Radunz, B. and Glanville, R.J. (2015) Lessons learned during the successful eradication of bovine tuberculosis from Australia. *Veterinary Record* 177(9), 224–232.

Nualláin, E.M., Davis, W.C., Costello, E., Pollock, J.M. and Monaghan, M.L. (1997) Detection of *Mycobacterium bovis* infection in cattle using an immunoassay for bovine soluble interleukin-2 receptor-alpha (sIL-2R-alpha) produced by peripheral blood T-lymphocytes following incubation with tuberculin PPD. *Veterinary Immunology and Immunopathology* 56(1–2), 65–76.

OIE Bovine tuberculosis (2009) *The Tuberculin Test. Manual of Diagnostic Tests and Vaccines for Terrestrial Animals* (6th ed.). OIE, Paris, France, pp. 6–7.

Olsen, I., Boysen, P., Kulberg, S., Hope, J.C., Jungersen, G., *et al.* (2005) Bovine NK cells can produce gamma interferon in response to the secreted mycobacterial proteins ESAT-6 and MPP14 but not in response to MPB70. *Infection and Immunity* 73(9), 5628–5635.

Palmer, M.V., Thacker, T.C. and Waters, W.R. (2015) Analysis of cytokine gene expression using a novel chromogenic *In-situ* hybridization method in pulmonary granulomas of cattle infected experimentally by aerosolized *Mycobacterium bovis*. *Journal of Comparative Pathology* 153, 150–159.

Parlane, N.A., Chen, S., Jones, G.J., Vordermeier, H.M., Wedlock, D.N., *et al.* (2015) Display of antigens on polyester inclusions lowers the antigen concentration required for a bovine tuberculosis skin test. *Clinical and Vaccine Immunology* 23(1), 19–26.

Phalane, K.G., Kriel, M., Loxton, A.G., Menezes, A., Stanley, K., *et al.* (2013) Differential expression of host biomarkers in saliva and serum samples from individuals with suspected pulmonary tuberculosis. *Mediators of Inflammation* 2013, 981984.

Pollock, J.M. and Andersen, P. (1997a) The potential of the ESAT-6 antigen secreted by virulent mycobacteria for specific diagnosis of tuberculosis. *Journal of Infectious Diseases* 175(5), 1251–1254.

Pollock, J.M. and Andersen, P. (1997b) Predominant recognition of the ESAT-6 protein in the first phase of interferon with *Mycobacterium bovis* in cattle. *Infection and Immunity* 65(7), 2587–2592.

Pollock, J.M., Buddle, B.M. and Andersen, P. (2001) Towards more accurate diagnosis of bovine tuberculosis using defined antigens. *Tuberculosis (Edinburgh)* 81(1–2), 65–69.

Pollock, J.M., McNair, J., Bassett, H., Cassidy, J.P., Costello, E., *et al.* (2003) Specific delayed-type hypersensitivity responses to ESAT-6 identify tuberculosis-infected cattle. *Journal of Clinical Microbiology* 41(5), 1856–1860.

Ravn, P., Demissie, A., Eguale, T., Wondwosson, H., Lein, D., *et al.* (1999) Human T cell responses to the ESAT-6 antigen from *Mycobacterium tuberculosis*. *Journal of Infectious Diseases* 179(3), 637–645.

Rhodes, S.G., Buddle, B.M., Hewinson, R.G. and Vordermeier, H.M. (2000) Bovine tuberculosis: immune responses in the peripheral blood and at the site of active disease. *Immunology* 99(2), 195–202.

Rhodes, S.G., McKinna, L.C., Steinbach, S., Dean, G.S., Villarreal-Ramos, B., *et al.* (2014) Use of antigen-specific interleukin-2 to differentiate between cattle vaccinated with *Mycobacterium bovis* BCG and cattle infected with *M. bovis*. *Clinical and Vaccine Immunology* 21(1), 39–45.

Rivière, J., Carabin, K., Le Strat, Y., Hendrikx, P. and Dufour, B. (2014) Bovine tuberculosis surveillance in cattle and free-ranging wildlife in EU Member States in 2013: a survey-based review. *Veterinary Microbiology* 173(3–4), 323–331.

Rizzi, C., Bianco, M.V., Blanco, F.C., Soria, M., Gravisaco, M.J., *et al.* (2012) Vaccination with a BCG strain overexpressing Ag85B protects cattle against *Mycobacterium bovis* challenge. *PLoS One* 7(12), e51396.

Rothel, J.S., Jones, S.L., Corner, L.A., Cox, J.C. and Wood, P.R. (1990) A sandwich enzyme immunoassay for bovine interferon-gamma and its use for the detection of tuberculosis in cattle. *Australian Veterinary Journal* 67(4), 134–137.

Rovina, N., Panagiotou, M., Pontikis, K., Kyriakopoulou, M., Koulouris, N.G., *et al.* (2013) Immune response to mycobacterial infection: lessons from flow cytometry. *Clinical and Developmental Immunology* 2013, 464039.

Salgame, P., Geadas, C., Collins, L., Jones-López, E. and Ellner, J.J. (2015) Latent tuberculosis infection – Revisiting and revising concepts. *Tuberculosis (Edinb)* 95(4), 373–384.

Schiller, I., Oesch, B., Vordermeier, H.M., Palmer, M.V., Harris, B.N., *et al.* (2010) Bovine tuberculosis: a review of current and emerging diagnostic techniques in view of their relevance for disease control and eradication. *Transboundary Emerging Diseases* 57(4), 205–220.

Seth, M., Lamont, E.A., Janagama, H.K., Widdel, A., Vulchanova, L., *et al.* (2009) Biomarker discovery in subclinical mycobacterial infections of cattle. *PLoS One* 4(5), e5478.

Shu, D., Heiser, A., Wedlock, D.N., Luo, D., de Lisle, G.W., *et al.* (2014) Comparison of gene expression of immune mediators in lung and pulmonary lymph node granulomas from cattle experimentally infected with *Mycobacterium bovis*. *Veterinary Immunology and Immunopathology* 160(1–2), 81–89.

Sidders, B., Withers, M., Kendall, S.L., Bacon, J., Waddell, S.J., *et al.* (2007) Quantification of global transcription patterns in prokaryotes using spotted microarrays. *Genome Biology* 8(12), R265.

Sidders, B., Pirson, C., Hogarth, P.J., Hewinson, R.G., Stoker, N.G., *et al.* (2008) Screening of highly expressed mycobacterial genes identifies Rv3615c as a useful differential diagnostic antigen for the *Mycobacterium tuberculosis* complex. *Infection and Immunity* 76(9), 3932–3939.

Skogstrand, K., Thysen, A.H., Jørgensen, C.S., Rasmussen, E.M., Andersen, A.B., *et al.* (2012) Antigen-induced cytokine and chemokine release test for tuberculosis infection using adsorption of stimulated whole blood on filter paper and multiplex analysis. *Scandinavian Journal of Clinical and Laboratory Investigation* 72(3), 204–211.

Streeton, J.A., Desem N. and Jones, S.L. (1998) Sensitivity and specificity of a gamma interferon blood test for tuberculosis infection. *International Journal of Tuberculosis and Lung Disease* 2(6), 443–450.

Tebruegge, M., Dutta, B., Donath, S., Ritz, N., Forbes, B., *et al.* (2015) Mycobacteria-specific cytokine responses detect tuberculosis infection and distinguish latent from active tuberculosis. *American Journal of Respiratory and Critical Care Medicine* 192(4), 485–499.

Thakur, A., Pedersen, L.E. and Jungersen, G. (2012) Immune markers and correlates of protection for vaccine induced immune responses. *Vaccine* 30, 4907–4920.

Tonby, K., Ruhwald, M., Kvale, D. and Dyrhol-Riise, A.M. (2015) IP-10 measured by dry plasma spots as biomarker for therapy responses in *Mycobacterium tuberculosis* infection. *Scientific Reports* 5, 9223.

van Pinxteren, L.A., Ravn, P., Agger, E.M., Pollock, J. and Andersen, P. (2000) Diagnosis of tuberculosis based on the two specific antigens ESAT-6 and CFP10. *Clinical and Diagnostic Laboratory Immunology* 7(2), 155–160.

Vordermeier, H.M., Cockle, P.C., Whelan, A., Rhodes, S., Palmer, N., *et al.* (1999) Development of diagnostic reagents to differentiate between *Mycobacterium bovis* BCG vaccination and *M. bovis* infection in cattle. *Clinical and Diagnostic Laboratory Immunology* 6(5), 675–682.

Vordermeier, H.M., Cockle, P.J., Whelan, A.O., Rhodes, S. and Hewinson, R.G. (2000) Toward the development of diagnostic assays to discriminate between *Mycobacterium bovis* infection and bacille Calmette-Guérin vaccination in cattle. *Clinical Infectious Diseases* 30 (Suppl 3), S291–298.

Vordermeier, H.M., Whelan, A., Cockle, P.J., Farrant, L., Palmer, N., *et al.* (2001) Use of synthetic peptides derived from the antigens ESAT-6 and CFP-10 for differential diagnosis of bovine tuberculosis in cattle. *Clinical and Diagnostic Laboratory Immunology* 8(3), 571–578.

Vordermeier, H.M., Chambers, M.A., Cockle, P.J., Whelan, A.O., Simmons, J., *et al.* (2002) Correlation of ESAT-6-specific gamma interferon production with pathology in cattle following *Mycobacterium bovis* BCG vaccination against experimental bovine tuberculosis. *Infection and Immunity* 70(6), 3026–3032.

Vordermeier, M., Whelan, A.O. and Hewinson, R.G. (2003) Recognition of mycobacterial epitopes by T cells across mammalian species and use of a program that predicts human HLA-DR binding peptides to predict bovine epitopes. *Infection and Immunity* 71(4), 1980–1987.

Vordermeier, H.M., Brown, J., Cockle, P.J., Franken, W.P., Drijfhout, J.W., *et al.* (2007) Assessment of cross-reactivity between *Mycobacterium bovis* and *M. kansasii* ESAT-6 and CFP-10 at the T-cell epitope level. *Clinical and Vaccine Immunology* 14(9), 1203–1209.

Vordermeier, H.M., Villarreal-Ramos, B., Cockle, P.J., McAulay, M., Rhodes, S.G., *et al.* (2009) Viral booster vaccines improve *Mycobacterium bovis* BCG-induced protection against bovine tuberculosis. *Infection and Immunity* 77(8), 3364–3373.

Vordermeier, M., Jones, G.J. and Whelan, A.O. (2011) DIVA reagents for bovine tuberculosis vaccines in cattle. *Expert Reviews of Vaccines* 10(5), 1083–1091.

Vordermeier, H.M., Hewinson, R.G., Wilkinson, R.J., Wilkinson, K.A., Gideon, H.P., *et al.* (2012) Conserved immune recognition hierarchy of mycobacterial PE/PPE proteins during infection in natural hosts. *PLoS One* 7(8), e40890.

Vordermeier, H.M., Jones, G.J., Buddle, B.M., Hewinson, R.G. and Villarreal-Ramos, B. (2016) Bovine tuberculosis in cattle: vaccines, DIVA tests, and host biomarker discovery. *Annual Reviews in Animal Biosciences* 4, 87–109.

Wallis, R.S., Kim, P., Cole, S., Hanna, D., Andrade, B.B., *et al.* (2013) Tuberculosis biomarkers discovery: developments, needs, and challenges. *The Lancet Infectious Diseases* 13, 362–372.

Walzl, G., Ronacher, K., Hanekom, W., Scriba, T.J. and Zumla, A. (2011) Immunological biomarkers of tuberculosis. *Nature Reviews Immunology* 11(5), 343–354.

Waters, W.R. (2015) Bovine Tuberculosis. In: Smith, B.P. (ed.) *Large Animal Internal Medicine – Fifth Edition*, Elsevier, St. Louis, Missouri, USA, pp. 633–636.

Waters, W.R., Palmer, M.V., Whipple, D.L., Carlson, M.P. and Nonnecke, B.J. (2003) Diagnostic implications of antigen-induced gamma interferon, nitric oxide, and tumor necrosis factor alpha production by peripheral blood mononuclear cells from *Mycobacterium bovis*-infected cattle. *Clinical and Diagnostic Laboratory Immunology* 10(5), 960–966.

Waters, W.R., Palmer, M.V., Thacker, T.C., Payeur, J.B., Harris, N.B., *et al.* (2006a) Immune responses to defined antigens of *Mycobacterium bovis* in cattle experimentally infected with *Mycobacterium kansasii*. *Clinical and Vaccine Immunology* 6, 611–619.

Waters, W.R., Palmer, M.V., Thacker, T.C., Bannantine, J.P., Vordermeier, H.M., *et al.* (2006b) Early antibody responses to experimental *Mycobacterium bovis* infection of cattle. *Clinical and Vaccine Immunology* 13, 648–654.

Waters, W.R., Palmer, M.V., Nonnecke, B.J., Thacker, T.C., Scherer, C.F., *et al.* (2009) Efficacy and immunogenicity of *Mycobacterium bovis* DeltaRD1 against aerosol *M. bovis* infection in neonatal calves. *Vaccine* 27(8), 1201–1209.

Waters, W.R., Buddle, B.M., Vordermeier, H.M., Gormley, E., Palmer, M.V., *et al.* (2011) Development and evaluation of an enzyme-linked immunosorbent assay for use in the detection of bovine tuberculosis in cattle. *Clinical and Vaccine Immunology* 18, 1882–1888.

Waters, W.R., Thacker, T.C., Nonnecke, B.J., Palmer, M.V., Schiller, I., *et al.* (2012) Evaluation of gamma interferon (IFN-γ)-induced protein 10 responses for detection of cattle infected with *Mycobacterium bovis*: comparisons to IFN-γ responses. *Clinical and Vaccine Immunology* 19(3), 346–351.

Waters, W.R., Maggioli, M.F., Palmer, M.V., Thacker, T.C., McGill, J.L., Vordermeier, H.M., Berney-Meyer, L., Jacobs, W.R. Jr. and Larsen, M.H. (2015a) Interleukin-17A as a biomarker for bovine tuberculosis. *Clinical and Vaccine Immunology* 23(2), 168–180.

Waters, W.R., Palmer, M.V., Stafne, M.R., Bass, K.E., Maggioli, M.F., *et al.* (2015b) Effects of serial skin testing with purified protein derivative on the level and quality of antibodies to complex and defined antigens in *Mycobacterium bovis*-infected cattle. *Clinical and Vaccine Immunology* 22(6), 641–649.

Waters, W.R., Vordermeier, H.M., Rhodes, S. Khatri, B., Palmer, M.V., *et al.* (2017) Potential for rapid antibody detection to identify tuberculous cattle with non-reactive tuberculin skin test results. *BMC Veterinary Research* 13 (1), 164–170.

Whelan, C., Shuralev, E., O'Keeffe, G., Hyland, P., Kwok, H.F., *et al.* (2008a) Multiplex immunoassay for serological diagnosis of *Mycobacterium bovis* infection in cattle. *Clinical and Vaccine Immunology* 15, 1834–1838.

Whelan, A.O., Wright, D.C., Chambers, M.A., Singh, M., Hewinson, R.G., *et al.* (2008b) Evidence for enhanced central memory priming by live *Mycobacterium bovis* BCG vaccine in comparison with killed BCG formulations. *Vaccine* 26(2), 166–173.

Whelan, A.O., Clifford, D., Upadhyay, B., Breadon, E.L., McNair, J., *et al.* (2010a) Development of a skin test for bovine tuberculosis for differentiating infected from vaccinated animals. *Journal of Clinical Microbiology* 48(9), 3176–3181.

Whelan, C., Whelan, A.O., Shuralev, E., Kwok, H.F., Hewinson, R.G., *et al.* (2010b) Performance of the Enferplex TB assay with cattle in Great Britain and assessment of its suitability as a test to distinguish infected and vaccinated animals. *Clinical and Vaccine Immunology* 17, 813–817.

Whelan, A.O., Villarreal-Ramos, B., Vordermeier, H.M. and Hogarth, P.J. (2011) Development of an antibody to bovine IL-2 reveals multifunctional CD4 T(EM) cells in cattle naturally infected with bovine tuberculosis. *PLoS One* 6(12), e29194.

Wilkinson, K.A. and Wilkinson, R.J. (2010) Polyfunctional T cells in human tuberculosis. *European Journal of Immunology* 40(8), 2139–2142.

Zak, D.E., Penn-Nicholson, A., Scriba, T.J., Thompson, E., Suliman, S., *et al.* (2016) A blood RNA signature for tuberculosis disease risk: a prospective cohort study. *Lancet* 387(10035), 2312–2322.

13 Biomarkers in the Diagnosis of *Mycobacterium tuberculosis* Complex Infections

Sylvia I. Wanzala[1] and Srinand Sreevatsan[2],*

[1]Department of Pathobiology and Diagnostic Investigation, Michigan State University, East Lansing, Michigan, USA; [2]Department of Veterinary Population Medicine, College of Veterinary Medicine, University of Minnesota, St Paul, Minnesota, USA

13.1 Introduction

Bovine tuberculosis (bovine TB) is a zoonotic infection in cattle caused by the intracellular bacterium, *Mycobacterium bovis* that belongs to the *Mycobacterium tuberculosis* complex (MTB complex), a group of related mycobacteria that cause TB in mammals. Bovine TB is the most prevalent infectious disease of dairy cattle worldwide (Cosivi *et al.*, 1998), causing a conservative annual loss of about US$3 billion (Palmer *et al.*, 2007). In the USA, the eradication programme of bovine TB uses a test-and-slaughter strategy that cost about $38 million between 1917 and 1992; the current programmes cost approximately $3.5–4 million annually (Charles and Theon, 2006).

Cattle of all ages are susceptible to infection with *M. bovis*; however, older animals appear to have greater susceptibility (Mackay and Hein, 1989; Thoen and Bloom, 1995; Munroe *et al.*, 2000). In most cases, *M. bovis* infection primarily leads to a subclinical disease (95%) with rapid onset in only 5% of the exposed animals. Thus, detection of subclinical infected animals with progressing granulomatous infection is critical in the control and eradication of bovine TB. Current USDA surveillance for bovine TB is a laborious multistep procedure involving the caudal fold test (CFT) and the comparative cervical test (CCT) or γ-interferon release assays. The current diagnostics are problematic: CFT lacks specificity for *M. bovis* and fails to detect all diseased cattle, while the γ-interferon assay is costly and requires blood samples to be processed within 24 hours of collection. Moreover, early detection of subclinical infection by serological tests is hindered, since the humoral immune response in bovine TB occurs at a late stage of disease progression. Early diagnosis of bovine TB is essential to prevent substantial losses of valuable resources, monetary and production losses, as well as to minimize the risk of human infection. Thus, there is a need to develop a low cost-effective, early detection assay for bovine TB.

Host macrophages are the main site for *M. bovis* infection in cattle. Infection is mainly transmitted via aerosols that are inhaled into the respiratory tract, and gross lesions involve granuloma formation in lungs and thoracic lymph nodes (Thoen and Bloom, 1995). The biology of the granuloma involves intense cellular and biological activity at the site of infection leading to 'leakage' of RNA, DNA and proteins into circulation that may serve as biomarker(s) for early detection of bovine TB. Recent advances in

---

* Email: sreevats@msu.edu

© CAB International 2018. *Bovine Tuberculosis*
(eds M. Chambers, S. Gordon, F. Olea-Popelka, P. Barrow)

genomics and proteomics have opened new robust means for biomarker discovery. Discovery of novel biomarkers is essential for developing new diagnostic tests to aid in identification of infected animals in disease surveillance for bovine TB.

13.1.1 Biomarkers of tuberculosis in animals

Bovine TB presents unique challenges in TB diagnostics and this is further exacerbated by the presence of wildlife reservoirs. Major reservoirs for bovine TB include white-tailed deer (*Odocoileus virginianus*) in the USA, the European badger (*Meles meles*) in the UK and Ireland, brush tail possum (*Trichosurus vulpecula*) in New Zealand, Cape buffalo (*Syncerus caffer*) and greater kudu (*Tragelaphus strepsiceros*) in southern Africa, elk (*Cervus canadensis*) and American bison (*Bison bison*) in Canada and wild boar (*Sus scrofa*) in Spain (Palmer *et al.*, 2000, 2001; Miller and Sweeney, 2013; Talip *et al.*, 2013). *M. bovis*, with the largest host range among the MTB complex organisms, also causes zoonotic TB in humans. In the USA, TB testing in wildlife is carried out with the *in vivo* tuberculin skin test together with the *in vitro* interferon γ assay (Palmer *et al.*, 2000, 2001, 2004; O'Brien *et al.*, 2009). These strategies identify bacteria in lesions or detect host immune responses, but they suffer from low sensitivity, are labour intensive, costly and not always readily available in crucial locations.

In cattle, bovine TB is a major welfare and economic challenge. Bovine TB reduces productivity in affected animals, with the identification of infected animals leading to movement controls, testing of herds, culling of affected animals, and trade restrictions (Humblet *et al.*, 2009; Rodriguez-Campos *et al.*, 2014). In countries that practice active bovine TB surveillance, the three main tests used are the CFT, CCT, and a gamma interferon release assay (IGRA). The primary test for screening for bovine TB is the century-old tuberculin skin test or CFT, whereby bovine purified protein derivative (PPD), prepared from a culture of *M. bovis*, induces a delayed-type hypersensitivity reaction when injected intradermally, resulting in skin swelling after 72 hours. These tests are all labour intensive, present logistical problems and have challenges with sensitivity and specificity (Lamont *et al.*, 2014a). The CFT is not very specific for *M. bovis* infection and does not detect all diseased cattle; co-infection with *Mycobacterium avium* subsp. *paratuberculosis* further confounds the results. The IGRA test is based on release of a cytokine IFN-γ, when sensitized lymphocytes are re-exposed *in vitro* to *M. bovis* antigens (Vordermeier *et al.*, 2014, 2016b). IGRA requires a very quick turnaround for sample processing that is not always possible when working with large herds in a remote location.

Although the tuberculin test is the most common for diagnosis of bovine TB, it has several limitations. The PPD used in the test contains more than 200 antigens that are shared between pathogenic mycobacterial species and other 'atypical' mycobacteria (Chaparas *et al.*, 1970). In the US, the estimated sensitivity of CFT and CCT are 80.4–88.4% and 75%, respectively, while specificity are 96% and 98%, respectively (Whipple *et al.*, 1995). These tests require accredited veterinarians for testing and the animal needs to be restrained at least twice for each test. Serological tests are not applicable in bovine TB surveillance programmes as the antibody titres rise very late in the *M. bovis* infection.

Thus, it is quite evident that the diagnosis of bovine TB can be extremely difficult. If missed, the consequences could be disastrous, including substantial loss of valuable resources, time (lengthy quarantine period of the animals for the diagnosis of disease in the area of bovine TB outbreak), money, emotional expense and trauma (slaughtering of 100–1000 animals for the identification of a single infected animal in the disease surveillance area) associated with the cattle owners, as well as the risk of human infection. Thus, the development of serological-based tests that are more sensitive and specific using novel approaches could be useful in slaughterhouse surveillance programmes.

There are several biomarkers related to bovine TB pathology and vaccine efficacy. For example, the *ex vivo* ESAT-6 induced production of IFN-γ from blood is correlated with the degree of pathology following experimental infection of cattle with *M. bovis*. Bacillus Calmette–Guérin (BCG)-vaccinated calves had lower or reduced responses as well as reduced gross pathology

(Vordermeier *et al.*, 2016a). Another marker investigated as a potential predictor of vaccine-induced protection and memory is IL-2. IL-2 production is also a potential biomarker for latency and different disease stages in cattle (Palmer *et al.*, 2000, 2001, 2004; O'Brien *et al.*, 2009; Vordermeier *et al.*, 2016b).

Mycobacteria have evolved an array of sophisticated mechanisms for evading the host immune system and defending itself in the harsh intracellular environment of the macrophage, some of which are well understood while others are yet to be discovered. In the 'dance of seduction' with *M. bovis*, the host has also evolved several responses to contain infection, and together with the pathogen mechanisms will make up the gist of our discussion.

13.2 Biomarkers Defined

A biomarker can be defined as a characteristic that can be measured and evaluated as an indicator of a normal biological process, a pathogenic process or pharmacologic responses to a therapeutic intervention (Biomarkers Definitions Working Group, 2001). Biomarkers can be used as diagnostic tools for the identification of patients with disease (e.g. elevated glucose concentration for diagnosis of diabetes mellitus), for disease staging (e.g. prostate specific antigen concentration in blood), as an indicator of disease prognosis (e.g. anatomic measurement of tumour shrinkage of certain cancers) or for prediction and monitoring of clinical response to an intervention (e.g. response to anti-tuberculosis drug treatment, vaccine efficacy, blood cholesterol concentration for determination of heart disease, etc.). Currently, the technologies used in biomarker discovery include in vitro analyses of DNA variation (disease susceptibility), circulating DNA or RNA (disease progression-apoptosis/proliferative pathways), transcriptomes (disease induced transcriptional alterations) and proteomics (disease progression).

Discovery of novel biomarkers is essential for developing new diagnostic tests to aid in identification of infected animals in disease surveillance for bovine TB, without necessarily slaughtering herds of 100s to 1000s of animals for identification of the single infected animal.

Early diagnosis is essential in bovine TB because clinical symptoms appear very late, when the disease has significantly advanced and the risk of infection being transmitted is high.

13.2.1 Characteristics of an ideal biomarker

For a biomarker to qualify as an ideal diagnostic tool it has to meet a minimum set of criteria or target product profiles (Gardiner and Karp, 2015). The ultimate diagnostic test for MTB complex infections would be one that is highly sensitive, specific and non-sputum-based with a clear predictive response to therapy, independent of the host response (Gardiner and Karp, 2015). An ideal biomarker-based assay should also have a very high degree of sensitivity and specificity (>98%), be non-invasive or minimally invasive, provide results rapidly, without the need for the cold chain and be affordable. Haas *et al.* (2016) argue that having a combination of biomarkers would enhance the diagnostic value in different settings: for instance, having one set of biomarkers for differentiating between active and latent TB (humans)/subclinical TB (animals) and another set to diagnose TB in comparison with other diseases. Such efforts are possible through collaboration between human and bovine tuberculosis researchers. The pathway taken for a prospective biomarker to reach the market is a tortuous one and potential biomarkers must progress through sequential testing to confirm their efficacy in an independent cohort, then they are further validated in a prospective study. The biomarkers are also required to undergo tests on a platform appropriate for their proposed use; such platforms include TB clinics in endemic countries (Gardiner and Karp, 2015).

Existing TB diagnostics are inadequate. Infection with MTB complex organisms presents unique challenges for diagnostic testing. Current diagnostics have several shortcomings; potential new diagnostics are explored below.

13.3 Circulating Biomarkers

The analysis of alterations in circulating protein profiles or circulating DNA or RNA (including microRNA and small RNAs) in plasma are promising diagnostic tools, requiring only a limited blood sample. Recently completed human and animal genomes have brought refinements in technology including nucleotide and protein sequencing, mass spectrometry and microarrays (nucleic acid and protein arrays), and these have allowed researchers to elucidate fundamental biological processes of chronic diseases such as cancers, neurological disorders, cardiovascular disease and several infectious diseases (Maruvada et al., 2005; Scaros and Fisler, 2005; Jacobsen et al., 2008).

13.3.1 Circulating nucleic acid approach

Circulating nucleic acids (CNAs) are segments of DNA and RNA that are devoid of cellular material and are detected in biological fluids. They are present in small amounts in the plasma of healthy individuals. However, their increased levels are associated with disease conditions. Mandel and Metais first reported CNA in 1948 in human plasma (Mandel, 1947; Anker, 2000). Later studies on CNA were mainly focused on autoimmune diseases like lupus erythematosus (Tan et al., 1966) and rheumatoid arthritis (Ayala et al., 1951). Thirty years later, the diagnostic implications of CNA were recognized by Leon et al. in 1977, when he reported high levels of CNAs in patients with pancreatic cancer and demonstrated that levels of plasma CNA decreased after chemotherapy (Leon et al., 1977). Since then, elevated levels of CNA have been reported in chronic illness (Lui et al., 2002; Schutz et al., 2005), trauma (Lo et al., 2000), acute stroke (Rainer et al., 2003), myocardial infarction (Chang et al., 2003), prenatal diagnosis (Lo et al., 1997; Chim et al., 2005) and various cancerous diseases (Sorenson et al., 1994; Vasioukhin et al., 1994; Hibi et al., 1998; Capone et al., 2000; Shao et al., 2002).

In the last decade, CNA has gained more attention because of its potential application as a non-invasive, rapid and sensitive tool for molecular diagnosis and monitoring of acute pathologies. Most CANA-based laboratory diagnosis involves amplification of either RNA or DNA with primers designed for single-copy coding regions. These CNA tests primarily detect the functional genes associated with exogenous nucleic acid (Lui et al., 2002), for example, those belonging to West Nile virus, parvovirus B-19, human immunodeficiency virus, hepatitis B virus, hepatitis A virus, etc. In addition to detecting single-copy exogenous nucleic acids, CNA diagnostics are being developed that detect endogenous, repetitive sequences (Stroun et al., 2001). Often chronic diseases that lead to cell stress and the release of nucleic acids into the blood show a consistent pattern of endogenous CNAs in serum.

Although most of the diagnostic CNA signatures are associated with human disease, a few researchers have detected CNA in cattle diseases (Brenig et al., 2002; Schutz et al., 2005; Shaughnessy et al., 2015). Researchers have studied repetitive sequences including short Alu repeat sequences (SINE-like sequence of primates) in bovine spongiform encephalopathy (BSE) where they identified the 3′ region of Bov-tA fragments in PCR products derived from the serum of confirmed BSE cases or BSE-exposed cohorts (Schutz et al., 2005). These repetitive elements identified in BSE and other infectious disease lead us to believe that a similar pattern may exist in a chronic infection such as bovine TB.

Mechanism for release of CNA into circulation

Various hypotheses have been proposed as to the mechanism of release of CNA in biological fluids. However, there are controversies related to these hypotheses and the actual origin of CNA still remains ambiguous. On the one hand, necrosis and apoptosis has been considered as major pathway for CNA release (Lo et al., 2000; Lichtenstein et al., 2001); in contrast, it has been reported that cellular necrosis may not be an important pathway as plasma DNA levels fall rather than rise following radiation therapy (Tan et al., 1966). Researchers have considered cellular apoptosis as a source of plasma CNA based on the fact that the electrophoretic pattern produced by plasma CNA is similar to that found with DNA extracted from apoptotic cells (Kamm and Smith, 1975). Apoptosis-induced increased CNA level has been demonstrated in the plasma of patients with lung cancer (Fournie et al., 1995). Several *in vivo* experiments in mice have demonstrated increased CNA levels in blood via apoptotic or necrotic pathways (Fournie *et al.*, 1995; Jiang *et al.*, 2003; Jiang and Pisetsky, 2005). Increased CNA levels have been documented in plasma as a result of apoptosis-induced oxidative stress on placental tissue (Tjoa *et al.*, 2006). Evidence for the active release of CNA from activated lymphocytes or other nucleated cells (Anker *et al.*, 1975; Stroun *et al.*, 2001) and lysis of tumour cells has also been reported (Sorenson, 2000). Apoptosis and necrosis are also associated with TB pathogenesis and are critical for mycobacterial killing, granuloma formation and chronic inflammatory condition induced by the pathogen (Cosivi et al 1997). Thus, an increase in CNA of *M. bovis*-infected animals is expected to occur as the disease progresses.

Methodologies used for CNA discovery

Although there has been a controversy about the use of serum or plasma for CNA discoveries, most of the CNA discoveries have been applied to serum (Leon *et al.*, 1977; Sorenson *et al.*, 1994; Nawroz *et al.*, 1996; Kopreski *et al.*, 1997; Lo *et al.*, 1997). It has been reported that CNA recovered from serum is several-fold higher than that in plasma. The difference in CNA levels have been considered due to the *in vitro* lysis of white blood cells during the process of clotting (Chen *et al.*, 1999; Lui *et al.*, 2002). Lui *et al.*'s study concluded that the serum CNA might not be a true representation of the biological condition of the patient.

Several groups have measured the levels of CNA in different diseases in search of diagnostic or prognostic markers (Ziegler *et al.*, 2002). Multiple techniques have been used in different studies for quantitative analysis of CNA post discovery using *de novo* sequencing of total circulating nucleic acids. These include radioimmunoassay (Leon *et al.*, 1977; Shapiro *et al.*, 1983), competitive PCR (Jahr *et al.*, 2001), quantitative real-time PCR (Thijssen *et al.*, 2002), fluorimetric quantification (Thijssen *et al.*, 2002), spectrophotometric determination (Shao *et al.*, 2001) and visual comparison with known standards (Sozzi *et al.*, 2001). To date, all the studies into CNA demonstrated a significant increase of CNA levels in the diseased condition irrespective of the use of serum or plasma.

13.3.2 Proteomics approach

The term proteome is derived from '*pro*tein and gen*ome*' and was first coined by Marc Wilkin in 1995. Proteome refers to all the proteins expressed by a genome at a given time within a given environment (Solassol *et al.*, 2006). With the completion of the genome sequences for many prokaryotic and eukaryotic organisms, researchers had to assign cellular and molecular functions to thousands of newly predicted gene products and explain how these products cooperate in complex physiological processes. This led to the emergence of a new field of research termed 'proteomics' that aims to characterize biological mechanisms by identifying different proteins involved.

In the last decade, proteomics has provided us with an ability to rapidly identify novel protein biomarkers for various cancerous and non-cancerous diseases. Several researchers have reported that not a single biomarker, but a battery of biomarkers is required to show the specificity and sensitivity for the detection or monitoring of most cancerous diseases (Petricoin *et al.*, 2002a, 2002b; Tirumalai *et al.*, 2003; Zhang *et al.*, 2004; Stone *et al.*, 2005). While substantial research on biomarker discovery exists in fields such as oncology, very few studies have investigated the utility in using the proteomic approach to understanding the pathogenesis of infectious diseases (Gravett *et al.*, 2004; Poon *et al.*, 2004; Yip *et al.*, 2005; Agranoff *et al.*, 2006; Pang *et al.*, 2006).

Nonetheless, several studies have looked at the diagnostic potential of proteomic fingerprinting to determine different disease states as well as monitor the treatment response in TB (Haas *et al.*, 2016). Early proteomic research showed that a combination of four biomarkers (serum amyloid A, transthyretin, neopterin and C-reactive protein) could distinguish between active pulmonary TB and non-TB disease and healthy controls (Agranoff *et al.*, 2006; Seth *et al.*, 2009). It was speculated that targeting specific protein variants rather than the total protein would improve the accuracy of the diagnosis. The translation of proteomic biomarkers into diagnostic tests has been faced with some challenges: the protein biomarker candidates reported by independent studies vary considerably and a universal proteomic profile of TB is yet to be agreed upon. In addition, varying results may be due to differences in proteomic techniques and their resolutions, study design, case definitions and statistical analyses (Haas et al., 2016). There are overlaps though, of serum proteins that are differentially expressed in active TB like CD14, S100A proteins, apolipoproteins, fibrinogen, orosomucoid and serum amyloid A. The challenge with proteomics research is that different investigators use different selection criteria when assessing common protein signatures and the identified proteins are not always evaluated for their diagnostic potential (i.e. with receiver operator curve analyses or decision trees); signatures may not be cross-validated in independent datasets or evaluated with external datasets (Scaros and Fisler, 2005).

A novel approach involves detecting circulating mycobacterial peptides and/or lipids or metabolites in the serum or plasma of infected animals. Research in the Sreevatsan laboratory has recently identified 16 M. bovis proteins including, MB2515c (transcriptional regulator, LuxR family), MB1895c (cell wall biosynthesis) and MB1554c or Pks5 (polyketide synthetase 5) in bovine TB-positive and -exposed cattle and deer (Lamont et al., 2014a; Wanzala et al., 2016). These proteins were first identified by gel-free multi-dimensional isobaric tag for relative and absolute quantitation (iTRAQ) proteomics and subsequently validated using a well-characterized cattle serum repository (Seth et al., 2009; Lamont et al., 2014a). An indirect ELISA using monoclonal antibodies synthesized against these peptides was developed to detect these biomarkers in serum and has been validated in bovine and primate TB (Sreevatsan, Kaushal and Lamont, unpublished data). Given that the current bovine TB diagnostics have a 'one-size-fits-all' testing method whereby disease prevalence status for a given region is not considered, these pathogen-specific biomarkers (Pks5, MB2515c and MB1895c) are unique in that they take the disease prevalence status into account and also detect TB.

Mechanisms of release of protein biomarkers into circulation

Peptide biomarkers are the low molecular, less abundant circulating proteome termed as 'peptidome' (Lai and Agnese, 2015). This peptidome may consist of many types of diagnostic information that may constitute the parent protein, the peptide fragment, the quantity of peptide or the nature of carrier protein to which it is bound (Petricoin et al., 2006). According to the peptidome hypothesis, many proteins and peptides are shed into the local circulation from the disease microenvironment. Apoptosis and necrosis of cells are considered as the main causes for release of proteins and peptides into circulation from the disease microenvironment. Mycobacterial lysis or its release into circulation (mycobacteremia), as has been recently proposed using a phage-based diagnostic test (Swift et al., 2016), can also lead to release of bacterial products into circulation. This is a phage-based test which has recently been commercialized. As a consequence, the blood peptidome could contain ongoing recordings of the molecular cascade of communication that takes place in the tissue microenvironment (Petricoin et al., 2006).

Researchers have explored all different kinds of biological matrices from cell cultures (lysates, supernatants) to clinical samples (serum, plasma, cerebrospinal fluid, bronchoaveolar lavage and urine) for protein biomarker discovery. Of these, serum has many attributes that make it preferable over others for biomarker discovery. Serum is readily available and has a dynamic range of proteins. Serum continuously perfuses through the tissues, and thus contains proteins and peptides secreted/released from cells and tissues from the disease microenvironment. However, there are many challenges associated with using serum for biomarker discovery. Candidate biomarkers are expected to exist in a very low concentration and are generally carried with high-abundant blood proteins like albumin, which exist in a billion-fold excess. Moreover, serum constitutes 65–97% of high-abundant proteins like albumin and immunoglobulins that mask the biologically significant variations among low-abundant serum proteins and prevents their detection and identification in proteomic studies (Govorukhina et al., 2003). Thus, there is a need for the depletion of these high-abundant proteins to enrich low-abundant biomarkers for the proteomic analysis. If not stored properly, serum protein may be depleted due to repeated freeze–thaw cycles.

13.4 Circulating microRNA

Biomarker research has also pointed to circulating microRNA (miRNA) as a potential prognostic and diagnostic biomarker (Farrell et al., 2015). MiRNAs are short (~22 nt), single-stranded, non-coding RNAs that regulate mRNA expression. MiRNAs are important regulators of gene expression and play a key role in regulating both the innate and adaptive immune responses. Recent work has shown that expression of miR-155 was more than 40 times higher in naturally infected cattle with visible pathology compared with infected animals that presented without visible pathology (Golby et al., 2014). This suggests that miR-155 could distinguish active from latent infection, and could be used as a diagnostic and prognostic biomarker to identify infected animals as well as be used for Differentiating Infected from Vaccinated Animals (DIVA) testing, although more research is still needed in this area (Abd-el-Fattah et al., 2013; Golby et al., 2014). What makes miRNAs particularly appealing as potential biomarkers is that they have tissue-specific expression patterns that can serve as a fingerprint for disease and also can be detected by RT-PCR assays and microarray techniques (Williams et al., 2013). In addition, it is hypothesized that different stages of mycobacterial infection have distinct miRNA signatures (Farrell et al., 2015). Another fascinating fact about them is that serum miRNA is stable to repeated freeze–thaw cycles as well as to heat, acidic and alkaline conditions.

13.5 Serum Cytokines

Alveolar macrophages and pulmonary dendritic cells represent the first line of defence against invading mycobacterial pathogens (Kaufmann, 2004). This process releases chemokines, which attract monocytes and other inflammatory cells to the lungs (Kleinnijenhuis et al., 2011). Chemokines are a form of cytokines – a group of mainly soluble proteins and glycoproteins that modulate the immune system. Examples include interleukins (ILs), interferons (IFNs), growth factors, colony stimulating factors, the tumour necrosis factor (TNF) family, and chemokines (Choi et al., 2016).

Phagocytic cells trigger the adaptive immune response by presentation of mycobacterial antigens to T cells. Once a macrophage is infected with mycobacteria, it releases interleukins 12 and 18 (IL-12 and IL-18). The released cytokines stimulate CD4, CD8 and natural killer cells to produce interferon gamma (IFN-γ) and TNF alpha (Villarreal-Ramos et al., 2003). T cells respond to the released IFN-γ in a positive feedback loop leading to the production of more IFN-γ. The IFN-γ activates macrophages to kill the invading mycobacteria by activating nitric oxide synthase, which produces nitric oxide while the TNF-α is critical for the initiation of the immune response against infection with mycobacteria (Kaufmann, 2004; Das et al., 2016). In a study published by Thacker et al. (2007), expression of IFN-γ, TNF-α, iNOS and IL-4 by peripheral blood mononuclear cells (PBMC) was increased in response to infection, whereas IL-10 expression decreased. There was also a positive association between Th1 responses and disease severity but as infection progressed, the differences in gene expression between the low and high pathology groups were indistinguishable, implying a possible influence of early Th1 response on pathology (Thacker et al., 2007). Characterization of the bovine immune response has been done by several research teams; examples include use of real-time PCR and bovine immune microarrays to characterize bovine cytokine/chemokine/transcription factor etc. responses to bovine TB (Schiller et al., 2010). Other cellular immunity-based tests include the development of bovine cytokine and chemokine multiplex systems detecting several parameters in a single sample, as well as the use of monoclonal antibodies that recognize bovine cytokines (Coad et al., 2010; Schiller et al., 2010).

A granuloma is a compact, organized collection of mature macrophages, which arises in response to persistent stimuli (Ramakrishnan, 2012). Necrotic areas called caesium occur within granulomas as a result of dying cells. Cells that make up the granuloma include neutrophils, dendritic cells, B and T cells, natural killer cells, fibroblasts and cells that secrete extracellular matrix components (Harding and Boom, 2010). After formation of granulomas, several scenarios may occur: cessation of infection or dormancy, progression of infection with dissemination to other organs, as well as reactivation, which may occur months or years after the initial infection due to a compromised immune system (van Crevel et al., 2002; Kaufmann, 2004; Kleinnijenhuis et al., 2011; Ramakrishnan, 2012). The various manifestations of infection with mycobacteria are a reflection of the delicate balance between the bacteria and the host defense mechanisms (van Crevel et al., 2002). Recent research by (Palmer et al., 2016) examined cytokine expression of TNF-α, IFN-γ, TGF-β, IL-17A and IL-10 in experimentally infected calves and found a moderate but positive correlation between the level of cytokine expression and cell size or number of nuclei in giant cells of granulomas. Their work demonstrated that these giant cells contribute to the 'cytokine milieu necessary to form and maintain granulomas' (Palmer et al., 2016).

Another cytokine is IL-17 (produced by Th17 cells), which has been demonstrated to play a role in tuberculosis immunopathology as well as other chronic illnesses. Antigen-specific in vitro expression of IL-17A has been correlated to both increased disease severity and vaccine-induced protection in cattle experimentally infected with M. bovis (Palmer et al., 2016). In tuberculosis, IL-17 cytokines play key roles in initiating both protective and harmful inflammatory responses and the use of Th17-associated cytokines have been suggested as possible biomarkers of infection and protection in the immune responses to bovine tuberculosis (Waters et al., 2015).

13.6. Cellular Immune Responses for Potential Biomarker Application

Mycobacteria are intracellular pathogens and the host mounts a successful response through a strong cell-mediated response by the adaptive immune system, which, in the case of bovine TB, also acts as the immunological diagnosis of infection (Vordermeier et al., 2000; Goosen et al., 2014). Several cellular immune responses have been the target for biomarker application. BCG vaccination is one example, though it has given variable responses in both humans and cattle and studies to improve the protection conferred by the BCG vaccine are in progress (Vordermeier et al., 2016b). One such method is the heterologous prime-boost strategy that involves use of supplemental or booster vaccine where the immune system is primed with BCG after which it is boosted with subunit vaccines containing protective antigens present in BCG (Vordermeier et al., 2016a). Other methods include complete replacement of BCG with attenuated M. bovis strains leading to overexpression of antigens or the use of genetically modified BCG strains with improved immunogenicity (Waters et al., 2009; Vordermeier et al., 2016a).

Identification of genes deleted in BCG when compared to M. bovis by comparative genomics identified key targets in cattle and humans, for example, the M. bovis proteins early secretory antigenic target (ESAT-6) and the culture filtrate protein (CFP-10) located on the RD1 region of M. bovis and in virulent strains of M. tuberculosis (Mahairas et al., 1996; Vordermeier et al., 2000, 2016a). In terms of diagnostics, ESAT-6 and CFP-10 can differentiate between M. tuberculosis-infected and BCG-vaccinated humans and ESAT-6 could differentiate between M. bovis-infected and BCG-vaccinated cattle; these peptides, through the Bovigam PC-EC assay (BEC) and the Bovigam PC-IHC (BHP), have been harnessed to improve the specificity of IGRAs, though the sensitivity of BTB diagnosis has been sub-optimal (Goosen et al., 2014). A study by Goosen et al. (2014) in African buffalo demonstrated that monocyte-derived chemokine IFN-γ-induced protein 10 (IP-10) was a useful marker of immune activation by M. bovis antigens when using the bovine IP-10 ELISA, and they recommended that the diagnostic potential of IP-10 for BTB in cattle be re-evaluated using species-specific reagents.

13.7 Human Tuberculosis

In humans, for MTB complex organisms to be detected from sputum, it implies that the airways are close to or have necrotic foci of infection (Gardiner and Karp, 2015). Thus, for diagnosis with sputum to be possible it means that most likely the patient has had active disease for quite some time, often with severe damage to the lungs (Gardiner and Karp, 2015). The most common method used is the direct detection of the pathogen via microscopy, culture or by PCR where the DNA is amplified. The presence of a sustained T-cell reactivity with *M. tuberculosis* complex antigens (tuberculin skin tests) or by use of interferon release assays of peripheral blood is also used to determine infection (Wallis et al., 2010). The gold standard for TB testing, culture, is lengthy due to the fastidious nature of MTB complex organisms with very slow generation time (20–22 hours for *M. tuberculosis*). Identification of *M. tuberculosis* therefore takes weeks and this delay also pushes back treatment of ill persons who may be actively infecting others. IGRAs are also used to detect infection, but they only have moderate predictive value, marginally higher than that of tuberculin skin test in low/middle income countries (Leung et al., 2013). IGRAs work by measuring the IFN-γ released by T cells in a blood sample after re-stimulation with specific *M. tuberculosis* complex (MTC) antigens. A positive outcome for IGRA gives an indication of infection but it cannot distinguish between active and latent TB.

Despite new automated molecular ways for TB detection and drug resistance, a simple, affordable point-of-care test for TB is still not available (Wallis et al., 2010). Low sensitivity is one of the biggest challenges facing microscopy, and one may miss diagnosis in more than 30% of samples tested. Research shows that use of matrix-assisted laser desorption ionization-time of flight (MALDI-TOF) mass spectrometry and nucleic acid amplification tests may soon accelerate this step for the identification of positive cultures (Wallis et al., 2010). The current molecular test (Xpert MTB/RIF) recommended by the World Health Organization has a sensitivity of 99.7% and specificity of 98.5% in smear-positive samples and is 76.1% sensitive and 98.8% specific in smear-negative samples (Boehme et al., 2010). The Xpert MTB/RIF test is expensive and not widely available in resource-limited settings where it is needed the most. In addition, it is not useful for testing extra-pulmonary manifestations of human and bovine TB (Wallis et al., 2010; Gardiner and Karp, 2015).

Biomarkers are unique because they provide prognostic information about the future health status of an individual; they can indicate normal or pathological states, as well as responses to anti-tubercular drug therapy. In TB diagnostics, biomarkers are required to detect active disease and latency as well as predict non-relapsing treatment success in humans. In addition, they would be useful in determining individuals that are protected from TB by new vaccines. Sputum-based biomarkers play a limited role in latent TB.

A simple, non-invasive test using urine, saliva or serum that can serve as both a diagnostic and prognostic test would greatly enhance TB diagnostics. Biomarkers in urine like lipoarabinomannan (a 17.3-kDa immunogenic glycolipid component of the mycobacterial cell wall or LAM) have been tested with varying results as well as detection of volatile organic compounds in patients with pulmonary tuberculosis though much more research needs to done to establish changes in these biomarkers during treatment or clinical outcome (Boehme et al., 2010). There is currently a commercially available urine LAM test, but use is limited due to sensitivity issues; however, it is useful if used in combination with other current testing methods (Leung et al., 2013; Lamont et al., 2014b; Gardiner and Karp, 2015).

Analyses to detect antibodies against antigen 85 have been carried out in blood and urine by mass spectrometry with promising results (Young et al., 2014). But in general, antibody analyses have not been very effective mainly due to the heterogeneity of the antibody response to *M. tuberculosis* and thus they have not been able to meet the requirements for a diagnostic test (Gardiner and Karp, 2015). Data from several researchers have concluded that antibody responses are unlikely to provide useful diagnostics for TB (Gardiner and Karp, 2015).

There are biomarkers that are increased at baseline in proportion to the degree of the disease and subsequently decline with treatment: these include soluble intercellular adhesion molecule (sICAM), C-reactive protein, soluble urokinase plasminogen activator receptor and procalcitonin (Eckersall and Bell, 2010; Wallis et al., 2010). Assays with these biomarkers are simple, affordable and can be carried out on frozen plasma samples so they can be incorporated into treatment protocols. Studies indicate that they have greatest prognostic value when measured at or near the completion of therapy (Wallis et al., 2010). Use of a panel of biomarkers gives a better response than just one marker. In addition, measuring multiple parameters by proteomics, transcriptomics, and metabolomics would greatly enhance the efficacy of biomarkers.

13.8 Biomarker Challenges

Major challenges in TB diagnostics include the absence of effective tools for appropriate and accurate TB diagnosis, as well as well-defined tools to monitor treatment response to enable shorter courses of chemotherapy for human patients and faster turnaround for farmers with a suspected cattle TB case. Although there is ongoing research on biomarkers in humans, new tools for TB diagnosis in animals are not as abundant (Vordermeier *et al.*, 2016a). There have been major issues with reproducibility in biomarker research and this has been put down to inattentiveness to methodological issues of study design and performance, which have been repeatedly claimed as a major reason for false-positive findings in biomarker research (Pesch *et al.*, 2014). Another significant challenge with biomarker research is the lack of a collaborative and systematic approach and this is the case for the development of biomarkers in both human and veterinary medicine (Kondo, 2014). Technical challenges such as low sensitivity, reproducibility and throughput have caused biomarker failures, but this has increasingly been overcome by use of DNA microarray technology that enables the measurement of the mRNA levels of thousands of genes in a quantitative and reproducible manner at relatively low cost (Kondo, 2014).

Market failure is another important challenge facing the development of new TB diagnostics like biomarkers. In the case of human TB, industry usually avoids developing and marketing products that will be mainly used by patients in resource-limited countries because such products do not generate profits (Wallis *et al.*, 2010). In addition, even if the products are available, neither their cost nor performance are adapted for developing countries, meaning that their potential benefits are unavailable to the patients and healthcare providers who need them most (Wallis *et al.*, 2010). For bovine TB, major strides have been made and the coming together of the bovine TB vaccine development programme with the international human TB vaccine programme has been beneficial and has led to development of platforms with DIVA capability to be applied in countries that plan to use vaccination together with test-and-slaughter (Vordermeier *et al.*, 2016b). The steps taken for a biomarker to be approved as a diagnostic test are rigorous before they can be approved for animal or human use (Pesch *et al.*, 2014).

13.9 Conclusions

For global bovine TB control to become a reality, there is need for a more accurate, affordable point-of-care diagnostic test. Biomarkers are key in this process, but it is important for researchers to harness the advantages of having multiple biomarkers. The bovine TB diagnostics pipeline has grown in recent years with many promising candidates. Biomarkers are among such candidates but there is need for improvements in standardization and validation procedures to increase reproducibility and accuracy and promote adoption of these biomarkers. Continuous improvement in our knowledge of these intriguing organisms is the best way of overcoming some of the knowledge gaps surrounding TB biomarkers. Knowledge about the biology of MTC organisms and their host–pathogen interactions is still incomplete thus research into these areas will greatly enhance the development of accurate, and safe biomarkers for bovine TB.

References

Abd-el-Fattah, A.A., Sadik, N.A., Shaker, O.G. and Aboulftouh, M.L. (2013) Differential microRNAs expression in serum of patients with lung cancer, pulmonary tuberculosis, and pneumonia. *Cell Biochemistry and Biophysics* 67, 875–884.

Agranoff, D., Fernandez-Reyes, D., Papadopoulos, M.C., Rojas, S.A., Herbster, M., *et al.* (2006) Identification of diagnostic markers for tuberculosis by proteomic fingerprinting of serum. *Lancet* 368, 1012–1021.

Anker, P. (2000) Quantitative aspects of plasma/serum DNA in cancer patients. *Annals of the New York Academy of Sciences* 906, 5–7.

Anker, P., Stroun, M. and Maurice, P.A. (1975) Spontaneous release of DNA by human blood lymphocytes as shown in an in vitro system. *Cancer Research* 35, 2375–2382.

Ayala, W., Moore, L.V. and Hess, E.L. (1951) The purple color reaction given by diphenylamine reagent. I. with normal and rheumatic fever sera. *The Journal of Clinical Investigation* 30, 781–785.

Biomarkers Definitions Working Group (2001) Biomarkers and surrogate endpoints: preferred definitions and conceptual framework. *Clinical Pharmacology and Therapeutics* 69, 89–95.

Boehme, C.C., Nabeta, P., Hillemann, D., Nicol, M.P., Shenai, S., et al. (2010) Rapid molecular detection of tuberculosis and rifampin resistance. *The New England Journal of Medicine* 363, 1005–1015.

Brenig, B., Schutz, E. and Urnovitz, H. (2002) [Cellular nucleic acids in serum and plasma as new diagnostic tools]. *Berliner und Münchener Tierärztliche Wochenschrift* 115, 122–124.

Capone, R.B., Pai, S.I., Koch, W.M., Gillison, M.L., Danish, H.N., et al. (2000) Detection and quantitation of human papillomavirus (HPV) DNA in the sera of patients with HPV-associated head and neck squamous cell carcinoma. *Clinical Cancer Research* 6, 4171–4175.

Chang, C.P., Chia, R.H., Wu, T.L., Tsao, K.C., Sun, C.F. and Wu, J.T. (2003) Elevated cell-free serum DNA detected in patients with myocardial infarction. *Clinica Chimica Acta* 327, 95–101.

Chaparas, S.D., Maloney, C.J. and Hedrick, S.R. (1970) Specificity of tuberculins and antigens from various species of mycobacteria. *The American Review of Respiratory Disease* 101, 74–83.

Charles, O., Theon, J.H.S. and Michael, F.G. (2006) Economics of bovine tuberculosis. In *Mycobacterium bovis Infection in Animals and Humans*. Blackwell Publishing, Hoboken, USA.

Chen, X., Bonnefoi, H., Diebold-Berger, S., Lyautey, J., Lederrey, C., et al.. (1999) Detecting tumor-related alterations in plasma or serum DNA of patients diagnosed with breast cancer. *Clinical Cancer Research* 5, 2297–2303.

Chim, S.S., Tong, Y.K., Chiu, R.W., Lau, T.K., Leung, T.N., et al. (2005) Detection of the placental epigenetic signature of the maspin gene in maternal plasma. *Proceedings of the National Academy of Sciences of the United States of America* 102, 14753–14758.

Choi, R., Kim, K., Kim, M.-J., Kim, S.-Y., Kwon, O.J., et al. (2016) Serum inflammatory profiles in pulmonary tuberculosis and their association with treatment response. *Journal of Proteomics* 149, 23–30.

Coad, M., Clifford, D., Rhodes, S.G., Hewinson, R.G., Vordermeier, H.M. and Whelan, A.O. (2010) Repeat tuberculin skin testing leads to desensitisation in naturally infected tuberculous cattle which is associated with elevated interleukin-10 and decreased interleukin-1 beta responses. *Veterinary Research* 41(2), 14.

Cosivi, O., Grange, J.M., Daborn, C.J., Raviglione, M.C., Fujikura, T., et al. (1998) Zoonotic tuberculosis due to *Mycobacterium bovis* in developing countries. *Emerging Infectious Diseases* 4, 59–70.

Das, K., Thomas, T., Garnica, O. and Dhandayuthapani, S. (2016) Recombinant *Bacillus subtilis* spores for the delivery of *Mycobacterium tuberculosis* Ag85B-CFP10 secretory antigens. *Tuberculosis* 101, S18–S27.

Eckersall, P.D. and Bell, R. (2010) Acute phase proteins: biomarkers of infection and inflammation in veterinary medicine. *Veterinary Journal* 185, 23–27.

Farrell, D., Shaughnessy, R.G., Britton, L., Machugh, D.E., Markey, B. and Gordon, S.V. (2015) The identification of circulating MiRNA in bovine serum and their potential as novel biomarkers of early *Mycobacterium avium* subsp *paratuberculosis* infection. *PLoS One* 10, e0134310.

Fournie, G.J., Courtin, J.P., Laval, F., Chale, J.J., Pourrat, J.P., et al. (1995) Plasma DNA as a marker of cancerous cell death. investigations in patients suffering from lung cancer and in nude mice bearing human tumours. *Cancer Letters* 91, 221–227.

Gardiner, J.L. and Karp, C.L. (2015) Transformative tools for tackling tuberculosis. *The Journal of Experimental Medicine* 212, 1759–1769.

Golby, P., Villarreal-Ramos, B., Dean, G., Jones, G.J. and Vordermeier, M. (2014) MicroRNA expression profiling of PPD-B stimulated PBMC from *M. bovis*-challenged unvaccinated and BCG vaccinated cattle. *Vaccine* 32, 5839–5844.

Goosen, W.J., Cooper, D., Warren, R.M., Miller, M.A., Van Helden, P.D. and Parsons, S.D. (2014) The evaluation of candidate biomarkers of cell-mediated immunity for the diagnosis of *Mycobacterium bovis* infection in african buffaloes (*Syncerus caffer*). *Veterinary Immunology and Immunopathology* 162, 198–202.

Govorukhina, N.I., Keizer-Gunnink, A., Van der Zee, A.G., De Jong, S., De Bruijn, H.W. and Bischoff, R. (2003) Sample preparation of human serum for the analysis of tumor markers. comparison of different approaches for albumin and gamma-globulin depletion. *Journal of Chromatography A* 1009, 171–178.

Gravett, M.G., Novy, M.J., Rosenfeld, R.G., Reddy, A.P., Jacob, T., et al. (2004) Diagnosis of intra-amniotic infection by proteomic profiling and identification of novel biomarkers. JAMA 292, 462–469.

Haas, C.T., Roe, J.K., Pollara, G., Mehta, M. and Noursadeghi, M. (2016) Diagnostic 'omics' for active tuberculosis. BMC Medicine 14, 37-016-0583-9.

Harding, C. and Boom, W.H. (2010) Regulation of antigen presentation by Mycobacterium tuberculosis: a role for Toll-like receptors. Nature Reviews Microbiology 8, 296–307.

Hibi, K., Robinson, C.R., Booker, S., Wu, L., Hamilton, S.R., et al. (1998) Molecular detection of genetic alterations in the serum of colorectal cancer patients. Cancer Research 58, 1405–1407.

Humblet, M.F., Boschiroli, M.L. and Saegerman, C. (2009) Classification of worldwide bovine tuberculosis risk factors in cattle: a stratified approach. Veterinary Research 40, 50.

Jacobsen, M., Mattow, J., Repsilber, D. and Kaufmann, S.H. (2008) Novel strategies to identify biomarkers in tuberculosis. Biological Chemistry 389, 487–495.

Jahr, S., Hentze, H., Englisch, S., Hardt, D., Fackelmayer, F.O., et al. (2001) DNA fragments in the blood plasma of cancer patients: quantitations and evidence for their origin from apoptotic and necrotic cells. Cancer Research 61, 1659–1665.

Jiang, N. and Pisetsky, D.S. (2005) The effect of inflammation on the generation of plasma DNA from dead and dying cells in the peritoneum. Journal of Leukocyte Biology 77, 296–302.

Jiang, N., Reich, C.F., 3rd, Monestier, M. and Pisetsky, D.S. (2003) The expression of plasma nucleosomes in mice undergoing in vivo apoptosis. Clinical Immunology 106, 139–147.

Kamm, R.C. and Smith, A.G. (1975) Plasma deoxyribonucleic acid concentrations of women in labor and umbilical cords. American Journal of Obstetrics and Gynecology 121, 29–31.

Kaufmann, S.H. (2004) New issues in tuberculosis. Annals of the Rheumatic Diseases 63(2), ii50–ii56.

Kleinnijenhuis, J., Oosting, M., Joosten, L.A.B., Netea, M.G. and Van Crevel, R. (2011) Innate immune recognition of Mycobacterium tuberculosis. Clinical & Developmental Immunology 2011, Article ID 405310.

Kondo, T. (2014) Inconvenient truth: cancer biomarker development by using proteomics. Biomedica Biochimica Acta 1844, 861–865.

Kopreski, M.S., Benko, F.A., Kwee, C., Leitzel, K.E., Eskander, E., et al. (1997) Detection of mutant K-ras DNA in plasma or serum of patients with colorectal cancer. British Journal of Cancer 76, 1293–1299.

Lai, Z.W.P. and Agnese, S.O. (2015) The emerging role of the peptidome in biomarker discovery and degradome profiling. Biological Chemistry 396, 185–192.

Lamont, E.A., Janagama, H.K., Ribeiro-Lima, J., Vulchanova, L., Seth, M., et al. (2014a) Circulating Mycobacterium bovis peptides and host response proteins as biomarkers for unambiguous detection of subclinical infection. Journal of Clinical Microbiology 52, 536–543.

Lamont, E.A., Ribeiro-Lima, J., Waters, W.R., Thacker, T. and Sreevatsan, S. (2014b) Mannosylated lipoarabinomannan in serum as a biomarker candidate for subclinical bovine tuberculosis. BMC Research Notes 7, 559.

Leon, S.A., Shapiro, B., Sklaroff, D.M. and Yaros, M.J. (1977) Free DNA in the serum of cancer patients and the effect of therapy. Cancer Research 37, 646–650.

Leung, C.C., Lange, C. and Zhang, Y. (2013) Tuberculosis: current state of knowledge: an epilogue. Respirology 18, 1047–1055.

Lichtenstein, A.V., Melkonyan, H.S., Tomei, L.D. and Umansky, S.R. (2001) Circulating nucleic acids and apoptosis. Annals of the New York Academy of Sciences 945, 239–249.

Lo, Y.M., Corbetta, N., Chamberlain, P.F., Rai, V., Sargent, I.L., et al. (1997) Presence of fetal DNA in maternal plasma and serum. Lancet 350, 485–487.

Lo, Y.M., Rainer, T.H., Chan, L.Y., Hjelm, N.M. and Cocks, R.A. (2000) Plasma DNA as a prognostic marker in trauma patients. Clinical Chemistry 46, 319–323.

Lui, Y.Y., Chik, K.W., Chiu, R.W., Ho, C.Y., Lam, C.W. and Lo, Y.M. (2002) Predominant hematopoietic origin of cell-free DNA in plasma and serum after sex-mismatched bone marrow transplantation. Clinical Chemistry 48, 421–427.

Mackay, C.R. and Hein, W.R. (1989) A large proportion of bovine T cells express the gamma delta T cell receptor and show a distinct tissue distribution and surface phenotype. International Immunology 1, 540–545.

Mahairas, G.G., Sabo, P.J., Hickey, M.J., Singh, D.C. and Stover, C.K. (1996) Molecular analysis of genetic differences between Mycobacterium bovis BCG and virulent M. bovis. Journal of Bacteriology 178, 1274–1282.

Mandel, P.M.P. (1947) Les acides nucleiques du plasma sanguin chez l'homme. *Comptes Rendus. Académie des Sciences Paris* 142, 241–243.

Maruvada, P., Wang, W., Wagner, P.D. and Srivastava, S. (2005) Biomarkers in molecular medicine: cancer detection and diagnosis. *Biotechniques* Suppl, 9–15.

Miller, R.S. and Sweeney, S.J. (2013) *Mycobacterium bovis* (bovine tuberculosis) infection in north american wildlife: current status and opportunities for mitigation of risks of further infection in wildlife populations. *Epidemiology and Infection* 141, 1357–1370.

Munroe, F.A., Dohoo, I.R. and Mcnab, W.B. (2000) Estimates of within-herd incidence rates of *Mycobacterium bovis* in Canadian cattle and cervids between 1985 and 1994. *Preventive Veterinary Medicine* 45, 247–256.

Nawroz, H., Koch, W., Anker, P., Stroun, M. and Sidransky, D. (1996) Microsatellite alterations in serum DNA of head and neck cancer patients. *Nature Medicine* 2, 1035–1037.

O'Brien, D.J., Schmitt, S.M., Lyashchenko, K.P., Waters, W.R., Berry, D.E., *et al.* (2009) Evaluation of blood assays for detection of *Mycobacterium bovis* in white-tailed deer (*Odocoileus virginianus*) in Michigan. *Journal of Wildlife Diseases* 45, 153–164.

Palmer, M.V., Whipple, D.L., Payeur, J.B., Alt, D.P., Esch, K.J., *et al.* (2000) Naturally occurring tuberculosis in white-tailed deer. *Journal of the American Veterinary Medical Association* 216, 1921–1924.

Palmer, M.V., Whipple, D.L. and Waters, W.R. (2001) Experimental deer-to-deer transmission of *Mycobacterium bovis*. *American Journal of Veterinary Research* 62, 692–696.

Palmer, M.V., Waters, W.R., Whipple, D.L., Slaughter, R.E. and Jones, S.L. (2004) Evaluation of an in vitro blood-based assay to detect production of interferon-gamma by *Mycobacterium bovis*-infected white-tailed deer (*Odocoileus virginianus*). *Journal of Veterinary Diagnostic Investigation* 16, 17–21.

Palmer, M.V., Waters, W.R. and Thacker, T.C. (2007) Lesion development and immunohistochemical changes in granulomas from cattle experimentally infected with *Mycobacterium bovis*. *Veterinary Pathology* 44, 863–874.

Palmer, M.V., Thacker, T.C. and Waters, W.R. (2016) Multinucleated giant cell cytokine expression in pulmonary granulomas of cattle experimentally infected with *Mycobacterium bovis*. *Veterinary Immunology and Immunopathology* 180, 34–39.

Pang, R.T., Poon, T.C., Chan, K.C., Lee, N.L., Chiu, R.W., *et al.* (2006) Serum proteomic fingerprints of adult patients with severe acute respiratory syndrome. *Clinical Chemistry* 52, 421–429.

Pesch, B., Bruning, T., Johnen, G., Casjens, S., Bonberg, N., *et al.* (2014) Biomarker research with prospective study designs for the early detection of cancer. *Biomedica Biochimica Acta* 1844, 874–883.

Petricoin, E.F., 3rd, Ornstein, D.K., Paweletz, C.P., Ardekani, A., Hackett, P.S., *et al.* (2002a) Serum proteomic patterns for detection of prostate cancer. *Journal of the National Cancer Institute* 94, 1576–1578.

Petricoin, E.F., Ardekani, A.M., Hitt, B.A., Levine, P.J., Fusaro, V.A., *et al.* (2002b) Use of proteomic patterns in serum to identify ovarian cancer. *Lancet* 359, 572–577.

Petricoin, E.F., Belluco, C., Araujo, R.P. and Liotta, L.A. (2006) The blood peptidome: a higher dimension of information content for cancer biomarker discovery. *Nature Reviews Cancer* 6, 961–967.

Poon, T.C., Chan, K.C., Ng, P.C., Chiu, R.W., Ang, I.L., *et al.* (2004) Serial analysis of plasma proteomic signatures in pediatric patients with severe acute respiratory syndrome and correlation with viral load. *Clinical Chemistry* 50, 1452–1455.

Rainer, T.H., Wong, L.K., Lam, W., Yuen, E., Lam, N.Y., *et al.* (2003) Prognostic use of circulating plasma nucleic acid concentrations in patients with acute stroke. *Clinical Chemistry* 49, 562–569.

Ramakrishnan, L. (2012) Revisiting the role of the granuloma in tuberculosis. *Nature Reviews Immunology* 12, 352–366.

Rodriguez-Campos, S., Smith, N.H., Boniotti, M.B. and Aranaz, A. (2014) Overview and phylogeny of *Mycobacterium tuberculosis* complex organisms: implications for diagnostics and legislation of bovine tuberculosis. *Research in Veterinary Science* 97(Suppl), S5–S19.

Scaros, O. and Fisler, R. (2005) Biomarker technology roundup: from discovery to clinical applications, a broad set of tools is required to translate from the lab to the clinic. *Biotechniques* Suppl, 30–32.

Schiller, I., Oesch, B., Vordermeier, H.M., Palmer, M.V., Harris, B.N., *et al.* (2010) Bovine tuberculosis: a review of current and emerging diagnostic techniques in view of their relevance for disease control and eradication. *Transboundary & Emerging Diseases* 57, 205–220.

Schutz, E., Urnovitz, H.B., Iakoubov, L., Schulz-Schaeffer, W., Wemheuer, W. and Brenig, B. (2005) Bov-tA short interspersed nucleotide element sequences in circulating nucleic acids from sera of cattle with bovine spongiform encephalopathy (BSE) and sera of cattle exposed to BSE. *Clinical and Diagnostic Laboratory Immunology* 12, 814–820.

Seth, M., Lamont, E.A., Janagama, H.K., Widdel, A., Vulchanova, L., et al. (2009) Biomarker discovery in subclinical mycobacterial infections of cattle. *PloS One* 4, e5478.

Shao, Z.M., Wu, J., Shen, Z.Z. and Nguyen, M. (2001) p53 mutation in plasma DNA and its prognostic value in breast cancer patients. *Clinical Cancer Research* 7, 2222–2227.

Shao, Z.M., Wu, J., Shen, Z.Z. and Nguyen, M. (2002) Retraction. *Clinical Cancer Research* 8, 3027.

Shapiro, B., Chakrabarty, M., Cohn, E.M. and Leon, S.A. (1983) Determination of circulating DNA levels in patients with benign or malignant gastrointestinal disease. *Cancer* 51, 2116–2120.

Shaughnessy, R.G., Farrell, D., Riepema, K., Bakker, D. and Gordon, S.V. (2015) Analysis of biobanked serum from a *Mycobacterium avium* subsp *paratuberculosis* bovine infection model confirms the remarkable stability of circulating miRNA profiles and defines a bovine serum miRNA repertoire. *PLoS One* 10, e0145089.

Solassol, J., Jacot, W., Lhermitte, L., Boulle, N., Maudelonde, T. and Mange, A. (2006) Clinical proteomics and mass spectrometry profiling for cancer detection. *Expert Review of Proteomics* 3, 311–320.

Sorenson, G.D. (2000) Detection of mutated KRAS2 sequences as tumor markers in plasma/serum of patients with gastrointestinal cancer. *Clinical Cancer Research* 6, 2129–2137.

Sorenson, G.D., Pribish, D.M., Valone, F.H., Memoli, V.A., Bzik, D.J. and Yao, S.L. (1994) Soluble normal and mutated DNA sequences from single-copy genes in human blood. *Cancer Epidemiology, Biomarkers and Prevention* 3, 67–71.

Sozzi, G., Conte, D., Mariani, L., Lo Vullo, S., Roz, L., et al. (2001) Analysis of circulating tumor DNA in plasma at diagnosis and during follow-up of lung cancer patients. *Cancer Research* 61, 4675–4678.

Stone, J.H., Rajapakse, V.N., Hoffman, G.S., Specks, U., Merkel, P.A., et al. (2005) A serum proteomic approach to gauging the state of remission in Wegener's granulomatosis. *Arthritis Rheum* 52, 902–910.

Stroun, M., Lyautey, J., Lederrey, C., Olson-Sand, A. and Anker, P. (2001) About the possible origin and mechanism of circulating DNA apoptosis and active DNA release. *Clinica Chimica Acta* 313, 139–142.

Swift, B.M., Convery, T.W. and Rees, C.E. (2016) Evidence of *Mycobacterium tuberculosis* complex bacteraemia in intradermal skin test positive cattle detected using phage-RPA. *Virulence* 7(7), 779–788.

Talip, B.A., Sleator, R.D., Lowery, C.J., Dooley, J.S. and Snelling, W.J. (2013) An update on global tuberculosis (TB). *Infectious Diseases(Auckl)* 6, 39–50.

Tan, E.M., Schur, P.H., Carr, R.I. and Kunkel, H.G. (1966) Deoxyribonucleic acid (DNA) and antibodies to DNA in the serum of patients with systemic lupus erythematosus. *Journal of Clinical Investigation* 45, 1732–1740.

Thacker, T.C., Palmer, M.V. and Waters, W.R. (2007) Associations between cytokine gene expression and pathology in *Mycobacterium bovis* infected cattle. *Veterinary Immunology and Immunopathology* 119, 204–213.

Thijssen, M.A., Swinkels, D.W., Ruers, T.J. and De Kok, J.B. (2002) Difference between free circulating plasma and serum DNA in patients with colorectal liver metastases. *Anticancer Research* 22, 421–425.

Thoentest, C.O. and Bloom, B.R. (1995) Pathogenesis of *Mycobacterium bovis*. In Thoen, C.O., Steele, J.H. and Gilsdorf, M.J. (eds) Mycobacterium bovis *Infection in Animals and Humans*. Blackwell Publishing, Hoboken, USA.

Tirumalai, R.S., Chan, K.C., Prieto, D.A., Issaq, H.J., Conrads, T.P. and Veenstra, T.D. (2003) Characterization of the low molecular weight human serum proteome. *Molecular and Cellular Proteomics* 2, 1096–1103.

Tjoa, M.L., Cindrova-Davies, T., Spasic-Boskovic, O., Bianchi, D.W. and Burton, G.J. (2006) Trophoblastic oxidative stress and the release of cell-free feto-placental DNA. *The American Journal of Pathology* 169, 400–404.

Van Crevel, R., Ottenhoff, T.H.M. and Van der Meer, J.W.M. (2002) Innate immunity to *Mycobacterium tuberculosis*. *Clinical Microbiology Reviews* 15, 294–309.

Vasioukhin, V., Anker, P., Maurice, P., Lyautey, J., Lederrey, C. and Stroun, M. (1994) Point mutations of the N-ras gene in the blood plasma DNA of patients with myelodysplastic syndrome or acute myelogenous leukaemia. *British Journal of Haematology* 86, 774–779.

Villarreal-Ramos, B., Mcaulay, M., Chance, V., Martin, M., Morgan, J. and Howard, C.J. (2003) Investigation of the role of CD8+ T cells in bovine tuberculosis in vivo. *American Society for Microbiology* 71, 4297–4303.

Vordermeier, H.M., Cockle, P.J., Whelan, A.O., Rhodes, S. and Hewinson, R.G. (2000) Toward the development of diagnostic assays to discriminate between *Mycobacterium bovis* infection and bacille Calmette-Guérin vaccination in cattle. *Clinical Infectious Diseases* Suppl(3), S291–8.

Vordermeier, H.M., De Val, B.P., Buddle, B.M., Villarreal-Ramos, B., Jones, G.J., *et al.* (2014) Vaccination of domestic animals against tuberculosis: review of progress and contributions to the field of the TBSTEP project. *Research in Veterinary Science* 97, S53–S60.

Vordermeier, H.M., Jones, G.J., Buddle, B.M. and Hewinson, R.G. (2016a) Development of immune-diagnostic reagents to diagnose bovine tuberculosis in cattle. *Veterinary Immunology and Immunopathology* 181, 10–14.

Vordermeier, H.M., Jones, G.J., Buddle, B.M., Hewinson, R.G. and Villarreal-Ramos, B. (2016b) Bovine tuberculosis in cattle: vaccines, DIVA tests, and host biomarker discovery. *Annual Review of Animal Biosciences* 4, 87–109.

Wallis, R.S., Pai, M., Menzies, D., Doherty, T.M., Walzl, G., *et al.* (2010) Biomarkers and diagnostics for tuberculosis: progress, needs, and translation into practice. *Lancet* 375, 1920–1937.

Wanzala, S.I., Waters, W.R., Thacker, T., Carstensen, M., Travis, D. and Sreevatsan, S. (2016) Pathogen specific biomarkers for the diagnosis of tuberculosis in deer. *American Journal of Veterinary Research* 78(6), 729–734.

Waters, W.R., Palmer, M.V., Nonnecke, B.J., Thacker, T.C., Scherer, C.F., *et al.* (2009) Efficacy and immunogenicity of *Mycobacterium bovis* DeltaRD1 against aerosol *M. bovis* infection in neonatal calves. *Vaccine* 27, 1201–1209.

Waters, W.R., Maggioli, M.F., Palmer, M.V., Thacker, T.C., Mcgill, J.L., *et al.* (2015) Interleukin-17A as a biomarker for bovine tuberculosis. *Clinical and Vaccine Immunology* 23, 168–180.

Whipple, D.L., Bolin, C.A., Davis, A.J., Jarnagin, J.L., Johnson, D.C., *et al.* (1995) Comparison of the sensitivity of the caudal fold skin test and a commercial gamma-interferon assay for diagnosis of bovine tuberculosis. *American Journal of Veterinary Research* 56, 415–419.

Williams, Z., Ben-Dov, I.Z., Elias, R., Mihailovic, A., Brown, M., *et al.* (2013) Comprehensive profiling of circulating microRNA via small RNA sequencing of cDNA libraries reveals biomarker potential and limitations. *Proceedings of the National Academy of Sciences of the United States of America* 110, 4255–4260.

Yip, T.T., Chan, J.W., Cho, W.C., Yip, T.T., Wang, Z., *et al.* (2005) Protein chip array profiling analysis in patients with severe acute respiratory syndrome identified serum amyloid a protein as a biomarker potentially useful in monitoring the extent of pneumonia. *Clinical Chemistry* 51, 47–55.

Young, B.L., Mlamla, Z., Gqamana, P.P., Smit, S., Roberts, T., *et al.* (2014) The identification of tuberculosis biomarkers in human urine samples. *The European Respiratory Journal* 43, 1719–1729.

Zhang, Z., Bast, R.C.J.R., Yu, Y., Li, J., Sokoll, L.J., *et al.* (2004) Three biomarkers identified from serum proteomic analysis for the detection of early stage ovarian cancer. *Cancer Research* 64, 5882–5890.

Ziegler, A., Zangemeister-Wittke, U. and Stahel, R.A. (2002) Circulating DNA: a new diagnostic gold mine? *Cancer Treatment Reviews* 28, 255–271.

14 Vaccination of Domestic and Wild Animals Against Tuberculosis

Bryce M. Buddle,[1],* Natalie A. Parlane,[1] Mark A. Chambers[2,3] and Christian Gortázar[4]

[1]AgResearch, Hopkirk Research Institute, Palmerston North, New Zealand; [2]Animal and Plant Health Agency – Weybridge, Addlestone, Surrey, UK; [3]School of Veterinary Medicine, Faculty of Health & Medical Sciences, University of Surrey, UK; [4]SaBio – Instituto de Investigación en Recursos Cinegéticos IREC, Universidad de Castilla-La Mancha & CSIC, Ciudad Real, Spain

14.1 Introduction

Mycobacterium bovis has a very wide host range and is the predominant cause of tuberculosis (TB) affecting domestic and wild animals, although tuberculosis in animals can also be caused by other members of the *Mycobacterium tuberculosis* complex. The disease in cattle, defined as bovine TB, continues to be a major economic animal health problem worldwide (Waters *et al.*, 2012). The test-and-slaughter bovine TB control programmes introduced in many countries in the mid-20th century achieved dramatic results and a number of countries were able to eradicate this disease. However, these control programmes have not been affordable or socially acceptable in many developing countries, and more than 94% of the world's population live in countries in which control of TB in cattle or buffaloes is limited or absent (Cousins, 2001). Furthermore, a confounding factor in the control of bovine TB in a number of countries is the existence of wildlife reservoirs of *M. bovis* infection. Wildlife serving as maintenance hosts for *M. bovis* includes the Australian brushtail possum (*Trichosurus vulpecula*) in New Zealand, the European badger (*Meles meles*) in UK and Ireland, white-tailed deer (*Odocoileus virginianus*) in Michigan, USA (reviewed by de Lisle *et al.*, 2001) and Eurasian wild boar (*Sus scrofa*) in the Iberian Peninsula (Naranjo *et al.*, 2008). In addition, red deer (*Cervus elaphus*) in several parts of Europe (Santos *et al.*, 2015a), African buffalo (*Syncerus caffer*) in South Africa (de Klerk *et al.*, 2010) and wood bison (*Bison athabascae*) and wapiti (*Cervus elephus manitobensis*) in Canada (Nishi *et al.*, 2006) serve as maintenance hosts for infection in hunting estates and national parks. These maintenance hosts act as sources of infection for domestic species, and in national parks, infection can spillover to other unique wildlife species including Iberian lynx (*Lynx pardinus*), lions (*Panthera leo*), cheetah (*Acinonyx jubatus*) and leopard (*Panthera pardus*). Partial control has been achieved for some of these maintenance hosts by reducing the density of animals or banning artificial feeding that causes local high densities of animals (Griffin *et al.*, 2005; O'Brien *et al.*, 2006; Livingstone *et al.*, 2015). However, few if any of these control measures can be implemented for some protected species or

---

* Email: bryce.buddle@agresearch.co.nz

where interference of a natural regulated ecosystem is deemed undesirable. For these reasons, the development and use of vaccines for control of TB in domestic and wild animals is very appealing.

Although no TB vaccines are currently registered for TB in cattle, there is renewed interest in their use from the realization of the financial impact of bovine TB on animal health and trade, and due to the difficulty controlling the disease. The major caveats that have restricted the use of TB vaccines in cattle have been that protection is not complete and vaccination can sensitize animals to respond in traditional TB diagnostic tests (Parlane and Buddle, 2015). These problems can now be potentially overcome by using a vaccination integrated with other control measures, revaccination with homologous or heterologous vaccines, and use of diagnostic tests that can differentiate infected from vaccinated animals (DIVA tests). Furthermore, experimental infection models of cattle with *M. bovis* and goats with *Mycobacterium caprae* are now being used to assess the efficacy of human TB vaccines (Vordermeier et al., 2009; Pérez de Val et al., 2013) with mutual benefits for both veterinary and medical applications. For wildlife, use of a vaccine to reduce or eradicate TB may be a cost-effective strategy, and vaccination has proven to be a successful method for control of rabies in wild foxes in Europe (Pastoret and Brochier, 1996). The focus of this chapter is to provide an update on the progress in vaccination of TB in domestic and wild animals. Reviews of the history of vaccination against TB in these animals can be found in Skinner et al. (2001), Waters et al. (2012) and Chambers et al. (2014).

14.2 Vaccination of Cattle

14.2.1 *Mycobacterium bovis* bacille Calmette–Guérin vaccine

The live, attenuated bacille Calmette–Guérin (BCG) vaccine strain of *M. bovis* is the only vaccine that is licensed for use in humans. There are many advantages for using BCG vaccine in domestic and wild animals as it is relatively inexpensive and proven safe for use in many animal species, is produced commercially for use in human application and DIVA tests to differentiate vaccinated animals from those infected with the wild-type strains are now available. BCG was first used in cattle by Calmette and Guérin in 1911, who showed that protection against *M. bovis* challenge was obtained by vaccination with relatively large (20 mg) doses of BCG (see Waters et al., 2012). Further BCG vaccination trials were undertaken by several other groups in the first half of the 20th century, and although experimental challenge trials provided encouraging results, more variable results were reported in field trials. Potential reasons for failure to protect include the administration of high doses of BCG (10^8–10^{10} colony-forming units [CFU] parenterally), very high level of *M. bovis* exposure, exposure of young calves to *M. bovis* through consumption of milk from infected cows prior to vaccination, lack of long-term protection and prior sensitization to environmental mycobacteria or helminths. Informative meta-analysis of these trials has been difficult as a number of different BCG strains, doses and vaccination routes were used, together with different methods to measure protection and varying levels of exposure to *M. bovis*.

Over the past 20 years a large number of vaccination/challenge trials have been undertaken in cattle using harmonized models, testing BCG alone or in comparative studies with other vaccines. Challenge models have focused on using a relatively low challenge dose of *M. bovis* (10^3–10^4 CFU) administered via endobronchial/intratracheal inoculation or by aerosol (Buddle et al., 1995; Palmer et al., 2002a). This has resulted in the development of tuberculous lesions mimicking those from natural disease in the lower respiratory tract. Similar BCG strains have been used (initially Pasteur, then BCG Danish 1331) and protection assessed by quantitative gross, histopathological and microbiological findings. Results from a number of studies have shown that doses of 10^4 to 10^6 CFU of BCG administered parenterally induced equivalent protection (Buddle et al., 1995), while higher doses (10^8 CFU) were required to induce protection when BCG was administered orally (Wedlock et al., 2011). Combinations of BCG by parenteral and mucosal routes has provided mixed results, with a small enhancement of protection observed when BCG was administered subcutaneously and endobronchially on the same day (Dean *et al.*, 2015), but not with the combination of subcutaneously and orally administered BCG (Buddle *et al.*, 2008). Pasteur and Danish strains of BCG induced similar protection, although the kinetics of the cellular immune response varied with the two strains (Wedlock *et al.*, 2007; Hope *et al.*, 2011). Neonatal or very young calves were protected at least as well as older calves (Buddle *et al.*, 2003; Hope *et al.*, 2005). Vaccination of cattle with BCG 3 weeks after an experimental challenge with *M. bovis* did not produce a beneficial effect, nor increased tuberculous pathology (Buddle *et al.*, 2016). Protection against experimental challenge was shown to be effective at ≤12 months post-vaccination, but had waned by 24 months post-vaccination (Thom *et al.*, 2012).

Two studies were undertaken to determine the effect of revaccination with BCG. In the first study, calves vaccinated within 8 hours of birth or at 6 weeks of age showed a high level of protection against *M. bovis*, while those vaccinated within 8 hours of birth and revaccinated at 6 weeks of age had a reduced level of protection (Buddle *et al.*, 2003). The revaccinated calves with the lowest level of protection had the strongest antigen-specific IFN-γ responses, suggesting that revaccination had induced an inappropriate immune response. In neonatal calves, antigen-specific IFN-γ responses remained at elevated levels for longer than those seen in older calves, possibly due to a more active BCG infection and BCG revaccination when immune responses were at high levels may be contraindicated. In contrast, calves vaccinated with BCG at 2 to 4 weeks of age and revaccinated at 2 years of age when immunity had waned, showed a significant level of protection when challenged 6 months later, while those receiving only the initial vaccine dose were not protected (Parlane *et al.*, 2014).

Trials in Ethiopia and Mexico that were undertaken in field conditions with exposure of vaccinated and non-vaccinated calves to in-contact, tuberculin-reactor cows, demonstrated a significant level of protection in the vaccinated calves (Ameni *et al.*, 2010; Lopez-Valencia *et al.*, 2010). In a large-scale field trial in New Zealand, cattle vaccinated orally with BCG and exposed to tuberculin-reactor cattle and a wildlife reservoir of infection had a significant level of protection compared to non-vaccinated cattle, with an estimated vaccine efficacy of 67% for preventing infection (Nugent *et al.* 2017).

14.2.2 New generation TB vaccines

In the past two decades, large amounts of funding have been provided to develop human TB vaccines and efforts to develop and evaluate cattle TB vaccines have greatly benefited from this research. The different types of TB vaccines that have recently been tested in cattle include live attenuated mycobacteria, which could replace BCG, and subunit TB vaccines such as DNA, protein, and virus-vectored vaccines, which could be used to boost immunity induced by BCG (Parlane and Buddle, 2015, summarized in Table 14.1).

Published reports evaluating live attenuated mycobacterial vaccines in cattle have included modified BCG strains, a *M. bovis* auxotroph and deletion mutants of *M. tuberculosis* and *M. bovis*. Significant protection against challenge with a virulent *M. bovis* strain combined with lower pulmonary histological scores was obtained by a BCG expressing Ag85B, in comparison with vaccination using BCG alone (Rizzi *et al.*, 2012). Additional modifications have been used, including a *zmp1* deletion, with the rationale that the Zmp1 protein in mycobacteria prevents activation of the inflammasome, thereby inhibiting maturation of the phagolysosome and MHCI and II dependent mycobacterial antigen presentation. Improved T-cell memory responses in comparison with BCG was obtained by vaccination involving either of two BCG *zmp1* deletants (Khatri *et al.*, 2014). Recent experiments to assess its protective efficacy have demonstrated a trend towards better protection against lesions in the thoracic lymph nodes (B. Khatri, unpublished data). Vaccination with a cocktail of four BCG Danish mutants (BCGΔ*leuCD*, BCGΔ*fdr8*, BCGΔ*mmA4*, BCGΔ*pks16*) induced significant protection in cattle against *M. bovis* challenge to a level comparable with wild-type BCG Danish (Waters *et al.*, 2015).

Vaccination with either of two attenuated *M. bovis* strains derived by UV irradiation, with deletions not defined, produced significant protection against challenge with *M. bovis* in calves naturally pre-sensitized to environmental

Table 14.1. Types of new TB vaccines tested in cattle.

Type of Vaccine	Vaccine	Protection against TB compared to BCG	Reference
Modified BCG	BCG over-expressing Ag85B	+	Rizzi et al., 2012
	BCG Δ zmp1	+	Khatri et al., 2014, and B. Khatri, unpublished data
	BCG mutants (BCGDleuCD, BCGDfdr8, BCGDmmA4, BCGDpks16)	=	Waters et al., 2015
Attenuated M. tuberculosis strain	M. tuberculosis ΔRD1 ΔpanCD	−	Waters et al., 2007
Attenuated M. bovis strain	UV-irradiated M. bovis	+	Buddle et al., 2002
	M. bovis Δ leuD	NT[b]	Khare et al., 2007
	M. bovis Δ RD1	=	Waters et al., 2009
	M. bovis Δ mce2	+	Blanco et al., 2013
DNA vaccine	Mycobacterial DNA	=	Maue et al., 2004; Cai et al., 2005
	Heterologous prime boost: mycobacterial DNA+BCG	+	Skinner et al., 2003, 2005; Maue et al., 2007
Adjuvanted protein vaccine	Simultaneous protein+BCG	+	Wedlock et al., 2005a, 2008
Virus-vectored vaccine	Heterologous prime boost: BCG+Ad85A	+	Vordermeier et al., 2009; Dean et al., 2014a

mycobacteria, in a study where BCG vaccine was shown to be ineffective (Buddle et al., 2002; Parlane and Buddle, 2015). Vaccination with a leucine auxotroph of M. bovis was shown to significantly reduce the bacterial burden and histopathology in calves following challenge with virulent M. bovis, compared to non-vaccinated controls (Khare et al., 2007). A comparison with BCG was not undertaken in this study. A double deletion mutant of M. tuberculosis, a region of difference 1 (RD1) knockout and pantothenate auxotroph, failed to protect calves from an aerosolised M. bovis challenge (Waters et al., 2007), while vaccination with a RD1 deletion mutant of M. bovis provided protection comparable to BCG (Waters et al., 2009). For cattle, an attenuated M. tuberculosis mutant may be less immunogenic as compared to those produced on a M. bovis or BCG background strain as cattle are not a natural host for M. tuberculosis. An attenuated M. bovis strain with a double deletion in the mce2 gene was shown to induce significant protection against an M. bovis challenge in cattle and significantly lower histopathological lesion scores in the lungs and pulmonary lymph nodes than those vaccinated with BCG (Blanco et al., 2013).

No subunit TB vaccine has been able to induce better protection in cattle than that induced by BCG, although they can produce a synergistic effect when used in combination with BCG. DNA vaccines have induced minimal protection against TB when used alone, although some protection has been observed when mycobacterial DNA was combined with DNA encoding co-stimulatory molecules CD80 and CD86 (Maue et al., 2004) or combined with an adjuvant (Cai et al., 2005). More encouraging results have been reported when DNA vaccines have been used in heterologous prime-boost regimes with BCG, and priming or boosting with mycobacterial DNA vaccines induced greater protection than with BCG vaccine alone (Skinner et al., 2003, 2005; Maue et al., 2007). Similarly, TB protein vaccines have induced little protection in cattle when used alone, whereas when co-administered at adjacent sites with BCG have induced protection that was better than that observed with BCG alone (Wedlock et al., 2005a, 2008). The major problem encountered using

TB protein vaccines in cattle has been the difficulty of inducing strong cellular immune responses with these vaccines, despite co-administration with a range of adjuvants and immunomodulators. The use of virally-vectored TB vaccines has shown considerable promise when applied in heterologous prime-boost approaches in which the bovine immune response is primed with BCG and then boosted with virally-vectored vaccines developed for use as human TB vaccines. Priming with BCG Danish and boosting with a replication deficient human adenovirus 5 expressing Ag85A (Ad85A) resulted in protection superior to that with BCG alone (Vordermeier et al., 2009). In a recent study, BCG-vaccinated calves were boosted with either Ad5 expressing Ag85A (Ad5-85A) or Ag85A, Rv0287, Rv0288 and Rv0251 (Ad5-TBF), but only those boosted with Ad5-85A induced a significantly lower histopathological lesion score than that for those vaccinated with BCG alone (Dean et al., 2014a). From an immunogenicity study, the optimal dose and route of immunisation of the Ad5-85A used as a boost following a BCG prime was determined to be 2×10^9 infectious units delivered intradermally (Dean et al., 2014b).

It has also been shown that Ad85A boosting of BCG delivered by mucosal (endobronchial) or systemic (intradermal) routes induced comparable peripheral blood responses, and bronchioalveolar lavage cells producing antigen-specific IFN-γ (Whelan et al., 2012). Furthermore, when calves were vaccinated at the same time with BCG via the systemic route and Ad85A via mucosal (endobronchial) application, there was a trend towards better protective efficacy than for vaccination with BCG alone (Dean et al., 2015).

14.2.3 Correlates of protection

An impediment in the development of improved TB vaccines for animals is that no single correlate of protection has been identified for TB, although a number have shown promise in this regard. Currently, it is still necessary to assess protection against TB by challenging animals with virulent mycobacteria. Protection against an intracellular pathogen such as M. bovis is largely dependent on a T-cell-mediated immune response, and the most promising correlates of protection include the quality of the immune response defined by the magnitude and profile of the cytokine response and induction of memory responses.

Early IFN-γ responses are required post-vaccination, so the timing of testing is important, but the magnitude of the IFN-γ responses does not always correlate with protection (Buddle et al., 2003; Wedlock et al., 2007). A search has been initiated for alternative or additional cytokines to serve as correlates for protection. In this regard, IL-17 and IL-22 responses to mycobacterial antigens have looked promising in cattle (Rizzi et al., 2012; Bhuju et al., 2012; Waters et al., 2015). IL-17 can be produced by a range of T cells (TH17, γΔ and NK cells) and is considered to be important for the accumulation of protective memory cells in the lungs and cross-regulation of T-cell subsets (Waters et al., 2015). Although the role of IL-22 has not been defined, one potential effector mechanism could be the production of beta-defensins. In small animal models, the numbers of polyfunctional T cells have been associated with protection (Aagaard et al., 2009; McShane, 2009). However, in cattle, the presence of IFN-γ, IL-2 and TNF-α or combinations of at least two of these markers did not predict vaccine efficacy when measured before challenge, but was associated strongly with increased pathology post-M. bovis challenge (Vordermeier et al., 2009; Whelan et al., 2011a). Detection of a delayed-type hypersensitivity response to tuberculin is the primary screening test for diagnosis of TB in cattle; however, it is not a consistent correlate for protection post-vaccination, particularly for the maintenance of protection (Whelan et al., 2011b). A confusing aspect is that many of these markers for protection also serve as indicators of disease post-challenge.

Measurement of T-cell memory responses in cattle using the cultured ELISPOT method has been recently shown to be a promising predictor of vaccine efficacy, with significantly elevated responses in vaccinated/protected animals compared to matched vaccinated/non-protected animals (Vordermeier et al., 2009; Dean et al., 2014a). In addition, maintenance of strong cultured ELISPOT responses was associated with the duration of immunity post-vaccination

(Thom et al., 2012). The T-cell subset involved in this response was almost exclusively CD4$^+$, particularly CD45RO$^+$CD62L^{high} 'central memory'-like phenotype. In contrast, the effector/effector memory T-cell phenotype (CD45RO$^+$CD62L^{low}) was the main contributor to *ex vivo* ELISPOT responses, not necessarily a predictor of vaccine protection (Blunt et al., 2015).

A number of immune parameters have been associated with pathology post-challenge, which indirectly correlates with vaccine efficacy. These include *ex vivo* ESAT-6-induced production of IFN-γ (Vordermeier et al., 2002) as well as IL-17A and IL-22 (Aranday-Cortes et al., 2012). In addition, a chemokine, IP-10 (CXCL10), was shown to be associated with up-regulation in infected versus non-infected animals (Aranday-Cortes et al., 2012). Micro-RNAs (miRNA) that serve as important regulators of gene expression and are known to play a role in both innate and adaptive immunity have been investigated as markers of pathology. The expression of mi155 following PPD-stimulation of PBMCs was shown to be associated with disease severity in *M. bovis*-infected cattle (Golby et al., 2014).

14.2.4 DIVA tests

Vaccination with TB vaccines can compromise the interpretation of the tuberculin skin test, which serves as the primary screening test for 'test-and-slaughter' bovine TB control strategies. Eighty per cent of BCG-vaccinated calves have been shown to react in the tuberculin skin test at 6 months post-vaccination, decreasing to 10–20% by 9 months post-vaccination (Whelan et al., 2011b). Alternative DIVA (differentiating infected from vaccinated animals) tests will be required for countries intending to use vaccination alongside conventional test-and-slaughter control strategies. DIVA tests have now been developed using antigens from the *M. tuberculosis* complex that are not expressed or secreted by BCG and can be used instead of bovine PPD in the whole-blood IFN-γ or skin tests. The first two antigens used in the DIVA IFN-γ test were the early secreted antigen target 6 kDa protein (ESAT-6) and culture filtrate protein 10 (CFP10), which are encoded in the RD1 region of *M. tuberculosis* and *M. bovis*, but not in BCG. This test had the added benefit of differentiating *M. bovis*-infected cattle from those infected with environmental mycobacteria or *M. avium* subsp. *paratuberculosis* (Buddle et al., 1999; Vordermeier et al., 2001). The sensitivity of this test was still lower than that for the IFN-γ test using avian and bovine PPDs and further antigen mining was required to identify additional antigens. Following comparative transcriptome analysis of *Mycobacterium* species, Rv3615c was added to the antigen-specific IFN-γ test to enhance sensitivity (Sidders et al., 2008). Although, this protein is not located in the RD1 region, its secretion is dependent on the esx-1 secretion system located in the RD1 region. A recent evaluation of the whole-blood IFN-γ test incorporating ESAT-6, CFP10 and Rv3615c in 75 BCG-vaccinated, *M. bovis*-infected cattle and 179 BCG-vaccinated, non-infected animals revealed estimates of 96% sensitivity and 95.5% specificity (Chambers et al., 2014).

The most efficient means of using a DIVA whole-blood IFN-γ test would be for re-testing tuberculin-positive cattle; however, a more cost-effective method would be to use the DIVA antigens in the primary screening skin test. Use of ESAT-6, CFP10 and Rv3615c in the DIVA skin test in cattle has now been shown to have a high sensitivity for *M. bovis*-infected cattle, while not compromised by vaccination with BCG or with vaccines against Johne's disease (Whelan et al., 2010; Jones et al., 2012). The cost of the reagents used in the test could be reduced by expression as a fusion protein and lowering the concentration of the antigens by display on nanoparticles such as polyester beads produced in bacteria (Parlane et al., 2016).

14.3 Vaccination of Goats

TB infection of goats is caused by *M. bovis* or *M. caprae* and in the natural disease, lesions are predominantly found in the lungs and associated lymph nodes, indicating an aerosol route of infection (Pesciaroli et al., 2014). The disease is responsible for economic losses in endemic areas and infected goats may be a source of TB for cattle or humans. Caprine TB is present in a number of European countries, but currently there are no caprine TB control campaigns in the

European Union. Recently, it was shown that infection of goats with a low dose of M. caprae (10^3 CFU) via the endobronchial route produced lesions in all infected animals at 14 weeks after infection, showing pathology reflecting the natural disease of caseous necrotic and cavitary lesions in the lungs (Pérez de Val et al., 2011). In contrast, aerosol infection of goats with a similar dose of M. bovis produced small pulmonary lesions (Gonzalez-Juarrero et al., 2013). This difference in pathology may have arisen from differences in routes of infection as in a subsequent study where groups of goats were challenged transthoracically with either M. bovis or M. caprae, the total lesion scores and culture results were higher for the M. bovis-challenged goats (Bezos et al., 2015). To determine protective efficacy of vaccines, gross and microscopic lesions have been assessed by qualitative and quantitative analyses, together with mycobacterial culture from lung-associated lymph nodes. The precise determination of the total lung lesion burden related to total lung volume has been achieved using multi-detector computed tomography (Pérez de Val et al., 2011).

BCG Danish vaccine administered subcutaneously at a dose of 5×10^5 CFU was shown to be safe and no shedding of BCG was detected in the faeces of vaccinated kids or in the milk of vaccinated, lactating goats (Pérez de Val et al., 2016). BCG was isolated from a lymph node draining the site of vaccination from one kid at 8-weeks post-vaccination, but not from any goats at 24-weeks post-vaccination. A single dose of BCG vaccine administered subcutaneously to goats was shown to significantly induce protection against challenge with M. caprae, with reductions in pulmonary pathology and bacterial load. The testing in goats of a heterologous prime/boost with BCG followed by virus-vectored vaccines, Ad5-Ag85A or Ad5-TBF, have provided encouraging results with significant protection against endobronchial M. caprae challenge compared to those receiving BCG vaccine alone or the non-vaccinates (Pérez de Val et al., 2012, 2013). Vaccination with BCG or BCG plus Ad5-Ag85A appeared to prevent haematogenous dissemination of mycobacteria with extra-thoracic TB lesions only found in non-vaccinated goats (Pérez de Val et al., 2012). Furthermore, use of mycobacterial DIVA reagents, ESAT-6 and CFP10, in the IFN-γ tests were able to differentiate TB-infected from BCG-vaccinated goats. In vaccinated goats, cultured IFN-γ ELISPOT responses against Ag85A correlated significantly with protection (Pérez de Val et al., 2013), concurring with results in cattle that measurement of specific IFN-γ-producing memory cells could be a predictor of TB vaccine efficacy.

Vaccination has been seen as a valuable long-term control prospect, reducing the TB prevalence prior to starting a test-and-slaughter eradication programme which would reduce economic costs for producers and the public sector. In addition, the goat model has considerable potential for testing candidate human TB vaccines and has a number of advantages including similar TB pathology such as the development of lung cavitary lesions and a lower cost compared to that for the model in cattle.

14.4 Vaccination of Deer

Vaccination studies of deer have been undertaken to assess whether vaccination could be an effective method of protecting farmed deer from TB and to develop a system for vaccinating feral deer to prevent re-infection back into cattle herds. TB in wild or farmed deer is predominantly caused by M. bovis, and commonly, tuberculous lesions are described as liquefied or abscess-like in contrast to the caseous nature of the lesions seen in cattle and goats (Beatson, 1985; Fitzgerald and Kaneene, 2013). The distribution of the tuberculous lesions also differs from those in cattle with the retropharyngeal lymph nodes being the most common site for lesions in deer, followed by lesions in the lungs and associated lymph nodes as well as in the mesenteric lymph nodes (Martín-Hernando et al., 2010). The primary lesion complex in deer appears to be tonsils and retropharyngeal lymph nodes, suggesting an oral or aerosol route of infection. To reproduce the typical pathology seen in natural infected deer, low doses of M. bovis (10^2 CFU) have been instilled into the tonsillar crypts with lesions developing in the tonsils and retropharyngeal lymph nodes (Griffin et al., 1995; Palmer et al., 2002b).

Studies of BCG vaccine in deer have shown that a single dose of BCG administered subcutaneously to 3-month-old deer could reduce disease severity, while re-vaccinating deer at intervals of 8- to 16-week intervals induced protection against infection, but not at an interval of 43 weeks (Griffin et al., 2006). Parenteral BCG administered to deer at a dose of 10^6 CFU and oral BCG at 10^8 CFU induced a similar degree of protection (Nol et al., 2008). Evidence has been provided of transmission of BCG by shedding of BCG from parenterally vaccinated deer to in-contact, non-vaccinated deer (Palmer et al., 2009, 2010; Nol et al., 2013). It is not known whether these non-vaccinated deer would be protected against TB. BCG was shown to persist for 3 to 9 months in lymphoid tissues of deer vaccinated parenterally or orally (Palmer et al., 2010). Oral bait vaccines would be the most feasible means to administer TB vaccines to large populations of wild deer. However, a complication can relate to vaccine bait delivery where there are bans in some TB-endemic areas (e.g. Michigan, USA) on the supplementary feeding of wild deer as a TB control measure to reduce deer congregation in large numbers. Secondly, there are concerns about non-target uptake of vaccine baits, particularly by cattle.

Simulation modelling has examined the potential role that vaccination could play in the eradication of TB in wild deer in Michigan, USA, and in control programmes to minimize cattle herd breakdowns (Ramsey et al., 2014). Using a vaccine with 90% efficacy, annual vaccination of 90% of susceptible deer was necessary to achieve a 95% probability of eradication within 30 years, whereas vaccination of 50–90% of susceptible deer within a 5-km radius of cattle farms could achieve a 95% probability of having zero cattle herd breakdowns in 15–18 years.

14.5 Vaccination of Wildlife

The requirements of a TB vaccine for wildlife are that the animals would only receive a single vaccination and, for practical purposes, the vaccine would be self-administered via an oral bait. For an oral bait vaccine to be left in the environment, the vaccine needs to be safe. These requirements can be met by using an attenuated mycobacterial vaccine such as BCG and a summary of studies undertaken with BCG vaccine in wildlife is shown in Table 14.2. The use of a killed M. bovis vaccine for wild boar has also shown promise.

14.5.1 Vaccination of brushtail possums

The brushtail possum is the major wildlife reservoir of M. bovis infection in New Zealand; it has been declared a noxious pest. Possums are highly susceptible to M. bovis infection and lesions are found predominantly in the lungs and superficial lymph nodes. Culling of possums by trapping and poisoning has been a major contributor in the dramatic reduction in the numbers of infected cattle over the past 20 years (Livingstone et al., 2015). Vaccination of possums against TB has the potential to be an effective TB control measure when it is not suitable to cull possums, for example, near urban areas. The key attribute of a successful wildlife TB vaccine would be to prevent the spread of M. bovis infection to other wildlife or domestic animals and prevention of infection is of lesser importance compared to that for domestic species. However, the major challenges for the vaccination of wildlife are vaccine delivery and need for a single dose vaccine. For the formulation of an oral bait BCG vaccine, the BCG bacilli have been encapsulated in a lipid matrix which protects the bacteria from degradation in the acidic stomach environment and enhances shelf life of the vaccine in the field. This vaccine was shown to protect possums against an experimental aerosol challenge with M. bovis, (Aldwell et al., 2003). Vaccine-induced immunity waned between 6 to 12 months post-vaccination following oral vaccination and there were no differences between BCG doses of 10^7 and 10^8 CFU or between Danish and Pasteur strains of BCG (Buddle et al., 2006). A more recent study indicated that protection against an experimental M. bovis infection extended out to 28 months post-vaccination (Tompkins et al., 2013). BCG bacilli were shown to be stable in the lipid matrix for 7 weeks under room temperature conditions and 3 to 5 weeks under field conditions in a forest/pasture habitat, when maintained in weather-proof, bait-delivery sachets (Cross et al., 2009). Uptake of oral bait placebo vaccines was shown to be high, with 85 to 100% of wild possums accessing baits at bait densities of 40–80 sachets/hectare (Cross et al., 2009).

Table 14.2. Summary of TB vaccine efficacy studies in wildlife.

Species/country	Vaccine/route[a]	Challenge type	Vaccine efficacy[b]	Notes/particular issues	Key references
Brushtail possum/New Zealand	BCG/O,M,P	Aerosol, natural exposure	+ +	High vaccine cost compared to that for poisons	Aldwell et al., 2003; Tompkins et al., 2009
European badger/UK, Ireland	BCG/O,M,P	Endobronchial, natural exposure	++	Parenteral vaccine licensed (BadgerBCG™) For an oral vaccine: demonstration of consistent protection and definition of minimal efficacious dose	Chambers et al., 2014 Murphy et al., 2014; Carter et al., 2012
White-tailed deer/USA	BCG/O,P	Intratonsilar	+	BCG persistence in tissues, bans on supplementary baiting, non-target update	Nol et al., 2008; Palmer et al., 2009
Eurasian wild boar/Spain	BCG/O,P Killed M. bovis/O,P	Oral Oral, Natural exposure	+ + +	Non-target bait uptake Regulatory issues	Gortázar et al., 2014 Beltrán-Beck et al., 2014a, 2014b; Díez-Delgado et al., 2016
Ferret/New Zealand	BCG/O,P	Oral	±	Rarely maintenance host for M. bovis	Qureshi et al., 1999; Cross et al., 2000
African buffalo/South Africa	BCG/P	Intratonsilar	–	Practicality of vaccine delivery in the field	De Klerk et al., 2010

[a] Vaccination route: O, oral; M, other mucosal; P, parenteral.
[b] Vaccine efficacy: +, protection; ±, partial protection; –, no protection

Consumption of oral bait BCG vaccine by possums resulted in the shedding of relatively low concentrations of BCG, 10^2–10^4 CFU/g faeces for up to a week (Wedlock et al., 2005b).

An encouraging result from a recent 2-year field trial involving oral vaccination of possums was that BCG vaccine had a 95% efficacy in prevention of TB (Tompkins et al., 2009). This result was different to that observed in experimental challenge studies where BCG vaccination resulted in a significant reduction in the severity of the pathology, but did not prevent infection (Aldwell et al., 2003; Buddle et al., 2006). These results indicated that the experimental challenge with M. bovis was more severe than that from natural exposure with M. bovis. There is potential for the development of new tuberculosis vaccines for wildlife that perform better than BCG. Collins et al. (2011) have produced a newly attenuated M. bovis vaccine that gave more measures of protection in possums against aerosol M. bovis challenge than BCG.

14.5.2 Vaccination of badgers

The European badger is the major wildlife reservoir of M. bovis infection in the British Isles due to their relative abundance and ecology, the prevalence of infection and presentation of TB pathology compared to other sylvatic species (Delahay et al., 2007; Godfray et al., 2013). Badgers are relatively resistant to the development of TB following infection with M. bovis, and latent infection without clinical signs or visible lesions at necropsy is not uncommon (Corner et al., 2011). In badgers, TB is a chronic, slowly progressing disease. As such its presentation can vary along a spectrum from latent infection through to lesions widely spread throughout the body (Corner et al., 2011). As lesions are found predominantly in the lungs it is believed that aerogenic acquisition and transmission of infection is the principal mode of transmission. More disseminated infection is thought to occur through bite wounding via the transmission of M. bovis within saliva.

Options for preventing the transmission of *M. bovis* from infected badgers to cattle are limited to minimizing the potential for contact between them (biosecurity), reducing the number and density of infected badgers via selective and non-selective culling, and vaccination, with the objective of reducing the force of infection within and between species (reviewed by Gormley and Corner, 2013). Badgers are protected by law in the UK and Ireland, which limits the public acceptability and practicality of disease control through culling. Trials to ascertain the impact of reducing badger populations of bovine TB in England and Ireland have delivered complex and sometimes conflicting results that likely reflect subtle differences in the epidemiology of the disease locally (O'Connor et al., 2012). Options for effective biosecurity may be limited by what is practical and feasible and the recognition that the environment may be contaminated by *M. bovis* leading to opportunities for indirect infection (King et al., 2015). Vaccination of badgers against TB has the potential to be an effective TB control measure, especially in combination with other control measures (Abdou et al., 2016). As in the case of possums in New Zealand, the key attribute of a successful TB vaccine for badgers would be to prevent the spread of *M. bovis* infection to other wildlife or domestic animals. Prevention of infection is of lesser importance compared to that for domestic species. At present, the developed vaccine agent for tackling TB in badgers is BCG.

The use of BCG to vaccinate badgers against TB in the UK was licensed by the UK Competent Authority (Veterinary Medicines Directorate) in 2010 as BadgerBCG™ and is available for use by vets and trained lay vaccinators under prescription from a veterinary surgeon. Licensing of BadgerBCG™ required evidence of vaccine safety and efficacy, obtained from laboratory and field studies. The laboratory studies showed that vaccination of badgers by injection with BCG was both safe and significantly reduced lesions of TB caused by *M. bovis* (Lesellier et al., 2006, 2011). Protection was incomplete, in that *M. bovis* infection of vaccinated badgers still produced either visible pathology or *M. bovis* was isolated from organs at necropsy. The problem with the experimental studies was that high challenge doses were necessary to ensure reproducible infection and therefore the protection produced by BCG vaccination may not reflect the level of protection against more natural challenge involving a range of infectious doses. When tested in a field study in wild badgers over 4 years, the level of protection using BCG was consistent with the protection induced directly by BCG in the experimental studies. Uninfected animals identified as negative in a range of diagnostic tests were less likely to become immunologically/serologically positive after vaccination than were non-vaccinated control badgers (Chambers et al., 2011; Carter et al., 2012). In addition, unvaccinated badger cubs taken from a vaccinated social group were much less likely to react to TB if more social group members had been vaccinated previously. This is remarkable and most likely an effect of herd immunity where transmission rates are effectively reduced in those groups of animals in which a higher percentage are vaccinated.

A practical limitation to the extensive use of BadgerBCG™ is the need to trap badgers before the vaccine can be injected. A form of BCG that could be delivered orally to badger populations via impregnated food baits would reduce this limitation and make more extensive vaccine deployment feasible. A wide variety of oral baits have been developed and assessed for their palatability and attractiveness to both captive and wild badgers (M. Chambers, unpublished results). BCG has been incorporated into the most promising of these, including encapsulation in the same lipid matrix used to deliver BCG orally to possums. BCG retains viability for prolonged periods in frozen baits and for sufficient time in simulated and actual environmental conditions (i.e. temperature and humidity) to make vaccination via bait feasible. Administration of BCG orally to captive badgers, either directly to the back of the throat, or indirectly via ingested bait has been shown to protect badgers against experimental challenge with *M. bovis* (Murphy et al., 2014; M. Chambers, unpublished results). A dose of 7.9×10^9 to 8.1×10^9 CFU BCG given to nine badgers orally was well tolerated. BCG was shed in faeces by two vaccinated badgers (372 CFU/g and 996 CFU/g) approximately 48 hours later (M. Chambers, unpublished results). The target dose of BCG for the oral vaccination of badgers is yet to be defined.

Assuming widespread annual deployment, the beneficial effects of badger vaccination should accrue over time as the proportion of the population vaccinated increases and animals with pre-existing infection die off naturally. There is currently no empirical evidence on the optimal size or duration for a badger vaccination programme. Benefits should start to accrue from the onset of immunity and most badgers (whether infected with TB or not) are expected to die off within 5 years (Wilkinson et al., 2000). A field trial was recently completed in Ireland that should provide the first estimate of BCG efficacy under field conditions. Lipid-encapsulated BCG was delivered to the back of the throat of anaesthetised badgers, while other badgers received only the lipid as placebo. The study area was divided into three equally representative zones with different proportions (0%, 50% and 100%) of the badger population in each zone being vaccinated with either BCG or placebo (Gormley and Corner, 2013). A secondary objective of the trial was to measure the effect of BCG vaccine in badgers with pre-existing *M. bovis* infection. When available, these data will add to those from the relatively small field study conducted in England with injectable BCG, in which no evidence was found of either a beneficial or detrimental effect of administering vaccine to badgers already harbouring TB. In addition to providing a measurement of protection and an estimate of vaccine efficacy, when published, the field trial in Ireland will also provide a practical basis for assessing the logistics of administering vaccine to wild badger populations annually on a large geographical scale.

14.5.3 Vaccination of wild boar

The wild boar is the main wildlife reservoir of the *M. tuberculosis* complex (MTC) in Mediterranean habitats of the Iberian Peninsula, where TB prevalence in wild boar is associated with TB occurrence on cattle farms (LaHue et al., 2016). The wild boar is also involved in MTC maintenance in many other regions (Gortázar et al., 2015a). This native suid is widespread in Eurasia and its populations are steadily growing despite legal hunting (Massei et al., 2015). Wild boar are highly susceptible to MTC infection and lesions are most frequently found in the mandibular lymph nodes, although over 50% of the cases generalize, affecting the lungs and thoracic lymph nodes (Martín-Hernando et al., 2007). Recent evidence shows that inter-species contacts involving wild boar are extremely rare in Mediterranean habitats (Cowie et al., 2016), and that transmission is most likely taking place indirectly, for instance at shared waterholes (Santos et al., 2015b; Barasona et al., 2016). While attempts to control TB in wild boar or at the wild boar–cattle interface through culling and farm biosafety have yielded some progress, vaccines will permit a more cost-effective and sustainable disease control (Gortázar et al., 2015b).

Both BCG and a heat-inactivated *M. bovis* vaccine yielded significant protection (70–80% lesion score reduction) in laboratory challenge trials (Garrido et al., 2011; Beltrán-Beck et al., 2014a; Gortázar et al., 2014). As mentioned above for other wild hosts, the key attribute of a successful TB vaccine would be to prevent the spread of MTC infection to other wildlife or domestic animals, with prevention of infection being less relevant. The major challenges for vaccinating wild boar are: (i) vaccine delivery including the selective targeting of (mostly uninfected) piglets while avoiding the risk of accidental live-vaccine uptake by cattle and subsequent positive TB-tests; (ii) vaccine safety for target and non-target species; and (iii) vaccine efficacy under field conditions. Regarding (i), selective wild boar piglet feeders, a patented bait and appropriate timing allowed delivery of oral baits containing TB vaccines in a safe manner (Beltrán-Beck et al., 2014b). Regarding (ii), recent research has focused on heat-inactivated *M. bovis* rather than on BCG. This implied full safety, since neither vaccine strain survival in host tissues nor vaccine strain transmission are possible after proper inactivation (Beltrán-Beck et al., 2014b). Finally, regarding (iii), two field trials tested the efficacy of parenteral vaccination and of oral vaccination, respectively. In the first one, 668 farmed wild boar piglets were parenterally (IM) vaccinated with heat-inactivated *M. bovis*, while 182 were not vaccinated and served as controls. In this low-prevalence setting, parenteral vaccination protected vaccinated individuals (66% reduction in lesion prevalence) against natural challenge

(Díez-Delgado et al., 2016). The second one (2012–2016) tested the uptake rates and efficacy of oral BCG and of oral heat-inactivated M. bovis in high prevalence settings (40–80% wild boar infection prevalence) in Montes de Toledo, Spain. Results are still in preparation, but preliminary analyses suggest that heat-inactivated M. bovis performed better than BCG, and that heat-inactivated M. bovis can significantly contribute to TB control in wild boar under field conditions (Díez-Delgado et al., unpublished data).

Ongoing laboratory research with heat-inactivated M. bovis is also targeting other hosts ranging from cattle, deer and goats (Roy et al., 2017; Thomas et al., 2017; van der Heijden et al., 2017). The multi-host nature and environmental survival of MTC generates complexity, a context where successful disease control strategies will need to integrate all available tools, including biosafety and prevention, population control where possible, and vaccination.

14.5.3 Vaccination of ferrets

In New Zealand, ferrets (*Mustela furo*) can become infected with M. bovis via feeding on tuberculous carcasses, particularly possums, and potentially can become a source of infection for other wildlife or cattle (Byrom et al., 2015). In most circumstances, ferrets are simply spill-over hosts, but on rare occasions may act as maintenance hosts when present in high densities. Vaccination has been considered as a possible control measure for ferrets and in the first of two vaccination trials, ferrets orally vaccinated with BCG incorporated into dietary meat were partially protected against oral challenge with virulent M. bovis (Qureshi et al., 1999). In the second trial, vaccination of ferrets with BCG by the subcutaneous route resulted in reduced severity of disease following experimental infection with M. bovis (Cross et al., 2000). Ferrets and badgers are members of the Mustelidae family and because of availability and ease of housing, ferrets may serve as a convenient model for evaluating tuberculosis vaccines designed for badgers. A new experimental infection model has been established in ferrets based on aerosolised M. bovis (McCallan et al., 2011),

but reports assessing vaccine efficacy using this model have yet to be published.

14.5.4 Vaccination of African buffalo

African buffaloes are the main wildlife reservoir of M. bovis in some South African game parks, and vaccination has been considered as one of the few ethically acceptable control measures that could be available. A vaccine trial was undertaken to assess the efficacy of BCG vaccine for buffaloes. Two doses of BCG were administered subcutaneously and the buffalo were challenged with virulent M. bovis via the intratonsillar route. The study did not reveal significant differences in the number of lesioned animals between the vaccinated and control groups (de Klerk et al., 2010). Delivery of a TB vaccine to large herds of buffalo continually on the move would be a considerable challenge.

14.6 Conclusions

Vaccination of cattle with BCG would have greatest application in countries where test-and-slaughter strategies are not affordable or socially acceptable, and in this situation reducing the spread of bovine tuberculosis would be very valuable. However, vaccination would need to be integrated with other control measures as vaccination alone is unlikely to induce complete protection. It is well recognized in humans that BCG confers some non-specific protective effects against other pathogens (Garly et al., 2003). This has yet to be evaluated in cattle, but could potentially have benefits in developing countries. It is important that BCG is field tested in different environments and husbandry systems as this may help explain any variations in vaccine efficacy. Collaborations with human TB research groups have resulted in the testing of a number of the new human TB vaccines in cattle. No single vaccine has been shown to be better than BCG, although combinations of various subunit TB vaccines and BCG have produced encouraging results. There has been encouraging progress on the development of DIVA tests, and these tests need to be evaluated in field situations and their use shown to be cost-effective.

The field testing of BCG vaccine in possums and badgers administered via oral or parenteral routes have resulted in the induction of significant levels of protection in these animals and a parenteral BCG vaccine has now been licensed for use in badgers in the UK. In wild boar, both BCG and killed *M. bovis* vaccines have been shown to protect these animals against TB and the killed *M. bovis* vaccine is in the process of being tested in other wildlife species as well. Oral bait TB vaccines have been shown to be effective in a number of wildlife species, but more research is necessary to improve formulations with appropriate attractants, systems for optimizing bait distribution and avoiding bait uptake by non-target species. In summary, there have been major advances in the development and testing of TB vaccines for domestic and wild animals in the past 5 to 10 years, and it is now becoming more certain that TB vaccines will play an important role in the control of bovine TB in the near future.

Acknowledgements

Funding has been received from AgResearch (New Zealand) and the Department of Environment, Food and Rural Affairs (UK). Research on heat-inactivated *M. bovis* is supported by Plan Nacional I+D+i grant AGL2014-56305 from MINECO, Spain and EU FEDER.

References

Aagaard, C., Hoang, T.T., Izzo, A., Billeskov, R., Troudt, J., *et al*. (2009) Protection and polyfunctional T cells induced by Ag85B-TB10.4/IC31 against *Mycobacterium tuberculosis* is highly dependent on the antigen dose. *PLoS ONE* 4, e5930.

Abdou, M., Frankena, K., O'Keeffe, J. and Byrne, A.W. (2016) Effect of culling and vaccination on bovine tuberculosis infection in a European badger (*Meles meles*) population by spatial simulation modelling. *Preventive Veterinary Medicine* 125, 19–30.

Aldwell, F.E., Keen, D., Parlane, N., Skinner, M.A., de Lisle, G.W., *et al*. (2003) Oral vaccination with *Mycobacterium bovis* BCG in a lipid formulation induces resistance to pulmonary tuberculosis in possums. *Vaccine* 22, 70–76.

Ameni, G., Vordermeier, M., Aseffa, A., Young, D.B. and Hewinson, R.G. (2010) Field evaluation of the efficacy of *Mycobacterium bovis* bacillus Calmette–Guérin against bovine tuberculosis in neonatal calves in Ethiopia. *Clinical and Vaccine Immunology* 17, 1533–1538.

Aranday-Cortes, E., Hogarth, P.J., Kaveh, D.A., Whelan, A.O., Villarreal-Ramos, B., *et al*. (2012) Transcriptional profiling of disease-induced host responses in bovine tuberculosis and the identification of potential diagnostic biomarkers. *PLoS One* 7, e30626.

Barasona, J.A., Torres, M.J., Aznar, J., Gortazar, C. and Vicente, J. (2016) DNA detection reveals *Mycobacterium tuberculosis* complex shedding routes in its wildlife reservoir the Eurasian wild boar. *Transboundary and Emerging Diseases* 64(3), 906–915.

Beatson, N.S. (1985) Tuberculosis in red deer. In: Brown, R.D. (ed.) *Biology of Deer Production*. Springer, New York, pp. 147–150.

Beltrán-Beck, B., De La Fuente, J., Garrido, J.M., Aranaz, A., Sevilla, I., *et al*. (2014a) Oral vaccination with heat inactivated *Mycobacterium bovis* activates the complement system to protect against tuberculosis. *PLoS ONE* 9(5), e98048.

Beltrán-Beck, B., Romero, B., Sevilla, I., Barasona, J.A., Garrido, J.M., *et al*. (2014b) Assessment of an oral *Mycobacterium bovis* BCG vaccine and an inactivated *M. bovis* preparation for wild boar in terms of adverse reactions, vaccine strain survival, and uptake by nontarget species. *Clinical and Vaccine Immunology* 21, 12–20.

Bezos, J., Casal, C., Diez-Delgado, I., Romero, B., Liandris, E., *et al*. (2015) Goats challenged with different members of the *Mycobacterium tuberculosis* complex display different clinical pictures. *Veterinary Immunology and Immunopathology* 167, 185–189.

Bhuju, S., Aranday-Cortes, E., Villarreal-Ramos, B., Xing, Z., Singh, M., *et al*. (2012) Global gene transcriptome analysis in vaccinated cattle revealed a dominant role of IL-22 for protection against bovine tuberculosis. *PLoS Pathogens* 8, e1003077.

Blanco, F.C., Blanco, M.V., Garbaccio, S., Meikle, V., Gravisaco, M.J., et al. (2013) *Mycobacterium bovis* Δmce2 double deletion mutant protects cattle against challenge with virulent *M. bovis*. *Tuberculosis* 93, 363–372.

Blunt, L., Hogarth, P.J., Kaveh, D.A., Webb, P., Villarreal-Ramos, B., et al. (2015) Phenotypic characterization of bovine memory cells responding to mycobacteria in IFNgamma enzyme linked immunospot assays. *Vaccine* 16, 7276–7282.

Buddle, B.M., de Lisle, G.W., Pfeffer, A. and Aldwell, F.E. (1995) Immunological responses and protection against *Mycobacterium bovis* in calves vaccinated with a low dose of BCG. *Vaccine* 13, 1123–1130.

Buddle, B.M., Parlane, N.A., Keen, D.L., Aldwell, F.E., Pollock, J.M., et al. (1999) Differentiation between *Mycobacterium bovis* BCG-vaccinated and *M. bovis*-infected cattle by using recombinant mycobacterial antigens. *Clinical and Diagnostic Laboratory Immunology* 6, 1–5.

Buddle, B.M., Wards, B.J., Aldwell, F.E., Collins, D.M. and de Lisle, G.W. (2002) Influence of sensitisation to environmental mycobacteria on subsequent vaccination against bovine tuberculosis. *Vaccine* 20, 1126–1133.

Buddle, B.M., Wedlock, D.N., Parlane, N.A., Corner, L.A., de Lisle, G.W., et al. (2003) Revaccination of neonatal calves with *Mycobacterium bovis* BCG reduces the level of protection against bovine tuberculosis induced by a single vaccination. *Infection and Immunity* 71, 6411–6419.

Buddle, B.M., Aldwell, F.E., Keen, D.L., Parlane, N.A., Hamel, K.L., et al. (2006) Oral vaccination of brushtail possums with BCG: investigation into factors that influence vaccine efficacy and determination of duration of immunity. *New Zealand Veterinary Journal* 54, 224–230.

Buddle, B.M., Denis, M., Aldwell, F.E., Vordermeier, H.M., Hewinson, R.G., et al. (2008) Vaccination of cattle with *Mycobacterium bovis* BCG by a combination of systemic and oral routes. *Tuberculosis* 88, 595–600.

Buddle, B.M., Shu, D., Parlane, N.A., Subharat, S., Heiser, A., et al. (2016) Vaccination of cattle with a high dose of BCG vaccine 3 weeks after experimental infection with *Mycobacterium bovis* increased the inflammatory response, but not tuberculosis pathology. *Tuberculosis* 99, 120–127.

Byrom, A.E., Caley, P., Paterson, B.M. and Nugent, G. (2015) Feral ferrets (*Mustela furo*) as hosts and sentinels of tuberculosis in New Zealand. *New Zealand Veterinary Journal* 63(1), 42–53.

Cai, H., Tian, X., Hu, X.D., Li, S.X., Yu, D.H., et al. (2005) Combined DNA vaccines formulated either in DDA or in saline protect cattle from *Mycobacterium bovis* infection. *Vaccine* 23, 3887–3895.

Carter, S.P., Chambers, M.A., Rushton, S.P., Shirley, M.D.F., Schuchert, P., et al. (2012) BCG vaccination reduces risk of tuberculosis infection in vaccinated badgers and unvaccinated badger cubs. *PLoS One* 7, e49833.

Chambers, M., Rogers, F., Delahay, R., Lesellier, S., Ashford, R., et al. (2011) Bacillus Calmette–Guérin vaccination reduces the severity and progression of tuberculosis in badgers. *Proceedings of the Royal Society B Biological Sciences* 278, 1913–1920.

Chambers, M.A., Carter, S.P., Wilson, G.J., Jones, G., Brown, E., et al. (2014) Vaccination against tuberculosis in badgers and cattle: an overview of the challenges, development and current research priorities in Great Britain. *Veterinary Record* 175, 90–96.

Collins, D.M., Buddle, B.M., Kawakami, P., Hotter, G., Mildenhall, N., et al. (2011) Newly attenuated *Mycobacterium bovis* mutants as vaccines for possums. *Veterinary Microbiology* 151, 99–103.

Corner, L.A., Murphy, D. and Gormley, E. (2011) *Mycobacterium bovis* infection in the Eurasian badger (*Meles meles*): the disease, pathogenesis, epidemiology and control. *Journal of Comparative Pathology* 144, 1–24.

Cousins, D.V. (2001) *Mycobacterium bovis* infection and control in domestic livestock. *Revue Scientifique et Technique (International Office of Epizootics)* 20, 71–85.

Cowie, C.E., Hutchings, M.R., Barasona, J.A., Gortázar, C., Vicente, J., et al. (2016) Interactions between four species in a complex wildlife: livestock disease community: implications for *Mycobacterium bovis* maintenance and transmission. *European Journal of Wildlife Research* 62, 51–64.

Cross, M.L., Labes, R.E., Young, G. and Mackintosh C.G. (2000) Systemic but not intraintestinal vaccination with BCG reduces the severity of tuberculosis infection in ferrets (*Mustela furo*). *International Journal of Tuberculosis and Lung Disease* 4, 473–480.

Cross, M.L., Henderson, R.J., Lambeth, M.R., Buddle, B.M. and Aldwell, F.E. (2009) Lipid-formulated BCG as an oral-bait vaccine for tuberculosis: vaccine stability, efficacy and palatability to New Zealand possums (*Trichosurus vulpecula*). *Journal of Wildlife Diseases* 45, 754–765.

Dean, G., Whelan, A., Clifford, D., Salguero, F.J., Xing, Z., et al. (2014a) Comparison of the immunogenicity and protection against bovine tuberculosis following immunization by BCG-priming and boosting with adenovirus or protein based vaccines. *Vaccine* 32, 1304–1310.

Dean, G., Clifford, D., Gilbert, S., McShane, H., Hewinson, R.G., et al. (2014b) Effect of dose and route of immunisation on the immune response induced in cattle by heterologous bacille Calmette–Guérin priming and recombinant adenoviral vector boosting. *Veterinary Immunology and Immunopathology* 158, 208–213.

Dean, G.S., Clifford, D., Whelan, A.O., Tchilian, E.Z., Beverley, P.C.L., et al. (2015) Protection induced by simultaneous subcutaneous and endobronchial vaccination with BCG/BCG and BCG/adenovirus expressing antigen 85A against *Mycobacterium bovis*. *PloS ONE* 10, e0142270.

de Klerk, L.M., Micel, A.L., Bengis, R.G., Kreik, N.P. and Godfroid, J. (2010) BCG vaccination failed to protect yearling African buffaloes (*Syncerus caffer*) against experimental intratonsilar challenge with *Mycobacterium bovis*. *Veterinary Immunology Immunopathology* 137, 84–92.

Delahay, R.J., Smith, G.C., Barlow, A.M., Walker, N., Harris, A., et al. (2007) Bovine tuberculosis infection in wild mammals in the South-West region of England: a survey of prevalence and a semi-quantitative assessment of the relative risks to cattle. *Veterinary Journal* 173, 287–301.

de Lisle, G.W., Bengis, R.G., Schmitt, S.M. and O'Brien, D.J. (2001) Tuberculosis in free-ranging wildlife: detection, diagnosis and management. *Revue Scientifique et Technique (International Office of Epizootics)* 21, 317–334.

Díez-Delgado, I., Rodríguiez, O., Boadella, M., Garrido, J.M., Sevilla, I., et al. (2016) Parenteral vaccination with heat-inactivated *Mycobacterium bovis* reduces the prevalence of tuberculosis-compatible lesions in farmed wild boar. *Transboundary and Emerging Diseases* 64, e18-e21.

Fitzgerald, S.D. and Kaneene, J.B. (2013) Wildlife reservoirs of bovine tuberculosis worldwide: hosts, pathology, surveillance, and control. *Veterinary Pathology* 50, 488–499.

Garly, M.-L., Martins, C.L., Balé, C., Baldé, M.A., Hedegaard, K.L., et al. (2003) BCG scar and positive tuberculin reaction associated with reduced child mortality in West Africa. *Vaccine* 21, 2782–2790.

Garrido, J.M., Sevilla, I.A., Beltrán-Beck, B., Minguijón, E., Ballesteros, C., et al. (2011) Protection against tuberculosis in Eurasian wild boar vaccinated with heat-inactivated *Mycobacterium bovis*. *PLoS ONE* 6(9), e24905.

Godfray, H.C., Donnelly, C.A., Kao, R.R., Macdonald, D.W., McDonald, R.A., et al. (2013) A restatement of the natural science evidence base relevant to the control of bovine tuberculosis in Great Britain. *Proceedings of the Royal Society B Biological Sciences* 280, DOI: 10.1098/rspb.2013.1634.

Golby, P., Villarreal-Ramos, B., Dean, G., Jones, G.J. and Vordermeier, M. (2014) MicroRNA expression profiling of PPD-B stimulated PBMCs from *M. bovis*-challenged unvaccinated and BCG vaccinated cattle. *Vaccine* 32, 5839–5844.

Gonzalez-Juarrero, M., Bosco-Lauth, A., Podell, B., Soffler, C., Brooks, E., et al. (2013) Experimental aerosol *Mycobacterium bovis* model of infection in goats. *Tuberculosis* 93, 558–564.

Gormley, E. and Corner, L.A. (2013) Control strategies for wildlife tuberculosis in Ireland. *Transboundary and Emerging Diseases* 60(1), 128–135.

Gortázar, C., Beltrán-Beck, B., Garrido, J.M., Aranaz, A., Sevilla, I., et al. (2014) Oral re-vaccination of Eurasian wild boar with *Mycobacterium bovis* BCG yields a strong protective response against challenge with a field strain. *BMC Veterinary Research* 10, 96.

Gortazar, C., Che-Amat, A. and O'Brien, D. (2015a) Open questions and recent advances in the control of a multi-host infectious disease: animal tuberculosis. *Mammal Review* 45, 160–175.

Gortazar, C., Diez-Delgado, I., Barasona, J.A., Vicente, J., De la Fuente, J., et al. (2015b) The wild side of disease control at the wildlife–livestock–human interface: a review. *Frontiers in Veterinary Science* 1, 27.

Griffin, J.F.T., Mackintosh, C.G. and Buchan, G.S. (1995) Animal models of protective immunity in tuberculosis to evaluate candidate vaccines. *Trends in Microbiology* 3, 418–424.

Griffin, J.M., Williams, D.H., Kelly, G.E., Clegg, T.A., O'Boyle, I., et al. (2005) The impact of badger removal on the control of tuberculosis in cattle herds in Ireland. *Preventive Veterinary Medicine* 67, 237–266.

Griffin, J.F., Mackintosh, C.G. and Rodgers, C.R. (2006) Factors influencing the protective efficacy of a BCG homologous prime-boost vaccination regime against tuberculosis. *Vaccine* 24, 835–845.

Hope, J.C., Thom, M.L., Villarreal-Ramos, B., Vordermeier, H.M., Hewinson, R.G., et al. (2005) Vaccination of neonatal calves with *Mycobacterium bovis* BCG induces protection against intranasal challenge with virulent *M. bovis*. *Clinical and Experimental Immunology* 139, 48–56.

Hope, J.C., Thom, M.L., McAulay, M., Mead, E., Vordermeier, H.M., et al. (2011) Identification of surrogates and correlates of protection in protective immunity against *Mycobacterium bovis* infection induced in neonatal calves by vaccination with *M. bovis* BCG Pasteur and *M. bovis* BCG Danish. *Clinical and Vaccine Immunology* 18, 373–379.

Jones, G.J., Whelan, A., Clifford, D., Coad, M. and Vordermeier, H.M. (2012) Improved skin test for differential diagnosis of bovine tuberculosis by the addition of Rv3020c-derived peptides. *Clinical and Vaccine Immunology* 19, 620–622.

Khare, S., Hondalus, M.K., Nunes, J., Bloom, B.R. and Adams, G.L. (2007) *Mycobacterium bovis* ΔleuD auxotroph-induced protective immunity against tissue colonization, burden and distribution in cattle intranasally challenged with *Mycobacterium bovis* Ravenel S. *Vaccine* 25, 1743–1755.

Khatri, B., Whelan, A., Clifford, D., Petrera, A., Sander, P., et al. (2014) BCG Δzmp1 vaccine induces enhanced antigen specific immune responses in cattle. *Vaccine* 32, 779–784.

King, H.C., Murphy, A., James, P., Travis, E., Porter, D., et al. (2015) The variability and seasonality of the environmental reservoir of *Mycobacterium bovis* shed by wild European badgers. *Scientific Reports* 5, 12318.

LaHue, N.P., Baños, J.V., Acevedo, P., Gortázar, C. and Martínez-López, B. (2016) Spatially explicit modeling of animal tuberculosis at the wildlife-livestock interface in ciudad real province, Spain. *Preventive Veterinary Medicine* 128, 101–111.

Lesellier, S., Palmer, S., Dalley, D.J., Davé, D., Johnson, L., et al. (2006) The safety and immunogenicity of bacillus Calmette–Guérin (BCG) vaccine in European badgers (*Meles meles*). *Veterinary Immunology and Immunopathology* 112, 24–37.

Lesellier, S., Palmer, S., Gowtage-Sequiera, S., Ashford, R., Dalley, D., et al. (2011) Protection of Eurasian badgers (*Meles meles*) from tuberculosis after intra-muscular vaccination with different doses of BCG. *Vaccine* 29, 3782–3790.

Livingstone, P.G., Hutchings, S.A., Hancox, N.G. and de Lisle, G.W. (2015) Toward eradication: the effect of *Mycobacterium bovis* infection in wildlife on the evolution and future direction of bovine tuberculosis management in New Zealand. *New Zealand Veterinary Journal* 63(1), 4–18.

Lopez-Valencia, G., Renteria-Evangelista, T., Williams, J.D.J., Licea-Navarro, A., Mora-Valle, A.D., et al. (2010) Field evaluation of the protective efficacy of *Mycobacterium bovis* BCG vaccine against bovine tuberculosis. *Research in Veterinary Science* 88, 44–49.

Martín-Hernando, M.P., Höfle, U., Vicente, J., Ruiz-Fons, F., Vidal, D., et al. (2007). Lesions associated with *Mycobacterium tuberculosis* complex infection in the European wild boar. *Tuberculosis* 87, 360–367.

Martín-Hernando, M.P., Torres, M.J., Aznar, J., Negro, J.J., Gandía, A., et al. (2010) Sampling strategy, lesion pattern and lesion distribution in naturally *Mycobacterium bovis* infected red deer and fallow deer. *Journal of Comparative Pathology* 142, 43–50.

Massei, G., Kindberg, J., Licoppe, A., Gacic, D., Šprem, N., et al. (2015) Wild boar populations up, numbers of hunters down? A review of trends and implications for Europe. *Pest Management Science* 71, 492–500.

Maue, A.C., Waters, W.R., Palmer, M.V., Whipple, D.L., Minion, F.C., et al. (2004) CD80 and CD86, but not CD154, augment DNA vaccine-induced protection in experimental bovine tuberculosis. *Vaccine* 23, 769–779.

Maue, A.C., Waters, W.R., Palmer, M.V., Nonnecke, B.J., Minion, F.C., et al. (2007) An ESAT-6:CFP10 DNA vaccine administered in conjunction with *Mycobacterium bovis* BCG confers protection to cattle challenged with virulent *M. bovis*. *Vaccine* 25, 4735–4746.

McCallan, L., Corbett, D., Andersen, P.L., Aagaard, C., McMurray, D., et al. (2011) A new experimental infection model in ferrets based on aerosolised *Mycobacterium bovis*. *Veterinary Medicine International* 2011, 981410.

McShane, H. (2009) Vaccine strategies against tuberculosis. *Swiss Medical Weekly* 139, 156–160.

Murphy, D., Costello, E., Aldwell, F.E., Lesellier, S., Chambers, M.A., et al. (2014) Oral vaccination of badgers (*Meles meles*) against tuberculosis: comparison of the protection generated by BCG vaccine strains Pasteur and Danish. *Veterinary Journal* 200, 362–367.

Naranjo, V., Gortázar, C., Vicente, J. and de la Fuente, J. (2008) Evidence of the role of European wild boar as a reservoir of tuberculosis due to *Mycobacterium tuberculosis* complex. *Veterinary Microbiology* 127, 1–9.

Nishi, J.S., Shury, T. and Elkin, B.T. (2006) Wildlife reservoirs for bovine tuberculosis (*Mycobacterium bovis*) in Canada: strategies for management and research. *Veterinary Microbiology* 112, 325–338.

Nol, P., Palmer, M.V., Waters, W.R., Aldwell, F.E., Buddle, B.M., et al. (2008) Efficacy of oral and parenteral routes of Mycobacterium bovis bacille Calmette–Guérin vaccination against experimental bovine tuberculosis in white-tailed deer (Odocoileus virginianus): a feasibility study. Journal of Wildlife Disease 44, 247–259.

Nol, P., Rhyan, J.C., Robbe-Austerman, S., McCollum, M.P., Rigg, T.D., et al. (2013) The potential for transmission of BCG from orally vaccinated white-tailed deer (Odocoileus virginianus) to cattle (Bos taurus) through a contaminated environment: experimental findings. PLoS ONE 8, e60257.

Nugent, G., Yockney, I.J., Whitford, J., Aldwell, F.E. and Buddle, B.M. (2017) Efficacy of oral BCG vaccination in protecting free-ranging cattle from natural infection by Mycobacterium bovis. Veterinary Microbiology 208, 181–189.

O'Brien, D.J., Schmitt, S.M., Fitzgerald, S.D., Berry, D.E. and Hickling, G.J. (2006) Managing the wildlife reservoir of Mycobacterium bovis: the Michigan, USA, experience. Veterinary Microbiology 112, 313–323.

O'Connor, C.M., Haydon, D.T. and Kao, R.R. (2012) An ecological and comparative perspective on the control of bovine tuberculosis in Great Britain and the Republic of Ireland. Preventive Veterinary Medicine 104, 185–197.

Palmer, M.V., Waters, W.R. and Whipple, D.L. (2002a) Aerosol delivery of virulent Mycobacterium bovis to cattle. Tuberculosis 82, 275–282.

Palmer, M.V., Waters, W.R. and Whipple, D.L. (2002b) Lesion development in white-tailed deer (Odocoileus virginianus) experimentally infected with Mycobacterium bovis. Veterinary Pathology 39, 334–340.

Palmer, M.V., Thacker, T.C. and Waters, W.R. (2009) Vaccination with Mycobacterium bovis BCG strains Danish and Pasteur in white-tailed deer (Odocoileus virginianus) experimentally challenged with Mycobacterium bovis. Zoonoses Public Health 56, 243–251.

Palmer, M.V., Thacker, T.C., Waters, W.R., Robbe-Austerman, S., Lebepe-Mazur, S.M., et al. (2010) Persistence of Mycobacterium bovis bacillus Calmette–Guérin in white-tailed deer (Odocoileus virginianus) after oral or parenteral vaccination. Zoonoses Public Health 57, 206–212.

Parlane, N.A., Shu, D., Subharat, S., Wedlock, D.N., Rehm, B.H., et al. (2014) Revaccination of cattle with bacille Calmette–Guérin two years after first vaccination when immunity has waned, boosted protection against challenge with Mycobacterium bovis. PLoS ONE 9, e106519.

Parlane, N.A. and Buddle, B.M. (2015) Immunity and vaccination against tuberculosis in cattle. Current Clinical Microbiology Reports 2(1), 44–53.

Parlane, N.A., Chen, S., Jones, G.J., Vordermeier, H.M., Wedlock, D.N., et al. (2016) Display of antigens on polyester inclusions lowers the antigen concentration required for a bovine tuberculosis skin test. Clinical and Vaccine Immunology 23, 19–26.

Pastoret, P.P. and Brochier, B. (1996) The development and use of a vaccinia–rabies recombinant oral vaccine for control of wildlife rabies; a link between Jenner and Pasteur. Epidemiology and Infection 116, 235–240.

Pérez de Val, B., López-Soria, S., Nofrarias, M., Martin, M., Vordermeier, H.M., et al. (2011) Experimental model of tuberculosis in the domestic goat after endobronchial infection with Mycobacterium caprae. Clinical and Vaccine Immunology 18, 1872–1881.

Pérez de Val, B., Villarreal-Ramos, B., Nofrarias, M., López-Soria, S., Romera, N., et al. (2012) Goats primed with Mycobacterium bovis BCG and boosted with a recombinant adenovirus expressing Ag85A show enhanced protection against tuberculosis. Clinical and Vaccine Immunology 19, 1339–1347.

Pérez de Val, B., Vidal, E., Villarreal-Ramos, B., Gilbert, S.C., Andaluz, A., et al. (2013) A multi-antigenic adenoviral-vectored vaccine improves BCG-induced protection of goats against pulmonary tuberculosis infection and prevents disease progression. PLoS ONE 11, e81317.

Pérez de Val, B., Vidal, E., López-Soria, S., Marco, A., Cervera, Z., et al. (2016) Assessment of safety and interferon-gamma responses of Mycobacterium bovis BCG vaccine in goat kids and milking goats. Vaccine 34, 881–886.

Pesciaroli, M., Alvarez, J., Boniotti, M.B., Cagiola, M., Di Marco, V., et al. (2014) Tuberculosis in domestic animal species. Research in Veterinary Science 97, S78–S85.

Qureshi, T., Labes, R.E., Cross, M.L., Griffin, J.F.T. and Mackintosh, C.G. (1999) Partial protection against oral challenge with Mycobacterium bovis in ferrets (Mustela furo) following oral vaccination with BCG. International Journal of Tuberculosis and Lung Disease 3(11), 1025–1033.

Ramsey, D.S.L., O'Brien, D.J., Cosgrove, M.K., Rudolph, B.A., Locher, A.B., et al. (2014) Forecasting eradication of bovine tuberculosis in Michigan white-tailed deer. Journal of Wildlife Management 78, 240–254.

Rizzi, C., Bianco, M.V., Blanco, F.C., Soria, M., Gravisaco, M.J., et al. (2012) Vaccination with a BCG strain overexpressing Ag85B protects cattle against *Mycobacterium bovis* challenge. *PLoS ONE* 7, e51396.

Roy, A., Risalde, M.A., Casal, C., Romero, B., de Juan, L., et al. (2017) Oral vaccination with heat-inactivated *Mycobacterium bovis* does not interfere with the antemortem diagnostic techniques for tuberculosis in goats. *Frontiers in Veterinary Science* 4, 124.

Santos, N., Almeida, V., Gortázar, C. and Correia-Neves, M. (2015a) Patterns of *Mycobacterium tuberculosis* complex excretion and characterization of super-shedders in naturally-infected wild boar and red deer. *Veterinary Research* 46, article 129, DOI: 10.1186/s13567-015-0270-4.

Santos, N., Santos, C., Valente, T., Gortázar, C., Almeida, V., et al. (2015b) Widespread environmental contamination with *Mycobacterium tuberculosis* complex revealed by a molecular detection protocol. *PLoS ONE* 10, e0142079.

Sidders, B., Pirson, C., Hogarth, P.J., Hewinson, R.G., Stoker, N.G., et al. (2008) Screening of highly expressed mycobacterial genes identifies Rv3615c as a useful differential diagnostic antigen for *Mycobacterium tuberculosis* complex. *Infection and Immunity* 76, 3932–3939.

Skinner, M.A., Wedlock, D.N. and Buddle, B.M. (2001) Vaccination of animals against *Mycobacterium bovis*. *Revue Scientifique et Technique (International Office of Epizootics)* 20, 112–132.

Skinner, M.A., Buddle, B.M., Wedlock, D.N., Keen, D., de Lisle, G.W., et al. (2003) A DNA prime-*Mycobacterium bovis* BCG boost vaccination strategy for cattle induces protection against bovine tuberculosis. *Infection and Immunity* 71, 4901–4907.

Skinner, M.A., Wedlock, D.N., de Lisle, G.W., Cooke, M.M., Tascon, R.E., et al. (2005) The order of prime-boost vaccination of neonatal calves with *Mycobacterium bovis* BCG and a DNA vaccine encoding mycobacterial proteins Hsp65, Hsp70, and Apa is not critical for enhancing protection against bovine tuberculosis. *Infection and Immunity* 73, 4441–4444.

Thom, M.L., McAulay, M., Vordermeier, H.M., Clifford, D., Hewinson, R.G., et al. (2012) Duration of immunity against *Mycobacterium bovis* following neonatal vaccination with bacillus Calmette–Guérin Danish: significant protection against infection at 12, but not 24 months. *Clinical and Vaccine Immunology* 19, 1254–1260.

Thomas, J., Risalde, M.Á., Serrano, M., Sevilla, I., Geijo, M., et al. (2017) The response of red deer to oral administration of heat-inactivated *Mycobacterium bovis* and challenge with a field strain. *Veterinary Microbiology* 208, 195–202.

Tompkins, D.M., Ramsey, D.S.L., Cross, M.L., Aldwell, F.E., de Lisle, G.W., et al. (2009) Oral vaccination reduces the incidence of bovine tuberculosis in a free-living wildlife species. *Proceedings of the Royal Society B: Biological Sciences* 276, 2987–2995.

Tompkins, D.M., Buddle, B.M., Whitford, J., Cross, M.L., Yates, G.F., et al. (2013) Sustained protection against tuberculosis conferred to a wildlife host by a single dose vaccination. *Vaccine* 31, 893–899.

van der Heijden, E.M.D.L., Chileshe, J., Vernooij, J.C.M., Gortazar, C., Juste, R.A., et al. (2017) Immune response profiles of calves following vaccination with live BCG and inactivated *Mycobacterium bovis* vaccine candidates. *PLoS One* 12(11), e0188448.

Vordermeier, H.M., Whelan, A., Cockle, P.J., Farrant, L., Palmer, N., et al. (2001) Use of synthetic peptides derived from the antigens ESAT-6 and CFP-10 for differential diagnosis of bovine tuberculosis in cattle. *Clinical and Diagnostic Laboratory Immunology* 8, 571–578.

Vordermeier, H.M., Chambers, M.A., Cockle, P.J., Whelan, A.O., Simmons, J., et al. (2002) Correlation of ESAT-6-specific gamma interferon production with pathology in cattle following *Mycobacterium bovis* BCG vaccination against experimental bovine tuberculosis. *Infection and Immunity* 70, 3026–3032.

Vordermeier, H.M., Villarreal-Ramos, B., Cockle, P.J., McAulay, M., Rhodes, S.G., et al. (2009) Viral booster vaccines improve *Mycobacterium bovis* BCG-induced protection against bovine tuberculosis. *Infection and Immunity* 77, 3364–3373.

Waters, W.R., Palmer, M.V., Nonnecke, B.J., Thacker, T.C., Scherer, C.F.C., et al. (2007) Failure of a *Mycobacterium tuberculosis* ΔRD1 ΔpanCD double deletion mutant in a neonatal calf aerosol *M. bovis* challenge model: comparisons to responses elicited by *M. bovis* bacille Calmette–Guérin. *Vaccine* 25, 7832–7840.

Waters, W.R., Palmer, M.V., Nonnecke, B.J., Thacker, T.C., Scherer, C.F.C., et al. (2009) Efficacy and immunogenicity of *Mycobacterium bovis* ΔRD1 against aerosol *M. bovis* infection in neonatal calves. *Vaccine* 27, 1201–1209.

Waters, W.R., Palmer, M.V., Buddle, B.M. and Vordermeier, H.M. (2012) Bovine tuberculosis vaccine research: historical perspectives and recent advances. *Vaccine* 30, 2611–2622.

Waters, W.R., Maggioli, M.F., Palmer, M.V., Thacker, T.C., McGill, J.L., *et al.* (2015) Interleukin-17A as a biomarker for bovine tuberculosis. *Clinical and Vaccine Immunology* 23, 168–180.

Wedlock, D.N., Vordermeier, H.M., Denis, M., Skinner, M.A., de Lisle, G.W., *et al.* (2005a) Vaccination of cattle with a CpG oligodeoxynucleotide-formulated mycobacterial protein vaccine and *Mycobacterium bovis* BCG induces levels of protection against bovine tuberculosis superior to those induced by vaccination with BCG alone. *Infection and Immunity* 73, 3540–3546.

Wedlock, D.N., Aldwell, F.E., Keen, D.L., Skinner, M.A. and Buddle, B.M. (2005b) Oral vaccination of brush-tail possums (*Trichosurus vulpecula*) with BCG: immune responses, persistence of BCG in lymphoid organs and excretion in faeces. *New Zealand Veterinary Journal* 53, 301–306.

Wedlock, D.N., Denis, M., Vordermeier, H.M., Hewinson, R.G. and Buddle, B.M. (2007) Vaccination of cattle with Danish and Pasteur strains of *Mycobacterium bovis* BCG induce different levels of IFN-γ post-vaccination, but induce similar levels of protection against bovine tuberculosis. *Veterinary Immunology and Immunopathology* 118, 50–58.

Wedlock, D.N., Denis, M., Painter, G.F., Ainge, G.D., Vordermeier, H.M., *et al.* (2008) Enhanced protection against bovine tuberculosis after coadministration of *Mycobacterium bovis* BCG with a mycobacterial protein vaccine-adjuvant combination but not after coadministration of adjuvant alone. *Clinical and Vaccine Immunology* 15, 765–772.

Wedlock, D.N., Aldwell, F.E., de Lisle, G.W., Vordermeier, H.M., Hewinson, R.G., *et al.* (2011) Protection against bovine tuberculosis induced by oral vaccination of cattle with *Mycobacterium bovis* BCG is not enhanced by co-administration of mycobacterial protein vaccines. *Veterinary Immunology and Immunopathology* 144, 220–227.

Whelan, A.O., Clifford, D., Upadhyay, B., Breadon, E.L., McNair, J., *et al.* (2010) Development of a skin test for bovine tuberculosis for differentiating infected from vaccinated animals. *Journal of Clinical Microbiology* 48, 3176–3181.

Whelan, A.O., Villarreal-Ramos, B., Vordermeier, H.M. and Hogarth, P.J. (2011a) Development of an antibody to bovine IL-2 reveals multifunctional CD4 T(EM) cells in cattle naturally infected with bovine tuberculosis. *PLoS ONE* 6, e29194.

Whelan, A.O., Coad, M., Upadhyay, B.L., Clifford, D.J., Hewinson, R.G., *et al.* (2011b) Lack of correlation between BCG-induced tuberculin skin test sensitisation and protective immunity in cattle. *Vaccine* 29, 5453–5458.

Whelan, A., Court, P., Xing, Z., Clifford, D., Hogarth, P.J., *et al.* (2012) Immunogenicity comparison of the intradermal or endobronchial boosting of BCG vaccinates with Ad5-85A. *Vaccine* 30, 6294–6300.

Wilkinson, D., Smith, G.C., Delahay, R.J., Rogers, L.M., Cheeseman, C.L., *et al.* (2000) The effects of bovine tuberculosis (*Mycobacterium bovis*) on mortality in a badger (*Meles meles*) population in England. *Journal of Zoology* 250, 389–395.

15 Managing Bovine Tuberculosis: Successes and Issues

Paul Livingstone[1],* and Nick Hancox[2]
[1]TB Consultant, Domestic Animals and Wildlife, New Zealand;
[2]OSPRI, New Zealand

15.1 Orientation

Infection with *Mycobacterium bovis* (TB) impacts on a wide spectrum of animals including man. The reality of managing *M. bovis*, wherever it is found, is that it requires adequate resources. These are either lacking or prioritized for other needs and wants for large sections of the world. The World Bank has categorized countries according to four income-related classes based on their gross national income (GNI) per capita in US dollars (The World Bank, 2016a). They are: low, low–medium, medium–high and high GNI economies. These categories provide an approach for proposing management options for bovine TB that take account of available resources. For the purpose of this chapter, countries in the low, low–medium and medium–high GNI economies will be considered together in one category (low to medium–high) with countries in the high GNI economy as a second category.

Analysis of data from the 168 OIE nations that reported on their bovine TB status in 2015 (OIE, 2016a; see also Chapter 1) found that 66 (39%) reported as either 'never had bovine TB', or their last reported case was prior to 2011. One hundred and two countries (60%) reported having had cases of bovine TB since 2010, and 90 (53%) reported infection in 2015. Of these 90, 23 (26%) reported presence of TB in wildlife (OIE, 2016a). Categorizing these responses by GNI economy groups identified bovine TB in 56% of the 54 high GNI countries, compared with 70% of the 100 countries in the low to medium–high GNI category.

From this it can be seen that high GNI economies have less *M. bovis* infection in livestock relative to low to medium–high GNI economies. Thus, a section has been devoted to features that appear important for successful management of TB in cattle, which is largely targeted at countries with a high GNI economy. The ability to successfully manage infection in some of these high GNI countries is being threatened by wildlife TB maintenance hosts. Therefore, a section provides a means of identifying and managing this exposure. Finally, and probably most importantly, there is a section that describes the largely under-diagnosed *M. bovis*-related problem facing people and livestock in low to medium–high GNI countries and identifies some actions that could be used to reduce the risk of exposure.

15.2 Features of Successful TB Cattle Programmes in High GNI Countries

15.2.1 Introduction

The effective management of bovine TB in cattle depends firstly on gaining agreement on the

* Email: consultantbtb@gmail.com

© CAB International 2018. *Bovine Tuberculosis*
(eds M. Chambers, S. Gordon, F. Olea-Popelka, P. Barrow)

overall purpose of the programme. This must then be underpinned by development of clear and achievable strategic objectives to meet this purpose. It is only in this context that the success or otherwise of management can be meaningfully evaluated.

This section seeks to identify the key technical and managerial issues that need to be addressed to effectively manage bovine TB in livestock. While the focus is on TB programmes involving only cattle, it addresses management issues that would apply equally to programmes for control or eradication of *M. bovis* from other domestic species, or for controlling other members of the *Mycobacterium tuberculosis* complex affecting domestic livestock. It is largely targeted towards national or countrywide TB freedom or eradication programmes, but would be suitable for regions or states to use. Similarly, the concept outline would provide guidance for a community wanting to develop a programme to manage TB in its livestock.

15.2.2 Defining programme purpose

The foundation of an effective TB programme is clarity of purpose. Historically, TB programmes have been introduced to reduce economic production losses due to *M. bovis* infection in cattle (Good and Duignan, 2011). For example, Olmstead and Rhode, cited by Palmer and Waters (2011) identified annual benefits from the United States Department of Agriculture (USDA) TB eradication programme as being 'equivalent to 12-times the annual costs' during the period 1917–1962. Later programmes were introduced to enable and facilitate international trade in live cattle or their products (Max *et al.*, 2011; Livingstone *et al.*, 2015a), or to meet international requirements such as conformity with EU policy (Reviriego Gordejo and Vermeersch, 2006).

While no TB programmes appear to have been introduced specifically to reduce the zoonotic risk of *M. bovis* infection in humans, which has largely been reliant on heat treatment of milk, effective TB control in cattle has nevertheless contributed to reduced bovine TB incidence in humans. Olmstead and Rhodes, cited by Palmers and Waters (2011) determined that together with pasteurization of milk, the USDA TB eradication programme 'prevented over 250,000 deaths annually'.

15.2.3 Strategic objectives

Once the overall purpose of TB management is established, clear strategic management objectives can then be set.

There has been a disparity in the terms used to apply to national objectives set for bovine TB programmes in high GNI economy countries. Essentially, these can be classified as control, freedom or eradication. TB control objectives are based on measures taken to reduce TB prevalence or incidence on a regional or national basis (Schwabe *et al.*, 1977). TB freedom is where a region or country has designed and implemented a programme to meet some international agreed prevalence target that is accepted as free from TB, such as that set by OIE (OIE, 2016b). TB eradication designates that *M. bovis* does not exist in a defined region or country. This may be a result of a fortuitous accident in that TB was never introduced, or as a result of a successful TB programme, leading to the extinction of *M. bovis* at a regional or national level (Schwabe *et al.*, 1977) as achieved by Australia (Cousins and Roberts, 2001). Even with adequate funding and a common purpose, as identified for Australia (Cousins and Roberts, 2001) and the ongoing programme in the USA (Palmer and Waters, 2011), regional eradication of *M. bovis* requires a realistic appreciation of a challenging, expensive and time-consuming objective to meet. Despite this, eradication may be the optimal objective, given that programme- and disease-related costs fall to zero once it has been achieved, whereas control costs continue indefinitely (TBfree NZ, 2009). Henceforth, the general term 'programme' will be used in this chapter instead of control, freedom and eradication, unless more detail is required.

Whatever objectives are chosen, they should meet SMART (specific, measurable, agreed/achievable, realistic and time-bound) criteria (Blanchard *et al.*, 1985) and be designed to 'stretch' administrators towards delivering an innovative and cost-effective programme. Long-term objectives should be supplemented by annual milestones to enable regular measurement of progress and performance. Where necessary, objectives or sub-objectives should apply to all domestic and wildlife species where intra- or interspecies transmission of *M. bovis* has been identified and where infection poses zoonotic, trade or production risks. For stakeholders to select the best strategy, they need to be presented with benefit–cost analyses for a range of programme options, to enable them to objectively choose the one that will most cost effectively meet desired SMART objectives. This may require development of a series of detailed and costed plans in an iterative process.

Regardless of the objectives of the TB programme, its effective implementation requires: (i) a sound understanding of the impacts and costs of both the disease itself and any planned control measure; (ii) sufficient technical, managerial and systems capacity for programme delivery; (iii) adequate and secure funding, and (iv) recognition of the needs of farmers, land users and stakeholders (Thrushfield, 2007; Osterholm and Hedberg, 2015).

15.2.4 Programme development

History has shown that developing and implementing an effective bovine TB programme at a national, regional or local level is no simple process. It may take some years to evaluate and address multiple technical, economic and policy considerations and to gain necessary stakeholder and political agreement (Palmer and Waters, 2011; Livingstone *et al.*, 2015b). Historically, this has usually been undertaken by government agencies, but increasingly there has been a shift to farmers and farmer organizations being involved with approving strategies and plans, as well as shouldering an increasing share of funding (Cousins and Roberts, 2001; Max *et al.*, 2011; Enticott, 2014; Livingstone *et al.*, 2015a).

A successful cattle TB programme normally goes through various phases. Most programmes have legacies of policy and knowledge derived from literature and local TB management history. Over time, experience, knowledge and research findings have honed these programmes such that it is possible to identify a range of factors that generally appear to be important in achieving success.

Following the identification of programme purpose and definition of strategic objectives to achieve that purpose, a successful bovine TB programme requires adequate funding, effective legal status, stakeholder support for the objectives based on a benefit–cost analysis, a sound science-based technical plan, and policies that take account of TB aetiology, epidemiology and costs, as well as consideration of farming, industry and societal contexts. Once agreed, the TB programme then needs to be delivered by a competent administrative organization or management agency, whose role is to ensure that an auditable, cost-effective and coordinated programme meets annual milestones, within budget.

15.2.5 Legal status

A number of national TB programmes began as regional or national voluntary programmes, with varying proportions of the cattle population being brought under TB testing regimes, assisted by surveillance of TB in cattle at abattoirs or slaughter plants (Livingstone *et al.*, 2015a). However, voluntary programmes have generally been found inadequate, leading to introduction of compulsory programmes (Cousins and Roberts, 2001; Palmer and Waters, 2011; Livingstone *et al.*, 2015a) supported by legislation to ensure farmer compliance with programme policies and rules. Legislation may also be required to secure programme funding, such as from taxes or levies. Ideally, such legislation should be enabling, rather than prescriptive, and be based around meeting strategic objectives, as well as setting out disease control policies, legal powers and funding responsibilities agreed to by stakeholders (Enticott, 2014; Livingstone *et al.*, 2015b).

15.2.6 Stakeholder support

Stakeholders for a TB programme could be defined as 'those groups without whose funding support the programme would cease to exist' (adapted from Freeman *et al.*, 2010). Under this definition, stakeholders control the strategic direction of the TB programme and its required revenue. A critical step in developing an effective TB programme is thus to identify and involve stakeholder leaders to ensure they understand the benefits for their members and the wider community.

15.2.7 Planning

Planning towards effective delivery of strategic objectives requires science-based tools, knowledge and understanding of TB epidemiology (including diagnostics, herd history analysis, cattle management factors and modelling capacity) supported by robust policy development and economic analysis. It is likely to require a number of years to develop the required level of local epidemiological and policy knowledge, data and financial information in order to develop fully costed plans. Guidance from epidemiologists and managers working in countries with well-developed plans could support new TB programme development elsewhere. Processes to develop and approve disease management plans may themselves be regulated (such as under New Zealand's Biosecurity Act 1993) (New Zealand Government, 2016), and this can provide for useful transparency, process discipline and public or stakeholder benefit and impact assessment.

15.2.8 Benefit–cost analysis

A benefit–cost analysis helps planners and stakeholders to evaluate identified strategic options for a proposed TB programme. This usually requires the development of epidemiological models, designed to represent the future outcomes (normally between 20 to 50 years) of selected strategic options. The models are used to calculate the future annual benefits and costs, based on present-day values, for the selected time period. For each option, the annual calculated cost is subtracted from the annual benefit for each year. The resulting value for each year is then discounted to the present-day value and summed for all years. This provides the net present value (NPV) as an option. Ideally the option of not having a TB programme, i.e. a 'do nothing' case or something similar, should also be modelled, together with its forecast annual costs, benefits, and resulting NPV. NPV provides a means of comparing the quantum difference of each of the options when compared with the 'do nothing' option and allows them to be ranked and evaluated (Livingstone et al., 2015b).

A major difficulty with TB benefit–cost analyses is obtaining or deriving a monetary value for the benefits. While programme costs can usually be estimated with some accuracy, benefits such as avoided disease-related productivity, product value or trade losses can be much harder to quantify. Approaches to this problem are likely to involve combinations of epidemiological, livestock production and economic modelling in order to project likely livestock infection levels, and the resulting production, value and trade losses, across a range of disease control options and scenarios over time, and compare these with projected programme delivery costs (including within-farm cost such as for mustering and yarding cattle for testing). Nevertheless, if it is possible to assess these costs or the costs of additional TB, then this provides a good basis for evaluating a TB programme (Zinsstag et al., 2006). The reliability of such comparisons may be limited by availability of data on likely impacts of various disease incidence levels on production value, which may require estimation by industry analysts (TBfree NZ, 2007).

A further problem arises through the long time frames required to achieve significant TB control or eradication objectives, which may span several decades. Most of the benefits of such programmes are only enjoyed well into the future, whereas costs are incurred from the outset. Discount rates used in conventional benefit–cost analysis tend to give strong effect to short-term costs while devaluing longer term benefits, which may result in a negative NPV (Livingstone et al., 2015b). In such situations, stakeholders will need to make judgements as to whether a programme will provide long lasting value, taking account of the time to reach objectives and the extent of the benefits when they eventually occur. This may result in choosing the modelled option with the least negative NPV. Stakeholders reviewing options and the outcomes of modelled benefit–cost analyses may seek a number of iterative changes to plans, which can have flow-on iterative effects on finalized strategic objectives and costs (Livingstone *et al.*, 2015b).

15.2.9 Agreement on funding

Gaining agreement as to who is responsible for funding a TB strategy is a major challenge for a sustained programme with a long time frame. Ideally, costs should be allocated to funders in proportion to the value of the benefits they receive. In practice this can be difficult to ascertain, the benefit proportions may change over time, and mechanisms to collect funds from certain beneficiaries may be cumbersome, avoidable or unavailable.

Regardless of the basis of apportioning funding, the method used needs to be transparent and agreed to by all funders. It should be seen to be fair and logical as well as simple and cost effective to implement. Where TB infection may affect export of cattle-derived products, export income may provide a means for allocating funding shares between export sectors such as dairy and beef industries. Where the benefit from a TB programme is an increase in animal or herd production, then individual farmers, or collectives representing them, should fund at least part of the programme directly, such as paying for certain TB tests or receiving reduced compensation for slaughter of test-positive cattle.

National or local government funding may be required in place of, or to augment, more targeted industry or stakeholder funding in situations where the latter beneficiaries are difficult to identify or raise funds from. Government funding may also be more secure, especially in the late stages of a programme when low disease incidence may lead farmers or industry to severely reduce TB programme expenditure. This ensures that when a programme is well advanced and immediate disease risks to industry stakeholders and farmers are minimal, government funding may enable the programme to be maintained to its desired conclusion. This protects against re-establishment of widespread infection which may occur if resources were withdrawn during the long end-phase of an eradication programme. Ideally, funding shares and mechanisms should be set out in legislation, based on negotiated agreements between funders. A range of funding options have been used, from total government funding (Enticott, 2014) to a mix of farmer/industry/government shares (Cousins and Roberts, 2001; Max *et al.*, 2011; Livingstone *et al.*, 2015a).

15.2.10 Programme policies

Given funding constraints, programme policies should be based on a mix of best technical knowledge and the practicality of applying disease control interventions across affected herds and areas, such that milestones and objectives will be met. Policies need to be clearly enunciated, unambiguous and compliant with legislation. They also need to meet the requirements of trading partners and as far as possible, farmer and stakeholder needs.

It is important that disease control policies take account of farming, industry and societal contexts. For example, when farmers have poor understanding of the disease and its control, they may mistrust what they see to be imposed control programmes. In particular, farmers may have concerns over the accuracy of TB tests, the impacts of reactor slaughter, adequacy of compensation and the effects of possible animal movement restrictions, all of which can reduce farming incomes. These concerns need to be identified and addressed through communication and consultation (see section 15.2.11), or otherwise they may lead to lack of compliance.

Funding arrangements and disease control policies that may impose costs or constraints on farmers need to be seen as fair in relation to benefits and cost. Policy impacts on different farming types need to be recognized and possibly ameliorated – for example, policies that constrain livestock movement may have little impact on farms that finish beef cattle for slaughter, but may be drastic for stock breeders reliant on live animal sales. Compensation payments can ease the impacts of necessarily restrictive disease control policies, but care must be taken to avoid perverse outcomes or wasted spending from overly generous compensation.

Mistrust or perception of unfairness can significantly affect programme acceptance by farmers, farming organizations, politicians and the general public (Moda, 2006; Palmer and

Waters, 2011; Livingstone et al., 2015b). Failure to address these issues in policy development and through clear, honest and ongoing communication may result in failure of a programme, as identified for the eradication of pleuropneumonia from Tanzania after it re-emerged in 1990 (Kusiluka and Sudi, 2003).

Proposed policies need to be communicated to farmers, funders and stakeholders during the strategic planning process so that they have an opportunity to raise concerns before policies are agreed and implemented.

15.2.11 Communication and consultation

Unless there is clear and open communication with the wider interest groups on the important aspects of a proposed strategic plan, it may incur unnecessary delays and costs once the programme is implemented. Therefore, once stakeholders have reached agreement on the strategic plan, then its objectives, essential components of the plan, major policies and how it will be funded need to be clearly and simply communicated to wider interest groups. These include farmers, members of the stakeholder organizations, industry leaders, government agencies and politicians, as well as the wider interested public who may be affected or impacted (New Zealand Government, 2016). Consultation with the main groups who may be affected by the strategy, its policies or funding should then follow. Individuals or groups should be provided with the opportunity to respond either orally or in writing, indicating their support for the proposed strategy design and funding or to note their concerns and suggest alternatives. Following consultation, written or oral submissions need to be reviewed by planners and stakeholders to determine whether the strategic plan needs to be revised to accommodate concerns raised. If it is decided to make changes to the strategy design, this may involve another iteration round, possibly leading to modified objectives, plans, costs and timelines.

15.2.12 Programme implementation

Implementing a TB programme should be the role of a management agency that is accountable to stakeholders. There are various models for such an agency. It may exist within government as in the UK (Enticott, 2014), or it may be an independent stakeholder-owned business structure as in New Zealand (Livingstone et al., 2015b). Stakeholder ownership may have advantages in ensuring acceptance and support from farmers and industry, but a stakeholder-owned agency will require access to legal powers and will need to be subject to regulated technical and managerial standards.

Whatever model is chosen or available, the management agency must be responsible for implementing the plan within budget, meeting all legislative requirements (including for health, safety and environmental management) and reporting to stakeholders against annual milestones and progress towards strategy objectives. The management agency must be equipped with or capable of providing: (i) a senior management group under a CEO responsible for a management structure that oversees the delivery of the plan within budget, maintains links with stakeholders and minimizes surprises; (ii) a TB surveillance capacity that would include recording, collation and analysis of a range of integrated activities and data such as herd and animal TB tests and results, post-mortem TB findings from slaughtered cattle, case management reports on infected or suspect herds, and tracing of cattle movements to and from suspect or infected herds; (iii) communication with stakeholders, farmers and farming organizations, industry leaders and government officials to support routine programme delivery, manage operational issues and report on performance and progress; (iv) appropriate financial management to provide annual income and expenditure plans, pay farmers and contractors as required, and keep senior management group updated on budget matters; and (v) effective delivery and monitoring of field services and operations.

There are two broad options for delivery of operational services such as TB testing of cattle, managing reactor slaughter, monitoring livestock movement controls and laboratory diagnostics. An agency may have capacity to deliver such services itself, or it may contract for delivery by other providers. External contracting may bring advantages through encouraging commercial competition between contractors, which may in turn drive innovation and cost savings. However, this requires management agency capacity for contract specification, tendering and audit to ensure contractors meet performance requirements. Direct operational service delivery by the management agency itself may offer greater management control, but may lead to unwanted agency expansion. In practice, a mix of contracted and direct service delivery may be appropriate.

15.2.13 Research

While there is an existing large body and literature of research on TB in cattle (some of which has been summarized in earlier chapters) further research may be required to address local technical or biological problems, to improve programme cost-efficacy, or to mitigate adverse operational or social impacts. Research requirements will vary from programme to programme – often reflecting programme maturity – but will likely be directed towards cost-effective applications of new diagnostic methods, animal recording, or control policies within existing TB programmes.

Research planning and delivery processes will need to reflect available institutional arrangements and structures. A management agency may have direct access to research capacity, or may need to utilize external capacity in institutes or universities. In either case the management agency should possess or be able to co-opt the expertise needed to identify research needs, develop and manage a research portfolio to meet these needs, and to oversee the planning and delivery of specific research projects. It may also need processes to deal with possible conflicts of interest between funders and research providers, and to ensure intellectual property rights and commercial interests are appropriately managed. Research projects must be designed to ensure delivery of clearly specified outcomes under fixed budgets.

Information derived from analysis of data, outcomes of relevant research, feedback from farmers and audit findings should be used to modify plans, policies and the implementation process to ensure these remain best-aligned to current programme objectives and are cost effective (Tweddle and Livingstone, 1994; Sheridan, 2011; Livingstone et al., 2015b).

15.3 Impact of Wildlife Reservoirs on Tuberculosis Strategies

The finding of TB in a reservoir or maintenance wild animal host (Morris and Pfeiffer, 1995; Palmer, 2013) in high GNI economy countries may initially be seen as scientifically interesting or a novel nuisance. Once both the full geographic distribution of the TB maintenance host and its impact as a source of infection for cattle have been determined, then the finding can range from minor inconvenience to a major setback. Where the maintenance host is of limited distribution, it may have a relatively minor impact on a TB programme, such as with infection of white-tailed deer in Michigan in the USA (Palmer, 2013) and in elk and white-tailed deer in Canada (O'Brien et al., 2011). However, where a maintenance host has a wide distribution and is an effective vector of infection for cattle, such as with badgers in the UK and Republic of Ireland (Abernethy et al., 2006; More and Good, 2006; Wilson et al., 2011), wild boar in Spain (Naranjo et al., 2008) and possums in New Zealand (Nugent et al., 2015a) this greatly increases both cost and time frames required to achieve TB freedom or eradication goals.

The presence of a significant wildlife maintenance host introduces ecological, environmental and possibly societal factors that extend beyond the immediate farming environment. These factors may vary greatly from situation to situation, and will require locally designed responses. Altogether, these will be more challenging and complex than the largely standard test, slaughter and quarantine processes that are sufficient for effective control where the disease is limited to farmed cattle. Controlling TB in wildlife requires different sets of knowledge and analysis of much more complex situations. A programme that requires disease management in wildlife as well as cattle is likely to impact on people who may have little interest in cattle TB control, whereas cattle farmers and TB control stakeholders may have little interest in wildlife management. This can lead to conflict based on differing attitudes towards controlling livestock disease and preferred treatment of wildlife (Bengis et al., 2002; Cassidy, 2012).

If wide-scale eradication of TB from cattle is an extraordinary goal as espoused by Miller et al. (2006), eradicating TB from a wildlife host as well as from cattle is much more so. Nevertheless, with the right research knowledge and detailed planning, costed strategic options should be able to be developed for stakeholders and the wider public to consider. This consideration needs to involve technical and operational validity, the concerns of affected parties and the wider public, and a realistic assessment of costs and benefits, which may fall much more widely than for a programme involving cattle TB control alone. This will take time.

15.3.1 Determining the presence of a tuberculosis in a wildlife maintenance host

Foremost in coming to grips with finding TB in wildlife is proving which species is acting as a maintenance host and whether it (or any other species) is acting as a TB vector or source of infection for cattle, as described by O'Brien et al. (2011). In some cases, a complex multi-host epidemiological situation may become apparent, which needs to be evaluated through detailed epidemiological research and modelling. This can be time-consuming and expensive. Figure 15.1 shows the level of interrelationships identified for transmission of bovine TB in New Zealand.

There are at least two alternative processes that can be used to determine the presence of a TB wildlife maintenance host. Firstly, the TB maintenance host may emerge through the accumulation of circumstantial evidence, anecdotal information and serendipitous findings that point to the culprit species, with knowledge gaps being filled in through later systematic work as happened in New Zealand (Livingstone et al., 2015a). Secondly, based on the New Zealand experience, the following describes a more efficient process that could be used to identify the presence of a TB maintenance host.

If a wildlife source of infection for cattle is suspected but not proven, an epidemiological review of all recent herd infections should be undertaken. This should aim to identify any geographic clustering of recent herd infections that are not clearly associated with livestock-only infection pathways or sources (such as cattle purchase or movement, mixing with infected stock, or undiagnosed residual infection). Significant clustering of herd infection that cannot be explained by livestock pathways would initially suggest wildlife involvement. Further evaluation of this would require investigation of the distribution and density of the suspected wildlife species in proximity to clusters of infected herds.

Irrespective of the suspect species, postmortem surveys of the most common wildlife scavengers in areas of concern will assist in determining the extent of wildlife TB presence (Byrom et al., 2015; Nugent et al., 2015b). As identified by Byrom (2015) and Nugent (2015b), scavenger species have relatively large home ranges over which they will scavenge wildlife carrion. If the carrion is from a TB-infected population, then over time the scavenger species will also become infected. This can provide a relatively quick way of determining the presence of wildlife infection around clusters of herd infection, although survey design and species targeting needs to take account of factors such as species longevity, population density, home range and likely TB prevalence, for both the scavenger species and the suspected maintenance host or hosts. (Byrom et al., 2015; Nugent et al., 2015b).

If TB is identified in a wildlife scavenger species, then further research will be required to identify its epidemiological role as described by Palmer (2013). It may turn out to be a maintenance host as, for example, wild boar in Spain (Boadella et al., 2012), or a spillover host such as wild pigs in New Zealand (Nugent et al., 2015b). If the infected scavenger species is deemed to be a spillover host, then the exact source of infection will need to be determined for the scavenger (i.e. which of its carrion source species was infected). Information on the distribution and home range attributes of the scavenger species will help to define the geographic area in which an intensified survey of other wildlife species would be undertaken. Such a survey would sample intensively all wildlife species that are likely to be carrion sources and are present in the probable home range of the spillover TB animal. If the likely maintenance host and vector for

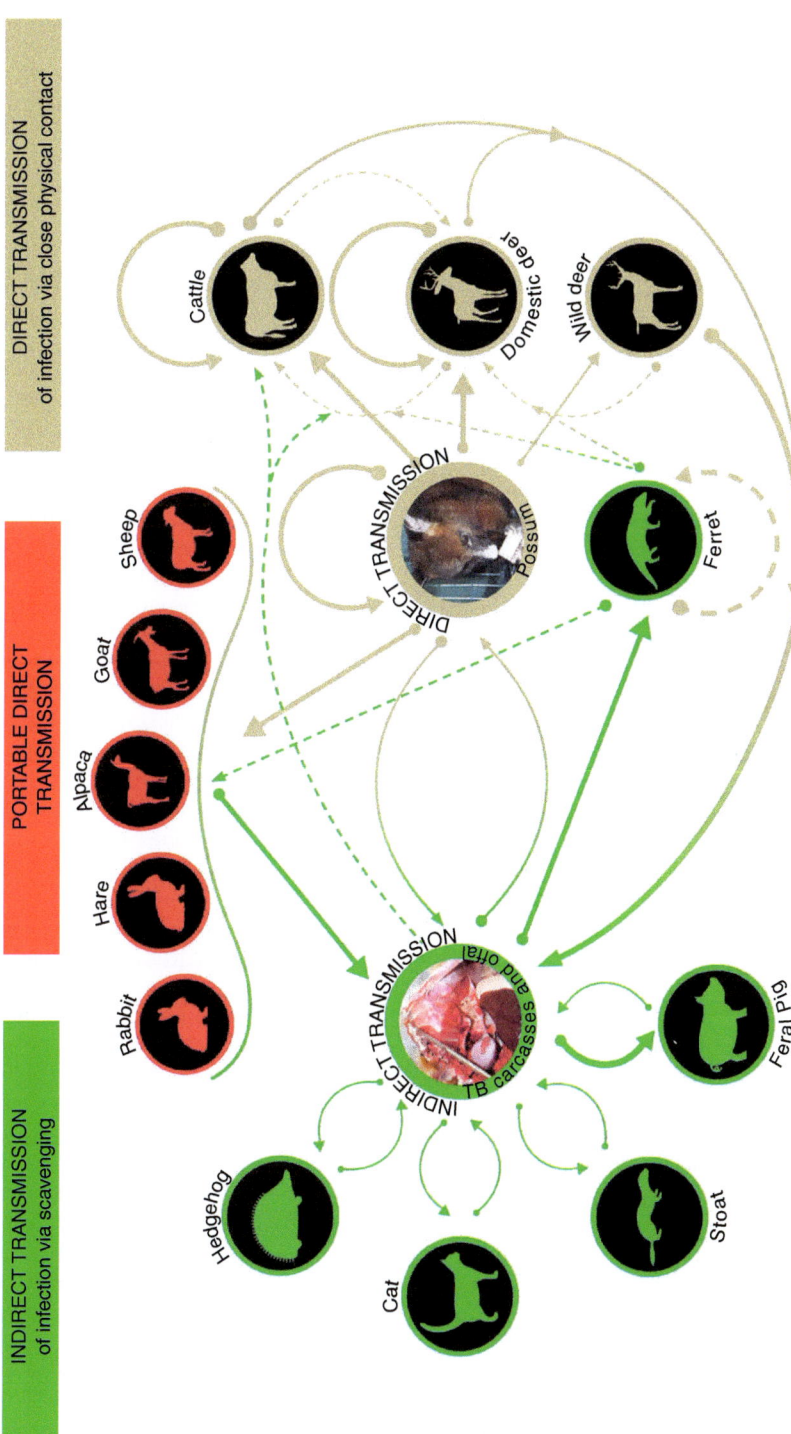

Fig. 15.1. Direct and indirect pathways for spread of bovine tuberculosis between and within species in New Zealand. Bold arrows indicate a main source or route of infection; brown depicts direct transmission, green depicts indirect transmission via scavenging or investigation of tuberculous carcasses and offal, red indicates that the source of infection is unknown but is likely to be by direct means. This figure is reproduced with permission of the Editor, *New Zealand Veterinary Journal*, where it was first published as Figure 2 in the following paper: P.G. Livingstone, N. Hancox, G. Nugent, G.W. de Lisle (2015) Toward eradication: the effect of *Mycobacterium bovis* infection in wildlife on the evolution and future direction of bovine tuberculosis management in New Zealand. *New Zealand Veterinary Journal* 63 (S1), p7.

livestock infection is not identified, additional surveys may need to be undertaken, as it is possible that the prevalence of infection in the maintenance host may vary over time.

Given there is sufficient ecological and epidemiological information to show an association between infection in a particular wildlife species and cattle that is indicative of a maintenance host, then this finding needs to be investigated further. It is likely to require undertaking a broader epidemiological and ecological investigation, concentrating on areas where there have been other unexplained TB breakdowns in cattle herds. In addition, areas where the wildlife species is present, but TB is absent from cattle herds, should also be investigated. These investigations will help to determine the distribution of infected wildlife species, their TB prevalence, their relationship to TB breakdowns in cattle herds, and the exact mode of disease transmission from wildlife species to cattle (and vice versa) as identified by O'Brien et al. (2011). Over time these surveys will also provide data to determine whether TB infection in wildlife is spreading geographically. It may be possible to undertake a longitudinal study to assist in proving that the infected wildlife is a maintenance host for TB (Morris and Pfeiffer, 1995).

Evidence from a number of studies indicates that for TB to be maintained in wildlife species – that is, when the basic reproduction rate of the disease R_0 is ≥ 1 (Palmer, 2013) – then the local density of the wildlife host reflects an elevation of environmental carrying capacity caused by some form of ecosystem disturbance or modification.

Thus, badger densities appear to have increased over time in Ireland following pasture improvement and abandonment of traditional game-keeping and hunting (Smal, 1995). An increase in badger density has also been reported in England, possibly due to climate change (Macdonald and Newman, 2002). As well as density effects, human activity may have inadvertently caused changes to a wildlife species social structure, enabling greater interspecies and possibly intraspecies interaction as suggested for badgers by Wilson et al. (2011). In New Zealand, the possum experienced ecological release from its natural controls when it was deliberately introduced from Australia and released into vacant mammalian browsing niches. Following release and redistribution of possums for their fur value, the species became ubiquitous at often high population densities due to its tolerance of a wide range of conditions, generalized omnivorous diet and freedom from predation or competition (Clout and Ericksen, 2000; Efford, 2000). In Michigan and Minnesota, supplementary feeding of white-tailed deer increased deer congregation and interaction at feed dumps, which has facilitated TB transmission (O'Brien et al., 2006; Palmer, 2013). In south-central Spain, wild boar aggregation at artificial watering or feeding sites has been associated with an increased risk of TB (Vicente et al., 2007).

Measures to manage or reduce infection levels in wildlife populations thus need to take account of factors such as increased densities and social interaction that appear to have facilitated some species becoming TB maintenance hosts with $R_0 \geq 1$. Management options may include density reduction by culling as for possums in New Zealand (Warburton and Livingstone, 2015) and badgers in Ireland (Sheridan, 2011). Vaccination to protect wildlife against TB has been investigated in a number of species including possums and badgers (Buddle et al., 2011) white-tailed deer (Waters and Palmer, 2015) and wild boar (Garrido et al., 2011). Combinations of testing, culling and vaccination are under consideration for badgers in Northern Ireland (Department of Agriculture, Environment and Rural Affairs, 2016). Consideration of wildlife management options requires engagement with farmers, wildlife organizations, interest groups and the wider public, who may all have relationships or concerns with the species under evaluation. Wildlife management also needs to be effectively integrated with cattle TB control measures. Failure to do so may lead to setback or collapse of a cattle TB programme (Wilson et al., 2011; O'Brien et al., 2011; Livingstone et al., 2015a).

TB programmes that include controlling infection in a wildlife source are subject to similar broad success factors as those identified for programmes where cattle are the sole functional disease host. Nevertheless, some changes in management approach and emphasis will be required to deal with the complications introduced by wildlife ecology, TB epidemiology and greater public interest in findings and outcomes.

Wildlife involvement also introduces some completely new management factors which must be addressed in a successful programme.

15.3.2 Purpose and strategic objectives

Depending upon its impact, the involvement of a TB wildlife maintenance host may force significant reappraisal of the achievable purpose, direction and objectives of a cattle TB programme. Strategic direction may switch towards emphasizing the control of TB infection in the wildlife maintenance host, in order to facilitate effective control of TB in the cattle population. If controlling infection in the wildlife maintenance host is not tenable, then the strategy may be directed towards excluding wildlife from contact with cattle or their feed, as has been proposed for badgers in England (Tolhurst et al., 2009) and white-tailed deer in Michigan (Walter et al., 2012). The finding of a TB wildlife reservoir may also pose an increased risk of transmission to humans. Unfortunately, the final purpose of the TB programme is unlikely to become clear until the extent of the wildlife–cattle relationship has been reviewed and the proposed programme and its costs undertaken.

The presence of a significant wildlife maintenance host and TB vector may initially force the adoption of disease containment objectives for cattle, based on continued and possibly intensified livestock test, slaughter and movement control programmes. In parallel with this, research and investigation should be undertaken to fully elucidate wildlife epidemiology and to identify possible measures to control TB in the wildlife maintenance host or otherwise prevent it from transmitting TB to cattle. This may involve long-term multifactorial research projects that will take considerable time (approximately 22 years for New Zealand; Livingstone et al., 2015a) to provide a realistic basis for setting more ambitious long-term objectives for TB freedom or eradication. This does not imply that nothing should be undertaken until the best solution has been identified and shown to work. It is far easier and cheaper to intervene and control new infection in a wildlife population before it becomes established and widespread. Therefore, identifying a more moderate objective and means of implementing within 3–5 years of finding TB infection in a wildlife maintenance host is preferable to waiting until all the research and analysis has been completed before beginning. Such a moderate programme will provide much needed information and data that can be used to improve its effectiveness and also identify important areas for future research.

For countries like New Zealand, UK and Ireland, national goals for TB freedom for cattle or eradication of *M. bovis* will not be achieved until transmission of *M. bovis* from the infected wildlife maintenance host to cattle permanently ceases (Livingstone et al., 2015a, 2015b).

15.3.3 Legal status

Controlling infection in wildlife is likely to involve or impact on a wider segment of the public than when the disease is functionally limited to cattle. Additional legal powers may be required to enable effective surveillance and control of TB in wildlife. This could include enabling vaccination of cattle, wildlife or both, or a requirement for physical exclusion of wildlife from farms or facilities. Further legal controls may also need to be applied to cattle farming practice, such as restricting livestock movement to and from areas of high wildlife TB prevalence or even excluding them from areas where TB wildlife is present or suspected. The need for such legal powers will not become clear until a wider strategic plan to control TB in both wildlife and cattle has been evaluated, costed, communicated and agreed with funding stakeholders, government agencies, affected interest groups, the general public and legislators.

15.3.4 Stakeholder support

Control or management of wildlife as part of a cattle TB programme will most likely impact on a wide range of people and organizations. Not all of these will be willing or able funders, and some may indeed be strongly opposed to the proposed programme. In such a situation, a process will be needed to manage this wider range of people and interests to gain agreement (or at least acceptance of) the programme and its funding.

In New Zealand, a significant share of government funding has been instrumental in the effective implementation of a programme requiring large-scale wildlife control and management affecting multiple interests and extending widely beyond cattle farming lands (Livingstone et al., 2015b).

15.3.5 Planning

In order to identify the most cost-effective strategy for controlling TB in both cattle and wildlife maintenance hosts, it is critical that a range of options is considered, modelled and costed. The ability to compare options will depend upon the availability and accuracy of a variety of information including: (i) research findings on the geographic and temporal distribution of infection in wildlife; (ii) an understanding of the relationships between population densities and TB prevalence levels in wildlife hosts, and the effects of this for cattle TB incidence rates; (iii) the feasibility and public acceptance of methods to control, contain or regionally eradicate infection from wildlife, or methods to prevent transmission between infected wildlife and cattle; (iv) modelling the interactions between wildlife and cattle, and the options for, and effects of, controlling infection in wildlife populations; (v) detailed costings for each control or management option; and (vi) economic assessment of the benefits to be gained under each option. Provided information of reasonable quality is available to model and cost these options, this will help to identify those that are not acceptable, and to clarify further research or data requirements for developing potentially acceptable strategic choices.

It is important at the initial planning stage to identify up to four possible options that span the control spectrum, together with associated policies, likely costs and possible implications. A summary of information on each option should be presented to stakeholders, farming and wildlife organizations, government agencies, politicians and the wider public for them to consider. At a point in time, however, a decision needs to be made on a strategic way forward, even without the unanimous agreement of affected parties. An extreme option may be to forego cattle farming in defined areas until TB can be eradicated locally from the wildlife maintenance host. An opposite extreme would be to eradicate the wildlife species regionally and with it the wildlife infection. After TB has also been eradicated from the cattle population, the wildlife species could be reintroduced from a known TB-free population. Where the wildlife host is an invasive exotic pest, such as the possum in New Zealand, lethal population control is more likely to be a favourable option with major conservation benefits. Where the host is a valued species, such as the badger in the UK, planning and option development will be more complex, but nevertheless, a range of options need to be fully analysed and costed. As identified earlier, presenting this information provides all stakeholders with an ability to see the modelled impacts of the costed options, likely issues that may arise and an insight as to how it will be financed. These can be considered together with proposals to mitigate any relatively short-term impacts for wildlife or cattle farmers.

15.3.6 Benefit–cost analysis

Compared with a cattle-only programme, modelling for benefit–cost analysis involving wildlife management will be more intricate and assumption-based, with likely longer time frames and higher costs. It will require comparing costs and benefits of various modelled options, including a 'no-control' option. Wildlife management in itself may have benefits or disbenefits that are quite separate from solely disease-related outcomes, but which also may be difficult to measure. Possum population control in New Zealand reduces commercial fur hunting opportunities but improves forest ecosystems and indigenous biodiversity (Warburton and Livingstone, 2015). The latter benefits were valued by public survey of individual willingness to pay for the recovery of selected native plant and animal species expected to occur as a result of reduced possum densities (Tait et al., 2017). Because of the likely longer time frame to achieve TB objectives when infection needs to be controlled in wildlife as well as cattle, benefit–cost analyses are likely to provide strongly negative NPV results.

15.3.7 Agreement on funding

The geographic extent of wildlife infection and the attributable fraction of cattle infection in these areas (Rockhill et al., 1998; Livingstone et al., 2015a), will help to determine whether wildlife is a major or minor factor affecting a cattle TB programme. If wildlife is a major disease factor, then research into related epidemiology and implementing measures to prevent transmission of infection from wildlife to cattle will add to programme costs. Gaining funding to meet these costs is likely to require input from government agencies, research establishments, the farming industry and possibly wildlife interest groups or managers. There is no simple formula as to how funding should be shared, except a commitment by all to contribute towards gaining greater knowledge and to identify, evaluate and agree on solutions to implement now, rather than leaving it to future generations to resolve. Where costly wildlife management is required, then government may elect to contribute funds on behalf of the wider public. Alternatively, wildlife organizations and groups together with farmer organizations and government may identify a means of shared funding, especially where TB management will lead to overall benefits for wildlife health, welfare and biodiversity. Before entering into funding commitments, potential funders will need to be satisfied that the programme will meet clear and measurable goals and objectives within an agreed funding term. Legal mechanisms such as levies or rates may be required to obtain funding from appropriately targeted but unwilling funders or to prevent cost avoidance by free-riding (Anonymous, 2016).

15.3.8 Programme policies

Given an enlarged TB programme that encompasses measures directed towards both wildlife and cattle, policies should be based on the best available technical, research and operational knowledge and be deliverable within an agreed plan and budget. Policies need to be clearly enunciated, unambiguous, readily available and compliant with legislation. Policies should also meet the requirements of trading partners and as far as possible, those of stakeholders, farmers, animal welfare and wildlife interest groups. To achieve this, policy development will need to be part of a wide consultative process.

15.3.9 Communication and consultation

Once funding stakeholders and representatives of wildlife organizations and other key affected parties have reached agreement on the strategic option, its objectives, policies, costs and funding, these need to be communicated widely to those parties likely to be affected by the programme (New Zealand Government, 2016). These include members of the stakeholder organizations, farmers and farming organizations, wildlife organizations, government agencies, politicians and the interested public. As identified previously, consultation with the main groups who may be impacted by the strategy, its policies or funding, should then follow. Consultation should provide opportunities for written or oral submissions on proposed strategy design, policies, costs and methods of funding. Submissions need to be reviewed by the stakeholders to determine whether the proposed plan needs to be revised to accommodate concerns raised, and submitters should be provided with a response to their concerns. Significant changes may involve another planning iteration, possibly leading to modified objectives, plans, costs and timelines. If these would result in materially changed impacts for groups or individuals, this would need to be communicated and may necessitate another round of consultation.

15.3.10 Implementation

Implementing a programme designed to achieve strategic objectives of TB freedom for cattle and regional freedom from TB in a wildlife maintenance host, is a major long-term undertaking. The effects on cattle TB incidence rates following progressive wildlife management interventions are likely to be dynamic, geographically variable and multifactorial. Programme management and administration will require the capability to understand and interpret these unfolding dynamics and be able to modify operations or policies in order to ensure strategic milestones are met within budget. As well as being accountable to direct funders and key stakeholders, programme managers will also need to be responsive to wider public concerns relating to wildlife disease control measures. Managers will need access to ecological and wildlife management expertise alongside veterinary and epidemiological capability, and programme delivery will need to be supported by ongoing effective communications.

15.4 Options for Managing *M. bovis* and its Transmission in Low to Medium–High GNI Economies

15.4.1 Background

In 2016, countries in the low to medium–high GNI economies contained 84% of the estimated 7.4 billion world population (Worldometers, 2016). Low to medium–high GNI populations tend to be young, poorly educated, rural dwelling and employed in agriculture (The World Bank, 2016b). Randolph *et al*. (2007) consider livestock to be an essential household asset in rural and peri-urban parts of the low to medium–high GNI economies. Livestock provide nourishment, traction power, manure, fuel and social status, and may even serve as banks. Nevertheless, because of factors such as close contact (often with shared housing), poor sanitation and consumption of raw milk, meat and blood from animals (Mfinanga *et al*., 2003), people living in these economies are exposed to a disproportionately high share of zoonoses (Randolph *et al*., 2007), including TB (Cosivi *et al*., 1998; Mfinanga *et al*., 2003). This can undermine the value of livestock as a means of reducing poverty.

The need and ability to manage zoonotic diseases such as TB is directly affected by health priorities and availability of local and international funding and resources. Over the last few decades, low to medium–high GNI economy countries have faced resource constraints and declines in funding. Under such circumstances, the type of veterinary and public health services otherwise used to manage zoonotic diseases in livestock in high GNI countries are not sustainable (Randolph *et al*., 2007). Furthermore, because of migratory lifestyles, illiteracy, fragile social contexts and remoteness, critical healthcare, veterinary services and information are often unavailable to rural populations (Randolph *et al*., 2007; The World Bank, 2016b).

Despite these obstacles, livestock ownership can offer pathways to alleviate poverty in low to medium–high GNI economies. Perry *et al*. (2002) provided a framework describing how livestock could contribute to poverty reduction by reducing the vulnerability of the household livestock asset base, and by improving both productivity and access to markets for produce. Using this framework, Perry and Grace (2009) forecast a reduction in livestock disease, and improved availability of food and marketable livestock products. They also identified that value-adding and selling produce from small-scale producers provided employment opportunities, especially in a vertically integrated system, all of which would assist in poverty reduction.

Perry and Grace (2009) strongly supported the reduction of zoonotic diseases, but noted that the role of zoonoses and their impact on poverty had not been investigated or evaluated in poorer countries. Given that disease impacts can be measured, this provides a means of determining the feasibility and costs of some form of disease control. Perry and Grace (2009) caution that the form of disease control must be socially acceptable to the livestock-keeping community, not impede farming systems and ideally be able to be implemented from within the community.

They further identify Ecohealth as a transdisciplinary system to approach disease issues that 'aims to integrate human, livestock, wildlife and ecosystem health, exploring their interdependence'. Ecohealth appears very similar to the current One Health concept that recognizes that the health of humans and animals is interdependent with one another and the ecosystem they live in (OIE, 2016c). Positive and meaningful collaboration between ecologists, sociologists, physicians, veterinarians, epidemiologists and microbiologists under a One Health programme provides the best chance of understanding and then controlling infectious zoonotic diseases such as TB in low to medium–high GNI economies.

In 2016, the World Health Organization (WHO) reported that 10.4 million people became ill and 1.8 million people died from TB (World Health Organization, 2016). Sixty percent of new TB cases occurred in just six countries: China, India, Indonesia, Nigeria, Pakistan and South Africa. In 2014 the WHO developed and accepted the 'End TB Strategy' (World Health Organization, 2014) which supports the UN's poverty reduction policy. The WHO strategy has targets for: (i) a 75% reduction in the number of tuberculosis (TB)-related deaths and a 50% reduction in the TB incidence rate over the period 2015–2025; and (ii) a 95% reduction in tuberculosis deaths and a 90% reduction in TB incidence by 2035.

The WHO End TB Strategy is targeted at reducing TB caused by *M. tuberculosis*, and recently, in 2016, for the first time recognized and included *M. bovis* as a cause of disease in humans. However, on a global level the causative organism is still not being differentiated to the species level for the vast majority of human TB cases. From a practical point of view, it is important to further investigate the consequences of misdiagnosing *M. bovis* infection and its implications for the outcome of any TB treatment regime.

Cosivi *et al.* (1998) reported that between 1954 and 1970, *M. bovis* was responsible for 3.1% of human TB cases worldwide. Since then, the percentage of human cases attributable to *M. bovis* in high GNI countries is likely to have fallen significantly. The trend in low to medium–high GNI countries is unknown, but widespread HIV/AIDS infection is likely to have exacerbated both *M. tuberculosis* and *M. bovis* infection levels. Snippets of data from these countries arising from targeted non-representative studies indicated that the proportion of *M. bovis* isolated from human TB cases in largely rural areas ranged between 3.9% and 10% in Nigeria, 0.4% and 45% in Egypt and up to 36% in Tanzania (Cosivi *et al.*, 1998), and between 16.3% and 29.2% in Ethiopia (Shitaye *et al.*, 2007) (see also Chapter 3). Cook *et al.* (1996) found that there was a seven times greater risk of TB in humans in households in Zambia possessing tuberculin-positive cattle (odds ratio of 7.6). Cosivi *et al.* (1998) also identified that in low to medium–high GNI economies in Africa and Asia, between 82% and 94% of the human population lived in rural areas where there was very little or no control or management of TB in cattle. Given the increased demand for local milk in these countries, the authors identified cattle as a potential source of TB for humans. This is supported by Shitaye *et al.* (2007) who indicated that due to widespread HIV/AIDS in Ethiopia and other African countries, affected humans may have an increased chance of becoming infected with *M. bovis* from consuming raw milk, raw meat and blood from potentially infected animals (Mfinanga *et al.*, 2003). Furthermore, Chen *et al.* (2009) reported finding *M. tuberculosis* in cattle in China that had an epidemiological link to human *M. tuberculosis* infection. *M. tuberculosis* and *M. bovis* have both also been isolated from TB lesions from goats in Nigeria (Cadmus *et al.*, 2009) and Ethiopia (Deresa *et al.*, 2013). Therefore, the finding of both *M. bovis* and *M. tuberculosis* in cattle and in goats in low to medium–high GNI economies poses a potential challenge to the WHO End TB Strategy unless TB in livestock is also addressed. Future reduction in levels of human TB is likely to depend upon identifying and controlling the source of infection, despite this being of low importance for treatment purposes.

In order for the WHO End TB Strategy targets to be met, it is likely that human *M. bovis* cases will need to be reduced in low to medium–high GNI countries. Despite the fact bovine TB no longer poses a zoonotic risk in most high GNI economies compared to low to medium GNI countries, because most milk is pasteurized, meat is inspected following slaughter, and national test-and-slaughter programmes for cattle are in place. It is worth noting that in the USA, *M. bovis* continues to be a source of human TB although it is possible that a considerable proportion of these cases may have been acquired abroad (Scott *et al.*, 2016).

In considering strategies to reduce the risk of *M. bovis* spreading within livestock and to humans in low to medium–high GNI economies, it is important to take account of available disease management resources and the willingness of cattle owners to accept disease control interventions. No single strategy will suit all situations, with feasible options ranging from simple information gathering and dissemination, through to a comprehensive test-and-slaughter programme. Primary goals should be to reduce the risks of *M. bovis* being transmitted from livestock (cattle, buffalo, goats or camels) to humans. If possible, TB management should also lead to reduced livestock TB incidence, providing for animal health, production and economic gains.

15.4.2 Options

Empowering people through knowledge

In some low to medium–high GNI communities, there is poor understanding of bovine TB and its risks to human health. A study in Arusha, Tanzania, found that in areas where the prevalence of TB herd infection was up to 50%, 75% of people surveyed had little knowledge of TB; 50% did not boil milk and 18% ate raw meat (Mfinanga *et al.*, 2003). In a similar study in Cameroon, Ndukum *et al.* (2010) found 'among cattle handlers, 81.9% were aware of BTB, 67.9% knew that BTB is zoonotic, and 53.8% knew one mode of transmission, but over 27% consumed raw meat and/or drank unpasteurised milk'. It has been estimated that in East Africa, more than 80% of milk is sold untreated (Kurwijila, 2006). This indicates a greater need for education of milk producers and consumers, and promotion of simple disease prevention measures such as boiling milk or cooking meat. This would also bring wider health benefits through killing other potential pathogens such as *Listeria monocytogenes*, *Staphylococcus aureus*, *Klebsiella pneumoniae* and other enterobacteria, as well as *Brucella* and *Yersinia* species (Rea *et al.*, 1992; Gran *et al.*, 2003). There is a consensus that villagers in low to medium–high GNI communities are better able to absorb and act on information when it is provided by someone with standing in the local community (O'Toole and McConkey, 1998). Mobile phones and other information and communication technologies offer increasingly cheap and available avenues for delivering key disease control and health protection messages to rural populations (Masuki *et al.*, 2010). Uptake of these messages may be enhanced if they are linked to other widely used information, such weather forecasts.

In addition to providing grass-roots information to rural villages, there is also a need to ensure politicians, government officials, health workers and community leaders understand that drinking raw milk or eating poorly cooked or raw meat can cause a range of diseases, including TB. The risk of catching any of these diseases can be greatly reduced by boiling milk and ensuring that meat is well-cooked before consumption.

Pasteurization of milk

There may be opportunities for collectives of small-scale cattle or goat farmers to limit transmission of *M. bovis* to humans by treating milk in small pasteurizers powered by wood or gas stoves (Kurwijila, 2006) or solar power (Wayua *et al.*, 2013). Pasteurization of raw milk before it is sold or made into products such as soured milk or cheese would reduce health risks to a broader cross-section of the community at low cost, and may increase the value of milk or milk produce sold by participating farmers or collectives.

Calves can become infected from drinking raw milk containing *M. bovis* (Doran *et al.*, 2009). Pasteurizing both colostrum and milk prior to feeding to calves and kids mitigates the risk of these animals becoming infected with *M. bovis* early in life. Some Chilean cattle owners used this sanitation process to assist them to clear TB infection from their herds (C. Cabrera, personal communication). Having young cattle that are TB free is a pre-requisite to a successful TB vaccination programme.

Slaughterhouse TB surveillance

Slaughterhouse inspection of carcasses has identified TB-infected livestock carcasses in a number of low to medium–high GNI African countries, including Nigeria (Cadmus *et al.*, 2009) and Cameroon (Ndukum *et al.*, 2010). However, routine slaughterhouse inspection correctly detected only 32% of infected cattle within a sample of 3322 cattle slaughtered at five abattoirs in Ethiopia (Biffa *et al.*, 2010). While possibly unreliable as a disease detection tool, finding TB at slaughterhouses may lead to reduced payment to the supplier of the animal. This in turn can provide a suitable opportunity for targeted communication to affected cattle-herders encouraging them to adopt improved disease control practices.

Vaccination of cattle

Vaccination of neonate calves with live *M. bovis* bacillus Calmette–Guérin (BCG) vaccine provided 56–68% protection against subsequent exposure to natural *M. bovis* infection (Ameni *et al.*, 2010; Lopez-Valencia *et al.*, 2010). Further to this Ameni *et al.* (2010) identified that more of the vaccinated cattle would have passed the standard meat inspection process. Lopez-Valencia *et al.* (2010) found that fewer vaccinated calves had positive PCR nasal swabs and suggested that they may pose a lower TB transmission risk. Buddle *et al.* (2005) identified that calves orally vaccinated with a lipid formulated BCG had a significant level of protection against TB compared with unvaccinated calves. Nugent *et al.* (2017) identified an efficacy of 64% for oral BCG vaccinated calves that were up to 9 months old and exposed to natural, mostly wildlife, TB infection.

Even if BCG vaccination effectively protects no more than about half of vaccinated cattle, this would still provide a significant advantage in reducing cattle TB incidence in low to medium–high GNI economies able to facilitate vaccination programmes. While vaccination with BCG sensitizes cattle to the tuberculin test, this would be immaterial for its use in these countries, as they are unlikely to be TB testing cattle on any large scale. Vaccinating female calves will reduce their later risk of passing *M. bovis* in milk, thereby potentially reducing the number of humans exposed to infection. Where resources are limited, vaccinating female calves alone may thus be a well-targeted strategy to reduce human health risks.

In order to maximize the efficacy of BCG vaccination, calves need to be TB free to start with. This means that before and for a period after calves are vaccinated, they should not have access to colostrum or milk that may contain *M. bovis*. At a practical level, this may be difficult to achieve unless colostrum and raw milk can be pasteurized before being fed to calves intended for vaccination, or ensuring that calves are not raised on TB test-positive cows.

TB testing

Exposure to *M. bovis* can be diagnosed in livestock by a range of *in vivo* (intradermal tuberculin) and *in vitro* (whole blood and serological) tests as outlined in Chapter 12. Serological tests work best if the animal's immune system has been stimulated with tuberculin some 10 to 14 days earlier. Milk can also be tested for TB using a serological test that provides similar result to that for sera, provided few animals are involved (Buddle *et al.*, 2013). Testing is better at diagnosing infection at a herd than animal level. Most test evaluations have been carried out in cattle, so the available data on diagnostic utility may not be equally applicable to other species such as goats, deer and camelids.

As identified in the Chapters 12 and 13 on diagnostic tests, evaluation is based on measures of sensitivity and specificity. Unfortunately, no diagnostic test has a sensitivity and specificity of 100%. Test measurement can be adjusted to increase either sensitivity or specificity, but an increase in one parameter will generally result in a decrease in the other. For disease control purposes, when TB prevalence is high, it is preferable to maximize test sensitivity. However, the consequent lower test specificity will lead to more non-infected animals giving false-positive test results. Livestock owners may have difficulty seeing the value in this, especially when cattle are their main asset and there is a reduction in value or a requirement to slaughter test-positive animals.

The other factor that needs to be considered is test cost. The intradermal tuberculin skin test is currently cheapest, but requires skill to apply, and animals need to be presented twice: first to inject the tuberculin, and then 3 days later to read the test by examining the injection site. This may not suit all grazing arrangements. Whole blood and serological testing only need animals to be presented once, for a blood sample. Testing milk samples may be simpler, but not all animals may be lactating. However, blood, sera and milk samples currently need to be sent to a laboratory with sophisticated equipment and trained staff to undertake the testing. Whole blood testing requires blood samples to be submitted to the laboratory within 24 hours. These factors need practical and logistic consideration before deciding upon which test to use for a particular situation.

Before introducing a testing programme, the proposed test and its implications need to be explained to livestock owners and agreement reached on how test-positive animals – and herds as a whole – need to be managed. Management options or requirements under a testing programme will depend on its ultimate purpose, but can include one or some combination of: (i) removal of all test-positive animals from the herd; (ii) separating test-negative animals from test-positive animals and managing each group separately; and/or (iii) managing the herd as one group, but vaccinating young stock with BCG. Ideally, the young stock would be TB free prior to being vaccinated.

Any testing programme also needs to be carried out in the context of appropriate wider herd and farm management to close off any infection pathways from livestock trading, movement or contacts with unmanaged sources of livestock infection. Cattle owners thus need to understand and accept the purpose of the programme and full range of its implications.

15.5 The Bigger Picture: Reducing Zoonotic Tuberculosis in Humans

For the WHO End TB Strategy targets to be achieved, then in at least some low to medium–high GNI countries, the transmission of either *M. bovis* or *M. tuberculosis* from infected livestock to humans will need to be prevented. This supports the views for a One Health system involvement as outlined by Olea-Popelka *et al.* (2016). This will require a coordinated process, to be funded by a combination of WHO, United Nations and other international aid organizations, supported by resources and where possible funding from individual programme countries. It should be based upon the One Health concept and involve the correct combination of knowledgeable people to ensure the goal of TB reduction is achieved. A suggested process is outlined as follows:

1. Identify for each low to medium–high GNI economy country the number of new human cases of TB and number of human deaths due to TB in 2016.
2. Undertake a modelling exercise based on previous TB annual rates and any proposed treatments for each country to forecast the expected annual number of new TB human cases and TB deaths through to 2035.
3. Calculate the difference between the sum of new cases and TB deaths forecast by modelling for 2025 and 2035, and the number determined by WHO 2025 and 2035 targets.
4. If the modelled new cases and deaths forecast for 2025 and 2035 exceed the number determined by WHO targets, then based on individual country new cases and death rates, identify which countries to prioritize for additional action to ensure targets are met.
5. Identify for the selected countries, the epidemiological characteristics of new TB cases and TB deaths.
6. For countries where rural or peri-urban location is identified as an important factor in new human cases or TB deaths, then:

    a. Determine at a species level, the mycobacteria responsible for the infection, based on an epidemiologically structured cross-section of new cases and deaths.

    b. Where greater than (a suggested) 10% of the sample cultured indicates infection due to *M. bovis*, then undertake the following programme:

        i. *Communication*

            1. Discuss with politicians, government agencies and village leaders and determine how best to inform villagers and livestock owners about the risks associated with consumption of TB-infected foodstuffs (raw milk and raw milk products, blood and undercooked meat).

            2. Undertake a communication programme using multimedia and local leaders to ensure that all rural and peri-urban inhabitants are continuously aware of the dangers of consuming TB-infected foodstuffs. Recommend all milk to be boiled or pasteurized prior to consumption and meat to be cooked through.

            3. Provide small pasteurizers to villages where there are relatively large numbers of livestock being milked and milk sold widely for human consumption. Provide guidance on the use of pasteurizers; ensure they are being used correctly and that all milk coming from the pasteurizer is bacteriologically safe and protein quality is unaffected.

ii. *Livestock TB surveillance*
1. Undertake surveys to identify at a herd and animal level the TB prevalence for each livestock species used for milk or meat.
2. Isolate the species of mycobacteria from a cross-section of samples cultured.
3. Ideally, the samples selected should be based on a test-and-slaughter programme where a geographically representative cross-section of stock ownership and types of livestock are tested. All test-positive animals should be slaughtered. Samples from all TB-like lesions found in carcasses at slaughter to be submitted for mycobacterial culture and mycobacteria isolates typed to species level. If a test-and-slaughter programme is not feasible, then the survey could be based on animals sent to an abattoir. However, unless the quality of inspection was high, this may provide a biased result.
4. Surveillance would provide, for each selected country, an indication of the countrywide TB prevalence for each livestock species sampled and it would determine the relative proportions of *M. bovis* and *M. tuberculosis* cases. It may also identify whether a particular livestock species or region of the country poses a greater threat of infection to humans. The surveillance results should assist in identifying a course of action that has the greatest probability of reducing transmission of *M. bovis* to humans and in-contact animals. This would include better targeting of communication and possibly introduction of other TB control methods.

iii. *Vaccination of livestock*
1. Given a particular livestock species or spatial distribution of infection in livestock is identified, targeted vaccination of young livestock could provide a way of reducing future infection in that species or area.

iv. *Test-and-slaughter of reactors*
1. If TB infection is identified to be particularly high at a herd or flock level as well as within herds or flocks, and there is a need to rapidly reduce the risk of livestock related human infection that cannot be achieved by pasteurization, then test-and-slaughter of the high-risk livestock species should be undertaken. This requires a TB programme to be developed and agreed to by representatives of livestock owners, government officials and knowledgeable veterinarians.
2. Implementation of such a programme is likely to require an ability to replace slaughtered test-positive livestock with equivalent TB-free animals at no cost to the owners.

References

Abernethy, D.A., Denny, G.O., Menzies, F.D., McGuckian, P., Honhold, N. and Roberts, A.R. (2006) The Northern Ireland programme for the control and eradication of *Mycobacterium bovis. Journal of Veterinary Microbiology* 112, 231–237.

Ameni, G., Vordermeier, M., Aseffa, A., Young, D.B. and Hewinson, R.G. (2010) Field evaluation of the efficacy of *Mycobacterium bovis* Bacillus Calmette–Guérin against bovine tuberculosis in neonatal calves in Ethiopia. *Clinical and Vaccine Immunology* 17(10), 1533–1538.

Anonymous (2016) Free Rider Problem. Available at: https://en.wikipedia.org/wiki/Free_rider_problem (accessed 17 December 2016).

Bengis, R.G., Kock, R.A. and Fischer, J. (2002) Infectious animal diseases: the wildlife/livestock interface. *Scientific and Technical Review of the Office International des Epizooties* 21(1), 53–65.

Biffa, D., Bogale, A. and Skjerve, E. (2010) Diagnostic Efficiency of Abattoir Meat Inspection Service in Ethiopia to Detect Carcasses Infected with *Mycobacterium bovis*: Implications for Public Health. *BMC Public Health* 10, 462.

Blanchard, K.H., Zigarmi, D. and Zigarmi, P. (1985) *Leadership and the One Minute Manger.* William Morrow & Company, New York, USA, p. 89.

Boadella, M., Vicente, J., Ruiz-Fons, F., de la Fuente, J. and Gortázar, C. (2012) Effects of culling Eurasian wild boar on the prevalence of *Mycobacterium bovis* and aujeszky's disease virus. *Preventive Veterinary Medicine* 107, 214–221.

Buddle, B.M., Aldwell, F.E., Skinner, M.A., de Lisle, G.W., Denis, M., et al. (2005) Effect of oral vaccination of cattle with lipid-formulated BCG on immune responses and protection against bovine tuberculosis. *Vaccine* 23, 3581–3589.

Buddle, B.M., Wedlock, D.N., Denis, M., Vordermeier, H.M. and Hewinson, R.G. (2011) Update on vaccination of cattle and wildlife populations against tuberculosis. *Journal of Veterinary Microbiology* 151, 14–22.

Buddle, B.M., Wilson, T., Luo, D., Voges, H., Linscott, R., et al. (2013) Evaluation of a commercial enzyme-linked immunosorbent assay for the diagnosis of bovine tuberculosis from milk samples from dairy cows. *Clinical and Vaccine Immunology* 20(12), 1812–1816.

Byrom, A.E., Caley, P., Paterson, B.M. and Nugent, G. (2015) Feral ferrets (*Mustela furo*) as hosts and sentinels of tuberculosis in New Zealand. *New Zealand Veterinary Journal* 63(S1), 42–53.

Cadmus, S.I., Adesokan, H.K., Jenkins, A.O. and van Soolingen, D. (2009) *Mycobacterium bovis* and *M. tuberculosis* in goats, Nigeria. *Emerging Infectious Diseases* 15(12), 2066–2071.

Cassidy, A. (2012) Vermin, victims and disease: UK framings of badgers in and beyond the bovine TB controversy. *Journal of the European Society for Rural Sociology* 52(2), 192–214.

Chen, Y., Chao, Y., Deng, Q., Liu, T., Xiang, J., et al. (2009) Potential challenges to the stop TB plan for humans in China: cattle maintain *M. bovis* and *M. tuberculosis*. *Tuberculosis* 89(1), 95–100.

Clout, M. and Ericksen, K. (2000) Anatomy of a disastrous success: the brushtail possum as an invasive species. In: Montague, T.L. (ed.) *The Brushtail Possum: Biology, Impact and Management of an Introduced Marsupial.* Manaaki Whenua Press, Lincoln, New Zealand, pp. 1–9.

Cook, A.J.C., Tuchilli, L.M., Buve, A., Foster, S.D., Godfrey-Faussett, P., et al. (1996) Human and bovine tuberculosis in the monze district of Zambia – a cross-sectional study. *British Veterinary Journal* 152, 37–46.

Cosivi, O., Grange, J.M., Daborn, C.J., Ravigliione, M.C., Fujikura, T., et al. (1998) Zoonotic tuberculosis due to *Mycobacterium bovis* in developing countries. *Emerging Infectious Diseases* 4(1), 59–70.

Cousins, D.V. and Roberts, J.L. (2001) Australia's campaign to eradicate bovine tuberculosis: the battle for freedom and beyond. *Tuberculosis* 81 (1–2), 5–15.

Department of Agriculture, Environment and Rural Affairs (2016) Bovine Tuberculosis Eradication Strategy for Northern Ireland: An Integrated Eradication Programme. Available at: https://www.daera-ni.gov.uk/sites/default/files/publications/daera/bovine-tuberculosis-eradication-strategy.pdf (accessed 20 December 2016).

Deresa, B., Conraths, F.J. and Ameni, G. (2013) Abattoir-based study on the epidemiology of caprine tuberculosis in Ethiopia using conventional and molecular tools. *Acta Veterinaria Scandinavica* 2013(55), 15.

Doran, P., Carson, J., Costello, E. and More, S.J. (2009) An outbreak of tuberculosis affecting cattle and people on an Irish dairy farm, following the consumption of raw milk. *Irish Veterinary Journal* 62(6), 390–397.

Efford, M. (2000) Possum density, population structure and dynamics. In: Montague, T.L. (ed.) *The Brushtail Possum: Biology, Impact and Management of an Introduced Marsupial.* Manaaki Whenua Press, Lincoln, New Zealand, pp. 47–61.

Enticott, G. (2014) Biosecurity and the bioeconomy. The case of disease regulation in UK and New Zealand. In: Morley, A. and Marsden, T. (eds) *Researching Sustainable Food: Building the New Sustainability Paradigm.* Earthscan, London, pp. 122–142.

Freeman, R.E., Harrison, J.S., Wicks, A.C., Parmar, B.L. and de Colle, S. (2010) *Stakeholder Theory: The State of the Art.* Cambridge University Press, Cambridge, UK, p. 26.

Garrido, J.M., Sevilla, I.A., Beltrán-Beck, B., Minguijón, E., Ballesteros, C., *et al.* (2011) Protection against tuberculosis in Eurasian wild boar vaccinated with heat-inactivated *Mycobacterium bovis*. *PLOS One* 6(9), e24905.

Good, M. and Duignan, A. (2011) Perspectives on the history of bovine TB and the role of tuberculin in bovine TB eradication. *Veterinary Medicine International* 2011, 410470.

Gran, H.M., Wetlesen, A., Mutukumira, A.N., Rukure, G. and Narvhus, J.A. (2003) Occurrence of pathogenic bacteria in raw milk, cultured pasteurised milk and naturally soured milk produced at small-scale diaries in Zimbabwe. *Food Control* 14(8), 539–544.

Kurwijila, L.R. (2006) *Hygienic Milk Handling, Processing and Marketing: Reference Guide for Training and Certification of Small-scale Milk Traders in East Africa*. Sokoine University of Agriculture, Morogoro, Tanzania, p. 102.

Kusiluka, L.J.M. and Sudi, F.F. (2003) Review of successes and failures of contagious bovine pleuropneumonia control strategies in Tanzania. *Preventive Veterinary Medicine* 59(3), 113–123.

Livingstone, P.G., Hancox, N., Nugent, G. and de Lisle, G.W. (2015a) Toward eradication: the effect of *Mycobacterium bovis* infection in wildlife on the evolution and future direction of bovine tuberculosis management in New Zealand. *New Zealand Veterinary Journal* 63(1), 4–18.

Livingstone, P.G., Hancox, N., Nugent, G., Mackereth, G. and Hutchings, S.A. (2015b) Development of the New Zealand strategy for local eradication of tuberculosis from wildlife and livestock. *New Zealand Veterinary Journal* 63(1), 98–107.

Lopez-Valencia, G., Renteria-Evangelista, T., de Jesús Williams, J., Licea-Navarro, A., De la Mora-Valle, A. and Medina-Basulto, G. (2010) Field evaluation of the protective efficacy of *Mycobacterium bovis* BCG vaccine against bovine tuberculosis. *Research in Veterinary Science* 88(1), 44–49.

Macdonald, D.W. and Newman, C. (2002) Population dynamics of badgers (*Meles meles*) in Oxfordshire, UK: number, density and cohort life histories, a possible role of climate change in population growth. *Journal of Zoology* 256(1), 121–138.

Masuki, K.F.G., Kamugisha, R., Mowo, J.G., Tanui, J., Tukahirwa, J., Mogoi, J. and Adera, E.O. (2010) Role of Mobile Phones in Improving Communication and Information Delivery for Agricultural Development: Lessons from South Western Uganda. Paper presented at ICT and Development – Research Voices, 22–23 March 2010. Available at: https://www.mak.ac.ug/documents/IFIP/RoleofMobilePhonesAgriculture.pdf (accessed 14 December 2016).

Max, V., Paredes, L., Rivera, A. and Ternicier, C. (2011) National control and eradication programme of bovine tuberculosis in Chile. *Journal of Veterinary Microbiology* 151, 188–191.

Mfinanga, S.G., Mørkve, O., Kazwala, R.R., Cleaveland, S., Sharp, J.M., Shirima, G. and Nilsen, R. (2003) Tribal differences in perception of tuberculosis: a possible role in tuberculosis control in Arusha, Tanzania. *International Journal of Tuberculosis and Lung Disease* 7(10), 933–941.

Miller, M., Barrett, S. and Henderson, D.A. (2006) Control and eradication. In: Jamison, D.T., Breman, J.G., Measham, A.R., Alleyne, G., Claeson, M., *et al.* (eds) *Disease Control Priorities in Developing Countries*. Copublication of The World Bank and Oxford University Press, New York, USA, p. 1163.

Moda, G. (2006) No-technical constraints to eradication: the Italian experience. *Journal of Veterinary Microbiology* 112(2–4), 253–258.

More, S.J. and Good, M. (2006) The tuberculosis eradication programme in Ireland: a review of scientific and policy advances since 1988. *Journal of Veterinary Microbiology* 112, 239–251.

Morris, R.S. and Pfeiffer, D.U. (1995) Directions and issues in bovine tuberculosis epidemiology and control in New Zealand. *New Zealand Veterinary Journal* 43, 256–265.

Naranjo, V., Gortázar, C., Vicente, J. and de la Fuente, J. (2008) Evidence of the role of European wild boar as a reservoir of *Mycobacterium tuberculosis* complex. *Journal of Veterinary Microbiology* 127(1–2), 1–9.

Ndukum, J.A., Kudi, A.C., Bradley, G., Ane-Anyangwe, I.N., Fon-Tebug, S. and Tchoumboue, J. (2010) Prevalence of bovine tuberculosis in abattoirs of the littoral and western highland regions of Cameroon: a cause for public concern. *Veterinary Medicine International* 2010, 495015.

New Zealand Government (2016) *Biosecurity Act 1993, version as at 18 October 2016*. Government Printer, New Zealand, Sections 61–65. Available at: http://www.legislation.govt.nz/act/public/1993/0095/latest/versions.aspx (accessed 6 December 2016).

Nugent, G., Buddle, B.M. and Knowles, G. (2015a) Epidemiology and control of *Mycobacterium bovis* infection in brushtail possums (*Trichosurus vulpecula*), the primary wildlife host of bovine tuberculosis in New Zealand. *New Zealand Veterinary Journal* 63(1), 28–41.

Nugent, G., Gortázar, C. and Knowles, G. (2015b) The epidemiology of *Mycobacterium bovis* in wild deer and feral pigs and their role in the establishment and spread of bovine tuberculosis in New Zealand wildlife. *New Zealand Veterinary Journal* 63(S1), 54–67.

Nugent, G., Yockney, I.J., Whitford, E.J., Aldwell, F.E. and Buddle, B.M. (2017) Efficacy of oral BCG vaccination in protecting free-ranging cattle from natural infection by *Mycobacterium bovis*. *Journal of Veterinary Microbiology* 208, 181–189.

O'Brien, D.J., Schmitt, S.M., Fitzgerald, S.D., Berry, D.E. and Hickling, G.J. (2006) Managing the wildlife reservoir of *Mycobacterium bovis*: the Michigan, USA, experience. *Journal of Veterinary Microbiology* 112, 313–323.

O'Brien, D.J., Schmitt, S.M., Rudolph, B.A. and Nugent, G. (2011) Recent advances in the management of bovine tuberculosis in free-ranging wildlife. *Journal of Veterinary Microbiology* 151, 23–33.

OIE (2016a) WAHIS Interface of the World Animal Health Information. Available at: http://www.oie.int/wahis_2/public/wahid.php/Countryinformation/Animalsituation (accessed 18 August 2016).

OIE (2016b) Terrestrial Animal Health Code, Chapter 11.5: Bovine Tuberculosis. World Organisation for Animal Health. Available at: http://www.oie.int/index.php?id=169&L=0&htmfile=chapitre_bovine_tuberculosis.htm (accessed 22 July 2016).

OIE (2016c) One Health at a Glance. Available at: http://www.oie.int/en/for-the-media/onehealth/ (accessed 20 December 2016).

Olea-Popelka, F., Muwonge, A., Perera, A., Dean, A.S., Mumford, E., *et al.* (2016) Zoonotic tuberculosis in human beings caused by *Mycobacterium bovis* – a call for action. *Lancet Infectious Diseases* 17(1), e21-e25.

Osterholm, M.T. and Hedberg, C.W. (2015) Epidemiologic principles. In: Bennett, J.E., Dolin, R. and Blaser, M.J. (eds) *Mandell, Douglas and Bennett's Principles and Practice of Infectious Diseases*, 8th edn, vol. 1. Elsevier, Philadelphia, USA, pp. 155–156.

O'Toole, B. and McConkey, R. (1998) A training strategy for personnel working in developing countries. *International Journal of Rehabilitation Research* 21, 311–321.

Palmer, M.V. (2013) *Mycobacterium bovis*: characteristics of wildlife reservoir hosts. *Transboundary and Emerging Diseases* 60(S1), 1–13.

Palmer, M.V. and Waters, W.R. (2011) Bovine tuberculosis and establishment of an eradication program in the United States: role of veterinarians. *Veterinary Medicine International* 2011, 816345.

Perry, B. and Grace, D. (2009) The impacts of livestock diseases and their control on growth and development processes that are pro-poor. *Philosophical Transactions of the Royal Society B* 364, 2643–2655.

Perry, B.D., Randolph, T.F., McDermott, J.J., Sones, K.R. and Thornton, P.K. (2002) *Investing in Animal Health Research to Alleviate Poverty*. International Livestock Research Institute, Nairobi, Kenya.

Randolph, T.F., Schelling, E., Grace, D., Nicholson, C.F., Leroy, J.L., *et al.* (2007) Role of livestock in human nutrition and health for poverty reduction in developing countries. *Journal of Animal Science* 85, 2788–2800.

Rea, M.C., Cogan, T.M. and Tobin, S. (1992) Incidence of pathogenic bacteria in raw milk in Ireland. *Journal of Applied Microbiology* 73(4), 331–336.

Reviriego Gordejo, F.J. and Vermeersch, J.P. (2006) Towards eradication of bovine tuberculosis in the European Union. *Journal of Veterinary Microbiology* 112(2–4), 101–109.

Rockhill, B., Newman, B. and Weinberg, C. (1998) Commentary: use and misuse of population attributable fractions. *American Journal of Public Health* 88, 15–19.

Schwabe, C.W., Reimann, H.P. and Franti, C.E. (1977) *Epidemiology in Veterinary Practice*. Lea & Febiger, Philadelphia, USA, pp. 34–35.

Scott, C., Cavanaugh, J.S., Pratt, R., Silk, B.J., LoBue, P. and Moonan, P.K. (2016) Human tuberculosis caused by *Mycobacterium bovis* in the United States, 2006–2013. *Journal of Clinical Infectious Diseases* 63(5), 594–601.

Sheridan, M. (2011) Progress in tuberculosis eradication in Ireland. *Journal of Veterinary Microbiology* 151, 160–169.

Shitaye, J.E., Tsegaye, W. and Pavlik, I. (2007) Bovine tuberculosis infection in animal and human populations in Ethiopia: a review. *Veterinarni Medicina* 52(8), 317–332.

Smal, C. (1995) The badger and habitat survey of Ireland. *Report Prepared for the Department of Agriculture, Food & Forestry*. Government Publications, Dublin, pp. 1–5.

Tait, P., Saunders, C., Nugent, G. and Rutherford, P. (2017) Valuing conservation benefits of disease control in wildlife: A choice experiment approach to bovine tuberculosis management in New Zealand's native forests. *Journal of Environmental Management* 189, 142–149.

TBfree NZ (2007) *Economic Analysis of the 2009 NPMS Review Options*. TB free New Zealand, New Zealand, p. 20. Available at: http://www.tbfree.org.nz/Portals/0/2014AugResearchPapers/Economic%20 analysis%20of%20the%202009%20NPMS%20review.pdf (accessed 6 December 2016).

TBfree NZ (2009) Review of the National Bovine Tuberculosis Pest Management Strategy: Future Options for Sustained Control or Eradication of Bovine TB from New Zealand. TBfree New Zealand, New Zealand, pp. 8–10. Available at: http://www.tbfree.org.nz/Portals/0/2014AugResearchPapers/NPMS_ Review_DDOC%20%20March%2009.pdf (accessed 6 December 2016).

The World Bank (2016a) How Does the World Bank Classify Countries. Available at: https://datahelpdesk. worldbank.org/knowledgebase/articles/378834-how-does-the-world-bank-classify-countries (accessed 2 December 2016).

The World Bank (2016b) Working for a World Free of Poverty: Overview. The World Bank, 2 October 2016. Available at: http://worldbank.org/en/topic/poverty/overview (accessed 13 December 2016).

Thrushfield, M.V. (2007) *Veterinary Epidemiology*, 3rd edn. Butterworth-Heinemann Ltd, Oxford, UK, p. 223.

Tolhurst, B.A., Delahay, R.J., Walker, N.J., Ward, A.I. and Roper, T.J. (2009) Behaviour of badgers (*Meles meles*) in farm buildings: opportunities for the transmission of *Mycobacterium bovis* to cattle? *Journal of Applied Animal Behaviour Science* 117(1–2), 103–113.

Tweddle, N.E. and Livingstone, P. (1994) Bovine tuberculosis control and eradication programs in Australia and New Zealand. *Journal of Veterinary Microbiology* 40(1–2), 23–39.

Vicente, J., Höfle, U., Garrido, J.M., Fernández-de-mera, I.G., Acevedo, P., Juste, R., Barral, M. and Gortázar, C. (2007) Risk factors associated with the prevalence of tuberculosis-like lesions in fenced wild boar and red deer in south central Spain. *Journal of Veterinary Research* 38(3), 451–464.

Walter, W.D., Anderson, C.W., Smith, R., Vanderklok, M., Averill, J.J. and VerCauteren, K.C. (2012) On-farm mitigation of transmission of tuberculosis from white-tailed deer to cattle: Literature review and recommendations. *Veterinary Medicine International* 2012, 616318.

Warburton, B. and Livingstone, P. (2015) Managing and eradicating wildlife tuberculosis in New Zealand. *New Zealand Veterinary Journal* 63(1), 77–88.

Waters, W.R. and Palmer, M.V. (2015) *Mycobacterium bovis* infection of cattle and white-tailed deer: translation research of relevance to human tuberculosis. *ILAR Journals* 56(1), 26–43.

Wayua, F.O., Okoth, M.W. and Wangoh, J. (2013) Design and performance assessment of a flat-plate solar milk pasteuriser for arid pastoral areas of Kenya. *Journal of Food Processing and Preservation* 37(2), 120–125.

Wilson, G.J., Carter, S.P. and Delahay, R.J. (2011) Advances and prospects for management of TB transmission between badgers and cattle. *Journal of Veterinary Microbiology* 151, 43–50.

World Health Organization (2014) The End TB Strategy: Global Strategy and Targets for Tuberculosis Prevention, Care and Control after 2015. World Health Organization, Geneva, p. 30. Available at: http:// www.who.int/tb/strategy/End_TB_Strategy.pdf?ua=1 (accessed 16 December 2016).

World Health Organization (2016) World TB Report 2016. Available at: http://www.who.int/tb/global-tb-report-infographic.pdf?ua=1 (accessed 17 December 2016).

Worldometers (2016b) Countries of the World by Population (2016). Available at: http://www.worldometers. info/world-population/population-by-country/ (accessed 8 December 2016).

Zinsstag, J., Schelling, E., Roth, M.A. and Kazwala, R. (2006) Economics of bovine tuberculosis. In: Thoen, C.O., Steele, J.H. and Gilsdorf, M.J. (eds) *Mycobacterium bovis Infection in Animals and Humans*, 2nd edn. Blackwell Publishing, USA, pp. 68–83.

16 Perspectives on Global Bovine Tuberculosis Control

Francisco Olea-Popelka,[1] Mark A. Chambers,[2,3] Stephen Gordon[4] and Paul Barrow[5],*

[1]*Department of Clinical Sciences, College of Veterinary Medicine and Biomedical Sciences, Colorado State University, Fort Collins, Colorado, USA;* [2]*Animal and Plant Health Agency – Weybridge, Addlestone, Surrey, UK;* [3]*School of Veterinary Medicine, Faculty of Health & Medical Sciences, University of Surrey, Guildford, UK;* [4]*UCD School of Veterinary Medicine, University College Dublin, Dublin, Republic of Ireland;* [5]*School of Veterinary Medicine and Science, University of Nottingham, Sutton Bonington, Loughborough, UK*

16.1 Introduction

In the preceding chapters the authors have distilled the current status of research on bovine tuberculosis (TB) and the challenges and opportunities that lie ahead on the path to disease control. In this final chapter, we present some of our own thoughts on the control of bovine TB, highlighting the relevant chapters where particular issues are dealt with in more depth. While great strides have clearly been made in our understanding of the fundamental pathogen biology of *Mycobacterium bovis* and its interaction with the bovine host, substantial challenges remain in diagnosis, vaccination, disease epidemiology, public health and ultimate eradication.

16.2 Epidemiology and One Health

As presented by Caceres *et al.* in Chapter 1, the OIE reported that over the past 30 years there was a consistent improvement in the global situation regarding bovine TB with the percentage of affected countries decreasing by about 30% during this period. However, in order to address current and future challenges posed by bovine TB, different countries and regions will need to adhere to high standards to improve the prevention, diagnosis, and control of the disease in cattle herds, using approaches and tools that are appropriate and effective under the field conditions in each country/region. It is also recognized that the prevention and control of *M. bovis* infection and TB in cattle by the veterinary sector (and other animal species, as described by Michel in Chapter 4) is crucial to prevent the spread of *M. bovis* to humans (zoonotic TB). In Chapter 2 Olea-Popelka *et al.* pointed out that the impact of zoonotic TB on the global burden of TB is unknown, poorly understood and most likely underestimated. This is due to the lack of systematic surveillance for *M. bovis* as a causal agent of human TB in low-income, high TB burden countries where bovine TB is also endemic, and because the tests most commonly used to diagnose human TB in many parts of the world, such as sputum smear microscopy or GeneXpert do not differentiate *M. bovis* from *Mycobacterium*

---

* Email: paul.barrow@nottingham.ac.uk

tuberculosis. However, current available estimates indicate that the global incidence of human TB caused by *M. bovis* in 2015 was approximately 149,000 new cases and 13,400 deaths. Thus, to achieve the ambitious goals of the WHO End TB strategy (http://www.who.int/tb/post2015_strategy/en/) and the STOP TB Partnership Global Plan for TB (http://www.stoptb.org/global/plan/) in which every single case of TB counts whether it is human or zoonotic TB, a comprehensive and multisectorial 'One Health' approach, including the veterinary and human health sectors, will be needed to better prevent, diagnose, and treat zoonotic TB in humans.

In this regard, the OIE (Chapter 1) is promoting a collaborative 'One Health' approach at international and national levels for the control of zoonotic diseases, including bovine TB. Specifically, Olea-Popelka *et al.* in Chapter 2 proposed three critical action points required to address the challenges posed by zoonotic TB. These are (i) governments must first acknowledge *M. bovis* in official national policies as a source of human TB and warranting attention; (ii) knowledge, attitudes and practices of both healthcare providers and communities at risk must be improved in order to identify gaps and develop appropriate interventions; and (iii) existing laboratory methods that differentiate *M. bovis* from *M. tuberculosis* should be more widely implemented.

With regard to a 'One Health' approach to control bovine TB, Azami and Zinsstag suggested, in Chapter 3, implementing and promoting dialogue between different stakeholders as well as creating a greater environment of trust between the different sectors (farmers, decision makers, scientists, the veterinary and human health sectors). Also, it is vital to inform farmers and decision makers about the economic losses (impact) caused by bovine TB and about the different approaches required to control this disease and minimize economic losses.

The importance and necessity of modelling the epidemiology of *M. bovis* in cattle is highlighted by Conlan and Wood in Chapter 4, who also show the gaps in our knowledge that contribute to the weaknesses of predictive modelling. The effects of herd size and age and the value of abattoir surveillance are well known. Although the current limitations reflect the huge variation in parameters required for incorporation into models, recently developed models provide guidance relating to inter-herd transmission and how much intervention might be required where sympatric host species might be involved in infection. Although these models have been developed for countries such as the UK, the inclusion of data pertaining to genetic resistance and additional information arising from a greater understanding of the host response (see Chapters 10 and 11) may increase value for countries where the pattern of transmission is very different.

As discussed by Skuce and colleagues in Chapter 5, the decreasing cost, increasing speed of turn-around and exquisite resolution offered by bacterial whole-genome sequencing (WGS) 'looks set to revolutionize the way we do veterinary bacteriology, much as it is doing for human medical microbiology'. A number of studies have highlighted the utility of WGS to resolve *M. bovis* transmission chains between wildlife and cattle populations and provide greater understanding of the epidemiology of infection. WGS data also provides a window into evolutionary analysis and dating of the most recent common ancestor (MRCA) of *M. bovis* populations. An example of such evolutionary analysis is that of Crispell *et al.* (2007) who used WGS to date the MRCA of *M. bovis* isolates sampled from New Zealand to approximately 1859, agreeing well with previous estimates that *M. bovis* has been circulating in New Zealand since the mid-19th century. WGS analysis of global *M. bovis* populations will also allow increased insights into the evolution of *M. bovis*, and to our mind there is no doubt that WGS will become the standard method of *M. bovis* molecular typing in the coming years.

Michel, in Chapter 6, summarized the current knowledge and challenges presented by *M. bovis* infection and as a cause of clinical disease in other domestic species such as sheep, goats, pigs, water buffalo, farmed deer and camel. There is a general paucity of information on the true prevalence and distribution of *M. bovis* infection in domestic species other than cattle, especially where they are farmed extensively or live under semi-free roaming conditions. Water buffalo and small ruminants have maintenance host potential and, given the high risk for economic losses and zoonotic *M. bovis* transmission, there is a need to integrate those species in national bovine TB control programmes. With regard to the potential zoonotic transmission from these domestic species, the risk profile should, in principle, be based primarily on utilization of milk and meat and, to a smaller extent, on close contact, indicating that these species should clearly be considered in future strategies to prevent and control zoonotic TB when local conditions and socio-cultural practices favour the transmission of *M. bovis* from these domestic species to humans.

16.3 Diagnosis and Immunology

Current approaches to diagnosing TB in the live animal rely on an immunological readout. This introduces the possibility that animals that have been exposed to the infection but have subsequently cleared it successfully will be killed unnecessarily. Indeed, we may unwittingly be removing animals with a degree of immunological resistance to infection. This could be avoided if there was a suitably accurate and cost-effective means of detecting bacilli within bodily excretions. This would also focus control on those animals at risk of infecting others. However, as pointed out by Waters in Chapter 12, agent-based strategies for the detection of tuberculous cattle are currently unreliable for use as antemortem tests, possibly due to the paucibacillary nature of the disease resulting in a transient and low level of bacterial shedding.

Although the existing immunological means of diagnosis, including the intradermal tuberculin test, remain the cornerstone of diagnosis and control for bovine TB, there is still a requirement for novel and improved antemortem tests and testing algorithms to be developed and implemented. These might be based on immunological and/or molecular markers identified in circulating T cells and/or monocytes in infected animals differentiating them from uninfected or even vaccinated animals. As discussed by Wanzala and Sreevatsan in Chapter 13, while the pipeline for new bovine TB diagnostics has shown some interesting new developments, 'improvements in standardization and validation procedures to increase reproducibility and accuracy and promote adoption of these biomarkers' is required. Emerging technologies developed for improved diagnosis of human *M. tuberculosis* infection, such as the GeneXpert (Stevens *et al.*, 2017), circulating nucleic acid (Miotto *et al.*, 2013) or breath analysis (McNerney *et al.*, 2010) will likely prove useful in time for the discovery and application of biomarkers of diagnostic relevance for bovine TB.

Underpinning the development of new or improved means of immunodiagnosis is an increased understanding of the immune response to vaccination and infection. The host immune response on exposure to mycobacteria is complex, as emphasized by Salguero in Chapter 9 and Hope and Werling in Chapter 11, and more work is needed to tease apart the nature of protective immunity from immune responses that are detrimental to the host together with information on the major bacterial antigens or combinations of antigens that stimulate these responses. It is likely that these differences are quantitative as well as qualitative, including a strong temporal component. While much has been learnt about the immune response of cattle to infection, supported by an increasing array of specific reagents with which to study it, the same cannot be said for other species.

The immune response of the host during mixed infection is also likely to become a major topic for further investigation, and this has implications not only for immunological diagnosis, but also for vaccination. We have seen in Chapters 11 and 12 that co-infection with *Fasciola hepatica* can confuse the response to *M. bovis*. *M. avium* subsp. *paratuberculosis* (MAP) is another pathogen causing a chronic infection in which an initial Th1 response can modulate to a Th2 response. This could also profoundly affect the response to *M. bovis*. The high prevalence of MAP in some countries suggests that this could be a real problem that will require addressing.

Tuberculins, including purified protein derivatives (PPDs), are a poorly defined and complex mix of proteins, lipids and carbohydrates of inherently poor specificity as many of the compounds within PPDs are antigenically cross-reactive amongst the various mycobacterial species. Efforts to replace tuberculin with defined proteins or peptides for immunodiagnosis are generating promising results, as reviewed by Waters in Chapter 12. It is hoped that advances in computational methods to predict which peptides bind to bovine histocompatibility antigen molecules will provide an unbiased, *in silico* means to define the *M. bovis* T-cell antigenome in cattle. Recent advances in this regard include the report by Farrell *et al.* (2016) who used three MHC-II-binding prediction methods to screen the *M. bovis* proteome for potential binders to the bovine BoLA-DRB3. Using this method, they demonstrated significant enrichment (>24%) for promiscuously recognized epitopes. Even so, it will remain a challenge to predict which antigens are specific for *M. bovis*. The absence of a particular protein within a genome does not guarantee that the short antigenic region it may contain is not shared with other intact antigens encoded elsewhere in the genome. *In silico* approaches need to be validated using the target species, in their natural setting.

Whole blood assays for the immunological detection of TB currently require live and fully functional leukocytes to be delivered to the laboratory for testing. This is a challenge, especially in large or resource-poor countries with diverse environmental conditions and under-developed transport networks. In these settings, improved methods to assure sample viability, or the development of improved assays not requiring live cells and with new fixation methods, are critical for the use of such tests. An 'in tube' approach for immediate antigen stimulation may overcome these challenges once the logistical and technical hurdles have been addressed for cattle blood, in the way they have been for human samples. Even better would be the development of accurate point of care assays for use in the field which might, for example, reflect cellular changes taking place early in infection (see Chapter 10).

Antibody-based assays are appealing due to ease and convenience of sample collection, storage and analysis. However, they generally have insufficient sensitivity for most applications. This has prevented widespread development and use of these assays for the diagnosis of TB in cattle. Currently, the best promise for developing an improved antibody-based test is the discovery of antigens that are recognized early after infection and preferably without the requirement for injection of PPD for skin test to achieve detectable levels. Proteome-wide antigen mining for sero-dominant antigens has yet to be undertaken in cattle but should yield additional relevant targets for sero-diagnosis that could increase the sensitivity of serology to detect tuberculous cattle.

A critical need for the next decade is to evaluate the emerging immunological approaches for diagnosis in practical platforms with a wide range of samples from naturally infected cattle for direct comparison to existing official tests (in particular, traditional TST and IGRAs). This crucial need for robust validation will require collaboration and investment from funding agencies, biologics companies, livestock stakeholders, policymakers and federal/regional veterinary field staff.

16.4 Vaccination

The multi-host nature (see Chapters 6 and 7) and environmental survival of pathogenic mycobacteria (see Chapter 4) generates complexity in a context where successful disease control strategies will need to integrate all available tools, including biosafety and prevention, population control where possible, and vaccination as a component intervention (see Chapter 15). While there has been progress in vaccine development, evaluation and licensing for TB control, there remain some considerable challenges (see Chapter 14). These relate to the immunogenicity and safety of the vaccine and to the practicalities of its delivery. Many of these challenges are overlapping.

16.4.1 Microbiological

Until recently, vaccine development has been largely empirical or involved introducing attenuations used with other classes of bacteria such as the Enterobacteriaceae. Identification of major immunogens is under way, but a greater in-depth analysis of the surface and other proteins, carbohydrates and complexes has not been undertaken with a view to modelling interaction with the MHC of cattle and other species, identifying those likely to initiate strong Th1 responses. While distinct genes have been suggested as *M. bovis* virulence factors (see Chapter 8), genome-wide approaches, such as those applied to reveal gene essentiality in *M. tuberculosis*

(DeJesus et al., 2017) will be required to expand the identification of *M. bovis* factors involved in host–pathogen interaction. A 2017 update to the annotation of the *M. bovis* AF2122/97 genome, the reference genome sequence for *M. bovis* (Malone et al., 2017), is welcomed; this annotation needs to be revised on a regular basis to ensure that functional information on antigens, virulence factors, biosynthetic pathways, etc. is collated into a single data source for the community.

16.4.2 Immunological

A significant impediment to the development of improved TB vaccines for animals is that no single correlate of protection has been identified for TB (as indicated in Chapters 11 and 14), although a number have shown promise in this regard. A confusing aspect is that many of these markers for protection also serve as indicators of disease post-challenge. This means that each vaccine type, dose and method of delivery must be tested empirically using a host challenge model before eventually being evaluated for efficacy in settings of natural infection acquisition. It is important that bacillus Calmette–Guérin is field-tested in different environments and husbandry systems as this may help explain any variations in vaccine efficacy. This makes vaccine research and development for animal TB both time-consuming and costly and places limitations on the statistical power to detect a protective effect, either due to constraints on the number of infected animals that can be held in biosecure laboratory facilities, or limitations posed by a comparatively low force of infection in the natural setting.

Another immunological consideration is the need to define the target dose of vaccine for each species and route of potential administration. In the case of an oral, bait-delivered vaccine for sylvatic species, the dose is impossible to control precisely and there is always the risk that non-target species may access the vaccine. At best, this results in vaccine wastage, at worst it could result in the induction of misdiagnosis of TB in livestock should they become exposed to sufficient quantities of the vaccine.

Finally, there is often little to no empirical data to inform the optimal size or duration of an animal vaccination programme, a fact exacerbated by the difficulty of defining the practical duration of immunity. This makes long-term commitment or buy-in from stakeholders difficult to secure.

16.4.3 Practical

Major challenges for the vaccination of wildlife, in particular, are the identification of the means for cost-effective and reproducible vaccine delivery coupled to the need for a single dose vaccine, as in many cases there will be no certainty of accessing the same animal to administer a second dose of the vaccine.

Oral bait TB vaccines have been shown to be effective in a number of wildlife species, but more research is needed to improve formulations with appropriate attractants, systems for optimizing bait distribution and avoiding bait uptake by non-target species.

16.4.4 Safety

Although the majority of vaccines under consideration for TB control in animals are likely to be safe, this cannot be assumed and needs to be demonstrated formally for at least the target species, in order for a licence to be granted from the national competent authority. Where there is the possibility of exposure of non-target species to the vaccine, e.g. for an oral, bait-delivered vaccine, it may prove necessary to evaluate the safety of the vaccine to each species that is at risk of exposure.

16.5 Challenges to Disease Control

In some countries, elimination of TB in livestock is unlikely to occur without some form of control targeted to wildlife vectors of the disease as highlighted by Fox and co-authors in Chapter 7. This raises the question as to who 'owns' or is ultimately responsible for wildlife? Is it the government, landowners or even the public? Where control options, such as culling, are constrained by national legislation, this is more than a philosophical question, and generates considerable obstacles to the development and implementation of national disease control policies.

As was noted in Chapters 6 and 7, the multi-host nature and environmental survival of pathogenic mycobacteria generates complexity in disease control. While there is much research on the infection in different species and even of multi-host epidemiology, the role played by an environmental component is sometimes ignored or over-simplified in its presentation. More research is justified on the ability of mycobacteria to survive outside of an animal host and the conditions that favour this. Greater understanding in this area will help epidemiological investigation, mathematic disease modelling, and ultimately which control options are developed and employed.

As noted by Livingstone in Chapter 15, the reality of managing *M. bovis*, wherever it is found, is that it requires adequate resources. These are either lacking or prioritized for other needs and wants for large sections of the world. To our knowledge there has been no systematic review of the international funding picture for *M. bovis*. This needs to differentiate between investment from international bodies such as the WHO and the proportion of gross national income (GNI) spent on TB control. Expenditure will need to be broken down into broad categories, such as surveillance, compensation or research. This is a prerequisite for understanding how impactful this expenditure is, or for conducting retrospective or prospective benefit–cost analyses. A major difficulty with TB benefit–cost analyses is obtaining or deriving a monetary value for the benefits. Gaining agreement as to who is responsible for funding a TB strategy is a major challenge for a sustained programme with a long time frame.

Infection of humans with *M. bovis* within countries of lower GNI is gaining greater recognition as a 'hidden zoonosis'. Beyond the ethical imperative to address this, further work is needed to understand the significance of the zoonosis as a driver of poverty itself. What is feasible in terms of TB control within low GNI countries will be very different to what is feasible within higher GNI countries, and must be developed as a collaboration between different disciplines and community representatives with a clear appreciation of what is socially acceptable and practical in each case. Effective communication and knowledge sharing is crucial to success. At the time of writing (August 2017) there were multi-institutional efforts from WHO, OIE, FAO and The Union to officially launch a 'Road Map' to address the global challenges posed by zoonotic tuberculosis.

16.6 Conclusion

In this book, leading researchers have provided an update on our knowledge of bovine TB and the many obstacles that remain to eradication of this disease as a threat to humans and animals. The goal of eradication can only be achieved through a holistic approach that integrates current thinking and translates it to novel modalities for disease control. This is a substantial challenge but inspired by the information contained herein, one that we strive to achieve.

References

Crispell, J., Zadoks, R.N., Harris, S.R., Paterson, B., Collins, D.M., *et al.* (2017) Using whole genome sequencing to investigate transmission in a multi-host system: bovine tuberculosis in New Zealand. *BMC Genomics* 18(1), 180.

DeJesus, M.A., Gerrick, E.R., Xu, W., Park, S.W., Long, J.E., *et al.* (2017) Comprehensive essentiality analysis of the *Mycobacterium tuberculosis* genome via saturating transposon mutagenesis. *MBio* 8(1), e02133-16.

Farrell, D., Jones, G., Pirson, C., Malone, K., Rue-Albrecht, K., *et al.* (2016) Integrated computational prediction and experimental validation identifies promiscuous T cell epitopes in the proteome of *Mycobacterium bovis*. *Microbiology Genomics* 2(8), e000071. doi: 10.1099/mgen.0.000071.

Malone, K.M., Farrell, D., Stuber, T.P., Schubert, O.T., Aebersold, R., *et al.* (2017) Updated reference genome sequence and annotation of *Mycobacterium bovis* AF2122/97. *Genome Announcements* 5(14), e00157-17.

McNerney, R., Wondafrash, B.A., Amena, K., Tesfaye, A., McCash, E.M. and Murray, N.J. (2010) Field test of a novel detection device for mycobacterium tuberculosis antigen in cough. *BMC Infectious Diseases* 10, 161.

Miotto, P., Mwangoka, G., Valente, I.C., Norbis, L., Sotgiu, G., *et al.* (2013) miRNA signatures in sera of patients with active pulmonary tuberculosis. *PLoS One* 8(11), e80149.

Stevens, W.S, Scott, L., Noble, L., Gous, N. and Dheda, K. (2017) Impact of the genexpert MTB/RIF technology on tuberculosis control. *Microbiology Spectrum* 5(1). doi: 10.1128/microbiolspec.TBTB2-0040-2016.

Index

Note: Page numbers in **bold** type refer to **figures**
Page numbers in *italic* type refer to *tables*

abattoirs 22, 32, 34–35, 67, 80, 124, 243
    Ethiopia 240
    Nigeria 22
    surveillance 38, 51, 249
abdominal tuberculosis 22
abscesses, deer 96
acid-fast bacilli (AFB) 124–125, **125**, 130, 131, 133, 134
adaptive immunity 154–172
aerosol transmission 80, 81, 86, 95, 191
Africa 5, 6, 13
    annual incidence 7, **9**
    camels 85
    European colonialism 64
    human tuberculosis 33
    imported cattle 34
    molecular typing 64
    zoonotic tuberculosis 19, 22
African buffalo 9, 98, 134, 180, 206
    vaccination 217
agent identification 12
agro-pastoral communities 85
agro-pastoral farming, South Africa 20
aid organisations 242
AIDS 162, 239
AIM2 inflammasome 145, 146–147
airborne transmission 34, 69
Algeria 64
    camels 85
alpacas 131, **132**
America, eradication programmes 8

Americas 5, 6
    annual incidence 6, **8**
    molecular typing 64
anergic animals 46, 47
animal welfare 9
animals
    diseases
        control 2
        reporting 2
    domestic 3–4, 8–9, **10**, 13, 16, 63, 80–92
    health 14, 31, 36, 59, 207
        authorities 13
        services 12, 14, 35
    management 17
    models 163
    movements 60
        restrictions 35, 229
    products 13, 17
    testing 12
    tuberculosis statistics 2, **3**
annual incidence 6, 13
    Africa 7, **9**
    Americas 6, **8**
    Asia 7, **9**
    Europe 6, **8**
    group C 6, **7**
    group D 6, **7**
    Oceania 6, **9**
    zoonotic tuberculosis 19
ante-mortem testing schemes 174–175
antelopes, *Mycobacterium orygis* in 106

anthrax 2
antibiotics 149
antibodies 47, 161, 162, 180, 199
antibody-based assays 183, 251
antigen mining 177–179, 183, 251
    hypothesis-driven approaches 177–178
    non-biased genome-wide approaches 178–179
antigen-presenting cells (APCs) 159
antigenicity, and gene expression 177
antigens 176, 181, 183, 184, 192, 197, 198, 250, 251
    microbacterial 210
    screening 183
antimicrobial resistance (AMR) 23–24, 69
antimicrobial therapy 23
apoptosis 145–146, 194, 195, 196
apoptosis inducing factor (AIF) 146
Argentina
    Mycobacterium bovis 65
    spoligotyping 67
Asia 5, 6, 13
    annual incidence 7, **9**
    eradication programmes 8
Asian water buffalo, *Mycobacterium bovis* in 84
audits 231
Australia
    bovids 98
    camels 85
    control programmes 38
    eradication 62, 65, 226
    human tuberculosis 33
    test-and-slaughter 38
    wild boar 95
autoimmune diseases 194
autophagy 144–145
avian influenza 32
avian tuberculosis 2
awareness campaigns 38

B cells 133, 134, 161–162, 183
B lymphocytes 126, **127**
Bacillus Calmette–Guérin (BCG) *see* BCG
bacteria 58–59
    shedding 45
bacterial cell biology 177–178
BadgerBCG™ 215
badgers 9, 32, 54, 63, 68, 82, 132, 192, 206, 231
    BCG 215–216, 218
    containment phase 132
    culling 53, 63, 100, 215
    England 234, 235
    foraging 99–100
    Ireland 99–100, 216, 234
    lesions 132, **133**, 214
    lymph nodes 132
    mobility 63

    Mycobacterium bovis in 93–94, 99–100
    pasture 99
    respiratory tract 94
    road-kill 67
    UK 99–100
    urine 94, 95
    vaccination 214–216, 234
badger–cattle transmission 69, 100
Bangladesh, milk production 33
basic reproduction number 48, 49, 50
BCG (Bacillus Calmette–Guérin) 109, 115, 143, 154, 158–163, 174, 176, 177, 179, 180, 182, 198, 242, 252
    badgers 215–216, 218
    buffaloes 217
    calves 144, 159, 192–193, 211, 241
    cattle 207–208, 209
    deer 212–213
    ferrets 217
    late strains 114
    possums 213, 218
    routes 210
    virulence 108
    wild boar 216, 218
beef industry 17
Belgium 23, 64
between-herd transmission 53–54
between-species infection 53
biodiversity 237
biomarkers 179–182, 250
    cellular immune responses 198
    challenges 200
    characteristics 193
    circulating 193–196
    CMI based assays 179–180
    definition 193
    hosts 174
    Mycobacterium tuberculosis complex (MTBC) 191–205
    peptide 196
    protein 195, 196
biosafety 35
biosecurity 83, 215, 228
birds 82
bison 33, 38, 192
black pigs, lesions 83
blood-based laboratory tests 12
border control 12
Bordetella pertussis, in mice 162
Bos
    indicus 148
    taurus 148
bovids 132
    Australia 98
Bovigam 181
Bovigam PC-EC assay (BEC) 198
Bovigam PC-IHC assay (BHP) 198

bovine spongiform encephalopathy (BSE) 194
bovine tuberculosis 122–123
    cost 35–36
    evolution 6
    notification 2–4
    pathogenesis 126–127
    progression model 44–46, **44**
    regional trends 5
    trends 4–5
    worldwide picture 1–15
bovine viral diarrhoea virus (BVDV) 162
Brazil 62
    buffalo 84
    Mycobacterium bovis 65
breath analysis 250
breeding 34, 148, 149
    selective 148, 149
bronchopneumonia, caseous 83
Brooks-Pollock model 53–54
Brucella abortus 69, 148
brucellosis 32, 148
brushtail possums 32, 93, 134, 192, 206
    New Zealand 97, 98
    vaccination 213–214
BSE (bovine spongiform encephalopathy) 194
buffalo 33, 38, 64, 98, 180, 192, 226
    BCG 217
    Brazil 84
    lesions 134
    see also African buffalo
Burkina Faso 64
Burundi, *Mycobacterium bovis* 64
BVDV (bovine viral diarrhoea virus) 162

calciferol 149
calves 207, 208
    BCG 144, 159, 192–193, 211, 241
    lesions 161
    Mycobacterium bovis in 155
    T cells 158
    transmission 123–124
        pseudo-vertical 47
camels 84–86, 131, 249
    Africa 85
    Algeria 85
    Australia 85
    Bactrian 84–85
    dromedary 84–85
    Egypt 85, 86
    Eritrea 85
    husbandry 86
    India 85
    lesions 85–86, 131
    lymph nodes 86
    milk 85, 86
    MTBC 85

    respiratory tract 85
    SCITT 85
    Somalia 85
    Sudan 85
Cameroon 22, 240
Canada, veterinarians 21
cancer, lungs 182, 194
cannibalism 84
carrion 83, 96, 232
caseation 129
caseous bronchopneumonia 83
caseous lymphadenitis 81
cats, lesions 130, **131**
cattle 68, 173, 236
    BCG 207–208, 209
    Brucella abortus in vivo 148
    deer–cattle transmission 100
    imported 34
    lesions 20–21, 159
    movements 54, 60, 65, 66, 230
        statutory reporting 53
    Mycobacterium bovis in 43–57, 63
    and *Mycobacterium tuberculosis* 209
    selective breeding 148, 149
    super-spreading 46
    sympatric 98
    T cells 158–159
    tracing systems 53, 60
    trade 173
    vaccination 207–211, 241
cattle–cattle transmission 45, 47, 65, 68
cattle–human transmission, Morocco 37, **37**
caudal fold test (CFT) 175, 191, 192
CD3+ T lymphocytes 126, **126**
CD4+ T cells 155, 156, 157
CD4+ T lymphocytes 126
CD8+ T lymphocytes 126, 161
CD68+ cells 125–126, **126**
CD79a+ cells **127**
cell envelope, mycobacteria 109–111, 113
cell-mediated immune (CMI) responses 154–158,
    173, 176, 179, 181
cells
    antigen-presenting (APCs) 159
    CD68+ 125–126, **126**
    CD79a+ **127**
    death mechanisms 144–146
    dendritic (DC) 140, 142–143, 146, 156, 197
    lipid-restricted 160–161
    multi-nucleated giant (MNGCs) 124, 125, 126,
        128, 133
    natural killer 140, 143
    peripheral blood mononuclear (PBMCs) 115,
        174, 180, 197
    phagocytic 197
    see also T cells
central memory T cells 157–158

cerebrospinal fluid (CSF) 24
cervical test, single intradermal comparative (SICCT)
    47, 52, 85, 175
cervids 12, 80, 97, 131, 132–133
Chad 64
    vaccination 32
channel proteins 110
cheese 33, 84
cheetah 206
chemokines 127, 129, 140, 143, 149, 179, 180,
    181–182, 197
children 44, 182
    Mycobacterium bovis disease 22
Chile 240
cholesterol 110
chromatin condensation 145, 146
circulating biomarkers 193–196
circulating microRNA 197
circulating nucleic acid 194–195, 250
climate change 31, 48, 234
clustered regularly interspersed polymorphic repeat
    (CRISPR) 61
CMI based assays 179–180
co-infection 34, 65, 162–163, 192, 250
colony forming units (CFU) 94
colostrum 240
communication 242, 253
communities, agro-pastoral 85
community leaders 240
companion animals, *Mycobacterium bovis* in 130
comparative cervical test (CCT) 175, 191, 192
comparative genomic analysis 177
comparative transcriptome analysis 177
compensation 35, 38, 229, 253
contagious pleuropneumonia 2
contracting 230–231
control 5, 8, 14, 18, 142, 173, 226, 228, 238, 239
    border 12
    challenges 252–253
    developing countries 37–38
    global 248–254
    measures 13, 206–207, 217
    mycobacteria 144–145
    Mycobacterium tuberculosis 147
    policies 229
    programmes 17, 33, 58, 70, 206
        Australia 38
        industrial countries 51
        Ireland 62
        UK 62
    strategies 36, 38, 99
    zoonotic tuberculosis 12–13
CpnT proteins 110
cryptic infection, wildlife 53–54
culling 98, 99, 192, 234, 253
    badgers 53, 63, 100, 215
    possums 213

cultural behavioural habits 34
culture 17
cutaneous tuberculosis 21
cynomolgus macaques 129
cytokines 127, 128, 129, 134, 135, 140, 142, 143,
    146–149, 155–158, 160, 161, 163, 174,
    179–182, 210
    serum 197–198

dairy industry 17, 34
    New Zealand 34
dairy products 21
    unpasteurised 17, 19–20, 23, 25
DALYs (disability-adjusted life-years) 19
DAMs (damage-associated molecular patterns) 140,
    144
Dassie bacillus 106
data 6, 19, 32
deaths, human tuberculosis 16, 32, 239, 249
decision makers 36, 38, 249
decision-support tools 70
deer 21, 63, 98, 183, 249
    abscesses 96
    BCG 212–213
    hunting 94
    lesions 96, 212
    lymph nodes 96
    lymphadenitis 96
    maintenance hosts 100
    Mycobacterium bovis in 96–97, 98
    New Zealand 96, 99, 101
    Spain 96, 101
    spillover hosts 97
    Sweden 64
    USA 100, 213
    vaccination 212–213
    see also fallow deer; red deer; white-tailed deer
deer–cattle transmission 100
delayed hypersensitivity test 12
delayed-type hypersensitivity (DTH) 174
dendritic cells (DC) 140, 142–143, 146, 156, 197
density-dependent transmission 48–50, **49**
developing countries 37–38
diabetes mellitus 193
diagnosis 23, 176, 184, 198, 250–251
    early 14, 191, 193
    human tuberculosis 24, 25
    immunological 173–190, 250
    rates 32
diagnostic tests 12, 24, 25, 43, 45, 46, 154, 163,
    193, 195, 199, 200, 207
    cost 241
    human tuberculosis 16–17, 18
    immunopathogenesis 174
    performance 47
    sensitivity 162, 241

serological 161
differentiate infected from vaccinated animals (DIVA) 176, 177, 200, 207, 211, 217
dimycocerosyl phthiocerol family (DIMs) 110
disability-adjusted life-years (DALYs) 19
disease
   animal 2
   autoimmune 194
   distribution 59
   foot and mouth 2, 35, 53
   infectious 68
   Johne's 211
   prevention 13
   prognosis 193
   pulmonary 82
   staging 193
   wildlife 2
disseminated tuberculosis 22
DIVA (differentiate infected from vaccinated animals) 176, 177, 200, 207, 211, 217
DNA 193, 194
   fragmentation 145, 146, 148
   vaccines 209
dogs 130
domestic animals 3–4, 8–9, **10**, 13, 16, 63, 80–92
domestic pigs 63
   Mycobacterium bovis in 82–84
dourine 2
drug resistance 23, 199
DTH assays 175
Dual-Path Platform VetTB Assay 183

earthworms 99
Ecohealth 238
ecological studies 66
ecology, and health 31
economic losses 13, 19, 35–36, *36*, 38, 81, 87, 106, 191, 211, 226, 249
   livestock 33
   pigs 82
economics 31–42
   One Health 36
ecosystems 32, 99, 101, 207, 238
ecotourism 31
ecotypes 59
education 22, 240
   health 36
effector memory T cells 157–158
Egypt
   camels 85, 86
   water buffalo 84
elephants 183
elimination, developing countries 37–38
ELISA 181, 183, 196
ELISPOT 157, 181, 182, 210–211
elk 21, 64, 65, 97, 192, 231

empowerment 240
endangered species 99
England, badgers 234, 235
Enterobacteriaceae 251
environmental reservoirs 54, 58
environmental transmission 47–48, 53
enzyme-linked immunosorbent assay 12
epi-systems 69, 70
epidemiological models 228
epidemiological typing 69
epidemiology 59–61, 61, 248–250
   genomic 67
   molecular 59–60, 67, 70
   Mycobacterium bovis 43–57
eradication 173, 191, 226, 228, 235, 253
   Australia 62, 65, 84, 226
   France 63–64
   Italy 63
   New Zealand 62, 65
   wildlife 232
eradication programmes 8, 9, 13, 14, 81, 82
Eritrea, camels 85
ethambutol 23
Ethiopia 38, 84, 208, 239
   abattoirs 240
   extra-pulmonary tuberculosis 24
   lesions 86
   livestock production 33
   meat 21
   milk 20, 22
   Mycobacterium bovis 64
   unmanaged herds 50
Europe 5, 6
   annual incidence 6, **8**
   molecular typing 62–64
European Economic Community (EEC) 3
exported repetitive proteins 110
exports 229
extra-pulmonary tuberculosis 18, 24, 34
   Ethiopia 24

fallow deer 96, 133, **133**
   lesions 133, **133**
farmers 38, 46, 80, 229, 230, 231, 237, 249
   aerosol infection 21
   Uganda 22
farming, agro-pastoral 20
farms 48, 227, 229
   cattle 236
   fragmentation 60
   profitability 58
Fasciola hepatica 162, 163, 250
feed, contaminated 122
ferrets 97
   BCG 217
   New Zealand 217

ferrets *continued*
    vaccination 217
fish 127
flow cytometry 181–182
food 22, 34, 238
    cultural 20
    safety 2, 31
Food and Agriculture Organisation (FAO) 3, 13, 14
foot and mouth disease 2, 35, 53
foraging 96
    badgers 99–100
France, eradication 63–64

game parks, South Africa 217
game-keeping 97, 234
gamma-interferon 157, 158, 160, 162, 163, 174, 179, 180, 181, 210, 211, 212
    assay 12, 191, 192
    tests 47
gastrointestinal tuberculosis 22
gene-expression
    and antigenicity 177
    profiling 181–182
genes
    PE/PPE 112–113
    polymorphisms 148, 149
    regulatory 113–115
genetic tests, molecular 61
genetics 107, 148
    diversity 60
GeneXpert 16, 248, 250
genomes 194
genomic epidemiology 67–70
genomics 67, 192
Ghon complex 123
glanders 2
Global Research Alliance for Bovine TB (GRAbTB) 18
glucose 193
goats 239, 249
    lesions 81, 82, 212
    milk 81
    Mycobacterium bovis in 63, 80–82, 130
    Mycobacterium caprae in 81, 106, 207, 211, 212
    Mycobacterium microti in 82
    Mycobacterium tuberculosis in 81
    Spain 81, 82
    vaccination 211–212
governments 249, 252
    agencies 227, 230, 235, 236, 237, 242
    funding 229, 236
granulomas 124–126, **125**, 127, 135, 156, 162, 191, 197–198
    cell composition 125–126
    fallow deer 133, **133**
    formation 158, 159, 195

guinea pigs 129, **130**
mice 129, **129**
red deer 133
stages 124–125, 127–128, **128**, 133, 134, 162
swine 134
granulysin 161
grazing 241
Great Britain (GB)
    herd breakdown 52–53
    testing 51
greater kudu 98, 192
gross national income (GNI) 225, 253
    economies 225–231, 238–242
guinea pigs 129, 163, 175
    granulomas 129, **130**

habitat destruction 31
Handistatus 2, 3, 4
health
    animal 12, 13, 14, 31, 35, 36, 59, 207
    care 25, 249
    and ecology 31
    education 36
    human 31, 33–34, 36, 59
    multidisciplinary approaches 17
    workers 240
    see also public health
hepatitis C 156
herds
    breakdown 51, 52–53, **52**, 54, 60, 234
    infection persistence 52
    prevalence 48
    reproduction ratio 54
    size 49, 50, 249
    tuberculin testing 51
    unmanaged 50
heterologous prime-boost strategy 198
HIV 18, 23, 32, 33, 34, 99, 113, 156, 162, 174, 182, 239
    non-human primates 155
Holstein Friesian cattle 148
horses, lesions 130
hosts 69, 97, 98, 106–107, 115
    biomarkers 174, 183–184
    damage 106–107
    deer 97, 100
    factors 148
    immune system 107
    preferences 108, 109
    reservoir 81
    resistance 145, 146
    role 93
    spillover 97, 98, 101, 106, 232
    susceptibility 48
    transitions 69
    wildlife 101

see also maintenance hosts
host–pathogen interactions 59, 109
human health 31, 33–34, 36, 59
human tuberculosis 35–36, 62, 178, 198–200,
    242–243, 250
    Africa 33
    Australia 33
    children 44
    clinical challenges 23–24
    clinical stages 182
    deaths 16, 32, 239, 249
    diagnostic tests 16–17, 18, 24, 25
    estimates 18–19
    incidence 239, 249
    incubation 43–44
    international epidemiological situation and
        control strategy 32
    Mexico 33
    mortality rates 23
    Mycobacterium bovis 16–30, 63, 65, 226, 239,
        240, 253
    Mycobacterium tuberculosis 173, 174, 179, 180
    occupational risks 34–35
    risk factors 12–13
    super-spreaders 66
    USA 16
human-to-human transmission, *Mycobacterium bovis*
    21, 23, 34
human–animal interface 14, 17
human–animal–ecosystem interface 13
humoral immunity 161–162
hunting 21, 206, 234, 236
    deer 94
husbandry 82, 217
    camels 86
    Cameroon 22
    pigs 82
hypersensitivity
    delayed test 12
    delayed-type (DTH) 174
hypoxia 176

Iberian lynx 206
IGRAs 175, 176, 178, 181, 184, 192, 198, 251
IHC techniques 134
immunity 148
    adaptive 154–172
    humoral 161–162
    in vivo studies 163
    innate 160, 161
    local 126–128
immunological diagnosis 173–190, 250
immunology 250–251
immunomodulatory proteins 114
immunopathogenesis, diagnostic tests 174
immunopathology 146

imported cattle, Africa 34
in-tube strategies 180–181
incidence
    age-dependent patterns 50–51, **50**
    within-herd 51, **52**
    see also annual incidence
India
    camels 85
    unmanaged herds 50
    water buffalo 84
industrial countries 51
industry 227, 229, 230
infection 45
    between-species 53
    cryptic 53–54
    dissemination 60
    force of 50
    hidden burden 46–47
    multiplicity of (MOI) 145
    sources 58
    super- 63
infectious diseases 68
infectiousness 45, 46, 48
inflammasome 146–147
inhalation model 129
innate immune system 140–153, 160, 161
inoculation 20, 45
inter-herd transmission 249
inter-species transmission 99
interferon release assays 199
interferon-?, *Mycobacterium bovis* 147
interleukins 143, 146
international trade 2, 3, 9, 12, 31, 32
intra-species transmission 83
Ireland
    badgers 99–100, 216, 234
    control programmes 62
    Food Safety Authority 20
    meat 20
    milk production 33
    Mycobacterium bovis 62–63
    Northern 65–67, 68
isobaric tag for relative and absolute quantitation
    (iTRAQ) 196
isoniazid resistance 24
Italy, eradication 63

Japan
    test-and-slaughter 37
    tuberculin skin test (TST) 37
Johne's disease 211

killer cells 140, 143
knowledge 240, 253
Kruger National Park 64, 99

laboratories 12, 35, 230, 249
laboratory animal models 128–130
laboratory tests, blood-based 12
landowners 252
laser-capture micro-dissection (LCMD) 127
latency 43, 45, 46, 132, 199, 214
lechwe 98, 134
    lesions 134
legislation 227, 229, 230, 237, 253
leishmaniasis 156
leopards 206
lesions 46, 47, 51, 52, 93, 135, 163, 174, 179, 243
    badgers 132, **133**, 214
    black pigs 83
    buffalo 134
    calves 161
    camels 85–86, 131
    cats 130, **131**
    cattle 20–21, 159
    deer 96, 212
    Ethiopia 86
    fallow deer 133, **133**
    feral pigs 95
    goats 212, 81.82
    guinea pigs 129
    horses 130
    lechwe 134
    mice 129
    Mycobacterium bovis 122–123, 124
    pigs 82, 83
    possums 94
    post-mortem 176
    reactor animals 44
    respiratory 123, **123**
    small ruminants 130
    wild boar 83, 95, 133, 134, **134**, 216
leukocytes 181, 182
life expectancy 48
lions 206
    Mycobacterium bovis in 98
lipid-responsive CD1-restricted T cells 154
lipid-restricted T cells 160–161
lipids 109–110, 113, 114, 160–161, 196
lipopolysaccharide (LPS) 142
liquifactive necrosis 81
live attenuated mycobacterial vaccines 208–209
liver fluke 162
livestock 3, 13, 34, 226, 238
    economic losses 33
    Ethiopia 33
    genetic improvement 58
    infection levels 228
    movement restrictions 99, 235
    Nigeria 21
    ownership 238, 242
    production 35, 80, 238
    productivity 19
    surveillance 243
    vaccination 243
livestock–wildlife transmission 99–100
llamas 131
losses *see* economic losses
LppA 110
lungs 127, 129, 156, 157, 198, 209, 212, 214
    cancer 182, 194
    lesions 127
    mice 162
lymph nodes 81, 122, 123, 124, 127, 156, 157, 209, 212, 216
    badgers 132
    camels 86
    deer 96
    pigs 83
    possums 94
lymphadenitis 82
    caseous 81
    deer 96
lymphocyte proliferation assay 12
lymphocytes 154, 181, 192, 195
    CD3+ T 126, **126**
    see also T lymphocytes
lynx 206
lysosomes 143

macaques 129
Mce proteins 109–110
macrophages 126, 127, 128, 133, 134, 140, 143, 145–146, 149, 156, 158, 163, 191, 197
    pro-inflammatory profile 148
maintenance hosts 97, 99, 106, 206, 231, 249
    deer 100
    wild boar 98, 101
    wildlife 225, 232, 234–235
major histocompatibility complex (MHC) 142
malaria 156
Mali 64
management 225–247
    agencies 230–231
    tools 38
market failure 200
marsupials 132
mass spectrometry 199
mathematical modelling 58, 69, 163
matrix-assisted laser desorption ionisation-time of flight (MALDI-TOF) 199
meat 17, 25, 31, 32, 80, 238, 250
    condemnation 35
    Ethiopia 21
    inspection 17, 51
    Ireland 20
    New Zealand 20
    production 33

raw 20–21, 240
UK 20
meerkats, *Mycobacterium suricattae* in 106
meningitis 22, 24
metabolites 196
Mexico 208
    human tuberculosis 33
    zoonotic tuberculosis 21
mice 129, 155, 159
    Bordetella pertussis in 162
    granulomas 129, **129**
    lesions 129
    lungs 162
    Mycobacterium tuberculosis in 146
    Salmonella enterica in 162
micro-epidemics 65, 68–69
micro-RNA (miRNA) 182, 194, 211
    circulating 197
microarray technology 177
microbacterial antigens 210
microscopy, sputum smear 16, 248
milk 16, 24, 31, 33, 47, 80, 239, 241, 250
    camels 85, 86
    Ethiopia 20
    goats 81
    heat treatment 20
    pasteurisation 17, 19, 20, 22, 33, 35, 36, 226, 239, 240, 242–243
    raw 20, 22, 238, 242
    temperature 20
    testing 241
    unpasteurised 22, 34, 37, 240
mitochondria 145
molecular epidemiology 17, 59–60, 65, 67, 70
molecular genetic tests 61
molecular patterns, damage-associated (DAMs) 140, 144
molecular surveillance 59–60
molecular typing 60, 61, 66
    Africa 64
    Northern Ireland 68
molecular virulence mechanisms 106–121
moose 96
Morocco 37
    cattle–human transmission 37, **37**
    stakeholders 38
mortality, *Mycobacterium bovis* 19
MPB70 proteins 112
mRNA 182, 200
mucosal invariant T cells (MAIT) 154, 160
multi-host complexes 97–99
multi-locus VNTR analysis (MLVA) 61, 62, 63, 64, 65, 66, 67, 69
multi-nucleated giant cells (MNGCs) 124, 125, 126, 128, 133
multi-species transmission 101
multidrug-resistant tuberculosis 24

multiplicity of infection (MOI) 145
muscle, *Mycobacterium bovis* 21
Mustelidae 132, 217
mycobacteria 70, 143, 144, 198
    cell envelope 109–111, 113
    control 144–145
    ecology 61
    environmental sources 46
    evolution 107, 193
    genomes 61
    in vitro 111
    molecular surveillance systems 68
    pathogenic 127
    proteins 115
    secretory systems 111–112
    twin arginine transporter (Tat) 112
    virulence 108, 109, 110–111
    virulent strains 147
mycobacterial interspersed repetitive units (MIRUs) 61
mycobacterial vaccines, live attenuated 208–209
Mycobacterium
    caprae 67, 81, 84, 114, 122
        in goats 81, 106, 207, 211, 212
    kansasii 176
    microti 82, 84, 106
    orygis 106, 114
    pinnipedii 106
    smegmatis 145
    suricattae 106
Mycobacterium avium 157, 162, 175, 176, 177, 192, 211, 250
    hominissuis 65
Mycobacterium avium complex (MAC) 82
Mycobacterium bovis
    Argentina 65
    in Asian water buffalo 84
    in badgers 93–94, 99–100
    beta-interferon 147
    Brazil 65
    Burundi 64
    in calves 155
    in camelids 84, 131
    in cattle 43–57, 63
    in children 22
    clinical challenges 23–24
    in companion animals 130
    in deer 96–97, 98
    in domestic pigs 82–84
    dynamics and persistence 97–99
    early generalisation 123
    epidemiology 43–57
    Ethiopia 64
    evolution 107
    in feral pigs 95–96
    foodborne 12
    genomes 69

Mycobacterium bovis continued
   genotyping 67
   in goats 63, 80–82, 130
   growth 143
   human-to-human transmission 21, 23
   in humans 16–30, 36–37, 63, 65, 226, 239, 240, 253
   intra-species transmission 83
   Ireland 62–63
   lesions 122–123, 124
   life history of infection and transmission 43–48
   in lions 98
   local immunity 126–128
   low to medium-high GNI economies 238–242
   macroscopic pathology 123–124
   molecular typing 58–79, 61–65, 67
      Africa 64
      Americas 64
      Europe 62–64
      Oceania 65
   molecular virulence mechanisms 106–121
   mortality 19
   most recent common ancestor (MRCA) 249
   multidrug-resistant strains 24
   muscle 21
   natural resistance 148–149
   New Zealand 99
   Northern Ireland 67
   occupational risk 21
   in Old World camelids 84
   Paraguay 65
   pasture 47
   patient demographics 22
   population structure 70
   in possums 93–94, 97, 99
   in predator species 98
   proteins 177–178, 198
   in road-kill badgers 67
   routes 122, 123
   seasons 47
   in sheep 80–82, 130
   in small ruminants 130
   South Africa 64, 99
   South America 65, 131
   Tanzania 64
   transmission 17
   Uganda 64
   UK 62–63
   vaccine 216, 217
   virulent strains 145, 146
   in white-tailed deer 69, 96–97
   in wild animals 131–134
   in wild boar 95–96, 97–98
   in wildlife 63, 93–105
   Zambia 64
Mycobacterium tuberculosis 16, 17, 59, 109, 135
   B cells 162
   in cattle 209
   control 147
   diagnosis 199
   four-drug treatment 23
   gene essentiality 251–252
   in goats 81
   host response 126
   in humans 173, 174, 179, 180
   immunological footprint 178–179
   in vitro 112
   in vivo 112
   in mice 146
   mutation rate 68, 69
   proteins 178
   virulent strains 143, 145, 146, 198
Mycobacterium tuberculosis complex (MTBC) 34, 58–59, 61, 67, 81, 82, 106, 122, 226
   biomarkers 191–205
   in camels 85
   genomic analysis 107–109
   secretion systems 112
mycomembrane 109

national parks 206
natural killer cells 140, 143
necrosis 129, 194, 195, 196
Nepal, water buffalo 84
net present value (NPV) 228
Netherlands 60
neutrophil extracellular traps (NETs) 143
neutrophils 140, 143–144, 146, 158
New Zealand 232, **233**, 235, 249
   Biosecurity Act (1993) 228
   brushtail possums 97, 98
   dairy herds 34
   deer 96, 99, 101
   eradication 62, 65
   feral pigs 83–84, 95
   ferrets 217
   government funding 236
   meat 20
   Mycobacterium bovis 99
   pigs 83
   possums 93–94, 98, 234, 236
   vaccination 208
   wild pigs 232
Nigeria 64, 84, 240
   abattoir workers 22
   Fuku elegusi 21
   livestock traders 21
nitric oxide 148
non-conventional T cells 158–161
non-human primates 129
   HIV 155
non-pulmonary tuberculosis 24
Northern Ireland 65–67, 68

nucleic acids 195
    circulating 194–195, 250

occult animals 47
occult periods 45
occupational risks 34–35
Oceania 5, 6
    annual incidence 6, **9**
    eradication programmes 8
    molecular typing 65
Old World camelids, *Mycobacterium bovis* in 84
One Health 13, 31–32, 36–37, 38, 238, 242, 248–250
Organisation for Economic Co-operation and Development (OECD) 3
overpopulation 31

Pakistan, water buffalo 84
Palestine, raw milk 20
Paraguay, *Mycobacterium bovis* 65
parasitic worms 162
parsimonious models 45
pasteurisation 17, 19, 20, 22, 33, 35, 36, 226, 239, 240, 242–243
pasture 83, 122
    badgers 99
    Mycobacterium bovis on 47
pathogen genomics revolution 59
pathogen genotype–phenotype associations 67
pathogen genotyping 70
pathogen-associated molecular patterns (PAMPs) 140, 143
pathogenesis 61, 115
pathogenic mycobacteria 126–127
PE/PPE genes 112–113
peptides 176, 178, 179, 196, 198, 250, 251
    biomarkers 196
peptidomes 196
peripheral blood mononuclear cells (PBMCs) 115, 174, 180, 197
perturbation effect 100
pets 22
phagocytic cells 197
phenolic glycolipids (PGL) 111
PhoPR 113–114
phthiocerol dimycocerosate (PDIM) 110–111
phylodynamics 69
pigs 65, 84, 134, 158, 249
    black 83
    domestic 82–84
    economic losses 82
    feral 83–84, 95, 98
    husbandry 82
    lesions 82, 83
    lymph nodes 83

Mycobacterium avium complex (MAC) in 82
Mycobacterium bovis in 95–96
Mycobacterium caprae in 84
    New Zealand 83, 95, 232
    Spain 83
    USA 84
pleurisy 130, 131
pleuropneumonia 2
pneumonia 182
policy 228, 230, 249, 253
politicians 229, 230, 236, 240, 242
polyfunctional T cells 155–156
polyketide synthases (PKS) 110
polymerase chain reaction 127
populations, rural 238, 240
possums 32, 83, 84, 99, 134, 192, 206
    BCG 213, 218
    culling 213
    lesions 94
    lymph nodes 94
    Mycobacterium bovis in 93–94, 97, 99
    New Zealand 93–94, 98, 234, 236
    vaccination 213–214
    see also brushtail possums
post-mortems 46, 47, 124
    wildlife 232
poultry 158
poverty 33, 238, 253
predators 98
prevention 18
primates 196
    non-human 129, 155
pro-apoptotic proteins 145
production animals 80
production risks 227
programmes
    benefit-cost analysis 228–229, 236, 253
    communication 230, 237
    compulsory 227
    costs 228
    development 227
    eradication 8, 9, 13, 14, 81, 82
    funding 227, 229, 230, 237
    high GNI countries 225–231
    implementation 227, 230–231, 237–238
    legal status 227, 235
    planning 228, 236
    policies 229–230, 237
    purpose 226, 235
    stakeholder support 227–228, 235–236
    strategic objectives 226–227, 230, 235
    voluntary 227
    see also control, programmes
protected species 100
protection
    correlates 210–211
    markers 252

proteins 112–113, 114, 115, 176, 178, 182, 250
   biomarkers 195, 196
   channel 110
   CpnT 110
   exported repetitive 110
   HLA binding 178, 179
   immunomodulatory 114
   Mce 109–110
   mycobacterial 115
   Mycobacterium bovis 177–178, 198
   Mycobacterium tuberculosis 178
   pro-apoptotic 145
   reported repetitive 110
   serum 196
   vaccines 209–210
proteome 195
proteomics 192, 195–196, 200
   fingerprinting 195
pseudo-vertical transmission 50
   calves 47
public health 3, 13, 14, 16–30, 24, 32–34, 36, 38, 61, 80, 122
   schools 31–32
   veterinary 9, 13
pulmonary disease 82
pulmonary tuberculosis 18, 21, 22, 34, 65
purified protein derivative (PPD) 175, 176, 183, 192, 250, 251
pyrazinamide, resistance 17, 23–24, 34
pyroptosis 146

Q-fever 32
Quantiferon 180, 181
quantitative data 6, 8, 13

rabbits 129
rabies 2, 32, 36
Randomised Badger Culling Trial (RBCT) 100
raw milk 238, 242
   Ethiopia 22
   Palestine 20
   Tanzania 20
re-infection 59
reactive latent period 45
reactor animals 50, 51, 66, 243
   herd breakdown **52**
   lesions 44
reagents, species-specific 163
recurrence 52–53
red deer 96, 133, 206
regions of difference (RD) 107, 108
   RD1-RD3 loci 108–109
regulatory genes 113–115
regulatory T cells (Tregs) 157

reindeer 96
reporting countries 4, **4**, 5, **5**
   groups A–D 6, **7**
research 231, 236, 253
reservoir hosts 81
resistance 23, 24, 34, 59, 148, 199
   antimicrobial (AMR) 23–24, 69
   host 145, 146
   isoniazid 24
   natural 148–149
respiratory tract 81
   badgers 94
   camels 85
   lesions 123, **123**
respiratory transmission 47
restriction enzyme analysis (REA) 61
restriction fragment length polymorphism (RFLP) 61, 63, 64, 65
revaccination 208
rhesus macaques 129
rhinoceros 21
rifampicin 23, 24
rinderpest 1, 2
risks
   factors 34–35, 59
   occupational 34–35
   production 227
RNA 193, 194
RskA-SigK regulon 113, 114–115
ruminants 158
   lesions 130
   Mycobacterium bovis in 130
rural populations 238, 240
Russia 85

Saharan West Africa 64
saliva 183–184, 199, 214
   wild boar 95–96
Salmonella
   Dublin 148
   enterica, in mice 162
   Typhimurium 148
sample viability 181
sarcoidosis 182
scavenger receptor cysteine rich (SCRC) superfamily 159
scavengers 84, 97, 98, 232
Scotland 48, 53
seals, *Mycobacterium pinnipedii* in 106
Sec secretion system 111–112
secretory systems, mycobacteria 111–112
seed management 12
serological tests 161, 183, 192, 241
serum 183–184, 199
   cytokines 197–198
   proteins 196

sheep 249
  Mycobacterium bovis in 80–82, 130
  pox 2
  Sudan 82
sigma K factor (SigK) 114
single intradermal comparative cervical test (SICCT) 47, 52, 85, 175
single intradermal test (SIT) 175
slaughter 37, 38, 54, 192, 193
  inspections 173, 175
  surveillance 124, 240
SMART objectives 226, 227
socio-economic impacts 3
Somalia, camels 85
South Africa 84, 98
  agro-pastoral farming 20
  game parks 217
  Mycobacterium bovis 64, 99
  national parks 98–99
South America 13
  camelids 131
  Mycobacterium bovis 65, 141
Spain 63
  deer 96, 101
  goats 81, 82
  Mycobacterium caprae 81
  pigs 83
  wild boar 95, 232
species-specific reagents 163
spillover hosts 97, 98, 101, 106, 232
  deer 97
  wild boar 101
spoligotyping 61, 62, 63, 64, 65, 67
sputum smear microscopy 16, 248
stakeholders 60, 227–229, 230, 232, 235, 236, 237, 238, 249
  Morocco 38
  transdisciplinary workshops 38
sterols 110
Stop TB Partnership 18
  Global Plan to End TB 24
Strategic and Technical Advisory Group 33
Sudan
  camels 85
  raw sheep 82
sulfolipids 111, 113
super-infection 63
super-spreading cattle 46
surveillance 12, 18, 24, 59, 68, 70, 175, 191, 192, 227, 230, 248, 253
  abattoirs 38, 51, 249
  gaps 46
  livestock 243
  molecular 59–60
  slaughter 124, 240
  wildlife 53, 66, 235
susceptibility 148

Sweden, deer 64
swine 82, 84, 132
  fever 2
  granulomas 134
Switzerland, test-and-slaughter 37–38

T cells 129, 142, 144, 154, 158–161, 174, 176, 177, 197, 199, 210–211, 250, 251
  calves 158
  cattle 158–159
  CD4+ 155, 156, 157
  central memory 157–158
  lipid-responsive CD1-restricted 154
  mucosal invariant (MAIT) 154, 160
  non-conventional 158–161
  polyfunctional 155–156
  regulatory (Tregs) 157
  responses 178, **178**
T lymphocytes 126, **126**, 127, 133, 161
Tanzania 240
  Mycobacterium bovis 64
  raw milk 20
test-and-cull 99
test-and-removal 180
test-and-slaughter 35, 37–38, 45, 191, 206, 212, 239, 243
test-insensitive animals 47
test-positive animals 51
testing 51, 53, 227, 241–242
  animal-level 60
  ante-mortem schemes 174–175
  effectiveness 52
  frequency 51
  tuberculin 51
tests
  blood-based laboratory 12
  molecular genetic 61
  serological 161, 183, 192, 241
  single intradermal comparative cervical (SICCT) 47, 52, 85, 175
  single intradermal (SIT) 175
  see also diagnostic tests
TH 1 immune response 127–128
therapy, antimicrobial 23
tissue responses 156–157
TLRs 143, 148
tonsils 122, 212
trade 58, 207, 227
  barriers 1, 9, 13, 14, 19
  cattle 173
  international 2, 3, 9, 12, 31, 32
transmission 34–35, 37, 43, 45, 49, 59, 66, 93, 97, 115, 216
  aerosol 80, 81, 86, 95, 191
  age-dependent patterns 50–51, **50**
  airborne 21, 34, 69

transmission *continued*
    between-herd 53–54
    calves 123–124
    cattle–cattle 45, 47, 65, 68
    cattle–human 37, **37**
    deer–cattle 100
    density-dependent 48–50, **49**
    direct 100
    dynamics 68, 70
    environmental 47–48, 53
    foodborne 34
    indirect 100
    inter-herd 249
    inter-species 99
    and life history of infection 43–48
    livestock–wildlife 99–100
    managed populations 51–54
    mathematical models 47
    models 44, 46
    multi-species 101
    multiple hosts 63
    Mycobacterium bovis 17
    pseudo-vertical 47, 50
    respiratory 47
    routes and mechanisms 47–48, 58
    unmanaged herds 48–51
transport networks 251
Tregs 157
Tripartite Alliance 13, 14
trojan horses 144
tuberculin 45, 46, 175, 210, 250
    testing 12, 46–47, 50, 54, 62, 67, 192, 241
        herds 51
tuberculin skin test (TST) 44, 173, 174–175, 176, 184, 199, 250, 251
    Japan 37
tuberculous meningitis 24
Tunisia 64

Uganda
    farmers 22
    Mycobacterium bovis 64
United Kingdom (UK)
    badgers 99–100
    control programmes 62
    Food Safety Agency 20
    meat 20
    Mycobacterium bovis 62–63
    zoonotic tuberculosis 22
United Nations (UN) 242
    Millennium Development Goals (MDGs) 17
    Sustainable Development Goals (SDGs) 17, 24
United States of America (USA) 60, 69
    deer 100
    Department of Agriculture (USDA) 226
    human tuberculosis 16

    pigs 84
    white-tailed deer 234
    wild deer 213
    zoonotic tuberculosis 22
unmanaged herds
    Ethiopia 50
    India 50
    transmission 48–51
urine 96, 183–184, 199
    badgers 94, 95
    LAM test 199

vaccination 14, 49, 62, 154, 155, 157, 158, 174, 179, 206–224, 235, 250, 251–252
    African buffalo 217
    badgers 214–216, 234
    brushtail possums 213–214
    cattle 207–211, 241
    Chad 32
    control 12
    deer 212–213
    delivery 216
    design 156, 157
    development 200
    DNA 209
    efficacy 163, 192, 207, 210–212, 216
    ferrets 217
    goats 211–212
    immunological 252
    livestock 243
    manufacturers 12
    microbiological 251–252
    Mycobacterium bovis 216, 217
    new generation 208–210, *209*
    oral 214, 252
        baits 216–217
    production 12
    protein 209–210
    safety 216, 252
    success 158
    trials 128
    virally-vectored 210
    wild boar 216–217
    wildlife 213–217, *214*, 234, 252
vaccines, live attenuated mycobacterial 208–209
variable number of tandem repeats (VNTRs) 61
veterinarians 2, 4, 25, 80, 248
    Canada 21
    protocol compliance 46
    public health 9, 13
    research laboratories 61
village leaders 242
virally-vectored vaccines 210
virulence 106–107, 113, 115, 145, 146, 163, 252
    BCG 108
viruses 143

vitamin D 148–149, 182
voles, *Mycobacterium microti* in 106

wapiti 206
water, contaminated 122
water buffalo 12, 84, 86, 87, 249
white-tailed deer 32, 100, 132–133, 192, 206, 231
    Mycobacterium bovis in 69, 96–97
    USA 234
whole blood
    assays 180–181, 251
    testing 241
whole-genome sequencing (WGS) 67–70, 249
wild animals 16
    Mycobacterium bovis in 131–134
wild boar 9, 32, 63, 133–134, 192, 206, 231
    Australia 95
    BCG 216, 218
    lesions 83, 95, 133, 134, **134**, 216
    maintenance hosts 98, 101
    Mycobacterium bovis in 95–96, 97–98
    piglets 95
    saliva 95–96
    Spain 95, 232
    spillover hosts 101
    vaccination 216–217
wildlife 3, 4, 13, 32, 48, 54, 59, 62, 65, 83
    cryptic infection 53–54
    diseases 2
    eradication 232
    health 237
    hosts 101
    maintenance hosts 225, 232, 234–235
    management 231–232, 234–235, 236, 238
    Mycobacterium bovis in 63, 93–105
    organisations 237
    population densities 236
    post-mortems 232
    prevalence 236
    reservoirs 35, 37, 173, 192, 206, 208, 231–238
    responsibility 252–253
    surveillance 53, 66, 235
    testing 192

vaccination 213–217, *214*, 234, 252
worldwide distribution 8–9, **11**
wildlife–cattle transmission 65, 249
within-herd incidence 51, **52**
wood bison 12, 206
World Animal Health 4
World Animal Health Information System (WAHIS) 2, 3, 4, 6, 8, 13
World Bank 13, 225
World Health Organisation (WHO) 13, 32, 199, 239
    End TB Strategy 17–18, 24, 32, 239, 242
    Global Burden of Foodborne Disease 19
    targets 242
World Organisation for Animal Health (OIE) 1, 13, 14
    data collection 6
    List A 3, 14n4
    List B 3, 14n3
    List of Notifiable Diseases 13
    Manual of Diagnostic Tests and Vaccines for Terrestrial Animals 12, 14
    Organic Statutes 2
    Scientific Commission for Animal Diseases 12
    standards 9, 12
    Terrestrial Animal Health Code 9, 12, 14, 80
World Trade Organisation (WTO) 1, 2
    Agreement on the Application of Sanitary and Phytosanitary Measures 12
worms, parasitic 162

Xpert MTB/RIF 199

Zambia, *Mycobacterium bovis* 64
zebra fish 127
zoo keepers 21
zoonotic tuberculosis 12–13, 16, 17, 18–19, 19–23, 25
    Africa 19, 22
    Belgium 23
    Mexico 21
    UK 22
    USA 22